# ASSISTIVE TECHNOLOGIES

*Principles and Practice*

SECOND EDITION

# ASSISTIVE
# TECHNOLOGIES

*Principles and Practice*

SECOND EDITION

**Albert M. Cook, PhD, PE**

Professor and Dean, Faculty of Rehabilitation Medicine
University of Alberta
Edmonton, Alberta


**Susan M. Hussey, MS, OTR**

Coordinator and Professor, Occupational Therapy Assistant Program
Sacramento City College
Sacramento, California

*with 265 illustrations*

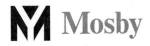

St. Louis   London   Philadelphia   Sydney   Toronto

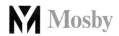 Mosby

*Publishing Director:* John Schrefer
*Editor:* Kellie Conklin
*Developmental Editor:* Christie M. Hart
*Project Manager:* Karen Edwards
*Design:* Judi Lang
*Cover Photography:* PhotoDisc and Clip Shots

SECOND EDITION

Mosby, Inc.
11830 Westline Industrial Drive
St. Louis, Missouri 63146

Printed in the United States of America

**Library of Congress Cataloging in Publication Data**
Cook, Albert M., 1943–
  Assistive technologies: principles and practice / Albert M. Cook, Susan M. Hussey.—2nd ed.
    p.  cm.
  Includes bibliographical references and index.
  ISBN 0-323-00643-4
  1. Self-help devices for the disabled.   I. Hussey, Susan M.   II. Title.
  RM698.C66 2002
  617′.03—dc21
                                                                    2001055837

01  02  03  04  05  GW/MV  9  8  7  6  5  4  3  2  1

*For giving us the reason and the direction for this work, we
dedicate this book to all of our students and to consumers of assistive
technologies, especially Elizabeth Cook, Brian Cook, and Rebecca Nemeth.*

*We hope that . . . "out of these vast warehouses of information
there constantly arise new possibilities for solving problems, for
discovering entirely new human capabilities."*

**H. Z. Bennett**

*The two most engaging powers of an author are to make*
***new*** *things* ***familiar*** *and* ***familiar*** *things* ***new.***
Samuel Johnson

The use of assistive technologies by persons with disabilities to pursue self-care, educational, vocational, and recreational activities continues to increase both in quantity and quality. The number of academic programs, clinical centers, schools, and hospitals applying these assistive technologies has increased dramatically.

When we wrote the first edition, there was a lack of carefully articulated *principles* as well as *practices* in the emerging assistive technology field, despite the growth in interest, application, and training. The common approach had been to focus on available devices with little synthesis of principles and practices. Some books focused on specialized areas (e.g., augmentative communication devices or seating systems) while others covered a broader range of devices. The first edition of this text was written to provide a framework for assistive technology application that was both *broad in scope* and *specific in content.* We are grateful for the extremely positive response to the first edition from an international audience of professionals, educators, and students.

In this second edition, we have taken several steps to increase the usefulness of this text to these audiences. Based on feedback from readers of the first edition, we have worked with our colleagues at Mosby to completely redesign the layout of the text, creating a much more friendly and accessible appearance. The changes to this edition are much more than cosmetic, however. All assistive technology device information has been updated, and new chapters have been added on funding, educational applications, and vocational applications.

Case examples and illustrations of devices in use have been added to each chapter. These additions foster the understanding of how assistive technologies are **used** as well as how they **function.** Readers of the first edition appreciated the inclusion of study questions; therefore we have increased the use of this feature by 25% throughout the text.

Also in response to requests from readers of the first edition, we have added a glossary for all key terms that appear in the text, and a list of resources which includes major conferences, professional associations, and manufacturers associations with Internet sites.

The primary audience for this book remains undergraduate and graduate university students. However, the first edition proved useful to assistive technology practitioners and assistive technology suppliers, many of whom used this text for RESNA certification examination review. These individuals represent a secondary audience: professionals who are practicing in this area even though they have had no formal training in this field while in school. Our intended audience is a transdisciplinary professional population including occupational therapists, speech-language pathologists, physical therapists, special educators, rehabilitation engineers, and vocational rehabilitation counselors.

The fundamental unifying concept in the text is a framework that describes the consumer participating in activities together with the assistive technologies and their contexts of use in a Human Activity Assistive Technology (HAAT) model. This model embodies the most fundamental of the concepts in the text (i.e., that assistive technologies represent someone [consumer with a disability] doing something [e.g., communicating, moving, manipulating] somewhere with someone [e.g., at home, at work, with peers, with strangers] through the use of assistive technologies). We use this model to develop principles for assistive technology application. These principles address everything from needs identification through system implementation to measuring outcomes. The book also provides the basis for discussion of current practices in this field and of the major technologies now in use across a wide range of specific application areas. This second edition includes updated information on all of the technologies discussed.

The book is organized into five main parts. Part One presents information on the assistive technology industry, including a historical perspective, relevant legislation, and issues of professional practices (Chapter 1). In Chapter 2, we develop the HAAT model from basic considerations of human performance and occupational science. Chapter 3 discusses the human operator in terms of the skills and abilities that are brought to assistive technology use. Part Two focuses on service delivery in assistive technologies. In Chapter 4 we focus on the service delivery system through which the consumer obtains assistive technologies. This chapter also includes a discussion of outcome measurement for assistive technologies. We have added an expanded discussion of assistive technology funding to this edition as a separate chapter (Chapter 5).

Part Three is devoted to general purpose assistive technologies, which apply across a wide range of areas. In Chapter 6 we develop basic concepts underlying seating and positioning. These concepts include pressure relief, positioning for function, and the achievement of comfort through proper positioning. Control interfaces for all applications are discussed in Chapter 7 with emphasis on the development of principles of selection and effective application. Computers play a large role in the lives of persons with disabilities, and in Chapter 8 we discuss both the major features of computers and how they are adapted for both input (alternatives to mouse and keyboard) and output (alternatives to visual display, sounds, and speech). This chapter includes a discussion of World Wide Web access for persons with disabilities.

In Part Four our emphasis shifts to a discussion of specific areas of application for assistive technologies. Selection and application of augmentative and alternative communication systems and their basic design principles are discussed in Chapter 9. Chapter 10 is devoted to manual and powered wheelchairs and driving aids. In Chapter 11 we discuss the use of assistive technologies to replace or augment manipulative ability. Also included are a wide variety of technologies, which range from simple, low technology aids (e.g., enlarged forks) to specialized electromechanical devices (e.g., feeders, electronic aids to daily living, robots). In Chapter 12 we focus on the need that individuals who have visual or auditory limitations have for assistance in obtaining information and moving freely in the world. Sensory aids that augment or replace visual or auditory function are presented in this chapter.

We have added Part Five to the second edition to allow consideration of two particularly significant contexts for assistive technology application. In Chapter 13 we describe educational applications; in Chapter 14 vocational applications. In writing these two chapters we have been able to bring together concepts, technologies, and strategies from the first 12 chapters and show how they are interrelated in these major areas of application.

The strength of our approach is that concepts are unified through the use of the HAAT model and reinforced as each specific application is presented. For each specific technology application we discuss assessment and training of the consumer, devices that are available, strategies for their use, and evaluation of outcomes. Learning objectives, key terms, study questions, and references are included for each chapter. Case studies have been added throughout the text. It is assumed that the reader will have a general understanding of normal human anatomy and physiology and disabilities.

It is our hope that those individuals familiar with assistive technologies will find something *new* in this text and that those readers who are new to this subject will develop *familiarity* with assistive technologies and appreciate their potential.

**Albert M. Cook**
**Susan M. Hussey**

# ACKNOWLEDGMENTS

The writing of a book is a huge and sometimes seemingly never-ending endeavor. The discussion that has ensued as a result of the first edition of this textbook and the constructive input we have received from many professionals in the assistive technology field has been inspiring. In this second edition of the book, Al and I learned how helpful technology could really be. When we wrote the first edition, the Internet was in its infancy. Since we ended up being miles apart for the writing of the second edition, the Internet became an invaluable tool. Throughout this process we have learned how to collaborate in new ways. Al continues to be a true mentor and friend and I am grateful for all of his patience and encouragement. I want to acknowledge my family and friends who supported me and had faith in me: my parents, Lois and Gary; Barb, Steve, Rob, and Maureen. I am so thankful to have friends and family like you. I also want to thank my colleagues in the Occupational Therapy Assistant Program and the Allied Health Division at Sacramento City College for their support and understanding. Two other colleagues who I wish to thank for their valuable feedback are Gordon St. Michel and Bob Cunningham, faculty members in the Occupational Therapy Department at Eastern Kentucky University. Finally, I want to thank and acknowledge my longtime feline companion (in memoriam), Cashflow, and my husband, Bruce, both of whom have sustained me throughout this process and shown me the meaning of unconditional love.

**Susan M. Hussey, MS, OTR**

In any creative effort, there are great demands placed on collaborators to give and take, to support and challenge, and to teach and learn. I am indebted to Sue for challenging me when I needed it, for supporting my ideas, for teaching me about many things, and for being willing to adapt her ideas to meet mutual goals. It has also been rewarding to share in the success of the first edition. As we began the revision of the text for this second edition we found ourselves separated by thousands of miles. We were able to take advantage of technology and the Internet to facilitate our continued collaboration, but this placed additional demands on our patience and understanding. Fortunately, Sue and I developed our skills at long-distance collaboration, and we found many ways to support each other. I continue to admire Sue's perseverance and dedication, and I thank her for her friendship. I am also indebted to Jim Vargo, Norma Harbottle, and Cheryl Taylor for friendship and support. A major undertaking such as this also requires large demands of time, and these are often taken away from family. I am grateful that my daughters, Barbara and Jennifer, supported my efforts through words of encouragement. I could not have completed this work without the continuing support, love, and understanding of my wife, Nancy. Finally, my son, Brian, gave me the inspiration to begin.

**Albert M. Cook, PhD, PE**

There are many individuals who have helped us with the preparation of this edition of our textbook, and we would like to acknowledge their valuable contributions. Sue Doessel, Barbara Kornblau, Simon Margolis, Larry Scadden, Elaine Trefler, and Gerry Weisman reviewed the first edition and provided many helpful suggestions for changes. Jim Geletka provided much assistance with the material on legislation in Chapter 1. Alexandra Enders convinced us to include personal assistant services as part of the AT continuum. Larry Scadden (Chapters 8 and 12) and Marion Hagler (Chapter 12) reviewed material for accuracy and provided many useful corrections and clarifications. Chris Beliveau of the Glenrose Rehabilitation Hospital I CAN Centre provided the pictures of devices in use, while Kathy Howery, also of the I CAN Centre, provided the framework for much of Chapter 13. Rob Hussey provided some of the original artwork for the first edition of the book. We are grateful for his creativity and his willingness to "make this one little change," even if it meant redrawing the entire figure. Kellie Conklin, editor, Christie Hart, developmental editor, and the editorial assistants at Mosby provided highly professional support and assistance in the production of this text.

**Albert M. Cook, PhD, PE, and Susan M. Hussey, MS, OTR**

# CONTENTS

## PART I
## Introduction and Framework

## ▦ 3 The Disabled Human User of Assistive Technologies *54*

# PART II
# Service Delivery in Assistive Technologies

## ▦ 4 Delivering Assistive Technology Services to the Consumer *91*

# PART III
# The Activities: General Purpose Assistive Technologies

# PART IV

# The Activities: Performance Areas

# PART V
# The Contexts for Assistive Technology Applications

# PART 1

# Introduction and Framework

# Introduction and Overview

## Chapter Outline

## Learning Objectives

Upon completing this chapter, you will be able to:

1. Define assistive technology
2. Delineate the characteristics of assistive technologies
3. Describe the history of assistive technology practice
4. List the major legislative initiatives that have affected the application of assistive technologies
5. Describe the components of the assistive technology industry
6. Explain the roles of the consumer

7. Identify several distinguishing features of service delivery programs
8. Identify the professionals who may work as assistive technology practitioners
9. Understand the transdisciplinary approach to assistive technology service delivery
10. Discuss the major professional issues in assistive technology practice

---

## Key Terms

| | | |
|---|---|---|
| Activity | Consumer of Assistive Technologies | Participation |
| Alpha Testing | Device | Prototype |
| Assistive Technology | Direct Consumer Services | Quality Assurance |
| Assistive Technology Practitioner (ATP) | Disability | Reasonable Accommodation |
| Assistive Technology Service | Handicap | Telerehabilitation |
| Assistive Technology Supplier | Impairment | Transdisciplinary Team Approach |
| Beta Testing | Least Restrictive Environment | Universal Design |

---

In the last 15 to 20 years there has been major growth in the application of technology in ameliorating the problems of persons with disabilities. Despite this growth, no unified set of principles for this application of technology has emerged, and one of the major goals of this text is to develop this set of principles. We begin in this chapter by providing an overview of assistive technologies and the industry that supports their development and distribution. We also present a brief historical perspective and a summary of the major United States federal legislation that provides the mandate for assistive technologies.

### ■ ASSISTIVE TECHNOLOGIES: A WORKING DEFINITION

In the document titled *International Classification of Impairments, Disabilities and Handicaps* (ICIDH), the World Health Organization (WHO) defines an **impairment** as "any loss or abnormality of psychological, physical or anatomical structure or function." A **disability** results when the impairment leads to an inability to "perform an activity in the manner or within the range considered normal for a human being" (e.g., difficulties in communicating, hearing, moving about, or manipulating objects). A **handicap** results when the individual with an impairment or disability is unable to fulfill his or her normal role. According to these definitions, a handicap is not a characteristic of a person; it is a description of the relationship between the person and the environment (World Health Organization, 1980). For example, an individual who is born without both upper extremities (the impairment) may not be able to write or complete self-care tasks in the normal fashion (the disability). If this person is prevented from participating in school or being em-

ployed by this impairment and disability, this is a handicap. In spite of this impairment, this individual may perform daily activities using his or her feet or mouth or may use prosthetic devices in order to overcome a handicapping condition. This approach, which shifts the handicap from the individual to the environment, provides an important perspective on the role of assistive technologies in reducing the handicapping effects of disabilities. Describing persons with disabilities in this way also emphasizes functional outcomes, instead of focusing on limitations, and assistive technologies are employed primarily to contribute to successful functional outcomes for persons with disabilities.

The WHO revised the original ICIDH into a new format titled *ICIDH-2: International Classification of Functioning, Disability and Health–ICF* (World Health Organization, 2001). This new framework substitutes **activity** for *disability* and **participation** for *handicap*. These terms are precisely defined in the ICIDH-2 guidelines in ways that differ from their everyday meanings. Developed in response to worldwide concern for the limitations of the original ICIDH, the new terminology has several benefits. First of all it recognizes that the limitations presented by an impairment are reflected in both the restrictions placed on the person's activities and in the barriers to participation created by society. The impairment, activity, and participation categories are viewed as distinct but parallel classifications. The ICIDH-2 document defines impairment as a loss or abnormality of body structure, physiology, or psychological function. Activity is the "execution of a task or action by an individual" (World Health Organization, 2001, p. 15). Participation is defined as "involvement in a life situation" (World Health Organization, 2001, p. 15). Contextual factors are referred to as environmental or personal. The latter are internal to the person and have an impact on how disablement is experienced. Examples include gender, age, other health conditions, fitness, lifestyle education, and similar factors. Environmental contextual factors are outside the individual (e.g., attitudes of society, architectural barriers, and legal factors). Both types of contextual factors can be influenced by assistive technologies, and Chapter 2 presents a model that includes these considerations. The ICF has great potential for influencing social policy, legislation, service delivery, and research in disability and assistive technologies. Fougeyrollas and Gray (1998) discuss the value of classification schemes like the ICIDH-2 and their implications for assistive technologies.

## Definition of Assistive Technology Devices and Services

Dictionaries provide the following definition of technology:

(1) The science or study of the practical or industrial arts, (2) applied science, (3) a method, process, etc. for handling a specific technical problem [McKechnie, 1983; Guralnik, 1979]

Surprisingly, none of these definitions says anything about a "device"; instead the emphasis is on the application of knowledge. This is an important concept, and we shall use the term **assistive technology** to refer to a broad range of **devices,** services, strategies, and practices that are conceived and applied to ameliorate the problems faced by individuals who have disabilities.

Within this framework there are many ways to define assistive technologies. One widely used definition is that provided in Public Law (PL) 100-407, the Technical Assistance to the States Act in the United States. The definition of an assistive technology device is as follows:

Any item, piece of equipment or product system whether acquired commercially off the shelf, modified, or customized that is used to increase, maintain or improve functional capabilities of individuals with disabilities.

This definition has several important components, and because we plan to use it as a working definition throughout this book, we need to examine these in some detail. First, the definition includes commercial, modified, and customized devices. By including all types of devices, we encompass an extremely wide range of applications. Second, this definition emphasizes *functional* capabilities of *individuals* with disabilities. Functional outcomes are the only real measure of the success of assistive technology devices, and throughout this text we stress the importance of providing technologies that result in increased functional capability. Finally,

the emphasis on individual persons with disabilities underscores the importance of treating each application of technology as a unique circumstance. No two applications are exactly the same in terms of the needs and skills of the person being served, the activities to be accomplished, and the context in which the application takes place.

Public Law 100-407 also defines an **assistive technology service** as

any service that directly assists an individual with a disability in the selection, acquisition or use of an assistive technology device.

The law also includes several specific examples that further clarify this definition. These include (1) evaluating needs and skills for assistive technology; (2) acquiring assistive technologies; (3) selecting, designing, repairing, and fabricating assistive technology systems; (4) coordinating services with other therapies; and (5) training both individuals with disabilities and those working with them to use the technologies effectively. This definition demonstrates the broad spectrum of services inherent in the delivery of assistive technologies.

## Characterization of Assistive Technologies

In this section we present a characterization of assistive technologies from several points of view. Each of these is a logical outgrowth of the definitions presented earlier, and each is useful in the process of applying assistive technologies. Box 1-1 shows several classifications used to distinguish different types of assistive technologies.

**Assistive versus rehabilitative or educational technologies.** Technology can serve two major purposes: helping and teaching (Smith, 1991). Technology that helps an individual to carry out a functional activity is termed *assistive technology.* Our emphasis in this text is on assistive technologies that serve a variety of functional needs. Technology

---

**BOX 1-1    Characterizations of Assistive Technologies**

Assistive versus rehabilitative or educational technologies
Low to high technology
Hard technologies and soft technologies
Appliances versus tools
Minimal to maximal technology
General versus specific technologies
Commercial to custom technology

---

Data from Odor, 1984; Rizer, Ourand, and Rein, 1990; Smith, 1991; Vanderheiden, 1987.

can also be used as part of an educational or rehabilitative process. In this case the technology is usually used as one modality in an overall education or rehabilitation plan. Technology in this sense is used as a tool for remediation or rehabilitation rather than being a part of the person's daily life and functional activities, and we refer to it as *rehabilitative* or *educational* technology, depending on the setting. Often rehabilitative or educational technology (e.g., cognitive retraining software) is employed to develop skills for the use of assistive technologies, and we discuss some of these applications in later chapters.

**Low to high technology.** The next of these distinctions is between low-technology devices and high-technology devices. Although this distinction is imprecise, we often describe inexpensive devices that are simple to make and easy to obtain as "low" technology and devices that are expensive, more difficult to make, and harder to obtain as "high" technology. According to this distinction, examples of low-technology devices are simple pencil and paper communication boards, modified eating utensils, and simple splints. Wheelchairs, electronic communication devices, and computers are examples of high-technology devices.

**Hard and soft technologies.** Odor (1984) has distinguished between *hard technologies* and *soft technologies*. Hard technologies are readily available components that can be purchased and assembled into assistive technology systems. This includes everything from simple mouth sticks to computers and software. The PL 100-407 definition of an assistive technology device applies primarily to hard technologies as we have defined them. The main distinguishing feature of hard technologies is that they are tangible. On the other hand, soft technologies are the human areas of decision making, strategies, training, concept formation, and so on. Soft technologies are generally captured in one of three forms: (1) people, (2) written, and (3) computer (Bailey, 1989). These aspects of technology, without which the hard technology cannot be successful, are much harder to obtain. Assistive technology services as defined in PL 100-407 are basically soft technologies. Soft technologies are difficult to acquire because they are highly dependent on human knowledge rather than tangible objects. This knowledge is obtained slowly through formal training, experience, and textbooks such as this one. The development of effective strategies of use also has a major effect on assistive technology system success. Initially the formulation of these strategies may rely heavily on the knowledge, experience, and ingenuity of the assistive technology practitioner. With growing experience, the assistive technology user originates strategies that facilitate successful device use. The roles of both hard and soft technologies as integral portions of assistive technology systems is discussed in the section on activities in Chapter 2.

**Appliances versus tools.** An appliance is a device that "provides benefits to the individual independent of the individual's skill level" (Vanderheiden, 1987, p. 705). Tools, on the other hand, require the development of skill for their use. Household appliances such as refrigerators do not require any skill to operate, whereas tools such as a hammer or saw do require skill. This same criterion applies to assistive technologies. The determining factor in distinguishing a tool from an appliance is that the quality of the result obtained using a tool depends on the skill of the user. For example, eyeglasses, splints, a seating system, or a keyguard for a computer are all appliances, since the quality of the functional outcome does not depend on the skill of the user. On the other hand, success in maneuvering a powered wheelchair does depend on the skill of the user; therefore the wheelchair is classified as a tool. Examples of assistive technology tools and appliances are shown in Table 1-1.

In some instances the device may be a tool or an appliance, depending on how it is set up to be used. For example, an environmental control system that controls lights or appliances (see Chapter 11) requires a relatively complex set of electronic circuits that most would agree are high tech. However, this system can be set up so that the only skill required to operate it is to turn it on or off, in which case it may be considered an appliance. In other instances this system may require the user to learn a sophisticated method of scanning in order to operate it; the system would then be considered a tool. It is important to note that an appliance that requires user skill because it is poorly designed is not considered a tool.

As Vanderheiden (1987) points out, the successful use of assistive technology tools requires training, strategies, and special skills. These are soft technologies. For example, learning aids that facilitate the use of an assistive device are tools that are employed only until the user gains sufficient skill to use the device independently. However, the use of the learning aid requires skill, and this aid is therefore a tool.

| Table 1-1 | Examples of Assistive Technology Tools and Appliances | |
|---|---|---|
| Topic (Chapter) | Appliances | Tools |
| Control interfaces (7) | Keyguards | Joystick |
| Computer access (8) | Enlarging lens | Enlarged keyboard |
| Augmentative communication (9) | — | Alphabet board |
| Manipulation (11) | Environmental control* | Electric feeder |
| Mobility (10) | Wheelchair armrest | Manual wheelchair push rims |
| Sensory (12) | Eyeglasses | Long cane |

*See text; classification depends on EADL (electronic aid for daily living) and its functions.

Strategies for the use of an assistive device require skill and are therefore properly categorized as tools. Both appliances and tools require careful assessment, recommendation, and fitting (see Chapter 4), but only the tool also requires skill development (Vanderheiden, 1987). If we include training of care providers, as well as the consumer of the technology, then training also may be necessary for appliances. For example, when a new seating system is provided (Chapter 6), the care staff must be trained in how to position the person in the seating system. By including soft technologies in our concept of a tool, we emphasize the importance of developing these skills together with the acquisition of the basic hard technology tool or appliance.

Another important point raised by Vanderheiden (1987) is that the tools used by persons with disabilities are often different from those used by the general population. This means that, in order to develop skill, the assistive technology user often cannot observe someone using the same device. People routinely use observation, such as watching someone using a hammer, as a means of learning how to use a tool. When the person with a disability is the only one in that environment who is using the tool, he or she must rely more heavily on personal experience and formal training to learn to use it effectively.

**Minimal to maximal technology.** Assistive technologies are specified and designed to meet a continuum of needs. At one extreme are devices that provide some assistance or augment the individual's ability to perform a task. For example, an individual with cerebral palsy may be able to speak, but on occasion his speech may be difficult to understand. In those instances the individual may clarify his speech using a letter board to spell out words not understood. Or a person with respiratory problems may be able to ambulate inside her house but, because of low endurance, may require a powered wheelchair to be able to do her grocery shopping independently. In fact, many grocery stores now provide powered carts for individuals who need this type of augmented mobility. At the other extreme are assistive technologies that replace significant amounts of ability to generate functional outcomes. For example, some individuals have no verbal communication ability and may require a device to be able to communicate. Likewise, some individuals are totally dependent on a manual or powered wheelchair for their personal mobility.

Minimal technologies generally *augment* rather than replace function. Classically, devices that augment have been termed *orthoses* or orthotic devices. Although this term originally referred to braces of various types, it has been broadened to include all devices that assist or augment function. The term *prosthetics* or prosthetic device originally was used to describe devices that replaced a body part both structurally and functionally. Now this term has also been broadened to include all devices that provide a *functional*

replacement. For example, augmentative communication systems that replace the function of speech are sometimes called *speech prostheses*.

**General versus specific technologies.** We differentiate between assistive technologies that are used in many different applications as general technology and those that are intended for a specific application. *General-purpose* assistive technologies include (1) positioning systems, (2) control interfaces, and (3) computers. These are classified as general purpose because they are used across a wide range of applications. Body position affects the way an individual uses the assistive technology. Frequently, external support systems, an assistive technology, are necessary to achieve a body position that facilitates functional activities. Control interfaces are the means by which the user interacts with any assistive technology. Examples include the joystick on a powered wheelchair, the keyboard on a computer, or the handle that operates the closing mechanism on a reacher. Virtually every electronic assistive technology has a computer incorporated into it. This enhances the flexibility and the breadth of application of these devices. Thus we also include computers as general-purpose technologies.

*Specific-purpose* assistive technologies facilitate performance in one unique application area. Examples include devices for communication, manual and powered wheelchairs, feeding devices, hearing aids, and mobility aids for persons with visual impairments. Because these devices are intended for a specific use, it is possible to design them to maximize their capabilities to meet a particular need.

**Commercial to custom technology.** Another distinction shown in Box 1-1 is between commercially available devices and those that are custom made for an individual person. There is actually a continuum from commercial devices (designed for the general public and designed for persons with disabilities), to modification of a commercial device, and finally to making a completely customized device.

Figure 1-1 illustrates the progression from commercially available devices to those that are completely customized for an individual. We use the term *commercially available* to refer to devices that are mass produced. These include commercial devices designed for the general population *(standard commercially available devices)* and assistive technologies *(special commercially available devices)*, which are mass-produced devices designed for individuals with disabilities. For example, standard personal computers designed for the general population are often used by persons with disabilities. Increasingly, commercial products are being designed according to the principles of **universal design:** the design of products and environments to be usable by all people, to the greatest extent possible, without the need for adaptation or specialized design (NC State

**BOX 1-2**   **Principles of Universal Design***

**ONE: EQUITABLE USE**
The design is useful and marketable to people with diverse abilities.

**TWO: FLEXIBILITY IN USE**
The design accommodates a wide range of individual preferences and abilities.

**THREE: SIMPLE AND INTUITIVE USE**
Use of the design is easy to understand, regardless of the user's experience, knowledge, language skills, or current concentration level.

**FOUR: PERCEPTIBLE INFORMATION**
The design communicates necessary information effectively to the user, regardless of ambient conditions or the user's sensory abilities.

**FIVE: TOLERANCE FOR ERROR**
The design minimizes hazards and the adverse consequences of accidental or unintended actions.

**SIX: LOW PHYSICAL EFFORT**
The design can be used efficiently and comfortably and with a minimum of fatigue.

**SEVEN: SIZE AND SPACE FOR APPROACH AND USE**
Appropriate size and space is provided for approach, reach, manipulation, and use regardless of user's body size, posture, or mobility.

From North Carolina State University, The Center for Universal Design, 1997.

*For complete guidelines, see www.design.ncsu.edu/cud/pubs/udprinciples.

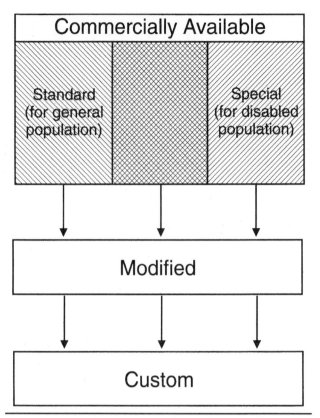

Figure 1-1   This diagram shows the progression from commercially available devices for the general population and commercially available devices for special populations to modified devices and custom devices.

University, The Center for Universal Design, 1997). In this approach, features that make a product more useful to persons who have disabilities (e.g., larger knobs; a variety of display options—visual, tactile, auditory; alternatives to reading text—icons, pictures) are built into the product. This is much less expensive than modifying a product after production to meet the needs of a person with a disability. In some cases (e.g., telecommunications equipment) this universal design approach is mandated by federal regulations. In some countries, universal design is known as "design for all." The North Carolina State University Center for Universal Design, in conjunction with advocates of universal design, have compiled a set of principles of universal design, shown in Box 1-2. This center also maintains a Web site on universal design (www.design.ncsu.edu/cud/pubs/udprinciples).

When an individual's needs for assistive technology cannot be met with a commercial device, we attempt to use special devices that are mass produced and commercially available for persons with disabilities. Examples include wheelchairs, augmentative communication systems, and many aids to daily living. In some cases a combination of standard and special-purpose technologies are used; this is represented by the crosshatched area of Figure 1-1. For example, a standard general-purpose computer may be used with special-purpose software to create an augmentative communication device (see Chapter 9).

If commercially available devices cannot meet an individual's needs, we may modify it. This modification can vary from simple to very complex. For example, if an individual has difficulty using the keys on a computer keyboard, we can purchase software that facilitates its use. In this case the most expensive and complex part of the system (the computer) is a standard commercial product, and the software is the simplest and least expensive portion of the system. However, the software may have a cost that is much higher than expected relative to its simplicity because it is a special product and all the costs of development must be recovered from the small production run. A special commercially available device may be modified as well. For example, a commercially available augmentative communication device may require modification so that it can be mounted on a user's wheelchair.

When no commercial device or modification is appropriate, it is necessary to design one specifically for the task at hand. This approach results in a *custom* device. Because they are mass produced, commercial devices have a lower per unit cost than do custom devices. For example, seating and positioning systems for persons with severe disabilities are often individually contoured to achieve the necessary functional result, and this can increase the cost (see Chapter 6).

Another important difference between modified or custom devices and commercial devices is the level of technical support that is available with each. A commercially produced device generally has written documentation and operator's manuals available. Although the quality of these written materials varies widely, some documentation is better than none, and modified or custom devices often have none. The manufacturer or supplier of commercial equipment provides technical support and repair. Because modified or custom devices are one of a kind, technical support may be hard to obtain, especially if the original designer and builder is no longer available (e.g., if the user moves to a new area).

## Summary

Assistive technology can be characterized in many ways. It is useful to realize, however, that yesterday's high tech is tomorrow's low tech, custom devices become commercial if more than a few people need them, and appliances often enable the use of tools. Thus no good categorization is perfect or is static. As the field advances, there will be new considerations that will further stretch our concepts and force new ways of categorizing and describing assistive technologies.

## ■ A HISTORICAL PERSPECTIVE ON ASSISTIVE TECHNOLOGY DEVICES AND SERVICES

### (Very) Early Developments in Assistive Technologies

Although it is tempting to view assistive technologies and the assistive technology industry as innovations that have occurred over the past 20 years, we must go back much further in time to really investigate the origins of this field. Imagine that we are in the Stone Age. Our friend Borg has broken his leg on a hunting expedition. Because there is no plaster yet available, his leg is not placed in a plaster cast, and when it heals he has a decided limp. Determined to continue providing for his clan, he reaches for the nearest stick to assist his walking. Thus one of the first assistive technology devices is conceived, fabricated, and put into use. At the time this custom device is referred to as "high tech" because of its advanced design and its use of state-of-the-art materials. As time moves on, Borg's descendants begin to realize that assistive technologies can help meet other needs. His great granddaughter, Myra, now in her later years, discovers that an empty animal horn can be used to make voices louder and help compensate for her fading hearing. One of the first uses of the wheel, a new invention that will be reinvented many times over the years, is to transport people. This key component of the current wheelchair is surprisingly similar to its predecessor. Most important, each version emphasizes function rather than form or style. Borg's walking stick also bears a strong resemblance to present-day canes and crutches. However, Myra's animal horn is only functionally related to the modern-day hearing aid. There is little structural relationship between these two devices, which brings us to the next major point in the history of assistive technologies.

### Evolution of State-of-the-Art Assistive Technology

Assistive technologies have always been based on the materials and state-of-the-art technology available to the practitioners. In assistive technologies we emphasize functional outcomes above all other considerations. For this reason, some applications have had little change for many years. Borg's cane is one example; although the structure has remained the same, the materials have changed. However, other applications have only been possible as technologies have advanced.

During the Civil War in the United States, great strides were made in the development of prostheses, especially for the lower limb. Sockets were improved, creating a better fit and more functional outcome. A socket developed by Parmelee in 1863 featured the first suction attachment of a lower limb prosthesis (Murphy, Cook, and Harvey, 1982). This type of socket, still used in modern prostheses, eliminated discomfort caused by pelvic attachment bands and reduced alignment problems and the risk of breakage at the joint. The materials used in 1863, however, bear little resemblance to those used today. Current prostheses use composite metals and plastics, whereas Parmelee's device was made of wood and leather.

Miniature electronic circuits only available in the past 20 years have replaced Myra's horn. However, hearing aids were first patented in the 1890s, and the major function of amplifying sound has not changed over the years. What has changed is the *structure* of these aids. Now they fit into the ear, amplify a wider range of sounds, and are generally more effective (see Chapter 12). In the 1890s these aids were bulky and produced much lower fidelity. It was a long time between Myra's horn and the first hearing aids in the 1890s, but in the last 100 years the state of the art in this field has changed dramatically.

In some cases, current assistive technology applications were not possible as few as 15 years ago. The well-documented revolution in electronics is the reason for most of these gains, and computers are the vehicle by which the advancements have been made. The single most important change in computer design and construction was the reduction in complexity brought about by the development of the microprocessor electronic circuit "chip." This innovation, the *microprocessor*, resulted in reduced size (from a room full of electronics to a typewriter-sized device), reduced cost (affordable by an individual), and greatly increased functional capabilities. Whereas we normally think of computers as stand-alone personal systems, microprocessors are built into a large number of devices, from computer printers to microwave ovens and other household appliances. These chips also make possible such important innovations as synthesized speech (see Chapters 8, 9, and 12), robotic aids (see Chapter 11), and computer graphics, all of which play major roles in assistive technology applications. It is difficult to find assistive technology applications in any functional performance area that have not been affected by microcomputer advances. Even in the area of seating and positioning, computer technology is being used for the design and manufacture of custom seat cushions (see Chapter 6). Throughout the remainder of this text we describe the most important of these applications.

## Federal Legislation Affecting the Application of Assistive Technologies*

Whereas industrial advancements and competition have driven the recent development of assistive technology devices, the development of assistive technology services and service delivery in the United States has been impacted significantly by federal legislation. In this section we discuss only the recent legislation that has most directly affected the development and application of assistive technologies. Each of the major pieces of legislation that we discuss is summarized in Table 1-2. For the complete text of any federal law, refer to the Library of Congress's "Thomas" Web site at www.thomas.loc.gov/. Specific information on United States legislation related to assistive technologies is available on the Rehabilitation Engineering and Assistive Technology Society of North America (RESNA) Web site at www.resna.org.

**Rehabilitation Act of 1973 (Amended).** The Rehabilitation Act establishes several important principles on which subsequent legislation has been based. One of the most important of these is the concept of **reasonable accommodation** in employment and in secondary education. The act mandates that employers and institutions of higher education receiving federal funds seek to accommodate the needs of employees and students who have disabilities. It

specifically prohibits discrimination in employment or admission to academic programs solely on the basis of a disability. This law originally described both reasonable accommodation and **least restrictive environment** (LRE), a term relating to the degree of modification that is acceptable in a job or academic program.

As a result of the Rehabilitation Act of 1973, many employers and universities made architectural changes to campuses and work settings to reduce barriers. Elevators were added to buildings, ramps and curb cuts were made to accommodate wheelchair users, and voice and Braille labels were added to signs (including elevators) to provide access for visually impaired persons. Many of the efforts to achieve accommodation in the least restrictive environment involved the use of assistive technologies.

The Rehabilitation Act Amendments of 1998, which are contained in the Workforce Investment Act of 1998 (PL 105-220), are the most recent amendments to the Rehab Act. This act was also amended in 1986 (PL 99-506), 1992 (PL 102-569), and 1993 (PL 103-73). Together they include several provisions involving assistive technology. First the amendments require that each state include within its vocational rehabilitation plan a provision for assistive technology (referred to in PL 99-506 as *rehabilitation engineering or technology* and in PL 105-220 as *rehabilitation technology*). PL 99-506 defined rehabilitation engineering as

> the systematic application of technologies, engineering methodologies, or scientific principles to meet the needs of and address the barriers confronted by individuals with handicaps in areas which include education, rehabilitation, employment, transportation, independent living and recreation (Enders and Hall, 1990, p. 460).

Because this plan is the basis by which states receive federal funding for vocational rehabilitation, there is a strong incentive to provide these technology-related services. The Rehab Act also requires that provision for acquiring appropriate and necessary assistive technology devices and services be included in Individualized Written Rehabilitation Programs (IWPs), which are written for individuals with disabilities.

An important provision of the Rehab Act is Section 508. First added in the 1986 amendments and later strengthened in the 1998 amendments, this section was developed to ensure access to "electronic office equipment" by persons with disabilities who work for the federal government. Although limitation to the federal government may seem to be so restrictive as to severely reduce the impact of the regulations, the federal government is such a large purchaser of computers and other office technology that any purchasing specifications it makes take on the role of informal standards. This legislation has had a significant impact on the design and manufacture of computers and their accessibility to persons with disabilities. Persons who are blind or

---

*Jim Geletka, former Executive Director of the Rehabilitation Engineering and Assistive Technology Society of North America, provided significant assistance in the preparation of this section.

**TABLE 1-2**    Recent Major U.S. Federal Legislation Affecting Assistive Technologies

| Legislation | Major Assistive Technology Impact |
| --- | --- |
| Rehabilitation Act of 1973, as amended | Mandated reasonable accommodation and LRE in federally funded employment and higher education; requires both assistive technology device and services be included in state plans and IWRP for each client; Section 508 mandates equal access to electronic office equipment for all federal employees; defines rehabilitation technology as rehabilitation engineering and assistive technology devices and services; mandates rehabilitation technology as primary benefit to be included in IWRP |
| Individuals with Disabilities Education Act Amendments of 1997 | Recognized the right of every child to a free and appropriate education; included concept that children with disabilities are to be educated with their peers; extended reasonable accommodation, LRE, and assistive technology devices and services to age 3-21 education; mandated IEP for each child, to include consideration of assistive technologies; also included mandated services for children from birth to 2 and expanded emphasis on educationally related assistive technologies |
| Assistive Technology Act of 1998 (replaced Technology Related Assistance for Individuals with Disabilities Act of 1988) | First legislation to specifically address expansion of assistive technology devices and services; mandates consumer-driven assistive technology services, capacity building, advocacy activities, and statewide system change; supports grants to expand and administer alternative financing of assistive technology systems |
| The Developmental Disabilities Assistance and Bill of Rights Act | Provides grants to states for developmental disabilities councils, university-affiliated programs, and protection and advocacy activities for persons with developmental disabilities; provides training and technical assistance to improve access to assistive technology services for individuals with developmental disabilities |
| Americans with Disabilities Act (ADA) of 1990 | Prohibits discrimination on the basis of disability in employment, state and local government, public accommodations, commercial facilities, transportation, and telecommunications, all of which affect the application of assistive technology; use of assistive technology impacts requirement that Title II entities must communicate effectively with people who have hearing, vision, or speech disabilities; addresses telephone and television access for people with hearing and speech disabilities |
| Medicaid | Income-based ("means-tested") program; eligibility and services differ from state to state; federal government sets general program requirements and provides financial assistance to the states by matching state expenditures; assistive technology benefits differ for adults and children from birth to age 21; assistive technology for adults must be included in state's Medicaid plan or waiver program |
| Early Periodic Screening, Diagnosis and Treatment Program | Mandatory service for children from birth through age 21; includes any required or optional service listed in the Medicaid Act (see Box 1-5); service need not be included in the state's Medicaid plan |
| Medicare | Major funding source for assistive technology (durable medical equipment); includes individuals 65 or over and those who are permanently and totally disabled; federally administered with consistent rules for all states |

*IWRP,* Individualized Written Rehabilitation Plan.

have low vision and those with difficulty in accessing the keyboard have benefited from standards derived as a result of Section 508, and several manufacturers have included in the basic designs of their computer systems technology that increases access. Many of these features are discussed further in Chapter 8.

The major intent of Section 508 is that electronic and information technology developed, procured, maintained, or used by the federal government be accessible to people with disabilities. Section 508 applies to federal departments and agencies. It covers access to electronic office equipment and electronic information services provided to the public by the federal government. This includes ensuring that end users with disabilities (1) have access to the same databases and application programs as other end users, (2) are supported in manipulating data and related information resources to attain equivalent end results as other end users, and (3) can

transmit and receive messages using the same telecommunication systems as other end users. The U.S. Architectural and Transportation Barriers Compliance Board is now developing standards for Section 508. The guidelines accompanying Section 508 also detail the functional performance specifications for electronic office equipment accessibility. Because of provisions in the former Tech Act, now the Assistive Technology (AT) Act of 1998 (see p. 12), states and territories that receive AT Act funding and all subrecipients must comply with Section 508.

**Individuals with Disabilities Education Act Amendments of 1997.** The Individuals with Disabilities Education Act Amendments of 1997 (IDEA 97), PL 105-17, recognized the right of every child with a disability to receive a "free and appropriate public education" (FAPE). This right to a public education was initially legislated under the Education for All Handicapped Children Act (EHA; PL 94-142), which was first passed by Congress in 1975. Before this law, more than 1 million children with disabilities were excluded from American public schools. Currently there are approximately 6 million children being served under IDEA.

IDEA includes the concept that children with disabilities are to be educated with their nondisabled peers to "the maximum extent appropriate." Children with disabilities are to be segregated or otherwise removed from the regular classroom "only when the nature or severity of the handicap is such that education in regular classes . . . cannot be achieved." Under the requirements of this law, an individual education program (IEP) must be written for each student. The IEP "sets out the child's present educational performance, establishes annual and short-term objectives for improvements in that performance, and describes the specially designed instruction and services that will enable the child to meet the objectives."

Special education, under IDEA, is defined as "specifically designed instruction . . . to meet the unique needs of a child with disabilities with the necessary supplementary aids and related services" needed for the child to benefit from educational services in the least restrictive environment. The 1997 amendments to IDEA stated that the goals of IDEA 97 are to make education of children with disabilities more effective through the following steps:

1. Strengthening the role of parents and fostering partnerships between parents and schools
2. Increasing expectations and ensuring access to the general curriculum to the maximum extent possible
3. Aligning Part B programs (those for children ages 3 to 21) with state and local improvement efforts so that students with disabilities benefit from them
4. Providing whole-school approaches and prereferral intervention to reduce the need to label children to address their learning needs
5. Focusing resources on teaching and learning and reducing paperwork burdens
6. Supporting high-quality, intensive professional development for all personnel working with children with disabilities

IDEA 97 includes positive changes regarding assistive technology. The assistive technology needs of a child with disabilities must be "considered" along with other special factors by the IEP team in formulating the child's IEP.

The terms *assistive technology devices* and *assistive technology services* were first included in IDEA in 1991. The definitions of "assistive technology device" and "assistive technology service" were the same as those found in the 1988 Technology Related Assistance for Individuals with Disabilities Act (Tech Act; PL 100-407). A policy statement on the right of a student with a disability to receive assistive technology under PL 94-142 was issued on August 10, 1990, by the federal Office of Special Education Programs (OSEP) (Button, 1990). This policy statement outlines a wide range of services and devices that may be included in an IEP and describes the process of developing the IEP to include them. Button presents guidelines to parents in the development of an appropriate IEP involving the use of assistive technologies. Desch (1986) describes the implications of PL 94-142 regarding the acquisition of assistive technologies by children with disabilities. The impact of this law has been far reaching. Devices ranging from sensory aids (visual and auditory) to augmentative communication devices to specialized computers have been utilized to provide access to educational programs for children with disabilities. Lack of local services or lack of funds are not sufficient reasons to deny services or devices justified in the IEP. If the IEP goals are not met, or if there are differences over what should be included in the IEP, there is a fair hearing process that may be pursued. IDEA also mandated that local educational agencies be responsible for providing assistive technology devices and services if these are required as part of the child's educational or related services or as a supplementary aid or service.

The focus of IDEA 97 is on improving results for children with disabilities. One major portion of the original act invited states to expand and improve services to infants and toddlers with disabilities and their families (Part H, the Infants and Toddlers with Disabilities Program). In 1997 Part H became Part C of IDEA 97.

Part C of IDEA 97 provides for services to infants and toddlers (birth through age 2). More than 177,000 children receive services under Part C, and of those, nearly 10,000 receive assistive technology devices and services. State AT Act projects have been active in promoting the use of assistive technology for the very young and have contributed to building the capacity to provide AT services under Part C. Technology provided includes battery-operated toys with easy-access switches, seating and positioning systems, computers and alternative access aids, communications software, and others. Adapted toys help the child learn the basic concept of cause and effect. Seating and positioning systems provide support and guide the growth of a child's body. They also allow the child to move about in his or her environment. Computers and alternate access aids, such as large keypads and touch screens, can help children use software that develops communication, perceptual skills, fine motor skills, and many other skills. Through annual grants beginning in 1987, financial support is provided to develop, establish, and maintain a statewide system that offers early intervention services to all eligible children. Although participation in Part H (now Part C) was always voluntary, each state has chosen to develop a statewide system and, as of October 1, 1994, has committed to seeing that services are available to every eligible child and his or her family. The U.S. Department of Education, through OSEP, distributes funds under Part C to the states to help them carry out collaborative systems planning, policy development, and implementation of needed services for infants and toddlers who have disabilities.

The number of very young children using assistive technology (AT) has increased dramatically over the past 4 years. Besides assistive technology devices and services, states provide a variety of other services to children from birth to 2 years old, such as special education; physical and occupational therapy; nutrition services; audiology; nursing services; speech-language pathology; family training, counseling, and home visits; and vision services. The services to be provided to the child with a disability and the family are documented in an Individualized Family Service Plan (IFSP). Development of the IFSP, as with the IEP, is based on assessments of a child's capabilities, skills, and needs and is constructed through a team approach that includes family members.

**Assistive Technology Act of 1998.** Designated as PL 105-394, the Assistive Technology Act replaced the Technology-Related Assistance for Individuals with Disabilities Act of 1988 (PL 100-407) and the amendments to that law (PL 103-218) enacted in 1994. The Tech Act, PL 100-407, which ended in 1998, was the first federal legislation that specifically addressed expansion of the availability of assistive technology devices and services to individuals with disabilities. The replacement, the AT Act, carries over many of the concepts of the Tech Act. It extends funding to the 50 states, the District of Columbia, Puerto Rico, and outlying areas (Guam, American Samoa, U.S. Virgin Islands, and the Commonwealth of the Northern Mariana Islands) that received support under the Tech Act. The purposes of the AT Act include the following:

1. Support states in sustaining and strengthening their capacity to address the assistive technology needs of individuals with disabilities
2. Support the investment in technology across federal agencies and departments that could benefit individuals with disabilities
3. Support microloan programs to individuals wishing to purchase assistive technology devices or services

The AT Act is divided into three parts: Title I, State Grant Programs; Title II, National Activities; and Title III, Alternative Financing Mechanisms.

Title I provides grants to states to support capacity building and advocacy activities designed to assist the states in maintaining permanent, comprehensive, consumer-responsive, statewide programs of technology-related assistance. These include public awareness, interagency coordination, technical assistance and training to promote access to assistive technology, and support to community-based organizations that provide assistive technology devices and services or assist individuals in using assistive technology. Title I also provides legal protection and advocacy services; funding for technical assistance, including a national public Internet site; and technical assistance to the states.

Title II provides for increased coordination of federal efforts related to assistive technology and universal design. It authorized funding for multiple grant programs from fiscal years 1999 through 2000, including grants for universal design research, Small Business Innovative Research grants related to assistive technology, grants to commercial or other organizations for research and development related to universal design concepts, grants or other mechanisms to address the unique assistive technology needs of urban and rural areas and of children and the elderly, and grants or other mechanisms to improve training of rehabilitation engineers and technicians.

Title III requires the secretary of education to award grants to states and outlying areas to pay for the federal share of the cost of the establishment and administration of, or the expansion and administration of, specified types of alternative financing systems for assistive technology for people with disabilities. These alternative-funding mechanisms may include a low-interest loan fund, an interest buy-down program, a revolving loan fund, a loan guarantee or insurance program, and others (RESNA Technical Assistance Project, 1999).

**The Developmental Disabilities Assistance and Bill of Rights Act.** The Developmental Disabilities program was originally enacted as Title I of the Mental Retardation Facilities and Construction Act of 1963 (PL 88-164) and has been amended eight times since then. This program provides grants to states for developmental disabilities councils (DD Councils), university-affiliated programs (UAPs), and protection and advocacy activities for persons with developmental disabilities (PADD). Grants to UAPs include grants for training projects with respect to assistive technology services for the purpose of assisting university-affiliated programs in providing training to personnel who provide, or will provide, assistive technology services and devices to individuals with developmental disabilities and their families. Such projects may provide training and technical assistance to improve access to assistive technology services for individuals with developmental disabilities and may include stipends and tuition assistance for training project participants.

**Americans with Disabilities Act (ADA) of 1990.** The Americans with Disabilities Act (ADA; PL 101-336) prohibits discrimination on the basis of disability in employment, state and local government, public accommodations, commercial facilities, transportation, and telecommunications. It also applies to the United States Congress.

To be protected by the ADA, one must meet the following ADA definitions of disability: a person who has a physical or mental impairment that substantially limits one or more major life activities, a person who has a history or record of such an impairment, or a person who is perceived by others as having such an impairment. The ADA does not specifically name all the impairments that are covered.

The ADA has four main titles: Title I (employment), Title II (state and local government agencies and public transportation), Title III (public accommodations), and Title IV (telecommunications), all of which affect the application of assistive technology.

The standards for determining employment discrimination under the Rehabilitation Act are the same as those used in Title I of the Americans with Disabilities Act. Title I requires employers with 15 or more employees to provide qualified individuals with disabilities an equal opportunity to benefit from the full range of employment-related opportunities available to others. For example, it prohibits discrimination in recruitment, hiring, promotions, training, pay, social activities, and other privileges of employment. It restricts questions that can be asked about an applicant's disability before a job offer is made. Many issues of employment involve the use and application of assistive technology, because Title I of the ADA requires that employers make reasonable accommodation to the known physical or mental limitations of otherwise qualified individuals with disabilities unless it results in undue hardship. Religious entities with 15 or more employees are also covered under Title I.

Title II covers all activities of state and local governments regardless of the government entity's size or receipt of federal funding. Title II requires that state and local governments give people with disabilities an equal opportunity to benefit from all their programs, services, and activities (e.g., public education, employment, transportation, recreation, health care, social services, courts, voting, and town meetings).

State and local governments are required to follow specific architectural standards in the new construction and alteration of their buildings. They also must relocate programs or otherwise provide access in inaccessible older buildings. In addition, the use of assistive technology such as specialized computer software impacts the requirement that Title II entities must communicate effectively with people who have hearing, vision, or speech disabilities; this includes screen readers, enlarged computer screens, and augmentative and alternative communication devices. Public entities are not required to take actions that would result in undue financial and administrative burdens. They are required to make reasonable modifications to policies, practices, and procedures where necessary to avoid discrimination, unless they can demonstrate that doing so would fundamentally alter the nature of the service, program, or activity being provided.

The transportation provisions of Title II cover public transportation services, such as city buses and public rail transit (e.g., subways, commuter rails, Amtrak). Public transportation authorities may not discriminate against people with disabilities in the provision of their services. They must comply with requirements for accessibility in newly purchased vehicles, make good faith efforts to purchase or lease accessible used buses, remanufacture buses in an accessible manner, and, unless it would result in an undue burden, provide paratransit where they operate fixed-route bus or rail systems. Paratransit is a service in which individuals who are unable to independently use the regular transit system (because of a physical or mental impairment) are picked up and dropped off at their destinations.

Title III covers businesses and nonprofit service providers that are public accommodations, privately operated entities offering certain types of courses and examinations, privately operated transportation, and commercial facilities. Public accommodations are private entities that own, lease, lease to, or operate facilities such as restaurants, retail stores, hotels, and movie theaters; private schools; convention centers; doctors' offices; homeless shelters; transportation depots; zoos; funeral homes; day care centers; and recreation facilities, including sports stadiums and fitness clubs. Transportation services provided by private entities are also covered by Title III.

Public accommodations must comply with basic nondiscrimination requirements that prohibit exclusion, segregation, and unequal treatment. They also must comply with specific requirements related to architectural standards for new and altered buildings and reasonable modifications to policies, practices, and procedures. In addition, public accommodations must utilize assistive technology for their requirement to offer effective communication for people with hearing, vision, or speech disabilities, as well as other access requirements. Additionally, public accommodations must remove barriers in existing buildings where it is easy to do so without much difficulty or expense, given the public accommodation's resources.

Courses and examinations related to professional, educational, or trade-related applications, licensing, certifications, or credentialing must be provided in a place and manner accessible to people with disabilities, or alternative accessible arrangements must be offered. For example, courses and examinations given via a computer should utilize appropriate computer assistive technology for people with vision, hearing, or cognitive disabilities.

Title IV addresses telephone and television access for people with hearing and speech disabilities; this has wide assistive technology implications, especially as emerging and developing technologies in the telecommunications and television fields are changing at a rapid pace. Title IV requires common carriers (telephone companies) to establish interstate and intrastate telecommunications relay services (TRS) 24 hours a day, 7 days a week. TRS enables callers with hearing and speech disabilities who use text telephones (TTYs) and callers who use voice telephones to communicate with each other through a third-party communications assistant. The Federal Communications Commission (FCC) has set minimum standards for TRS services. Title IV also requires closed captioning of federally funded public service announcements.

Widely hailed as a major civil rights bill for the disabled, the ADA has the potential of removing many of the barriers that have kept individuals with disabilities from engaging in all aspects of society. Assistive technologies surely play a major role in this process.

**Medicaid.** Medicaid is a federal and state program authorized under Title XIX of the Social Security Act of 1965 (42 U.S.C. §§1396. et. seq.). It is an income, or "means-tested," program, so eligibility depends on a person's income level. Although the program was established by federal legislation, eligibility and services differ from state to state. The federal government (through the Health Care Financing Administration [HCFA]) sets general program requirements and provides financial assistance to the states by matching state expenditures. This match is based on the relative wealth of each state, ranging from an 80% federal match to the poorest state down to 50% for the wealthiest.

The states are responsible for administering the program consistent with a State Plan submitted to HCFA. Although states do not have to participate in the plan, all 50 states do so. The State Plan specifies who is eligible for services and what services are covered. The Medicaid program neither provides services directly nor pays cash assistance directly to individuals who need medical care. Rather the program reimburses providers (e.g., doctors, pharmacies, hospitals, therapists) for covered supplies and services rendered to qualified recipients.

An individual who seeks Medicaid funding for AT must generally meet a three-part test: (1) The individual must be eligible for Medicaid; (2) the specific device requested must be one that can be funded by the Medicaid program; (3) the individual must establish that the device requested is medically necessary.

As Medicaid-funded AT is considered, it is important to distinguish benefits available to adults age 21 or older from those available to children up to age 21 under the Early Periodic Screening, Diagnosis and Treatment (EPSDT) program (42 U.S.C. §1396[a][4][B]; 42 C.F.R. §§441.50-441.62).

In order to qualify for AT as an adult, the device in question must be available under the state's Medicaid plan or it must be available under a specific Medicaid waiver program (such as the home or community-based waiver).

These waivers allow states to provide services that are not otherwise furnished under the Medicaid plan to a specific population within the state. However, under the law, certain Medicaid services are mandatory; that is, they must be made available to Medicaid beneficiaries, whereas others are optional. As shown in Box 1-3, there are 11 separate Medicaid service categories that have been identified for funding assistive technology or durable medical equipment

Each service category is specifically defined in the federal regulations. For example, 42 C.F.R. §§440.70(b)(3) defines medical supplies, equipment, and appliances as mandatory items under home health services; 440.110 defines physical therapy, occupational therapy, and speech, hearing, and language therapy; 440.120(c), prosthetic devices; 440.130(c), preventive services; and 440.130(d), rehabilitation services.

Persons with disabilities who are seeking to use Medicaid as a source of funding for assistive technology must navigate a cumbersome process that usually requires both their specific conditions and needs to be expressed in language designed to fit program criteria. The Medicaid law and its implementing regulations do not provide for the funding of any particular AT devices, nor do they spell out a specific test of medical necessity or other criteria governing when a person is eligible for a specific device. The federal law provides a general framework, and the individual federal regulations often spell out in detail what a particular category contemplates. For example, the federal law indicates that the primary goal of Medicaid is to provide medical assistance to persons in need and to furnish them with rehabilitation and other services to help them "attain or retain capability for independence or self-care" (42 U.S.C. §1396). The federal regulations provide that "each service must be sufficient in amount, duration and scope to

---

**BOX 1-3    Categories of Medicaid Funding for Assistive Technologies**

**MANDATORY SERVICE CATEGORIES FOR AT FUNDING**
- Home health care services (medical supplies, equipment, and appliances)
- Early Periodic Screening, Diagnosis and Treatment (for children)

**OPTIONAL SERVICE CATEGORIES FOR AT FUNDING**
- Home health care (home health aide and personal care services)
- Intermediate care facilities
- Occupational therapy
- Physical therapy
- Preventive services
- Private duty nursing
- Prosthetic devices
- Rehabilitation services
- Speech, hearing, and language therapy

reasonably achieve its purpose" (42 C.F.R. §440.230[b]). The law of each state may also provide language that can be referenced for interpretive guidance.

### Early Periodic Screening, Diagnosis and Treatment Program.

EPSDT is a mandatory service under Medicaid (42 U.S.C. §§1396a[a][10A]; 1396d[a][4][B]; 1396d[r]). EPSDT services are available for children from birth through age 21. A state must provide Medicaid beneficiaries under age 21 any service among those listed in the Medicaid Act, including optional services, whether or not the service is included in the state's Medicaid plan. Screenings include a physical examination; assessment of developmental, nutritional, and mental health; and vision, hearing, and dental examinations. According to federal law, if a condition is identified at an EPSDT screening, Medicaid must then cover all follow-up care that is medically necessary regardless of any limits a state might impose on such services. The EPSDT program offers a significant opportunity for funding of assistive technology that is not otherwise provided by Medicaid.

### Medicare.

The Medicare Program was authorized under Title XVIII of the Social Security Act of 1965. Medicare is administered by the federal government, and the rules are the same for every state in the nation. Medicare is another major funding source for assistive technology, which in the language of both the Medicare and Medicaid systems is called *durable medical equipment* (DME).

Medicare is a health insurance program for (1) individuals age 65 or older, (2) people of all ages who are permanently and totally disabled, and (3) people with end-stage renal disease. It is divided into two parts. Part A, known as "hospital insurance," covers inpatient services, posthospital care in skilled nursing homes, hospice care, and home health care. Home health care includes durable medical equipment, occupational and physical therapy, and speech-language pathology (SLP) services. Part B, known as "supplemental medical insurance," covers physician's services; laboratory services; durable medical equipment; medical supplies; prosthetic devices; rehabilitation therapy services, including SLP services; and home health care for beneficiaries not covered by Part A.

The Medicare program is a cost-sharing one in which both beneficiary and federal contributions are used. Beneficiary contributions include cash deductions and coinsurance requirements under Parts A and B and monthly premiums for Part B. State Medicaid programs can assume the Medicare cost-sharing requirements for those individuals who qualify for both Medicare and Medicaid.

Assistive technology items are categorized by Medicare as durable medical equipment. Medicare defines DME as equipment that (1) can withstand repeated use, (2) is primarily and customarily used to serve a medical pur-

pose, (3) generally is not useful to a person in the absence of illness or injury, and (4) is appropriate for use in the home.

Certain items that do not meet the criteria listed above may be covered under a special exception when the items clearly serve a therapeutic purpose. To establish the medical necessity for the item, it must be included in the physician's treatment plan and a physician must supervise its use.

Payment for DME items is subject to the requirement that the equipment be necessary and reasonable for the treatment of an illness or injury or will improve the functioning of a malformed body member. Although an item may be medically necessary, it may not be covered by Medicare if (1) the cost of the item is disproportionate to the therapeutic benefits derived from its use, (2) the item is more expensive than an appropriate alternative, or (3) the item serves the same purpose as equipment already available to the beneficiary.

Medicare excludes many items for coverage. Although there are many specific bases for such exclusions, they generally are based on the principle that Medicare is a program, like insurance, to provide "medical care." Therefore items are excluded if used for "personal comfort" or "custodial care."

## ■ THE ASSISTIVE TECHNOLOGY INDUSTRY TODAY

Now that we have defined assistive technology and reviewed historical and legislative factors affecting the delivery of assistive technology, we can describe the structure of the assistive technology industry. Figure 1-2 depicts the components of the assistive technology industry and how they are interrelated. It is important to be aware of the function of each component, its contribution to the industry, and the necessary interaction among these components.

### The Consumer and Direct Consumer Services

Without a consumer who uses the assistive technology devices and services, all the components in Figure 1-2 are unnecessary. Likewise, without a delivery system that actually provides the technology to the consumer, the supporting components in Figure 1-2 are ineffective. For this reason, we have shown the consumer and direct consumer services at the center of the figure. However, it is important to note that the consumer may be involved in all aspects of the industry.

**Direct consumer services** is the component in which a consumer's need for assistive technology is identified, an evaluation is completed, recommendations are made, and the system is implemented. The steps in providing these services are described in Chapter 4.

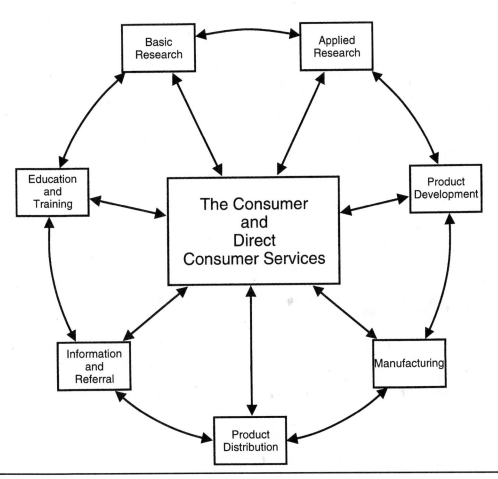

**Figure 1-2**  The assistive technology industry. The components center around the delivery of devices and services to consumers through direct services. The other industry components are arranged to illustrate their relationships to each other. (Modified from Smith RO: Models of service delivery in rehabilitation technology. In Perlman LG and Enders A: *Rehabilitation service delivery: a practical guide,* Washington, DC, 1987, RESNA.)

**The consumer.** The **consumer of assistive technologies** is viewed primarily as the recipient, or end user, of assistive technology. With this in mind, the industry components should be responsive to the consumer, his or her needs, and recommendations based on utilization of assistive technology services and products. As assistive technology systems are applied in the "real world," information from the consumer (and direct service providers) flows out to the other components so that changes in products and services can be made. Likewise, the other components interact among themselves and ultimately affect the consumer and the direct consumer service providers through research, new product development, and dissemination of information.

The consumer should not, however, be viewed solely as the recipient of the technology. The consumer must be considered an active participant in the other industry components as well if the application of assistive technologies is to be effective and the industry is to grow. A number of sources recognize the many roles of the consumer in the assistive technology industry. Corthell (1986) used the term *consumer as co-developer* to describe a philosophy wherein the consumer is involved in all aspects of the assistive technology industry. The National Institute on Disability and Rehabilitation Research (NIDRR) furthers this concept by stressing the importance of *participatory research* in assistive technology. As Graves (1993) points out, it is people with disabilities, their families, and the professionals serving them who are the customers of NIDRR. It is imperative that the research activities be responsive to the needs of these individuals. Therefore projects funded by NIDRR must be participatory in nature and involve individuals who will benefit from the research (e.g., persons with disabilities) in all phases of the project. This includes involvement in designing and conducting, as well as disseminating, the research.

Consumers can also be effective in training others in how to use a particular device and in assistive technology education. For example, the Empowering End Users through Assistive Technology (EUSTAT) project in Europe has developed guidelines for trainers, a set of critical factors for assistive technology training and descriptive information on programs that provide assistive technology training for consumers (www.siva.it/research/eustat). One of the documents developed by EUSTAT is written for consumers of AT services and gives practical guidance regarding how to access these services. Keep in mind, as you read about each component of the assistive technology industry, that there are many ways in which consumers can be and are involved.

**Characteristics of direct consumer service programs.** Assistive technology systems and services are delivered to the consumer through a variety of models and in different types of settings. There are several attributes that set direct consumer service programs apart from one another. The primary distinguishing factor, and the one most commonly used, is the type of administrative setting in which the service delivery program exists (Smith, 1987). Based on Smith's classification, Box 1-4 describes models of service delivery programs according to their administrative setting.

Smith (1987) also identifies several distinguishing features of service delivery programs. The *purpose and mission* may differ among service delivery programs. The purpose of some programs may be only to provide one-time evaluations, whereas other programs may provide comprehensive assistive technology services. The *functional areas,* or types of services, provided by assistive technology service delivery programs is another variable. Augmentative communication, seating and mobility, orthotics and prosthetics, sensory aids, computer access, robotics, and driving are some of the functional areas in which services are rendered. One program is unlikely to provide services in all these areas. Programs usually focus on a few of these functional areas.

The *type of population* served by an assistive technology program may be another distinguishing feature. For example, the United Cerebral Palsy Association (UCPA) supports a number of programs involving assistive technology that serve adults with cerebral palsy. The requirement for a military service-connected disability distinguishes the population served by the Veterans' Administration. Service delivery programs also differ depending on the *geographical area* that they serve. Some programs are community based in that they are set up strictly to serve individuals in their community. Other programs provide specialized evaluation services to a large geographical region. On a larger scale, there are also providers such as national equipment distributors that have offices throughout the nation. Whether the program is in a rural or an urban area is another geographical factor reflected in the types of services provided. For example, programs in rural service delivery areas need to be able to provide services to farmers who have work-related injuries and require adaptation of their farm machinery in order to continue their livelihood.

In order to serve consumers who do not live in urban areas, some assistive technology service delivery occurs through **telerehabilitation** programs. *Telerehabilitation* refers to the use of telecommunications technologies to capture and transmit visual and audio information, biomedical data (e.g., electroencephalograms [EEGs], x-ray films, ultrasound data), and consumer information (Kim, 1999). In assistive technology service delivery, telerehabilitation (telerehab) is used for preassessment screening, postassessment training in device use, and the provision of follow-up services. Transmission of telerehab data may be via computer interfaces over the Internet, via telephone lines, or via satellite. For home use there are small units that resemble fax machines (Kim, 1999). These portable units allow follow-up in a consumer's home. Scheck (1998) describes several examples of the use of telerehab for assistive technology service delivery, one of which is the use of telerehab for training in augmentative and alternative communication (AAC; see Chapter 9). In this application the speech-language pathologist uses a small "document camera" (typically used for projecting images onto a screen or photographing them for transmission) to visualize the symbol display on the AAC device. Another camera focuses on the consumer, and a microphone picks up the synthesized speech produced by his AAC device. The speech-language pathologist can provide both instruction and evaluation from her office while the consumer remains in his home.

Burns et al (1998) describe four case studies that illustrate the application of telerehabilitation to support the use of assistive technologies in the home. The four cases are (1) seating evaluation (see Chapter 6), (2) setup of a computer access system (see Chapter 8), (3) home accessibility evaluation (see Chapter 4), and (4) training in the use of an augmentative communication system (see Chapter 9). As Burns et al point out, telerehabilitation can overcome some of the difficulties faced by individuals who live at a distance from centers that provide assistive technology services. Low-cost video telephone technology was utilized in these studies. This technology, which has some limitations for studies involving full motion, was chosen because it depends only on standard telephone lines for implementation. For cases in which a family did not have a phone, cellular telephone transmission was used. Each of the cases described by Burns et al was initiated by the delivery of the telerehabilitation technology to the patient's home (often by mail). The family was then instructed in the use of the equipment (by telephone from the rehabilitation center), and the consultation was conducted remotely. The results that they obtained, although preliminary, are encouraging,

## BOX 1-4    Direct Consumer Service Delivery Settings

### REHABILITATION SETTING

- Assistive technology services are part of a comprehensive rehabilitation program; may be a part of one of the therapy departments or its own department.
- The primary purpose is to support the other services of the rehabilitation setting; therefore there is usually multidisciplinary team involvement.
- Typical populations served are persons with spinal cord injuries, head injuries, cerebral vascular accidents, and amputations.
- Services are usually billed to third-party health insurance payers.

### UNIVERSITY BASED

- Programs in this setting have largely evolved from a research component and may provide direct consumer services, as well as education and training.
- Staff usually consists of personnel capable of performing clinical, research, and educational duties. The types of professionals involved in the team depend on the functional areas addressed by the setting.
- Those settings conducting research provide a national service. The direct consumer service component is usually regionally oriented.
- Funding is largely grant and contract related (particularly for the research component), although portions of the direct consumer services may be billed to third-party payers.

### STATE AGENCY PROGRAM BASED

- State agency-based programs are usually a part of vocational rehabilitation departments or special education departments.
- Those programs based in vocational rehabilitation departments are statewide programs developed for the purpose of providing assistive technology services to individuals who need it for attaining or sustaining employment.
- The purpose of programs within special education departments is to facilitate the education of school-aged children. In some instances, school districts have their own multidisciplinary team. In other cases there may be a team that covers the entire state.
- Administration of these programs varies and may be statewide or on a local level.
- Funding is usually mandated at the state or federal level and designated for these agencies.

### PRIVATE PRACTICE

- A small number of assistive technology providers have gone into private practice. They may provide consultation to state agencies or rehabilitation centers.
- The population and functional service area varies and depends upon the professional backgrounds of those involved in the business.
- Operated as a for-profit, small-business venture with fees for service charged. Usually based in one local area.

### DURABLE MEDICAL EQUIPMENT SUPPLIER

- Usually these suppliers are for-profit agencies that addresses a range of equipment needs. Typically they provide walking aids, bathing and toileting aids, wheelchairs, and seating systems. Some suppliers may provide communication and environmental control equipment.
- DME suppliers are reimbursed by third-party payers.
- DME suppliers are known for their technical resources and ability to provide repair and maintenance services.
- There are some DME suppliers that operate on a nationwide basis; others are local operations.

### VETERANS' ADMINISTRATION (VA)

- Assistive technology services are provided at many of the Veterans' Administration hospitals. There is usually a multidisciplinary team approach.
- Research in the field of assistive technology is a large component of the services provided by the VA, and significant contributions have been made in this area.
- The population served is restricted to veterans with service-related disabilities. Veterans with spinal cord injury have been a major group served by the VA.

### LOCAL AFFILIATE OF A NATIONAL NONPROFIT DISABILITY ORGANIZATION

- National organizations such as the United Cerebral Palsy Association (UCPA), Easter Seal Society, Muscular Dystrophy Association (MDA), Association for Retarded Citizens (ARC), and American Foundation for the Blind provide assistive technology services through their local affiliates.
- The purpose of these organizations is often to serve individuals with a particular disability; therefore the populations served and the functional areas are geared primarily toward that disability group.
- Programs of the local chapters are usually administered at the local level, and assistive technology services vary among affiliates. Some local chapters may have a complete assistive technology team to provide services, whereas other chapters may only loan equipment.
- Funding for these agencies is through grants, contracts, donations, and fundraising events.

### VOLUNTEER PROGRAMS

- Volunteer organizations in the United States that provide assistive technology services include groups such as the Telephone Pioneers of America, the Volunteers for Medical Engineering, and Rehabilitation Volunteer Network.
- Most of these groups have developed out of private industry and have as their purpose the provision of a philanthropic service.
- These groups usually provide services on a local or regional basis.
- The functional areas served depends on the expertise of the volunteers involved.

Data from Hobson and Shaw, 1987; Smith, 1987.

and they provide useful information regarding the pros and cons of distance consultation through the use of telerehabilitation technology.

The *internal operations* of a service delivery program are another characterization. These include the structure of the organization (from large corporation to small, privately owned company), the number and type of professionals employed to provide the services, and whether the consumer must come in to the center for services or a van or mobile unit goes out to see them.

The final descriptor of service delivery programs is how the services are funded. Some assistive technology service delivery programs are funded under the general overhead of a larger organization, such as programs based within a rehabilitation hospital. Some programs are supported by grant funding, whereas others rely on a fee for service charged to third-party payers. Sources of third-party funding and mechanisms for obtaining funding for individual consumer services and equipment are discussed in detail in Chapter 5.

## Basic Research

The major goal of basic research is the generation of new knowledge. Research hypotheses are posed that address fundamental questions regarding physical or biological phenomena. There are basic research questions that underlie the successful application of assistive technologies. For example, basic neuroscience studies that help to describe movement patterns in persons with disabilities provide the fundamental basis on which new control interfaces can be designed (see Chapter 7).

The single most distinguishing feature of basic research in assistive technologies is that the outcomes are not known beforehand, although hypotheses are proposed. By carrying out basic investigations, we can begin to better understand how the presence of a disability affects functional performance and how this may be taken into account when designing an assistive device. Throughout this text we describe basic research studies that underlie the successful development and application of assistive technologies.

## Applied Research

The distinction between basic and applied research is not precise, and there is some overlap. However, in the area of assistive technology application the distinction between these two types of research is clearer than in the general case. There are many types of applied research studies in assistive technology. We can group them as follows: (1) testing of assistive devices under various operating conditions to answer a performance question; (2) development of new assistive devices based on clinical need, basic research findings, or both; (3) research on the use of assistive technologies by persons with disabilities; and (4) research studies designed to develop new assessment or training approaches or materials.

An example of the testing of devices is the use of performance standards to test wheelchairs or other devices (Axelson and Phillips, 1989). In some cases, such as wheelchairs, there are accepted standards against which devices are tested (see Chapter 10). In other cases, such as augmentative communication systems (Chapter 9), there is no generally accepted standard, but a device or series of devices can be evaluated against operational characteristics developed specifically for the research study (Dahlquist et al, 1981). Another example of an applied or clinical research study related to assistive technology use is the study of the effects of adaptive seating on eating and drinking of disabled children (Hulme et al, 1987). The purpose of this study, and of studies like it, was to determine whether positioning had any effect on the oral-motor functions of children with multiple handicaps. The results also advance the state of the art in adaptive seating systems (see Chapter 6) by providing insight into what these systems must do to facilitate positioning for functional activities.

The development of new devices may occur in a university or other research laboratory setting or in industry. In either case the objective is to design and build at least one copy of a device that will perform a specific function. In general, engineers (electrical or electronic, mechanical, or industrial) create the design and technicians carry out fabrication of the devices. The initial new device that is produced is referred to as a **prototype**. Consumers are involved in the design process, as well as in trial testing the prototype.

Applied research studies that focus on the use of assistive technologies are abundant. Often these studies involve assistive technologies that rely on user strategies for success. For example, augmentative communication systems used for conversation employ many different types of symbol systems. An applied research study might have a goal of comparing the effectiveness of these different symbol systems in facilitating conversation (see, for example, Burroughs et al, 1990). Another example is the use of computer adaptations that replace the keyboard with devices that recognize spoken words, known as automatic speech recognition (ASR). There are several different ways of accomplishing this same function, and applied research studies are carried out to compare them (Snell and Atkinson, 1987). A related example is the study of the effects of ASR on the vocal system (Kambeyana, Singer, and Cronk, 1997). Because ASR systems require abnormal speech patterns for recognition, there is concern that this might damage the vocal folds. Studies to determine the actual effects of prolonged usage of ASR systems contribute to both our knowledge of ASR use and to basic speech science.

Finally, some applied research has been carried out to improve the process of assessment, recommendation, and implementation for assistive technologies. Because the assistive technology field is so diverse, individuals from a variety of disciplines may conduct these studies. For example, Lee and Thomas (1990) conducted extensive research on the assessment of individuals for control interfaces suitable for accessing computers and other assistive devices. Their research resulted in an assessment protocol, a set of data collection forms, and a series of case studies usable by others. In another study, Cook and Coleman (1987) developed an assessment protocol for augmentative communication that included a hierarchy for relating the skills and needs of a person with a disability to the characteristics of devices. The research carried out to develop this hierarchy involved assessment and analysis of results from 40 children with disabilities. In both these studies the emphasis was on better application of assistive technologies as a result of improvements in the assessment process.

## Product Development

Product development involves the engineering and industrial design that must be applied to a prototype device to convert it to a version that can be fabricated in small quantities and tested with potential users. Testing of this "production prototype" is commonly referred to as **alpha testing** and is normally conducted in-house by manufacturers. Once the device appears to be functioning properly, several (as few as 5 or as many as 100) additional replicas are fabricated. There are several goals to be achieved by this procedure. First, by making more than one copy of the same device, the manufacturer can determine what potential problems may develop during the manufacturing phase (see the next section). Second, several individuals simultaneously can engage in more extensive evaluation of this set of prototypes. This phase of evaluation is often referred to as **beta testing**. Often manufacturers of assistive devices carry out beta testing with clinicians, consumers, and others who can give the preproduction prototypes a thorough evaluation. This accomplishes several things: (1) identification of as many potential product failures as possible, (2) evaluation of product documentation (e.g., user's manual) to ensure that it is clear and useful, and (3) evaluation of the product with a variety of disabled consumers to identify the target population as accurately as possible. The latter is important, since new products may be developed because one individual person with a disability has an unmet need, and it is not known how widely applicable the device will be. This situation is relatively unique to assistive technologies and is one of the reasons that new product development is

slower in this industry than in others such as consumer electronics.

## Manufacturing

Manufacturing is the process by which a working prototype can be converted into a device that is then mass produced. Although, in the case of assistive technologies, "mass production" may mean production runs of only a few hundred units or less, this is still quite different from producing a few beta-test prototype devices that function correctly. It is at this stage that production techniques become important. There are many fabrication techniques that are suitable for use only when many copies of an item are made. Several of these are based on the fabrication of a mold from which parts are formed. This technique can be used for polymer (plastic), metal, and ceramic materials. The cost of making the mold can often be very high ($50,000 to $200,000 or more) if the part is complex. However, once the mold is made, the individual copies of the item are quite inexpensive (from a few cents to a few dollars). This process is not feasible unless there are large numbers of parts manufactured; the cost of the mold is then amortized over the total number of parts produced. In assistive technologies this process is most often used for low-tech products such as reachers and eating utensils. Certain parts of some high-tech devices, such as wheelchair casters or the cases for augmentative communication devices, are also molded. Because the mold is a one-time cost, the size of the production run determines the cost of each part. The more pieces that are produced, the lower the cost per item. Because the cost of the molds is often very high, changes in design can also be expensive and may not be made until the original cost of the first model is recovered.

When manufacturing parts from molds, the major cost is in the production equipment; labor costs are relatively low. Other types of manufacturing are much more labor intensive. At one extreme are fabrication methods that rely exclusively on hand assembly. For example, most augmentative communication devices are fabricated one at a time by hand. There are no economies of scale in this type of process. Each device requires a certain amount of time to assemble, and the only savings in manufacturing cost are derived from the increased skill and speed of the individual worker doing the assembly. Thus production labor costs are a significant part of the cost of a manufactured item.

Both parts (materials) costs and labor costs are components of any manufacturing process. Savings in materials costs can be made by producing more units, even if they are hand assembled, since many suppliers give volume discounts for a larger order of the same part. In some assistive technologies, production runs are substantially below a level that generates a discount; for others they are much higher.

At the other extreme from hand assembly is a totally automated production process in which all fabrication and assembly is performed by dedicated machines. This ideal situation does not really exist, because some human intervention in the process is necessary for all manufacturing. However, many commercial products are produced using a great deal of automated manufacturing. Because the automated production machines do not require a salary, the cost per item is reduced as more copies are made, that is, as the production runs get larger. The production runs necessary for true production automation are approximately 100,000 and higher. This rarely occurs in the production of assistive technology devices.

The assistive technology market is diverse. The range of disabilities and the effects of those disabilities is extremely large, and this results in many needs that can be served by assistive devices. Unfortunately, the number of people who have exactly the same need, and for whom the same device will meet the need, is small. This leads to small volumes of production and increased costs per device. It also has the effect of making a device seem more expensive, because it is less complex but costs the same as a consumer device that is more flexible.

Many of the commercial general use devices that we employ as assistive technologies are produced using these automated manufacturing techniques. For example, personal computers often have production runs of 100,000 or greater. Thus the cost per unit for a system of this type is lower than for a device specifically designed and built for use by persons with disabilities.

We can draw several conclusions from this discussion. The volume in which devices are produced is directly related to their cost. This is reflected in two ways in assistive technologies. First there is the direct relationship between cost and volume of production. This is why certain low-tech devices such as mouth sticks may cost in the hundreds of dollars and a high-tech electronic calculator costs less than $20. Second, the difference between devices produced in large volumes and those produced in smaller volumes is sometimes reflected in overall sophistication and capability rather than directly in price. For example, a personal computer that is capable of performing a wide variety of tasks and that employs sophisticated and complex components is often comparable in price to a much less sophisticated but more specialized assistive device. Thus we often get more function for the price in a device produced in larger quantities.

## Distribution of Hard Technologies

Manufacturing a device is not worthwhile if consumers and service providers are not aware of its existence. Therefore marketing is an important part of the assistive technology distribution process. In contrast to consumer products, assistive technologies must be marketed and distributed to a highly specialized audience of providers (therapists, engineers, vocational rehabilitation counselors) and consumers. Marketing of assistive technologies involves significant costs, which must be recovered from the selling price of the device.

Distribution of manufactured assistive technologies can occur in several different ways. The major distribution options are (1) mail order, (2) direct sales by company representatives, and (3) distribution through a dealer or supplier. The choice of one or more of these is highly dependent on the type of product. For wheelchairs, seating and positioning systems, aids to daily living, and home care products, most distribution is through **assistive technology suppliers** (ATS). Most of these suppliers do not handle communication, environmental control, or computer access technologies.

For many low-tech devices, computer software, and some computer hardware, distribution is via mail order. This is an advantage in areas where there are no suppliers providing the needed equipment. This method of distribution is most effective for products for which there is no fitting or need for a prepurchase trial by the consumer. In some cases an evaluation center has devices to try, which can eliminate some limitations. Mail-order distribution can have significant costs for preparation and distribution of catalogs and brochures and for processing orders. Another limitation to this approach is that maintenance and repair is harder to obtain for high-tech devices, such as computer systems, purchased this way.

Relatively few assistive technology products are distributed through direct, company-employed representatives. Some exceptions are augmentative communication systems and aids for persons with visual impairments. Some of these have direct sales staffs, whereas others utilize dealers who carry several related products. In either case, this distribution network is not adequate to cover all geographical areas equally, and mail-order sales typically supplement the direct representative network. Electronic products such as augmentative communication systems, environmental control units, and feeders are often outside the range of capabilities of the standard rehabilitation equipment supplier. This has led to the development of more direct sales in these product areas.

## Information and Referral

The ability to readily obtain current information on assistive technology services and products is essential for both service provider and consumers. With the development of the Internet, there has been a dramatic increase in the amount of available information in many areas, including assistive technologies. This is the good news; the bad news is that much of this information is not validated by an independent source, so both the quality and accuracy of the information accessed must be carefully evaluated. The Appendix found at the end of this book contains a list of Web sites that is intended to provide some initial information; it is not meant to be all-inclusive.

ABLEDATA is the largest and most well known general source of information on products for individuals with disabilities. It contains more than 25,000 listings of devices (of which 17,000 are currently available). The ABLEDATA database also contains information on noncommercial prototypes; customized, one-of-a-kind products; and do-it-yourself designs. The scope of ABLEDATA listings is broad, encompassing sensory and motor aids, low- and high-tech devices, and applications from home care to employment. The ABLEDATA Web site (www.abledata. com) offers four different methods of searching the database: (1) by keyword or phrase, (2) by brand name of an assistive device, (3) by name of manufacturer or distributor, and (4) by Boolean search (specifying multiple features to be included in the search). If World Wide Web access is not available, an ABLEDATA search can be requested from their information specialists via phone, fax, or mail.

ABLEDATA also publishes *Informed Consumer Guides* that include information on product selection and purchase of a particular type of device. References to product write-ups, standards, or comparative studies on that product class are also included. Fact Sheets and Informed Consumer Guides can be viewed and downloaded from the ABLEDATA Web site. *The Guide to ABLEDATA Indexing Terms* lists terms used to index the products in the database and can be used to assist in a search. The *Assistive Technology Directory* lists companies with products included in the database.

Figure 1-3 shows several sample screens that represent each of the four types of searches. In Figure 1-3, *A*, we have searched by keyword ("feeding" in this case). The result, shown in Figure 1-3, *B*, list 66 records, of which only the first is shown. Figure 1-3, *C*, shows a manufacturer search. This search yielded 681 products and thus would not be the best choice. If we know the brand name, we can use the search shown in Figure 1-3, *D*. In this case we get the same result as the first entry in Figure 1-3, *B*. To narrow our choices from the 681 when we used only the manufacturer, we can use a Boolean search as shown the Figure 1-3, *E*. In this case we enter both the manufacturer and the keyword. Once again the result is the same as shown in Figure 1-3, *B*. Thus we can search by different methods depending on what we know about the product for which we are searching. Because the searches are all of the same database, the results are equivalent. Note that in Figure 1-3, *B*, the manufacturer's Web site is listed. In ABLEDATA a user can click on this Web address and go to that site for more information.

Written publications such as conference proceedings, periodicals, directories, and catalogs are another way to find information on assistive technology services and products. Most manufacturers have catalogs, and it is easy to be placed on their mailing lists so that you receive updated information. In addition to their catalogs, manufacturers may also publish regular newsletters of product updates and applications, and many also have their own Web sites that are updated frequently and provide instant information regarding their products. In some cases it is possible to purchase the product directly through the company Web sites. Many of the centers that provide services in assistive technology publish newsletters and maintain Web sites as well.

Electronic listservs are formed by individuals with common interests. Each user accesses the information from their own e-mail system, and all messages are available to all members of the list. There are many listservs that address various areas of assistive technology applications. Some are maintained by professional associations (e.g., RESNA, American Occupational Therapy Association [AOTA], American Speech-Language Hearing Association [ASHA], American Physical Therapy Association [APTA]), whereas others are established and maintained by rehabilitation centers or universities. There are also user- or consumer-oriented listservs, which address either specific issues (e.g., one particular disability) or general issues. These listservs are often useful places to gain information regarding specific assistive technology questions.

As discussed in the *Assistive Technology Sourcebook* (Enders and Hall, 1990), the method used to locate information does not matter as much as knowing what questions to ask and being as specific as possible. A good system for locating information assists the user in delineating the problem. When selecting a system from which to obtain information, it is important to remember that the information, including product and service information and manufacturers addresses and phone numbers, is constantly changing. Some resources used for obtaining information may update their information more frequently than others.

## Education

As previously stated, the growth of the assistive technology industry has meant an increased availability of devices and services for individuals with disabilities. However, it is necessary that competent professionals be involved in the delivery of these devices and services. It is also necessary that these professionals come from a variety of clinical and technical backgrounds. Until very recently, individuals practicing in the area of assistive technologies received their information on the job or through in-service training such as conferences or workshops. No formal training courses or programs existed as part of undergraduate or graduate educational programs. This has changed in the past few years, and current educational activities involving the

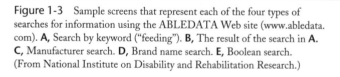

**Figure 1-3**    Sample screens that represent each of the four types of searches for information using the ABLEDATA Web site (www.abledata. com). **A,** Search by keyword ("feeding"). **B,** The result of the search in **A. C,** Manufacturer search. **D,** Brand name search. **E,** Boolean search. (From National Institute on Disability and Rehabilitation Research.)

assistive technology industry vary widely in terms of format, location, content, and specific intent.

For professionals currently in practice, *in-service* educational activities in assistive technologies that supplement the individual's professional training and experience are available. Typically this type of educational activity is very focused and of short duration. In-service programs have been the major type of formal educational activity for professionals applying these technologies. The variety of in-service opportunities in assistive technology applications is extremely large, and it is growing yearly. Some workshops are offered by industry, and they focus on a specific product or product line. Others are offered by rehabilitation centers or universities. These workshops may include one area of application (e.g., seating and positioning or augmentative communication), or they may be broader. Often workshops are offered in conjunction with major conferences of professional associations (e.g., AOTA, ASHA, RESNA). This can be a convenient way for conference participants to obtain in-service education in a cost-effective manner.

A major source of in-service education is conferences that focus on assistive technologies. These conferences provide a wealth of opportunities for education (see Enders and Hall, 1990). Many are regional, which makes them more financially accessible than the national meetings. Another source of continuing education is professional journals. Some professions have journals that occasionally publish articles on assistive technology; other journals are solely dedicated to assistive technology (see Appendix). Some professional associations and other organizations offer home self-study material in assistive technologies (Enders and Hall, 1990). With the growth of the Internet, there are an increasing number of assistive technology courses and educational programs offered at a distance (including online and teleconference formats). These often involve multiple institutions (both rehabilitation centers and universities) and international linkages.

*Preservice* educational activities are part of professional preparation at the undergraduate or graduate level for practice in specific disciplines such as occupational therapy, physical therapy, recreation therapy, rehabilitation engineering, special education, speech-language pathology, and vocational rehabilitation counseling. In recent years the number of programs that offer instruction in assistive technology topics has increased, particularly in occupational therapy, rehabilitation engineering, and speech-language pathology (focusing on augmentative and alternative communication) programs. Ratcliff and Beukelman (1995) and Blockberger and Haff (1995) describe AAC instruction in speech-language programs in the United States and Canada, respectively. The scope of assistive technology instruction in preservice educational programs varies widely. There may be an assistive technology specialization within another

discipline, required or elective courses or subjects in assistive technology, assistive technology material included within another course, or, at the graduate level, assistive technology projects or theses. The most common programs are those that include some assistive technology material in other courses; the least common are full specializations. With the increasing role of technology in the lives of individuals with disabilities, it is crucial that newly trained professionals entering their respective fields have some level of formal training in assistive technology applications.

Traditionally, academic programs in occupational therapy have included training in the application of low-technology devices (those without electronics) such as reachers, splints, and aids for daily living. However, in a 1989 survey, Kanny, Anson, and Smith (1991) found that training in the application of high technology, such as environmental control units, computers, and specialized power wheelchairs, was limited in occupational therapy preservice programs. In a follow-up study in 1995, Kanny and Anson (1998) found that assistive technology education in occupational therapy programs had increased in all areas. In the 1989 study, 50% of the programs surveyed had less than 20 hours of assistive technology education. When Kanny and Anson (1998) replicated their study 6 years later, this number had dropped to 10%. These changes reflect the increasing role that technology plays in the lives of individuals with disabilities. Most professional rehabilitation educational programs have recognized the importance of having some level of formal assistive technology applications training for newly trained professionals as they enter their respective fields.

In rehabilitation engineering, the entry level for professional practice is the master's degree. There are few universities that offer degrees in rehabilitation engineering at this level. More often, it is a subspecialization within another engineering discipline (e.g., biomedical engineering). In some cases a certificate of completion is presented to the student in addition to the master's degree in his or her field of specialization.

Rawley, Mitchell, and Weber (1997) described their experience over 6 years with one model master's level program in rehabilitation engineering. This program's curriculum has four areas of emphasis for student acquisition of knowledge and skills: (1) disability and technology, (2) major rehabilitation systems, (3) applied skills, and (4) lifelong learning.

The major impact of preservice educational programs is that more individuals than ever before are entering practice in their professional field with knowledge of assistive technologies and their application. This will have a major positive influence on the effectiveness of these technologies, the development of new and innovative devices, and the impact that these systems have on the lives of persons with disabilities.

## PROFESSIONAL PRACTICE IN ASSISTIVE TECHNOLOGY

This section describes the person who provides assistive technology and the issues surrounding his or her professional practice. Three broad issues are discussed in this section: (1) ethics of practice, (2) quality assurance, and (3) liability. Each of these has implications both for the individual practitioner and for organizations involved in the assistive technology industry. We begin with a description of the person providing assistive technology services and devices.

### Providers of Assistive Technology Services

The **assistive technology practitioner (ATP)** typically has a professional background in one of several areas, including engineering, occupational therapy, physical therapy, recreation therapy, special education, speech pathology, or vocational rehabilitation counseling. Each professional has a contribution to make to the industry based on his or her unique background. Therefore ATPs should be well grounded in their disciplines. It is equally important for each ATP to have knowledge and skills in assistive technology and familiarity with the scope of the assistive technology industry. RESNA has developed an assistive technology certification program to address this issue; it's discussed further in a later section.

Any of these professionals may be involved in any of the components of the assistive technology industry. For example, occupational or physical therapists with expertise in the area of seating may be found providing direct consumer services, consulting with manufacturers on the use and function of wheelchairs and seating systems, educating others on the prescription of seating systems, or working in research on the effect of certain body positions on functional activities. Likewise, speech pathologists may be involved in augmentative communication as a member of an evaluation team, may function as a representative for a manufacturer's particular products, or may conduct research on interactions among users of communication devices. These are just some examples of the ways in which ATPs can be involved. A similar variety of roles in the assistive technology industry are available to ATPs from other disciplines.

Having described the ATP's position in the industry as a whole, let us now look at his or her role in direct service delivery. ATPs are involved in the needs assessment, evaluation, implementation, training, and follow-up of assistive technology services in various functional areas. Examples of these areas are augmentative communication, seating and mobility, orthotics and prosthetics, sensory aids, computer access, robotics, and driving.

Because of the number of factors and the complexity involved in the delivery of assistive technology systems to the consumer, a team approach is desirable. This team may consist of as few as two professionals working together. Each individual team member brings knowledge and skills from his or her area of expertise that can be applied to the assistive technology service delivery process. Although it is tempting to view each functional service area (e.g., augmentative communication, seating, mobility) as being in the domain of one or two specific disciplines, service delivery is most effective when a **transdisciplinary team approach** is used.

In a transdisciplinary team approach, there is crossing over of professional boundaries and sharing of roles and functions. All individual team members must be well grounded in their profession but also feel comfortable enough to extend their role beyond that profession (Pronsanti, 1991). This can be seen, for example, during an augmentative communication assessment performed by a team consisting of a speech pathologist, an occupational therapist, and a rehabilitation engineer. Traditional roles may dictate that the occupational therapist perform an assessment of the consumer's pointing ability, the speech pathologist evaluate language skills, and the rehabilitation engineer design the mounting of the device. In contrast, with a transdisciplinary team all three disciplines contribute to identification of a good control site for the individual or to mounting the device in the most appropriate location. A team discussion may also form the basis for the type of vocabulary to include in the augmentative communication device. As a result of this team collaboration, a more thorough assessment of the individual's needs and skills is likely to occur.

Although some practitioners may feel threatened that the transdisciplinary approach takes away part of their professional identity, Kangas (quoted by Mastrangelo, 1992) points out that her experience has been that this approach improves the assessment process and actually strengthens each person's professional identity through the giving and confirmation of information. This approach also encourages support, creativity, and honesty among the disciplines (Mastrangelo, 1992).

### Ethics and Standards of Practice

*Ethics* is defined as "the study of standards of conduct and moral judgment . . . and the system or code of morals of a particular . . . profession" (McKechnie, 1983, p. 627). When applied to a field of professional endeavor such as assistive technology delivery or a profession such as occupational therapy or rehabilitation engineering, the ethical conduct of practitioners is embodied both in a code (or canons) of ethics and in standards of practice. Each assistive technology practitioner must comply with the code of ethics for his or her discipline (e.g., rehabilitation engineering, occupational or physical therapy, speech-language pathology, or vocational rehabilitation counseling). The code of

> ### RESNA Code Of Ethics
>
> *RESNA is an interdisciplinary association for the advancement of rehabilitation and assistive technology. It adheres to and promotes the highest standards of ethical conduct. Its members:*
>
> . *Hold paramount the welfare of persons served professionally.*
>
> . *Practice only in their area(s) of competence and maintain high standards.*
>
> . *Maintain the confidentiality of privileged information.*
>
> . *Engage in no conduct that constitutes a conflict of interest or that adversely reflects on the profession.*
>
> . *Seek deserved and reasonable remuneration for services.*
>
> . *Inform and educate the public on rehabilitation/assistive technology and its application.*
>
> . *Issue public statements in an objective and truthful manner.*
>
> . *Comply with the laws and policies that guide the profession.*

Figure 1-4    RESNA code of ethics. (Modified from RESNA Ethics Committee: *RESNA code of ethics,* Arlington, VA, 1991, RESNA.)

ethics for a discipline is typically developed by the professional association serving it. As we have discussed, ATPs have responsibilities in assistive technology service delivery that are not specified by their individual discipline's code of ethics. For this reason, it is important to have a code of ethics that addresses the specific issues related to the application of assistive technologies. Standards of practice differ from codes of ethics in that they describe more specifically what is and is not considered to be good practice in a given discipline.

**A code of ethics for assistive technologies: the RESNA Code of Ethics.** RESNA is an interdisciplinary professional association whose activities focus on assistive technologies. Its members come from many disciplines and a variety of settings, and their activities involve the full scope of assistive technology applications. In 1991 the RESNA Board of Directors adopted the code of ethics shown in Figure 1-4. This code is similar to those of other disciplines involved in rehabilitation and is based on several of them. However, it includes issues related to the provision of technology. It is presented as a reminder of the obligations that a practitioner in the assistive technology industry has to his or her consumers, others who work with and care for them, the general public, and the profession as a whole.

**Standards of practice.** Because each assistive technology practitioner belongs to his or her own discipline, it is important that the standards of practice pertaining to that specialty be adhered to. These standards are often the basis for professional certification programs. RESNA has developed the standards of practice shown in Box 1-5 for assistive technology practitioners and suppliers.

## Quality Assurance

**Quality assurance** is a broad area of fundamental importance to the safe and effective application of assistive technologies. It involves two basic considerations: (1) the quality of the services rendered, and (2) the quality of the devices supplied (Enders and Hall, 1990). Quality assurance is closely tied to reimbursement, and as the number of devices and practitioners increase, third-party payers are requiring some indication that the services and devices are necessary, safe, and effective. A comprehensive quality assurance program addresses these issues. The quality of services can be measured and evaluated by certification (of individual practitioners) and accreditation (of facilities and programs). The efficacy of devices is measured by adherence to device performance standards and good manufacturing practices (GMPs). Ultimately the quality of assistive technology services and devices is determined by measurement of outcomes resulting from both the provision of the services and devices and the utilization of the technologies to facilitate functional improvement and quality of life for the individual consumer.

## BOX 1-5 RESNA Standards of Practice for Assistive Technology Practitioners and Suppliers

These Standards of Practice set forth fundamental concepts and rules considered essential to promote the highest ethical standards among individuals who evaluate, assess the need for, recommend, or provide assistive technology. In the discharge of their professional obligations assistive technology practitioners and suppliers shall observe the following principles and rules:

1. Individuals shall keep paramount the welfare of those served professionally.
2. Individuals shall engage in only those services that are within the scope of their competence, considering the level of education, experience and training, and shall recognize the limitations imposed by the extent of their personal skills and knowledge in any professional area.
3. In making determinations as to what areas of practice are within their competency, assistive technology practitioners and suppliers shall observe all applicable licensure laws, consider the qualifications for certification or other credentials offered by recognized authorities in the primary professions which comprise the field of assistive technology, and abide by all relevant standards of practice and ethical principles, including RESNA's Code of Ethics.
4. Individuals shall truthfully, fully and accurately represent their credentials, competency, education, training and experience in both the field of assistive technology and the primary profession in which they are members. To the extent practical, individuals shall disclose their primary profession in all forms of communication, including advertising, which refers to their credential in assistive technology.
5. Individuals shall, at a minimum, inform consumers or their advocates of any employment affiliations, financial or professional interests that may be perceived to bias recommendations, and in some cases, decline to provide services or supplies where the conflict of interest is such that it may fairly be concluded that such affiliation or interest is likely to impair professional judgments.
6. Individuals shall use every resource reasonably available to ensure that the identified needs of consumers are met, including referral to other practitioners or sources which may provide the needed service or supply within the scope of their competence.
7. Individuals shall cooperate with members of other professions, where appropriate, in delivering services to consumers, and shall actively participate in the team process when the consumer's needs require such an approach.
8. Individuals shall offer an appropriate range of assistive technology services that include assessment, evaluation, recommendations, training, adjustments at delivery, and follow-up and modifications after delivery.
9. Individuals shall verify consumer's needs by using direct assessment or evaluation procedures with the consumer.
10. Individuals shall assure that the consumer fully participates, and is fully informed about all reasonable options available, regardless of finances, in the development of recommendations for intervention strategies.
11. Individuals shall consider future and emerging needs when developing intervention strategies and fully inform the consumer of those needs.
12. Individuals shall avoid providing and implementing technology [that exposes] the consumer to unreasonable risk, and shall advise the consumer as fully as possible of all known risks. Where adjustments, instruction for use, or necessary modifications are likely to be required to avoid or minimize such risks, individuals shall make sure that such information or service is provided.
13. Individuals shall fully inform consumers or their advocates about all relevant aspects, including the financial implications, of all final recommendations for the provision of technology, and shall not guaranty the results of any service or technology. Individuals may, however, make reasonable statements about prognosis.
14. Individuals shall maintain adequate records of the technology evaluation, assessment, recommendations, services, or products provided and preserve confidentiality of those records, unless required by law, or unless the protection of the welfare of the person or the community requires otherwise.
15. Individuals shall endeavor, through ongoing professional development, including continuing education, to remain current on all aspects of assistive technology relevant to their practice including accessibility, funding, legal or public issues, recommended practices and emerging technologies.
16. Individuals shall endeavor to institute procedures, on an ongoing basis, to evaluate, promote and enhance the quality of service delivered to all consumers.
17. Individuals shall be truthful and accurate in all public statements concerning assistive technology, assistive technology practitioners and suppliers, services, and products dispensed.
18. Individuals shall not invidiously discriminate in the provision of services or supplies on the basis of disability, race, national origin, religion, creed, gender, age, or sexual orientation.
19. Individuals shall not charge for services not rendered, nor misrepresent in any fashion services delivered or products dispensed for reimbursement or any other purpose.
20. Individuals shall not engage in fraud, dishonesty or misrepresentation of any kind, or any form of conduct that adversely reflects on the field of assistive technology, or the individual's fitness to serve consumers professionally.
21. Individuals whose professional services are adversely affected by substance abuse or other health-related conditions shall seek professional advice, and where appropriate, withdraw from the affected area of practice.

From Resna, 1700 North Moore Street, Suite 1540, Arlington, VA 22209-1903; phone: (703) 524-6686 (www.resna.org).

**Overview.** Patterson (1989) presented the following overview of quality assurance from the perspective of the Joint Commission on Accreditation of Healthcare Organizations (JCAHCO). The consumer, practitioner, and purchaser (of services or devices) each has a unique view of what constitutes quality. The consumer views it from his or her own point of view and, in the case of assistive technologies, judges the quality on how daily performance is improved in the specific areas of application. The practitioner generates measures of performance and then attempts to judge the quality of the services and devices against these measures. The practitioner evaluates both the technologies and the consumer, since motivation, amount of effort spent on training, and so on can impact success of any device or service. The purchaser of services or devices asks the most basic of questions: Are the services and devices cost effective? This question also implies the existence of a measurable outcome, and often purchasers require the practitioner to develop such measures before funding is approved.

Patterson cites several reasons why quality assurance programs are necessary. The most important is to ensure that practice is effective and appropriate to the consumer's needs. A good quality assurance program improves practices and outcomes, as well as consumer satisfaction. In addition, quality assurance programs are necessary to ensure accountability to the public and conformance with codes of ethics.

Quality assurance programs are implemented through both internal and external factors. Organizations that provide assistive technology services and equipment must have a philosophical commitment to quality assurance that is reflected in their mission statements, and there must be internal monitoring and evaluation. External monitoring is also important to ensure objectivity in meeting quality assurance goals. External monitoring can be accomplished through standards required by organizations that accredit the facility (such as JCAHCO); certification of individual practitioners; standards developed by third-party reimbursement organizations; and local, state, or federal legal requirements.

**Standards for service providers.** *Professional certification* is a voluntary process in which a professional organization measures and reports the degree of competence of an individual practitioner (Warren, 1991). In order to establish a certification program, there must be an agreed upon body of knowledge unique to the practitioners in the area to be certified. Once the body of knowledge is adequately described, a set of professional competencies must be established and a method for evaluating an individual's knowledge in these competency areas (usually a written examination) must be developed and implemented. As Warren points out, the examination process must be developed in such a way as to reflect how a person performs on the job, and it must reflect knowledge actually required for

satisfactory job performance. Within the assistive technology field, the challenge of establishing a valid and useful certification program is complicated by the great diversity of disciplines involved. RESNA has developed a certification program in assistive technologies that addresses the special requirements of this field and that builds on other disciplines' certification and licensure, such as registered occupational therapist (OTR), registered physical therapist (RPT), professional engineer (PE), or certificate of clinical competence-speech pathology (CCC-SP). RESNA offers a voluntary credentialing program; upon passage of an examination, one of two types of credentials are currently awarded. The *assistive technology practitioner certificate* is intended for service providers primarily involved in analysis of a consumer's needs and training in the use of a particular device. The *assistive technology supplier certificate* is intended for service providers involved in the sale and service of commercially available devices. The assistive technology certification focuses on the skills and knowledge required to deliver assistive technologies, assuming that the individual has already established disciplinary competence via certification or licensure. The certification process is further described on the RESNA Web site (www.resna.org).

The National Association of Medical Equipment Suppliers (NAMES), an association of suppliers of rehabilitation and home health care equipment, has established a national registry for rehabilitation technology suppliers. The NAMES National Registry of Rehabilitation Technology Suppliers (NRRTS; www.nrrts.org) has a goal of providing a mechanism for consumers, clinicians, and third-party payers to identify qualified suppliers in order to ensure provision of high quality rehabilitation technology and related services to people with physical disabilities. NRRTS defines a rehabilitation technology supplier as one who provides enabling technology in the areas of wheeled mobility, seating and alternative positioning, ambulation assistance, environmental control, and activities of daily living. To become a certified rehabilitation supplier, an individual must first join NRRTS. NRRTS membership "confirms that an RTS has demonstrated work experience, received recommendations from professional associates, adheres to a stringent 'Code of Ethics' and commits to participate in ongoing continuing education to remain a NRRTS member." NRRTS awards the Certified Rehabilitation Technology Supplier certificate to a NRRTS member in good standing who has successfully completed the RESNA assistive technology supplier credentialing examination.

Whereas certification programs address the qualifications of individual practitioners, *accreditation* addresses the quality of services provided by facilities. The Rehabilitation Accreditation Commission* (CARF) accredits organizations in

---

*4891 East Grant Road, Tucson, AZ, 85712, (520) 325-1044 (www.carf.org).

the rehabilitation field. This accreditation is based on the results of the organization's service delivery program, which includes hospitals, home care, mental health, long-term care, and ambulatory care. CARF views its activities as a quality improvement mechanism based on an external, impartial peer observation of current service practice. An organization's practices are measured against internationally developed and accepted quality indicators that focus on consumer-driven results, stakeholder satisfaction, and quality improvement. A CARF quality audit for accreditation serves as a framework for quality improvement, with a focus on individual consumers' outcomes and satisfaction. CARF accreditation is widely viewed as a mark of quality achievement. CARF accredits more than 20,000 service programs in the United States and Canada, and this accreditation is accepted or required for rehabilitation organizations in more than 40 states.

CARF includes standards for assistive technologies in both the employment and community services categories of their accreditation program (CARF, 1999). Standards for assistive technology services are included in the "principle standards," which apply to all types of accredited services, as well as in specific types of community and employment services. Principal CARF standards require that each person served must have access to assistive technologies to meet his or her identified needs. If an organization cannot provide the assistive technologies required, referrals must be made to providers who can meet the needs of the persons who are served by the organization. In addition, each person's exit report must contain a description of the assistive technology services provided. CARF also has specific standards for employment assistive technology services and community assistive technology services. These services focus on achievement of employment, community access, inclusion, and independence goals. Assistive technology services may include selection, acquisition, or use of assistive technologies; information, referral, or observation of AT; and exploration of alternative AT strategies. CARF standards also emphasize that the accredited organization should clearly tell people what it can and cannot do to help them regarding access to assistive technologies. In addition, the organization's services should be focused on helping people get and keep a job or on community access, inclusion, and interdependence, as appropriate. Appropriate staff knowledge, training, and experience are also evaluated.

**Standards for devices.** There are several types of standards that can be developed for assistive devices. The manufacture and production of assistive technologies and other medically related equipment is regulated by federal legislation in the United States (PL 94-295). These regulations include specification of good manufacturing practices and classify devices based on the risk of their use.

The FDA classifies medical devices in these categories. Class I devices (e.g., wheelchair accessories) are minimal risk. Class II devices require performance standards to be met (e.g., powered wheelchairs, standup wheelchairs, and special grade wheelchairs, as well as motorized three-wheel vehicles). Class III devices require premarket approval (e.g., a stair-climbing wheelchair ) (21 C.F.R. 890.3890). The Canadian system for medical devices is almost identical to this, with the same risk-based classification system, I through IV.

Two types of submissions may be made to the FDA for medical devices. The premarket approval (PMA) is the process that the FDA uses to evaluate the safety and efficacy of new products that pose a significant risk to the patient. A 510(k) notification is submitted for a change to an existing device that is already on the market or for a new device that is "substantially equivalent" to a preamendment device. Further information may be obtained from the FDA Web site (www.fda.gov/cdrh).

Most assistive technologies are judged to be minimal risk (Class I or Class II), and this reduces the restrictions on their development and testing, as well as on their approval for sale by prescription. However, in addition to paperwork and delays, there are costs associated with obtaining approval for a device at any level of risk, and these costs must be recovered from the sale of the product.

Third-party reimbursement may be refused for a device that is not FDA compliant. Repeated violations can result in fines and even jail for manufacturers who continue to market products after being informed that they needed to undergo FDA review; imported devices are often barred at the border by Customs officials if not cleared. AT providers and suppliers may also be at risk, from a legal perspective, if they use products that are not approved.

Devices can also be rated by development of compatibility and performance standards. *Compatibility standards* are developed to ensure that devices from different manufacturers can be used together. In assistive technologies, compatibility standards exist for control interfaces, computer emulating interfaces, powered wheelchair controllers, and other devices. For example, control interfaces have connectors on the end of their cables that allow them to be plugged into electronic assistive technologies. In order for a control interface from one manufacturer to be used with a device from another manufacturer, they must both adhere to a compatibility standard that specifies the type of connector, which pins have which functions, and so on. These standards are voluntary, but it is in the best interest of a manufacturer to adhere to them to maximize the use of its products.

*Performance standards* are also voluntary. These standards specify how a device should perform and provide a set of tests to be used for comparing similar products from different manufacturers (Enders and Hall, 1990). For example, wheelchair performance standards specify durability, maneuverability, dynamic stability, and energy consumption (Axelson and Phillips, 1989). In some cases, such as wheelchairs, the standards become formalized and adopted by the American National Standards Institute (ANSI) or the International Standards Organization (ISO). Approval by one or more of these bodies indicates that the standards have received a careful and thorough review, that they embody reasonable expectations of performance, and that they address issues of safety and efficacy. There are also less formal performance standards, which may be developed by an industry or an agency. The Veterans' Administration (VA) develops standards for their purchase of medical and assistive devices. Because the VA purchases large quantities of devices, manufacturers adhere to their standards and these purchase specifications serve as informal performance standards.

Whether standards are informal or formal, compatibility or performance, they have an impact on the success of assistive technology utilization only to the degree that they are voluntarily adopted by industry. The motivation for this adoption is both economic (e.g., increased sales) and altruistic (e.g., concern for safety and functional improvement). Assistive technology practitioners need to work with industry to ensure that standards are meaningful. They also need to insist that products they recommend have met applicable standards. These activities help to ensure that meaningful product standards are developed and used.

**Outcomes of assistive technology delivery.** Assistive technologies create unique challenges in quality assurance. For many therapies, a service is provided in a clinical rehabilitation setting and the success of the outcome is based on measures such as functional improvement, reduced hospitalization, or ability to work at average productivity. It is not possible to apply these measures directly to assistive technology services and devices because the goals of the service are different. In assistive technology service delivery, the selection of a device is based on what a person is able to

do now, not what she or he will be able to do upon completing a program of therapy. A device that is expected to meet the needs of the person is then recommended, and the individual consumer decides whether to use it or not. The device is used not in a well-controlled clinical environment, but in the larger context of employment, school, and community. To evaluate the effectiveness of this entire process, we must focus not on the service or device individually, but on the entire assistive technology system, which includes the user, the technology, the activities being carried out, and the context (environment) in which the system is being used. The determination of the "success" of the service delivery process is based on measurement of outcomes related to the success the consumer achieves using the assistive technology system. *Outcome measures* are objective criteria, usually developed during the assessment and recommendation process, that can be used to judge the effectiveness of both devices and services during the training and follow-up phases of the service delivery process. In Chapter 2 we develop a framework for assistive technologies that provides the basis for outcome measures. In Chapter 4 we discuss the development and application of outcome measures for assistive technology services and devices.

## ■ SUMMARY

The definitions, history, legislation, industry, and professional issues presented in this chapter provide the foundation for our discussion of assistive technologies and their application. In the remainder of this text, we present a set of principles, some of which are general and some of which apply to a specific need. In addition, the practices that underlie successful application are described in detail. Many specific assistive devices are also characterized in succeeding chapters.

## Study Questions

1. Distinguish between the WHO ICF and the 1980 ICIDH from the point of view of assistive technologies.
2. What is meant by a "low-tech" and a "high-tech" assistive device? Give an example of each.
3. Distinguish between hard and soft technologies.
4. Give three examples of assistive technology appliances and three examples of assistive technology tools.
5. What is the difference between minimal and maximal technology? Give an example of each.
6. Refer to Figure 1-1. Why are standard commercially available products less expensive than special commercially available products? Why are the latter less expensive than modified or custom-designed devices? Give examples of all four classes.

7. Why do we distinguish assistive technologies from rehabilitative and educational technologies? Can one device play a role in both areas?
8. Distinguish between specific purpose and general purpose technologies.
9. What has been the impact of federal legislation on the availability of assistive technology devices and services?
10. List at least four ways in which U.S. federal legislation has impacted the practice of assistive technology service delivery.
11. Compare the situation today regarding assistive technologies with that in 1972.
12. What is at the focal point of the industry of assistive technology? What are the other industry components?
13. Pick any one piece of legislation shown in Table 1-2

and describe its impact on the development and application of assistive technologies.

14. Why should the consumer be considered a "co-developer"?
15. Assistive technology practitioners may have a background in a variety of disciplines. List some typical disciplines.
16. Define the characteristics of direct consumer service settings in assistive technology.
17. Describe how you would carry out an ABLEDATA search if (1) you know the manufacturer, (2) you know the name of the device, and (3) you only know the general name of a device.
18. Describe the benefits of a transdisciplinary team.
19. Why is it necessary to have codes of ethics?
20. How does a code of ethics differ from standards of practice?
21. What are the major elements of a quality assurance program?
22. Describe how certification and accreditation differ. What is the purpose of each?
23. What are the major features of the CARF standards in assistive technology?
24. What is the difference between a performance standard and a compatibility standard?
25. What are the two kinds of liability with which assistive technology practitioners must be concerned?

## References

*Access to information technology by users with disabilities, initial guidelines,* U.S. Department of Education, Washington, DC, October 1987, U.S. Office of Education.

Axelson P, Phillips L: Wheelchair standards: Pushing for a new era, *Homecare Magazine,* pp 142-147, October 1989.

Bailey RW: *Human performance engineering,* ed 2, Englewood Cliffs, NJ, 1989, Prentice Hall.

Blockberger S, Haff R: Professional preparation in augmentative and alternative communication in Canadian speech-language pathology programs, *J Speech-Lang Pathol Audiol* 19:241-249, 1995.

Bryant L: Wheelchair standards ready to roll, *Team Rehabil Rep* 2(3):44-45, 1991.

Burns RB et al: Using telerehabilitation to support assistive technology, *Assist Technol* 10:126-183, 1998.

Burroughs JA et al: A comparative study of language delayed preschool children's ability to recall symbols from two symbol systems, *Augment Altern Comm* 6(3):202-206, 1990.

Button C: Fast facts on individualized education programs, *AT Q RESNA* 2(5):5-6, 1990.

CARF: *1999 Employment and community services standards manual,* Tucson, 1999, CARF.

Cook AM, Coleman CL: Selecting augmentative communication systems by matching client skills and needs to system characteristics, *Semin Speech Lang* 8(2):153-167, 1987.

Corthell D: *Rehabilitation Technologies 13th Institute on Rehabilitation Issues,* Research and Training Center, University of Wisconsin–Stout, 1986.

Dahlquist DL et al: Characterization and evaluation of augmentative communication systems, *Proc 4th Annu Conf Rehab Engr,* pp 185-187, June 1981.

Desch LW: High technology for handicapped children: a pediatrician's viewpoint, *Pediatrics* 77(1):71-87, 1986.

Enders A, Hall M: *Assistive technology sourcebook,* Washington, DC, 1990, RESNA Press.

Fougeyrollas P, Gray DB: Classification systems, factors and social change: the importance of technology. In Gray DB, Quatrano LA, and Lieberman ML, editors: *Using, designing and assessing assistive technology,* Baltimore, 1998, Brookes Publishing.

Graves WH: NIDRR plans for the future, *Assist Technol* 5(1):3-6, 1993.

Guralnik DB, editor: *Coles Concise English Dictionary,* Toronto, 1979, Coles Publishing.

Hall M: Microcomputer versions of AbleData, *Team Rehabil Rep* 1(2):27-28, 1990.

Hobson DA, Shaw CG: Program development and implementation. In *Rehabilitation technology service delivery: a practical guide,* Washington, DC, 1987, RESNA Press.

Hulme JB et al: Effects of adaptive seating services on the eating and drinking of children with multiple handicaps, *Am J Occup Ther* 41:81-89, 1987.

Kambeyana D, Singer L, Cronk S: Potential problems associated with the use of speech recognition products, *Assist Technol* 9:95-101, 1997.

Kanny EM, Anson DK: Current trends in assistive technology education in entry-level occupational therapy curricula, *Am J Occup Ther* 52(7):586-591, 1998.

Kanny EM, Anson DK, Smith RO: A survey of technology education in entry-level curricula: quantity, quality and barriers, *Occup Ther J Res* 11(5):311-319, 1991.

Kim, H: The long view: selling providers on telerehab, *Team Rehabil Rep* 10(4)15-19, 1999.

Lee KS, Thomas DJ: *Control of computer-based technology for people with disabilities,* Toronto, 1990, University of Toronto Press.

Mastrangelo R: Transdisciplinary treatment: crossing a bridge to better care. In *Advance for Occupational Therapists,* October 12, 1992.

McKechnie JL: *Webster's new twentieth century dictionary of the English language,* New York, 1983, Simon and Schuster.

Murphy EF, Cook AM, Harvey RF: Neuromuscular prosthetics and orthotics. In Cook AM, Webster JG, editors: *Therapeutic medical devices: application and design,* Englewood Cliffs, NJ, 1982, Prentice Hall.

Patterson C: *Overview of accreditation and certification.* Presented at the RESNA Annual Conference Quality Assurance Forum, Washington, DC, June 1989.

*Principles of universal design,* North Carolina State University, The Center for Universal Design, Raleigh, NC, 2001.

Pronsanti MP: Treating across role barriers. In *Advance for Occupational Therapists.* March 1991.

Public Law 94-256: *Medical device amendments of 1976.*

Odor P: Hard and soft technology for education and communication for disabled people, *Proc Int Comp Conf,* Perth, Australia, 1984.

Ratcliff A, Beukelman D: Preprofessional preparation in augmentative and alternative communication: state-of-the art report, *Augment Altern Commun* 11:61-73, 1995.

Rawley BA, Mitchell DF, Weber C: Educating the rehabilitation engineer as a service provider, *Assist Technol* 9:62-69, 1997.

RESNA Technical Assistance Project: *TAP Bull,* January 1999.

Rizer B, Ourand P, Rein J: *How adapted microcomputer technology contributes to successful educational and vocational outcomes.* Presented at Closing the Gap Conference, October 1990, Minneapolis.

Scheck A: Going the distance: developments in communications technology bring telemedicine to rehab, *Team Rehabil Rep* 9(11):30-40, 1998.

Smith RO: Models of service delivery in rehabilitation technology. In *Rehabilitation technology service delivery: a practical guide,* Washington, DC, 1987, RESNA.

Smith RO: Technological approaches to performance enhancement. In Christiansen C, Baum C, editors: *Occupational therapy: overcoming human performance deficits,* Thoroughfare, NJ, 1991, Slack.

Snell E, Atkinson C: Comparison of three PC-XT based voice recognition systems, *Proc 10th Annu Conf Rehab Engr,* pp 717-719, June 1987.

Vanderheiden GC: Service delivery mechanisms in rehabilitation technology, *Am J Occup Ther* 41:703-710, 1987.

Warren CG: Quality assurance: credentialing providers of assistive technology services, *RESNA News* 3(1):8, 1991.

World Health Organization: *International classification of impairments, disabilities and handicaps,* Geneva, 1980, WHO.

World Health Organization: *International classification of functioning disability and health–ICF,* Geneva, 2001, WHO.

# CHAPTER 2

# A Framework for Assistive Technologies

---

## Chapter Outline

---

## Learning Objectives

Upon completing this chapter you will be able to:

1. Define human behavior and contrast it with human performance
2. Describe the components of an assistive technology system
3. Distinguish between human performance and system performance
4. Describe and discuss the Human Activity Assistive Technology (HAAT) model
5. List the major performance areas in which assistive technology systems are applied
6. Discuss the contexts in which assistive technologies are used
7. Delineate the major considerations in designing an assistive technology system

## Key Terms

| | | |
|---|---|---|
| Activity | Human Activity Assistive Technology | Life Roles |
| Assistive Technology System | (HAAT) Model | Performance Areas |
| Contexts | Human Behavior | Setting |
| Extrinsic Enablers | Human Performance | System Performance |
| Function Allocation | Intrinsic Enabler | Tasks |

In Chapter 1 we defined an assistive technology *device* as "an item, piece of equipment, or product system . . . that is used to increase, maintain, or improve functional capabilities of individuals with disabilities" (Public Law 100-407). In this chapter we build on this base by defining an **assistive technology system** as consisting of an assistive technology device, a human operator who has a disability, and an environment in which the functional activity is to be carried out. In this chapter we formalize this concept of a system and lay the groundwork for applying it to specific applications in later chapters.

## ■ HUMAN PERFORMANCE AND ASSISTIVE TECHNOLOGIES

At the most fundamental level, assistive technology systems represent someone (person with a disability) doing something (an activity) somewhere (within a context). A major goal of the assistive technology practitioner (ATP) is to recommend an assistive device that meets an individual disabled person's specific needs, is consistent with his or her skills, and accomplishes unique functions within the contexts of that person's daily life. This assistive technology system selection process has as its emphasis using what function is available (human component) to accomplish what is desired (activity) in a given context (place, environment, people). We are not concerned as much with remediation of a disability as we are with enabling functional results and helping the individual to achieve what he or she wants to accomplish. Functional results require that we maximize the skills of the person with a disability. This places human performance at the center of our system.

## Human Performance

**Human performance** can be defined as "the result of a pattern of actions carried out to satisfy an objective according to some standard" (Bailey, 1989, p. 4). In an assistive technology system, this performance is that of the total system. This makes it important to observe and measure the performance of the human operator. Whereas performance

is a result, behavior is the pattern of actions leading to the result (Bailey, 1989). We can observe both **human behavior** and performance, but we can measure only performance. To illustrate the difference between behavior and performance in an assistive technology system, consider the following case study. Marian is a teenage girl with spastic cerebral palsy affecting all four of her limbs. Because of these motor impairments, she is unable to speak or write. She is also unable to control her facial expressions. When we observe Marian's motor behavior, it appears that her arm movements are random. When we converse with her, we see that her facial expressions do not appear to mirror her feelings, and it is difficult to interpret what she is feeling from either her arm movements or her facial expressions. Fortunately, Marian has a language board (an assistive device), similar to the one shown in Figure 2-1, which she uses to spell out words by pointing to the letters. As we observe her arm movements while she uses this system, it becomes clear that she is pointing to specific letters and that she is quite capable of carrying on an intelligent conversation. Marian's behaviors are the movements and facial expressions that we observe. If we attempt to measure these movements, we are limited by the lack of a standard. If our standard is that of a nondisabled person, we will misinterpret Marian's movements and facial expressions.

Our situation improves, however, if we measure Marian's *performance* rather than her behavior. Kondraske (1990) defines a measurement as "a process in which an absolute standard is used to quantify a single dimension of an object or event" (p. 104). If we look at the performance as conveying a message (communicating), we can establish a standard of performance and measure it. For example, we may decide on a specific rate of communication, such as so many words per minute (wpm). (As we discuss in Chapter 9, this may not be the best standard for determining Marian's ability to convey a message.) We can then determine how many words per minute Marian is generating— let's say 10 wpm. This measurement can then be assessed to determine the quality of Marian's performance. Kondraske (1990) defines assessment as the process of determining the worth of a measurement in a specific context. If our standard is human speech (approximately 150 wpm),

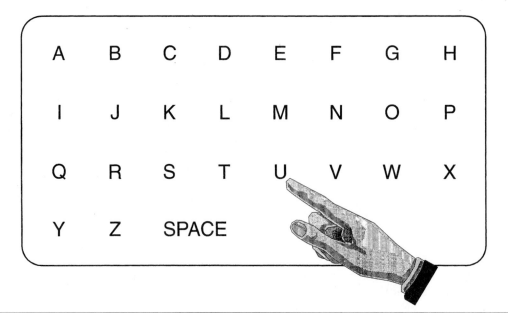

**Figure 2-1**    A common language board. The user points to letters in sequence and the listener puts them together as words to receive the communication.

Marian's rate will be assessed as slow and inadequate. If, on the other hand, we use language board performance as the standard (5 to 15 wpm), then Marian's performance will be assessed as good. Thus we can draw more useful conclusions by measuring Marian's performance than we can by only observing her behavior.

To continue this example, assume that Marian is assessed for augmentative communication (see Chapter 9), and an electronic device is selected for her. Let's say that with this device, similar to the one shown in Figure 2-2, Marian has a way of selecting whole words with one pointing action rather than requiring that they be spelled letter by letter. Now we can repeat our experiment and observe Marian's behavior and her performance. In this case, Marian's rate of communication goes up to 15 words per minute as a result of using whole words. Does this mean that her performance has improved? Actually, the performance of the entire assistive technology system, including Marian, has improved, but the measurement of words per minute does not allow us to determine the role of Marian's performance in the total system. This illustrates an important distinction: measuring **system performance** as compared with measuring *human* performance. In general, when we assess persons with disabilities for the use of assistive technologies, we want to measure *human* performance. However, when we want to determine the effectiveness of an assistive technology *system*, we must measure performance that is a combination of the human, the activity being performed, the environment in which it is performed, and the assistive technology (e.g., a communication device) being used. Focusing on system performance can lead to some surprising results. In Marian's case, if she is using her language board with a friend and the context of the communication is well

defined, she may not have to spell all words completely. For example, if she and her friend are thinking about what to do for the day and Marian begins typing *s-h-o-*, her friend will likely anticipate that she is spelling "shopping." This will save Marian five selections, and her rate will suddenly go up. Alternatively, if the electronic device is being used and she is spelling, her friend will have to wait until the whole word is entered into the device to speak the word. This makes it harder for her friend to anticipate what Marian is saying and compile the words for her. Thus the manual communication board may have advantages over the electronic device when system performance is considered. If Marian and her friend are out in a rainstorm, then the language board will be better than the electronic device because it will not be damaged as severely by the rain. We refer to the roles of her friend and the environment as **contexts;** these are described more fully later in this chapter.

We can measure Marian's *human* performance in the case of either the electronic or the manual communication device by, for example, measuring the time to make a selection with each system (see Chapters 4 and 9). The measurement of her rate of making selections using her upper extremity is an application-specific measurement. Alternatively, we may measure her range of motion, her reaction time, and so on. These measures can then be applied to a wider range of applications, and they are referred to as application-independent measures (Kondraske, 1990).

## A Human Activity Assistive Technology Model

Now that we have looked at human performance and system performance, we can develop a general model for an assistive technology system that clearly shows the interrelationship

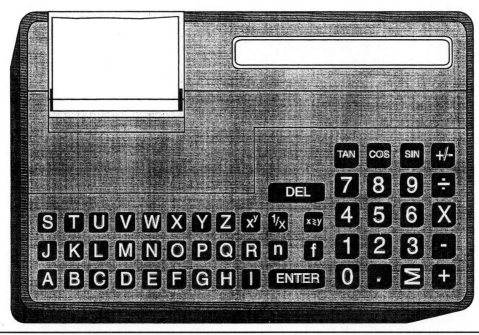

**Figure 2-2**    A generic electronic communication device in which the user types in words or codes and the device provides a written or synthetic speech output.

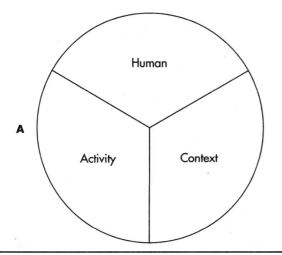

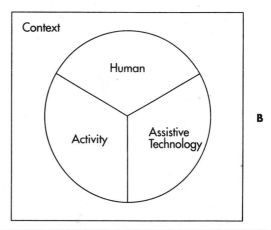

**Figure 2-3    A,** A human performance model. (Modified from Bailey RW: *Human performance engineering: using human factors/ergonomics to achieve computer system usability,* ed 2, Englewood Cliffs, NJ, 1989, Prentice Hall.) **B,** The human activity assistive technology (HAAT) model. This model shows assistive technologies incorporated into the basic human performance model.

between the system components. Bailey (1989) presents the model of human performance shown in Figure 2-3, *A.* This model is a framework for studying human performance in tasks involving technology, and it is typically employed to describe the performance of a human operator in a given task (activity) within a given situation (context). Human factors engineers and psychologists have developed this model to assist in the design and application of technology in a wide range of areas, including computers, telecommunications equipment, industrial processes, and vocational tasks. This model is most valuable in the design of mass-produced, commercially available devices that are intended for use by nondisabled persons.

When a person with a disability is faced with an activity in a given context, he may require assistive technologies to facilitate his performance. The model shown in Figure 2-3, *A,* does not take this component into account. Neither assistive technology nor standard technology (e.g., computer, automobile, microwave oven) is explicitly shown in Bailey's model. In order to describe the assistive technology system, we have adapted Bailey's model, as shown in Figure 2-3, *B.* Two major changes are necessary in order to create this **human activity assistive technology (HAAT) model.** First, the context is broadened to include social and cultural aspects, as well as environments and physical conditions (e.g., temperature, noise level, lighting), and its relationship to the other system components is altered. Second, assistive technologies are specifically shown, and their relationship to the other three components is illustrated. The HAAT model is ideally suited to the discussion of assistive technology systems as we have defined them.

Each of the components shown in Figure 2-3, *B,* plays a unique part in the total system. The specification of a system begins with a need or desire by the person to perform an **activity.** The activity (e.g., cooking, writing, playing tennis) defines the goal of the assistive technology system. This activity is accomplished by completing a set of tasks. Each activity is carried out within a *context.* The combination of activity and context allows specification of the *human* skills required for attainment of the goal. If the person lacks the necessary skills to accomplish the activity, *assistive technologies* may be used. This use still requires skills. However, they are adapted to the individual capabilities of the person and then matched to an assistive technology system, the function of which is to accomplish the desired activity.

The interaction among the components of the HAAT model can be illustrated by an example. Tony needs to write reports. Thus writing is his activity. He is required to accomplish this as part of his work, and this specifies part of the context. Because of a spinal cord injury, Tony is unable to use his hands, but he is able to speak clearly. A speech recognition system (the assistive technology) is obtained for him. This system allows Tony to use his skills (speaking) to accomplish the activity (writing) by translating what Tony says into computer-recognizable characters. As Tony speaks, the assistive technology recognizes what he says and sends it to the computer as if it has been typed. Because there are other workers in the office, Tony uses a noise-canceling microphone to avoid errors in speech recognition, and he works in a cubicle to avoid bothering other workers. These further define the context of this system. Tony's assistive technology system consists of the activity (writing), the context (at work in a noisy office), the human skills (speaking), and the assistive technology (speech recognition system). For another individual, one or more parts of this system may be different. For example, another person may be able to type, but only with an enlarged keyboard. A third person may need to write at home, rather than at work. Thus each assistive technology system is unique.

### ■ THE ACTIVITY

The *activity* is the fundamental element of the HAAT model shown in Figures 2-3, *B,* and 2-4 and defines the

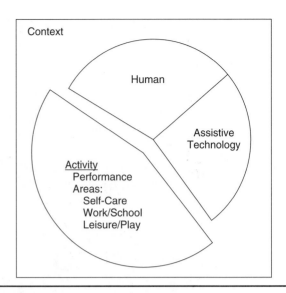

Figure 2-4   The activity component of the HAAT model.

overall goal of the assistive technology system. The activity is the process of doing something, and it represents the functional result of human performance. Activities are carried out as part of our daily living, are necessary to human existence, can be learned, and are governed by the society and culture in which we live (Cynkin, 1979).

The profession of occupational therapy is based on the use of occupation, or activity, and there is a significant amount of work that has been done in this area. In *Uniform Terminology for Occupational Therapy,* third edition (American Occupational Therapy Association, 1994), activities are categorized within three basic **performance areas:** activities of daily living, work and productive activities, and play and leisure. Activities of daily living include dressing, hygiene, grooming, bathing, eating, personal device care, communication, health maintenance, socialization, taking medications, sexual expression, responding to an emergency, and mobility. Included in work/productive activities are home management activities, educational activities, vocational activities, and care of others. The play and leisure area includes activities related to self-expression, enjoyment, or relaxation. Although some activities are unique to a specific performance area, other activities are carried out in all three performance areas. For example, reading is an activity that is accomplished in all three areas. We read for the purpose of relaxation or enjoyment, for work, and for self-care (e.g., reading a prescription). Therefore the performance area in which it is carried out further delineates the activity of reading.

The activities an individual performs are determined by the **life roles** that individual fulfills. Christiansen and Baum (1997) define roles as "positions in society having expected responsibilities and privileges" (p. 54). They go on to relate roles to tasks, actions, and occupational performance. Christiansen also notes that, "although roles are occupied by persons, they define performance expectations and are viewed as attributes of performance and not of individuals" (Christiansen, 1991, p. 28). A person can have multiple roles simultaneously, and roles change throughout the person's life span. Examples of roles we hold during our lifetime include student, parent, son or daughter, sibling, employee, friend, and homemaker. The life role of the individual influences the activities performed by the individual. By identifying the various life roles held by an individual, activities and tasks related to these roles can be defined. For example, let us return to the activity of reading. A mother reading to her 5-year-old child performs this activity differently than if she were in the role of an employee reading a report at work. Obviously the content of the reading materials will be different, as, most likely, will be the print size. Reading to her child requires a spoken output (typically with different intonation than regular conversational speech), whereas reading the report at work does not. She may also need to make notations while reading the report. This illustrates how activities change depending on the person's life roles.

Activities can be broken down into smaller **tasks.** For example, the activity of paying bills typically includes a series of tasks such as opening the bill, reading the amount, writing a check for the appropriate amount, putting the check in the envelope with the bill, recording the check in the check register, sealing the envelope, placing a stamp on the envelope, and putting the envelope in the mailbox. The skills and abilities intrinsic to the human allow the individual to complete a series of tasks to produce the functional outcome of the activity. For the tasks outlined above, requisite skills include fine motor dexterity, visual acuity, decision making, and oral motor function. An individual with a disability that limits his ability to manipulate objects with his hands still needs to perform the activity of paying his bills. However, the way in which the tasks are completed and the tools uses may need to change.

It is important that the ATP be aware of these different components of the activity. By identifying the life roles an individual has, activities carried out by that individual can be determined. Viewing the activity in terms of the underlying tasks allows us to see whether the individual has the required intrinsic skills and abilities or whether alternative approaches are necessary.

## THE HUMAN

The model in Figure 2-3, *B,* represents someone doing something someplace. Who is doing it? The individual with a disability is "operating" the system. By thinking of the person with a disability who needs assistive technology as the operator, we can utilize the concepts of human performance described earlier in evaluating the effectiveness of the assistive technology system. Christiansen and Baum (1997)

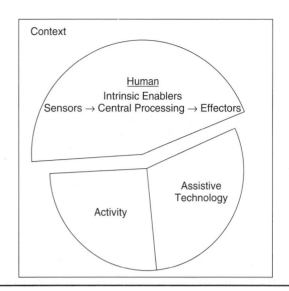

**Figure 2-5** The human component of the HAAT model showing the major intrinsic enablers normally used in assistive technologies.

use the term **intrinsic enabler** to describe general underlying abilities that individuals use to perform activities and tasks. In Figure 2-5, we group these intrinsic enablers into three categories: (1) sensory input, (2) central processing, and (3) effectors (motor).

In order to accomplish goals defined by activities, the motor outputs of communication, mobility, and manipulation are required. These three areas require that the human operator possess motor output skills. However, there are also sensory tasks that are required in performing these activities. For example, visual or auditory input is typically required for communication. If these skills are impaired, assistive technology systems can provide assistance by requiring different skills. For example, when a hearing aid compensates for reduced hearing thresholds or a braille output system avoids visual reading, the assistive technology provides replacement or augmentation of a sensory system. Finally, central processing is required for the successful completion of activities. Components of central processing include perception, motor control, cognition, and psychological function. If the human's capabilities are limited, then assistive technology systems can often provide assistance in this area as well. For example, procedures for device operation may be simplified for an individual who experiences difficulty in sequencing tasks, or recall aids may be incorporated to assist someone who has memory deficits. These human performance components of the HAAT model are examined in detail in Chapter 3.

### Skills and Abilities

We can distinguish between a person's skill and his or her ability. An *ability* is a basic trait of a person, what a person brings to a new task, whereas a *skill* is a level of proficiency

(Bailey, 1989). In assistive technology applications, this distinction is important. It is usually possible to obtain an assessment of a person's abilities, but it is difficult to predict the level of skill that she will develop using the technology. Ability can also mean transferring a skill from a related area and applying it to a new task. For example, a person with a disability might develop skill in the use of a joystick as a computer interface and then transfer this motor skill to the use of a powered wheelchair. In this type of situation, the acquired skill in the first task becomes an ability that can be used in the second task.

Although it is possible for most humans to *perform* more than one task at a time, it is generally necessary to concentrate on one task in order to *learn* it. For example, a beginning user of an augmentative communication system may need to concentrate initially on the development of motor skills necessary to make selections using a keyboard. Eventually, he will have mastered this motor task sufficiently that he can perform it reliably while also concentrating on the language content of his message.

In Chapter 1 we defined soft technologies as "the human areas of decision making, strategies, training, and concept formation." In particular, strategies are part of the human skills required for the success of an assistive technology system. As Enders (1999) has pointed out, people who have disabilities use strategies to complete tasks. These can often either replace assistive technologies completely or compensate for deficiencies in the technology. For example, Marion uses strategies to enhance her augmentative communication system functionality. She may wave instead of typing "hi," or she may use prestored words to increase her speed at times and spell other times to increase the participation of her communication partner. As in other aspects of the assistive technology system, the strategies used are highly dependent on all the other aspects of the assistive technology (AT) system. The context determines which strategies are important and useful, the characteristics of the technology affect which strategies are important to success, and the activity dictates the choice of strategies. Enders has proposed that strategies make up one side of a three-pronged approach to assistive technology applications that she calls "a human accomplishment support system." This framework is consistent with the HAAT model. The other two aspects of the framework are personal assistants and assistive technology devices. We discuss the role of personal assistants as part of the context in the next section.

### Novice versus Expert User

We use the term *novice* to describe a user of an assistive technology system who has little or no experience with that particular system or the task for which it is used. As the user gains more experience, she may become an *expert* user. This means that through practice and experience she has demon-strated a high degree of skill in the use of the system. She may be an expert in some tasks and in using some assistive technology systems, but she may also be a novice in other areas. This allows us to develop training programs and strategies (soft technologies) that take a user from novice to expert in a focused area.

### ▦ THE CONTEXTS

Over the past several decades the models used to describe disability and the disablement process have changed dramatically (Pope and Brandt, 1997). In the 1950s the focus was on the "problem" of an inability to participate in work, play, education, and daily activities of living by the disabled person; this problem was "in the person"; that is, it was strictly the result of the impairment. More recently, there has been an increasing awareness that the difficulties experienced by individuals with disabilities result as much from environmental factors as from the impairment itself. Initially the focus was on the physical or built environment, with much effort to make curb cuts, install elevators, and so on. As individuals with disabilities began to participate more fully in society, it became evident that the social and attitudinal barriers were just as great as the physical ones. A "minority group model" of disability emerged in which the attention was shifted away from the impairment to the social, political, and environmental disadvantages forced on people who have disabilities (Brooks, 1998). With this new perspective, problems of societal participation were no longer attributed to the impairment of the person with a disability. Rather, lack of participation in society was viewed as resulting from limitations in the social and physical environments. The emphasis on participation in the revised World Health Organization model (see Chapter 1) is indicative of the move away from a "problem in the person" concept to a "problem in the environment" model. In the HAAT model we have captured these external influences in the *context*.

As shown in Figure 2-6, the context includes four major considerations. These are (1) setting (e.g., at home, at work, in the community); (2) social context (with peers, with strangers); (3) cultural context; and (4) physical context, measured by temperature, moisture, light, and so on. The contexts in which the human carries out the activity are frequently forgotten when assistive technology application is considered. However, the context is often the determining factor in the success or failure of the assistive technology system.

### Setting

The first context is the **setting** in which the assistive technology is used. Setting is more than just location. It is a combination of an environment, tasks to be done (e.g.,

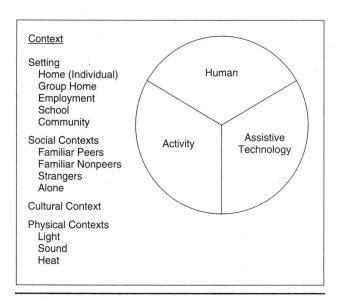

Context

Setting
   Home (Individual)
   Group Home
   Employment
   School
   Community

Social Contexts
   Familiar Peers
   Familiar Nonpeers
   Strangers
   Alone

Cultural Context

Physical Contexts
   Light
   Sound
   Heat

**Figure 2-6**   The four primary contexts considered in assistive technology use.

study, eat, shop), a set of rules governing the tasks (e.g., "Be on the job by 8:30 AM," "Lights out at 10:00 PM," "No talking in class"), and a level of comfort (formal, informal, playful, serious). The settings listed in Figure 2-6 have all these aspects. Many individuals who have disabilities live in *individual homes.* This setting may be an apartment or house, and it may be owned or rented. Individual home settings may need to be modified to accommodate for the special needs of a person with a disability. For example, a ramp may need to be added for a wheelchair user or a visual telephone (TTY) may be required for a person with a hearing impairment. Ownership of the building may dictate how some of these modifications are made. Also, a person living in an individual home setting may need an attendant or assistive technologies in order to perform tasks of daily living.

A *group home* setting differs from the individual home in that there are several (as few as 2 to more than 100) individuals with similar needs living together. Typically, because the individuals living in such homes have similar needs and disabilities, accessible facilities and appropriate programs are already in place. There are other differences between these two living situations, such as lack of privacy, degree of interaction with other consumers who can help in developing strategies of use, and the availability of organized recreational and educational activities. It is implicit in group home living situations that there be more structure and a set of rules to be followed (e.g., meals are served at a specific time, the bus arrives at 3:00 PM). Other factors to consider are noise, security and maintenance of equipment, and safe use of equipment.

In addition, it is sometimes difficult for individuals living in group homes to get funding for assistive devices, because

there is a perception that the technology is not needed or the consumer is not capable of using it. For example, a powered wheelchair may be deemed unnecessary because the home provides 24-hour attendant care and the user can be pushed in a manual wheelchair. However, this rationale does not take into consideration issues of independence and quality of life.

*Institutional settings* were more prevalent in the past. These are large group facilities that often lack a homelike atmosphere. Although the number of institutional facilities is decreasing, a significant number still exist. Many of the considerations for use of assistive technologies in group homes apply to institutional settings as well. However, because they are larger and are therefore often less personal, the routine setup, maintenance, and cleaning of assistive technologies may not occur as often as necessary.

Outside the living situation, we distinguish three settings important to the application of assistive technologies: employment, school, and community. In a vocational or educational setting, work needs to be completed in a timely and accurate manner, and assistive technologies can significantly affect the outcome for a given individual with a disability. The *community* setting encompasses all those places where recreation, leisure, shopping, and entertainment occur. Because this setting is so varied, it is difficult to characterize it specifically. This diversity also leads to greater demands being placed on the assistive technology used in this setting. For example, mobility by a person who is blind depends on the use of an assistive device (cane or electronic travel aid) to obtain some understanding of the type of terrain and presence of obstacles. It is relatively easy to obtain this orientation in a home or employment setting in which objects are relatively fixed and travel paths are used repeatedly (e.g., from a work station to the restroom or coffee machine). However, in a shopping mall, restaurant, or theater that is not visited often by the person who is blind, there is no detailed knowledge of the environment and travel is more difficult. The assistive technology must therefore be more flexible as well. This flexibility may be in the person's strategies (soft technology) or in the device itself (hard technology).

The type of setting dictates the characteristics of the assistive technology system, and a system that is successful in one environment may not be in another. For example, systems that replace the computer screen with a voice synthesizer may be used in the home without affecting other people, but their use in a work setting may require headphones for the operator. Likewise, a manual wheelchair that has hard rubber tires may work well around the house but not on rough outdoor terrain. In some cases the number of settings in which the system is to be used is limited to one or two. But often the system will need to function across all these settings, and flexibility in the system is absolutely necessary.

## Social Context

For assistive technology use, the social aspects of the context can be the most important. Because we are concerned with aiding human performance in communication, mobility, and manipulation, we must be concerned with the *social context* in which this performance takes place. As Fougeyrollas (1997) points out, social influence on individuals is related to what is considered normal or expected. Individuals who have disabilities may be stigmatized because of their disability. The use of assistive technologies can contribute to this labeling and lead to further isolation. The degree to which assistive technologies contribute to stigmatization differs. For example, an individual who has difficulty hearing may be resistant to wearing a hearing aid, but the same individual is unlikely to have the same resistance to wearing glasses for reading. Because the social context plays such a major role in assistive technology use, it is important to conduct assessments and technology trials in the environments where the activity will ultimately be performed (Fougeyrollas, 1997).

Fougeyrollas and Gray (1998) describe three levels of environmental interaction that must be considered in deciding on assistive technologies for a given individual in a given activity: macrosystemic, mesosystemic, and microsystemic. The macrosystemic analysis is at the level of society as a whole. This area includes policies relating to assistive technology use, funding levels (which can be a barrier to participation if a device is unfunded), and obstacles such as curbs, stairs, and so on. In this case the problem is not with the individual, but society as a whole. The mesosystemic level is the person's local environment—the community or neighborhood in which the person lives and functions. Analysis of the situation at this level takes into account the actual tasks and activities in which the person will engage. This includes the accessibility of the buildings in which the individual works and lives and the attitudes and policies of the school, employer, landlord, and others. Environmental concerns at the macro and meso levels include the "built environment." This includes aspects that affect mobility (e.g., curb cuts or elevators), communication (e.g., public telephone access for persons who are deaf), and business services (e.g., automatic teller systems that provide spoken output for those who are blind). Public transportation systems, theaters, schools, hospitals, government offices, and other parts of the infrastructure of society are also parts of the built environment that can influence the effectiveness of assistive technologies. At the microsystemic level, the analysis is of the person's immediate environment, including such factors as the existence of specific assistive technologies. This is the level at which the ATP typically functions in carrying out assessments, making recommendations and supporting users of assistive technologies. This is also the level at which *personal assistant services (PAS)* are considered and applied.

Another dimension of the social context is the types of relationships we have with people and how they affect our interactions. For instance, Marian may use her communication systems with her friends (familiar peers) or with her teacher (familiar nonpeer) or with a salesperson at the shopping mall (stranger). In each case her choice of vocabulary, her use of slang, and the ease with which she communicates is different. In Marian's case, she may have some stored slang words or phrases that are typically used by her friends. She may also have some more formal stored phrases that she can use in class or in a store. Additionally, because Marian and her communication partner know each other well, her friend anticipates what she is spelling, which increases Marian's rate of communication, as well as her effectiveness. A stranger who is unfamiliar with Marian's system would not anticipate, and the overall rate of communication would be slower. The social context directly affects total system performance. The effectiveness of her communication system is measured by the degree to which it accommodates these varied needs. Effective assistive technology systems are flexible and accommodating.

Communication systems are not the only type of assistive technology affected by social context. Brooks (1990) asked 595 disabled scientists and engineers to evaluate the assistive devices they used. She found that users applied devices in a variety of social settings, but use varied depending on the specific setting. For example, intimate, essential devices, such as those for personal hygiene, are not as frequently used as are those devices that assist in employment. Brooks interpreted this result as a reflection of the complex ties between the human (especially self-esteem), the technology, the activity, and the social setting. It is not possible, nor is it desirable, for us to separate the contexts (social and physical) from the other components of the assistive technology system.

## Cultural Context

The effectiveness of assistive technology systems is closely related to and influenced by the *cultural context*. Krefting and Krefting (1991) define culture based on three concepts: (1) "culture is a system of learned patterns of behavior"; (2) it is "shared by members of the group rather than being the property of an individual"; and (3) it includes effective mechanisms for interacting with others and with the environment (p. 102). The first of these is closely related to our definition of activity as a pattern of behaviors and our emphasis on human performance in the use of assistive technologies. The social aspect of culture is underscored by the second of the three concepts, and it emphasizes the interdependence of all of us regardless of disability. The third concept, interaction with the external world both socially and physically, illustrates the relationship of culture to the social and physical aspects of assistive technology context. Thus these three elements of culture clearly couple it with the HAAT model and emphasize the importance of cultural considerations in the design and implementation of assistive technology systems.

Krefting and Krefting (1991) point out that we all view the world through a "cultural screen" (p. 105) that is the product of our experiences, family relationships, heritage, and many other factors. This cultural screen differs for each of us, and it biases the way we interact with others and the ways in which we perceive various activities, tasks, and life roles. For example, in some cultures leisure is recognized as a desirable and socially acceptable pursuit. However, in other cultures pursuit of leisure time is thought to indicate laziness and lack of productivity. If the ATP and the consumer have differing cultural screens, they may have difficulty establishing and achieving mutual goals. For example, if the ATP views leisure as a desirable and satisfying occupation, she may recommend assistive technology systems that enable leisure activities to take place. This could include modified computer or video games, an adapted wheelchair for tennis or other sports, or adaptations of board games. However, if the consumer is from a culture in which leisure is viewed as being nonproductive, he may reject these assistive technology systems as frivolous.

There are many cultural factors that must be considered when applying assistive technology systems. Box 2-1 lists factors that affect how assistive technology systems are perceived and used by consumers from different cultures (Krefting and Krefting, 1991). These factors must be kept in mind by the ATP throughout the assistive technology delivery process. For example, consider three of these: importance of appearance, independence and its impor-

tance, and family roles. Wheelchair manufacturers now fabricate their products in a variety of colors. This allows a choice and avoids the "institutional chrome" appearance for those who care about such things.

Another example involves Frank, an adult male with amyotrophic lateral sclerosis (ALS) (Murphy and Cook, 1985). Before his disability, Frank was dominant as head of his family. He was fiercely independent, and he valued his role as provider. As he lost the ability to speak because of his ALS, he used a small typewriter-like device to interact with his family. This allowed him to retain his head-of-household role, and he used his communication device to make investment decisions, plan legal affairs, and make shopping lists. His family provided the legwork to carry out his directions. As his ALS progressed, his motor control deteriorated until he could only raise his eyebrows. A new communication device, which utilized this limited movement, was obtained for him, but he was uninterested in using it. After repeated unsuccessful attempts to provide support for the use of this new device, those working with Frank began to realize that his role in the family had changed. Because of his dependence on aides and the difficulty in communicating with the new device, he lost all interest in his family role. His wife became the family leader, and she began to make decisions that had always been reserved for him. These changes in the family, a difficult concept for Frank because of his cultural perception of family roles, led to his withdrawal and the failure of the assistive technologies to meet his needs.

## Physical Context

We call the environmental conditions that exist where the system is being used the *physical context*. Three commonly measured parameters—heat (related to temperature), sound, and light—most directly affect the performance of assistive technologies. Many materials are sensitive to temperature and affected by excessive heat or cold. For example, the properties of foams and gels used in seat cushions can change under conditions of very high or very low temperatures. Liquid crystal displays are affected by temperature, as well as by ambient (existing) light.

Ambient light in classrooms or work environments can affect the use of assistive technologies. Some displays emit light and are better in conditions of reduced ambient light, whereas others reflect light and are better used in bright light. For example, lighting that is appropriate for normal classroom work may be too bright for the use of some displays such as computer screens because of glare.

Ambient sound (including noise) can have a major effect on the intelligibility of voice synthesizers or voice recognition systems. Sounds generated by such devices as printers, powered wheelchairs, voice output communication aids, and auditory feedback from computer programs can be

---

| BOX 2-1 | Cultural Factors That Affect Assistive Technology Delivery |
|---------|------------------------------------------------------------|

1. Use of time
2. Balance of work and play
3. Sense of personal space
4. Values regarding finance
5. Roles assumed in the family
6. Knowledge of disabilities and sources of information
7. Beliefs about causality
8. View of the inner workings of the body
9. Sources of social support
10. Acceptable amount of assistance from others
11. Degree of importance attributed to physical appearance
12. Degree of importance attributed to independence
13. Sense of control over things that happen
14. Typical or preferred coping strategies
15. Style of expressing emotions

Modified from Krefting LH, Krefting DV: Cultural influences on performance. In Christiansen C, Baum C, editors: *Occupational therapy*, Thoroughfare, NJ, 1991, Slack, p 107.

disruptive in a classroom. Church and Glennen (1992) discuss ways of controlling sound and lighting to avoid interference in the classroom while still facilitating the functional gains provided by the assistive technology. Taken together, these three parameters describe the physical context in which assistive technologies are used.

## ■ EXTRINSIC ENABLERS: THE ASSISTIVE TECHNOLOGIES

The final component shown in Figure 2-3, *B,* is the assistive technology. We presented a detailed characterization of this component in Chapter 1 (see Box 1-1). We also describe assistive technologies as **extrinsic enablers** because they provide the basis by which human performance is improved in the presence of disability. The components shown in Figure 2-7 represent the flow of information and forces among the assistive technologies and the other components of the HAAT model. Interaction with the human is via the *human/technology interface*

component of the assistive technology. This component represents the boundary between the human and the assistive technology. This interaction is two way; that is, information and forces may be directed from the human to the technology or vice versa. In order for the technology to contribute to functional performance, it must provide an output. This is accomplished by the *activity output* component. The human/technology interface and activity output are linked by the *processor,* which translates information and forces received from the human into signals that are used to control the activity output. Finally, some assistive technologies (e.g., sensory aids) must also be capable of detecting external environmental data. The *environmental interface* accomplishes this function. Once the external data are detected, the *processor* interprets and formats them so they can be provided to the user through the human/technology interface. Not all assistive technologies have all the components of Figure 2-7. However, all of them have at least one of the components, and most have two or three.

Different sets of the components shown in Figure 2-7 are required to meet the needs of different consumers. These

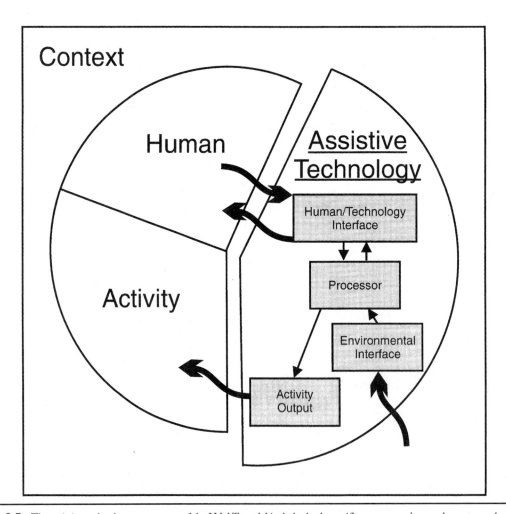

Figure 2-7 The assistive technology component of the HAAT model includes both specific purpose and general purpose technologies.

components function together to facilitate the completion of tasks that underlie specific activities. Because the use of assistive technologies has the effect of adapting the skills required for the task to match those of the human, these technologies enable the human operator. The specific characteristics of the assistive technology components are determined by the person's needs and skills together with the goals determined by the activities to be performed. This process is described in Chapter 4 as part of the needs assessment procedures.

## Hard Technology Components

Each of the components shown in Figure 2-7 can be implemented with hard technologies. These are discussed next.

**Human/technology interface.** All the interactions between the human user of the technology and the device occur through the human/technology interface. As we have said, these interactions can occur in either direction (e.g., from human to technology or from technology to human), and they include both forces and information. Sometimes separate components are used to provide input to the device and output from the device. For example, a computer keyboard can be used for typing, and a video monitor can be used for providing feedback to the typist. Sometimes bidirectional interaction occurs in one component. For example, the computer keyboard provides tactile, auditory, and visual feedback to the typist.

*Positioning devices,* or *postural support systems,* are one type of human/technology interface. Any person must be stable and in a position that allows interaction with his or her environment in order to carry out functional tasks. Some individuals with disabilities lack the capability to stabilize their bodies enough to produce the efficient and effective movements needed for this interaction. In many cases, providing a comfortable chair helps. However, in other situations, complex seating and positioning systems are needed. As we discuss in Chapter 6, the human exerts forces on the postural support system, and the postural support system exerts forces on the human. This two-way interaction also involves the human sensory system. For example, if paralysis causes absence of sensation, the human may not detect the forces exerted by the human/technology interface (e.g., a seat cushion). If the pressures exerted on the human user by the human/technology interface are too high, they can lead to tissue damage. Likewise, if the human user reduces the forces that her body exerts on the device's human/technology interface (e.g., by doing hand pushups), this also reduces the total pressure at the human/technology interface and decreases the possibility of tissue damage.

Another commonly employed human/technology interface is called the *control interface.* The control interface is the boundary between the user and an electronic or mechanical assistive technology device. This is what allows the individual to operate, or control, the device. For electronic assistive technology systems, control interfaces include joysticks for powered wheelchairs, keyboards for computers and communication devices, and single switches used to control household devices such as lights or radios. In addition to the motor output to the control interface exerted by the human user, sensory feedback is provided to the user during operation. This bidirectional interaction is essential to effective performance, and we discuss it in Chapter 7. The ways in which persons with disabilities are assessed for control interfaces, how they are selected, how they are used, and how training can be accomplished are also described in Chapters 4 and 8.

*Displays* that provide information to the human user are another type of *human/technology interface.* Displays are used in a wide range of technology, from powered wheelchairs, to computers, to augmentative communication devices, to environmental control systems, to sensory aids. Examples include the lighted display of remaining battery energy on a powered wheelchair and the lights used in a scanning display for augmentative communication. The major types of displays are visual, auditory (including synthesized speech), and tactile (e.g., braille). Visual and tactile output modes are discussed further in Chapters 8 and 12. Speech output is discussed in Chapter 9.

**Processor.** Many assistive technology devices require control and processing of data in order to accomplish the desired functional task. The processor, often a computer, performs these actions. Many assistive devices (e.g., powered wheelchairs, environmental control units) contain computers as integral components. This greatly increases flexibility and adaptability in performing functional tasks, and it also allows systems to be tailored to individual needs much more readily. Stand-alone personal computers also play an important role in increasing access to education, work, financial management, and recreation for persons with disabilities. Chapter 8 is devoted to the role of computers in assistive technology systems. The processor in an assistive technology device may also be a simple mechanical component that links the control interface to the activity output. A common manipulation device is a mechanical reacher, which is used to obtain objects from shelves that are too high. The user controls the reacher through a hand grasp, which is coupled with a mechanical linkage that closes a gripper to reach and carry the object. In this case the mechanical linkage is the processor.

**Activity outputs.** The *activity outputs* include communicating, moving from place to place, and manipulating objects for self-care, work, school, or recreation. Each of these activities can be either replaced by a functional equivalent (e.g., a computer word processor for someone who cannot use a pencil and paper) or augmented (e.g., a holder that allows someone with limited grip to manipulate the pencil). Assistive technology systems may provide one or more activity outputs that facilitate performance. These outputs include communication, manipulation, and mobility. The activity output for communicating is transmission of information, usually provided via voice synthesis, visual display, or printed copy. Devices for manipulation are either special purpose (e.g., a modified spoon, brush, or shoe horn) or general purpose (e.g., environmental control units or robotic systems). Mobility outputs are provided by wheelchairs, modified driving aids for vehicles, and similar devices.

**Environmental interface.** The final component of the assistive technology, the environmental interface, provides the link between the device and the external world, represented by the context. This interface supports sensory performance: seeing, hearing, and feeling. For augmentation or replacement of vision, the environmental sensor is a camera capable of imaging the information to be input to the human. Two broad classes of performance are typically aided: reading and orientation and mobility for persons with visual impairments. Systems for aiding hearing often use a microphone as an environmental interface. Finally, systems designed to assist with tactile input (feeling) use transducers to detect external pressures or forces. The environmental interface is linked to the human/technology interface by a processor, often a computer.

## Soft Technologies As Extrinsic Enablers

The extrinsic enablers that we have described for general and specific purposes are hard technologies. Soft technologies can serve as extrinsic enablers, in addition to their role as strategies that we include as part of the human component of the HAAT model. For example, performance aids, written instructions, and training are all extrinsic enablers. Performance aids are often conceptual (e.g., a method of remembering vocabulary in a communication system by using pictures that can have multiple meanings). Marian, our augmentative communication system user, can also benefit from the use of soft technologies. With the electronic communication system, Marian must use codes to represent words or phrases. If she has a lot of codes or difficulty in remembering the codes, a list of the codes can be displayed on the device. This is referred to as a *performance aid.*

Training is often required in order to make a system useful. Not only the user but also the caregivers and family must be included in this training process. Finally, written instructions and other documentation can make the difference between success and failure in the use of an assistive device. The quality of these materials varies widely. Performance aids, training, and development of written documentation are discussed in Chapter 4.

## Assistive Technology Devices for Specific Applications

Specific application devices for mobility, communication, or manipulation have a *human/technology interface,* a *processor,* and an *activity output.* For example, for a manual wheelchair system, the human/technology interface includes positioning components and the push rims used for turning the wheels. The processor consists of the mechanical linkages between the push rims and wheels, and the activity output is mobility. For augmentative communication, the human/technology interface has two parts: a control interface and a user display. The processor is typically a computer with a software program that relates the control interface to stored vocabulary and controls the outputs. The output is synthetic speech, print, or visual display. An environmental control unit for television, lights, telephone dialing, and other appliance control typically has a keypad or single switch and display as the human/technology interface. The processor is an electronic circuit, possibly a computer. The output is a signal or signals used to control the appliance and replace direct physical manipulation of its controls (e.g., television channel change or volume control).

Sensory aids have an *environmental interface,* a *processor,* and a *human/technology interface.* For example, a hearing aid uses a microphone as an environmental sensor, an amplifier as a processor, and a speaker (often called a receiver) as a human/technology interface. A reading machine for persons with severe visual impairments uses a camera as an environmental sensor, a computer as a processor, and a speech synthesizer as the human/technology interface.

## ■ DESIGNING ASSISTIVE TECHNOLOGY SYSTEMS FOR SUCCESSFUL OUTCOMES

In order to meet the needs of an individual person, we must design an *assistive technology system.* An assistive technology system is designed through the process of assessing a consumer's needs, goals, and skills; using these to determine the necessary characteristics that an assistive technology system must have; conceiving of and planning the system for that individual; delivering the device and training in its use; and following up to evaluate success. This total process represents a design activity, because each resulting system is uniquely configured to meet the person's needs and to make use of his or her skills and abilities. In this section we define the assistive technology system and discuss the important considerations in designing such systems.

## The Assistive Technology System

In the previous sections we have discussed each of the four components of the assistive technology human performance model. We define the assistive technology system to be the four components shown in Figure 2-3, *B*. Needs arise from all aspects of a person's life, and the assistive technology system goals are defined by the chosen activities (see Figure 2-5). The tasks required by the activity, together with the contexts of use (see Figure 2-6) and the human operator's skills, determine the characteristics of the assistive technologies. For the tasks dictated by the activity to be completed successfully, they must be matched to the human operator's abilities and skills. Facilitation of this match is accomplished through the assistive technologies, which enable the consumer to complete tasks that would be precluded by his disability. The choice of the assistive technology characteristics (see Figure 2-7) and the matching of them to the skills and needs of the consumer complete the design process and the specification of the assistive technology system.

## Integration of the Human with the Assistive Technologies

In order to design assistive technology systems effectively, we must carefully consider the interaction between the human and the technology. One way to do this is to consider how the human perceives the assistive technology she is using. Assistive devices are often perceived by the person with a disability as becoming part of her body. People working in prosthetics have long been aware of this phenomenon. In one study, individuals who wore artificial arms tended to overestimate the length of their residual limb (McDonnell et al, 1989). Subjects were asked to place their upper limb in an opaque tube. They were then instructed to point to where they thought the end of the limb (or limb plus prosthesis) was for a series of locations. When wearing their prostheses, subjects began to overestimate the end of their own limb by as much as 20% of the length of the prosthesis. When the prosthesis was removed, the subjects tended to estimate the length of the residual limb much more accurately. These results indicate that these subjects had adapted to the prosthesis and that they had perceptually incorporated it as part of their own limb.

Although we might expect an artificial limb system to result in very close perceptual coupling between the human and the device, this situation is not limited to artificial limbs. Ragnarsson (1990) points out that wheelchairs become a part of the user's self-image, and this image is significantly influenced by the characteristics of the wheelchair itself. For example, ultralight wheelchairs, which were originally designed for athletes, carry a much more positive image than bulkier and heavier types of chairs, and they are preferred by many users for daily use. The wheelchair user cannot be separated from the wheelchair and the context in which he uses it. The assistive technology system is the sum of all these components. We need not look even as far as a wheelchair to see examples of very close coupling between humans and the devices that they use. Gibson (1979) has

proposed that all tools may become part of the user. If this is true, it certainly applies to assistive technology "tools" that are used daily for functional tasks. As a final example, consider the case of a nonspeaking teenage boy with whom we worked. He had been provided with a communication system that had both a visual display and a small printer, but at the time he received his device, synthetic speech output was not available. He became quite skilled at using this system for communication, but it wasn't until someone told a joke that we really appreciated how much he had assimilated the device into his communicative functioning. After the punch line, he typed "ha ha" while everyone else was laughing. The human, technology, activity, and context had become inseparable, and they had become a single assistive technology system.

## The Role of Personal Assistants

Virtually all the functions carried out by assistive technology devices can also be accomplished by human attendants. With the current state of assistive technology devices, there are many things the device cannot do that require personal assistant services. This may involve setup of a system or transfer and positioning of a person in a wheelchair. In other cases, personal care (e.g., dressing, bathing) must be accomplished by PAS. There is often a tension between PAS and assistive technology device-based solutions (Enders, 1999). It is sometimes stated that an assistive technology device can replace PAS, thereby saving costs. Although this is sometimes the case, the most common situation is that a combination of AT and PAS is required. As we have stated in regard to AT systems in general, the relative amount of PAS and AT, coupled with strategies of the user, varies across contexts and activities. It is important to recognize the synergy among strategies, personal assistants, and assistive technology devices in developing any assistive technology system to meet the specific needs of a person with a disability (Enders, 1999). Verbrugge, Rennert, and Madans (1997) evaluated data provided from a national epidemiological study in the United States to determine how often PAS or AT enhances individuals' abilities to carry out everyday tasks. They chose 12 everyday tasks involving either upper or lower extremity function. Their findings indicate that personal assistance is used for upper extremity (e.g., eating, self-care) and body transfer tasks and assistive technologies are used more commonly for lower extremity tasks (e.g., mobility). They conclude that the use of AT allows the individual to maintain a greater sense of autonomy than does personal assistance, and they recommend a hierarchy of preference for assistance, with equipment first, then personal assistance. In developing such solutions, it is also important to take into account personal choice by the person. For example, some individuals may prefer to have PAS for eating, whereas others may want to use a feeding aid (see Chapter 11). This preference may change with the context. For example, some individuals may prefer to have PAS for the task of eating in public places and a device for eating in private (or vice versa).

## Allocation of Functions

In any human/device system we can allocate some functions to the human, some to the device, and some to the PAS. Bailey (1989) defines several approaches to **function allocation** that are used in general human factors design. Several of these are applicable to the design of assistive technology systems. The simplest approach is *comparison allocation.* Here each task to be carried out is assigned completely to the human or the device. The user's skills define the task that can be assigned to her, and the characteristics of the technology determine which capabilities are assigned to it. For example, a standard telephone is designed with the assumption that the user can hold the handset, press the buttons to dial, hear the other person, and speak into the telephone. These are all functions assigned to the user. However, if the user cannot perform any of these tasks, the assistive technology must provide an alternative set of tasks. For example, assume that a particular consumer is able to carry out all the functions except holding the handset and dialing. A speaker phone, which avoids the need to hold the handset, together with a mouth stick for dialing, could be used. These constitute the assistive technology component of this system. The setting (context) also affects the allocation of functions. For example, a speaker phone may work very well in a home setting, but in an office environment it can interfere with other workers and prevent the user from having private conversations. In this case an additional assistive technology characteristic (e.g., a headset) is required. We often use comparison allocation when matching characteristics of technology to a consumer's skills.

A second allocation approach is *leftover allocation,* in which as many functions as possible are assigned to the human and the device carries out the remainder. In assistive technology system design, this approach is often followed to give the consumer as much natural control over his activities as possible, but to provide assistance when needed. For example, some manual wheelchairs are equipped with a small motor that provides a powered assist when necessary. An individual may be able to power the manual chair on flat, level surfaces with little difficulty; however, going up hills or ramps may require too much effort. This type of wheelchair provides power to climb the hills, but the motor is not used on level surfaces. Thus a person who has limited strength and endurance can propel the wheelchair manually on flat surfaces but use the power assist unit to climb hills. This represents an allocation of the "power" function to the human part of the time and to the wheelchair part of the time. Alternatively, the leftover functions (e.g., assistance in climbing a hill) could be allocated to a personal assistant.

A third approach is *economic allocation,* in which the basic consideration is whether it is cheaper to select, train, and pay a personal assistant to do the activity or to design an assistive technology system for this purpose. Often the economic analysis initially favors the personal assistant because the purchase cost of the technology is relatively high. However, if the technology cost is amortized over its useful life, the technological approach may be significantly less expensive, since the personal assistant cost (salary) remains the same or rises over time. As we have discussed, though, the economic consideration must be coupled with other considerations relative to personal assistant services.

The final approach that we use when designing an assistive technology system is *flexible allocation.* In this approach the consumer can vary his or her degree of participation in the activity based on skills and needs. Whenever possible, we use this approach in assistive technology systems, and we couple the use of the AT system with PAS. The human and technology components are not fixed in scope; they change based on the specific activities and tasks to be carried out. Initially the novice operator may rely more heavily on intuitive skills to perform the desired tasks. As knowledge of the device operation increases and strategies are developed, the tasks carried out by the human operator change and system operation becomes more efficient. The role of PAS may also change over time. As an example, consider the case of Pat. He sustained a high-level spinal cord injury that resulted in quadriplegia. He has good control of his head, but he has no use of his arms or legs. He uses an electronic pointing device attached to a headband to substitute for using his fingers to type on the computer keyboard. This device must be placed on his head, and the computer must be set up by a personal assistant. Because of his underlying abilities, Pat will always need to rely on PAS to place the device on his head. Pat will also rely on PAS as a backup if his electronic pointing system becomes inoperative. The particular device that Pat is using is equipped with a word prediction feature, which presents a choice of words based on the keys he enters. Pat's assistant may also help with some system functions as Pat is learning to use the system. As Pat gains more skill in using the system, this assistance will not be necessary. Initially Pat will use just the letter-by-letter input mode, since he is familiar with that method from previous use of a keyboard. However, as he begins to learn what words are likely to be predicted when he types certain sequences of keys, he'll start using the word completion feature to speed up his selections. The advanced features of his system—in this case, word prediction—are not used until the basic features have become familiar. As Pat learns to use the advanced features, he will

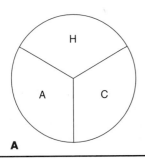 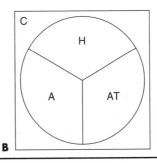 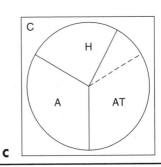

**Figure 2-8**    The allocation of functions among the components of an assistive technology system changes with the severity of disability and the need for more adaptations. **A,** Function allocation for a nondisabled person. **B,** Function allocation for a person with moderate disabilities. **C,** Function allocation for a person with more severe disabilities (see text). *H,* Human; *A,* activity; *C,* context; *AT,* assistive technology.

need to make fewer entries because the device has taken over a larger portion of the total system functions. If, as is often the case, the device also learns which words Pat uses most often and presents those to him as first choices, then his ease of entry will improve further. As Pat becomes more and more skilled, he will be able to allocate more functions to the system and reserve his own energy for thinking and decision making.

Flexible allocation also allows for the system to change to account for decreasing human function, as in the case of degenerative disease. For example, an individual with muscular dystrophy generally regresses from walking to using a manual wheelchair and then to a powered wheelchair as his disease progresses. This often requires two new systems, a manual and a powered wheelchair. However, there are add-on powered units that can be attached to a manual wheelchair. The use of an add-on unit makes the basic manual wheelchair more flexible and allows the transfer of functions from the human (upper body strength to propel a manual wheelchair) to the device (an electric motor to power the wheelchair). Similar considerations apply to individuals whose abilities, and resulting performance, fluctuate throughout the day or from day to day because of changing neuromuscular capabilities (e.g., muscle tone, strength, attention) or fatigue. Often this fluctuation in abilities is great, and the system must compensate for these changes. If the system is able to reallocate functions flexibly, the consumer will be able to accomplish tasks with greater device assistance when she is tired, and she will be able to exert more control and independence when she is well rested. The case of Frank, the individual with ALS, described earlier in this chapter provides an additional example of flexible allocation.

Some extrinsic enablers are more flexible than others, and they allow continual alteration in the allocation between the human and technology. For example, computer-based devices can be altered by software to perform many functions with the same control interface. On the other hand, some extrinsic enablers, including some seating and postural support systems, are less flexible, and

they must be redesigned or adjusted if the human component changes significantly (e.g., when a child goes through a growth phase).

In many ways the design of an assistive technology system is a process of function allocation. The total system performs a given activity, and it is not important how the functions are allocated within the system. Thus we refer to the sum of the four components as the *system.* Every assistive technology system is unique. This is because every person with a disability is unique, and the characteristics of assistive technologies that meet one person's needs differ from those that meet another's needs. When we begin to look at specific individuals with disabilities and certain tasks to be accomplished, the boundaries of the four areas shown in Figure 2-3, *B,* become quite flexible. For example, John and Sarah are co-workers in data entry for a public agency. Both have been evaluated as performing the tasks required for their positions at an acceptable level. The similarity ends there, however, because Sarah was born without a left hand. Her motor function is otherwise within normal limits. John has cerebral palsy, which limits the size of the target he can hit. If a human factors engineer were to allocate functions for the job to be performed among the human, activity, and context, it might look like Figure 2-8, *A.* The relative roles of the three components are balanced, and this allocation would apply to an average nondisabled worker. In Sarah's case, she needs only one adaptation to the standard data entry terminal, and that is to move one key (similar to a shift function) from the right side to the left side of the keyboard so she can press it with her residual limb while she hits other keys with her right hand. Figure 2-8, *B,* shows the addition of assistive technologies that modify the allocation of functions for Sarah's case. John's adaptations are more elaborate. He needs an expanded keyboard, which has larger keys that require less precise control for activation. His allocation of functions is shown in Figure 2-8, *C.* The human *(H)* component is reduced and the assistive technology *(AT)* is increased in size. This example illustrates the dynamic nature of the boundaries between the four components of the assistive technology system.

## The Effects of Time and Space on Allocation of Functions

A system can be defined generally as consisting of a group of objects that can interact with each other and are assembled in a way intended to achieve a desired goal (Cooper and McGillem, 1967). Systems are further described as being either open or closed. An *open system* exchanges matter, energy, and information with the external environment and is dynamic. A closed system does not exchange with the environment and is static. Because our system is dynamic and interacts with the environment, it is an open system; however, since the context (environment) is included as a component of the system, we change the system each time the context changes. Figure 2-9 illustrates the consideration of both time and space (location) as additional variables in the definition and design of the assistive technology system. In Figure 2-9, time is shown as a single line and the system at various times is represented by the boxes. At any time, the system has specific human, technology, activity, and context components; however, the allocation of functions between these four components may vary. This formulation allows us to take into account skill acquisition and degenerative conditions, as well as changing environmental conditions over time. Changes in location also result in alterations in the system, as shown in Figure 2-9. As the human and the other parts of the system move from one location to another, the context changes. The activity may also change, as well as the relative roles of the human and the technology within the system.

## The Effects of Errors in Assistive Technology Systems

An important operational characteristic of assistive technology systems is the way in which they deal with errors. This can be addressed through careful design. There are two types of errors that are of concern in assistive technology systems. *Random errors* are infrequent and are generally chance occurrences. An example of a random error is the inability to understand a voice synthesizer because of high amounts of ambient noise. If the noise is not present, there is no error, and even if there is noise it may not lead to an error in interpretation. It is only the random co-occurrence of the need to use the voice synthesizer, the presence of noise, and a listener who doesn't understand that creates the error. Random errors such as this can reoccur, but they are not consistently present in the system. We can do very little to avoid this type of error in the assistive technology system design process.

Of greater concern are *periodic,* or regular, *errors,* which occur under predictable conditions. These errors may also be infrequent, but they are foreseeable. As an example, many letter-to-speech software programs make mistakes in pronunciation when used with voice synthesizers. The mispronunciation always occurs whenever the particular word is entered. This does not mean that this is a frequent error, however, since the offending words may not be used often. Because it is predictable, this type of error can be dealt with in the design process. For our example of mispronunciation, exception tables are typically used so that the utterance sounds correct even though the letter-to-speech rule makes

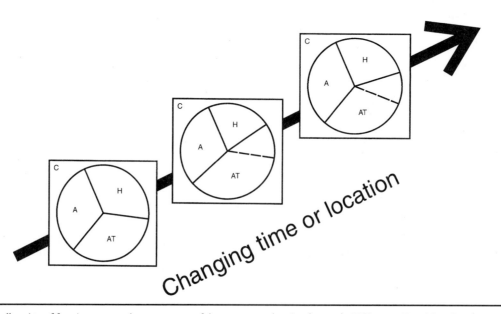

**Figure 2-9**   The allocation of functions among the components of the HAAT model of an assistive technology system may change with time or location (see text). *H,* Human; *A,* activity; *C,* context; *AT,* assistive technology.

an error. In some systems the word "breakfast" must be spelled "brekfast" in order to be pronounced correctly. This is because the rules for converting letters to sounds are inadequate for this case. An exception table would translate the typed spelling of "breakfast" into "brekfast" before sending it to the speech synthesizer, and the user would not have to spell it phonetically. This can be very important for young children learning to spell and for anyone whose input is also displayed visually.

There are several effects of errors on assistive technology system performance, including loss of information, injury, and embarrassment. All three of these can occur in the same system, and they may be due to the human, the activity, the context, or the assistive technology. A powered mobility system can have any of these errors. If the batteries are not charged and the human operator does not pay attention to them, the wheelchair will fail to operate. This is a loss of information caused by system error. More serious consequences of physical injury can occur if the motors fail to stop when the human operator turns them off (e.g., by releasing the joystick). However, even if the motors do stop as they are supposed to, a slippery surface (context) could lead to injury, and of course a fully functional set of motors is of no value if the user fails to release the joystick in time. Finally, if the horn malfunctions on the wheelchair, this can lead to embarrassment whether the operator inadvertently hits the horn button or the system fails.

Loss of information is a common effect associated with augmentative communication systems (see Chapter 9) and sensory aids (see Chapter 12). It can occur because the human operator makes an error in motor, sensory, or cognitive performance, or as a result of a device error. Although the net effect on system performance of either of these errors (human or device) may be the same, it is important to distinguish between them to correct the problem. If the errors are made by the human operator, we can determine whether the cause is lack of capability (e.g., excessive tremor resulting in erroneous selections or visual limitations in reading a display) or lack of skill (inadequate experience or practice in using the device). If the problem is the basic capability of the user, then modifications must be made in the system (e.g., using a keyguard to prevent erroneous entries or an enlarged display screen to improve visibility). If the problem is one of skill, training may help reduce the number of errors.

Physical injury is a more serious effect of a system error. This type of error can occur in a mobility system (see Chapter 10) if, for example, a braking system fails or a motor fails to turn off. Consideration of this type of error leads us to the concept of "failsafe" design. The objective of this approach is to attempt to anticipate the types of errors (termed *failures* when caused by the device) and to ensure that if they do occur the probability of injury is minimized. For example,

if a powered wheelchair controller fails, it should fail in the off state. If it fails in the full on state, the user is subject to injury because the chair is then out of control. Human errors can lead to injury also. If a powered wheelchair user cannot control the joystick adequately, he may drive into traffic or hit an obstacle, and this could cause injury.

A final general effect of assistive technology system errors is embarrassment. This effect is somewhat unique to assistive technologies, and it is a direct result of the role that assistive technology systems play in the daily life of the user who has a disability. Because the tasks being performed cannot be accomplished without the system, its use is continual throughout the day. Over a long period, system errors leading to embarrassment are inevitable. The embarrassment may be relatively minor, such as a manipulation system dropping a spoonful of food, it may be much more significant. For example, an augmentative communication device may fail and produce the wrong utterance. If the context is a presentation in an important meeting and the mistaken utterance is an obscenity, the consequences are potentially very negative. To place the importance of this type of error in perspective, recall that the device is often perceived by both the user and other people as being a part of the user. Thus the user is held responsible for an inappropriate utterance just as if she had used her own voice to produce it. The errors and their resulting effects may arise from any of the components of the assistive technology system. The human may make an error of capability or skill, or the device may malfunction. Alternatively, the temperature (physical context) may be so high or so low that the system cannot function as designed. One of our major goals in designing assistive technology systems is to minimize the occurrence and impact of system errors.

## The Importance of Measuring Assistive Technology System Effectiveness

Once we have designed an assistive technology system in conjunction with the consumer of the system, it is necessary to measure the performance of the system and determine whether it is functioning effectively. The HAAT model provides the basis by which system performance can be evaluated.

Because the assistive technology system consists of the four components of the HAAT model (see Figure 2-3, *B*), all four must be considered when we measure system effectiveness. The *activity*, based on the individual's life roles and performance areas, defines the goals of the system. The achievement of these goals is what we use to determine the success of the system. The *context* is the physical and social environments in which the system needs to function. There are *constraints* imposed on system performance by the given context. The ability of the system to function within these constraints is an important variable that is measured to determine system effectiveness. An evaluation of the human operator defines the *skills* available to meet the desired goals. It is critical that the ATP accurately evaluates the user's skills and generalizes their use with assistive technologies in everyday applications. *Assistive technology* is indicated when there is a disparity between the skills of the human operator and the skills required to complete the goals. The specific *characteristics* of the assistive technology are delineated by the combination of the goals, constraints, and available human skills in order to achieve the desired level of performance. If the assistive technology system is functioning effectively, the human operator can use his available skills to achieve the desired goals in the relevant contexts with the assistive technology chosen. If the system is not functioning effectively, we can reevaluate each of the HAAT model components to determine the nature of the failure. The system can then be revised, and the overall system performance can be reevaluated. A major role of the ATP is to develop and apply specific means of measuring system performance, and the HAAT model provides a basis for this measurement. We develop approaches to the process and application of measurement of system performance in Chapter 4.

## ■ SUMMARY

In this chapter we have presented the HAAT model for application of assistive technologies and analyzed its various component parts. We have also looked at the ways in which assistive technology systems change with varying conditions of use, and we have discussed the necessity for measuring effectiveness. This information forms the basis for much of the remaining chapters. In succeeding chapters we use this model to discuss specific applications of assistive technologies.

## Study Questions

1. Distinguish between human behavior and human performance. Which can be measured, and what is required for assessment of that measurement?
2. What are the components of the human performance model, and how do they relate to each other?
3. Describe the difference between *A* and *B* in Figure 2-3.
4. How is the model shown in Figure 2-3, *B*, affected by the presence of disability?
5. List at least three reasons why assistive technology systems are defined to include all four parts of Figure 2-3, *B*.
6. What are the three basic performance areas defined in the HAAT model? Give an example of each.
7. Define life roles. How do these relate to assistive technology use?
8. How are *tasks* related to *activities* in assistive technology application?
9. Why are the characteristics of the human user defined as *intrinsic enablers*?
10. What is the role of personal assistant services (PAS)? How do PAS complement the use of assistive technology systems to meet the needs of persons who have disabilities?
11. Describe the role that strategies play in the use of assistive technology systems. How can strategies compensate for the absence or inadequacy of an assistive technology?
12. Describe the four major parts of the context and how each can affect overall assistive technology system performance.
13. How do cultural considerations affect the application of assistive technology systems?
14. Explain the shift in thinking regarding societal participation by persons who have disabilities; that is, where is the "problem" with this participation thought to lie? What implications does this have for assistive technology applications?
15. What is meant by the terms *macrosystemic, mesosystemic,* and *microsystemic* in relation to considerations of the context of assistive technology application?
16. What are the four components of the assistive technology portion of the HAAT model?
17. What is meant by the terms *novice* and *expert,* and how do they affect assistive technology application?
18. Distinguish between *ability* and *skill.* How do abilities and skills relate to the concepts of novice and expert?
19. Why do we refer to assistive technologies as *extrinsic enablers*?
20. What are the three common effects of assistive technology system errors? Give an example of each type.
21. Why do we say that each assistive technology system is unique?
22. What is meant by the term *function allocation,* and how is it applied to assistive technology systems?
23. What are the major approaches to function allocation? What are the strengths and weaknesses of each approach when used in assistive technology system design?
24. What is the role of personal assistant services in allocation of functions?
25. How do time and location affect the makeup of an assistive technology system?
26. Describe how the HAAT model can be used to generate the basis for measuring assistive technology system effectiveness.

## References

American Occupational Therapy Association: Uniform terminology for occupational therapy, third edition, *Am J Occup Ther* 48:1047, 1994.

Bailey RW: *Human performance engineering,* ed 2, Englewood Cliffs, NJ, 1989, Prentice Hall.

Brooks NA: Models for understanding rehabilitation and assistive technology. In Gray DB, Quatrano LA, Lieberman ML, editors: *Designing and using assistive technology: the human perspective,* Baltimore, 1998, Paul H Brookes Publishing.

Brooks NA: User's perceptions of assistive devices. In Smith RV, Leslie JH, editors: *Rehabilitation engineering,* Boca Raton, Fla, 1990, CRC Press.

Christiansen C: Occupational therapy, intervention for life performance. In Christiansen C, Baum C, editors: *Occupational therapy,* Thoroughfare, NJ, 1991, Slack.

Christiansen C, Baum C: Person-environment occupational performance: a conceptual model for practice. In Christiansen C, Baum C, editors: *Occupational therapy: enabling function and well being,* ed 2, Thoroughfare, NJ, 1997, Slack.

Church G, Glennen S: *The handbook of assistive technology,* San Diego, Calif, 1992, Singular Publishing Group.

Cooper GR, McGillem CD: *Methods of signal and system analysis,* New York, 1967, Holt, Reinhart.

Cynkin S: *Occupational therapy: towards health through activities,* Boston, 1979, Little, Brown and Company.

Enders A: *Technology for the next millennium: building a framework for collaboration.* Presented at the 1999 conference of the Association for the Advancement of Assistive Technology in Europe (AAATE), Dusseldorf, Germany, November 1999.

Fougeyrollas P: The influence of the social environment on the social participation of people with disabilities. In Christiansen C, Baum C, editors: *Occupational therapy: enabling function and well being,* ed 2, Thoroughfare, NJ, 1997, Slack.

Fougeyrollas P, Gray DB: Classification systems, environmental factors and social change. In Gray DB, Quatrano LA, Lieberman ML, editors: *Designing and using assistive technology: The human perspective,* Baltimore, 1998, Paul H Brookes Publishing.

Gibson J: *The ecological approach to visual perception,* Boston, 1979, Houghton Mifflin.

Kondraske GV: Quantitative measurement and assessment of performance. In Smith RV, Leslie JH, editors: *Rehabilitation engineering,* Boca Raton, Fla, 1990, CRC Press.

Krefting LH, Krefting DV: Cultural influences on performance. In Christiansen C, Baum C, editors: *Occupational therapy,* Thoroughfare, NJ, 1991, Slack.

McDonnell PM et al: Do artificial limbs become a part of the user? New evidence, *J Rehab Res* 26(2):17-24, 1989.

Murphy JW, Cook AM: Limitations of augmentative communication systems in progressive neurological diseases, *Proc 8th Ann Conf Rehabil Technol,* pp 120-122, Washington, DC, June 1985, RESNA.

Pope A, Brandt E, editors: *Enabling America. Assessing the role of rehabilitation science and engineering,* Washington, DC, 1997, National Academy Press.

Ragnarsson KT: Prescription considerations and a comparison of conventional and lightweight wheelchairs, *J Rehabil Res Dev Clin Suppl* 2:8-16, 1990.

Verbrugge LM, Rennert C, Madans JH: The great efficacy of personal and equipment assistance in reducing disability, *Am J Pub Health* 87:384-392, 1997.

## CHAPTER 3

# The Disabled Human User of Assistive Technologies

---

### Chapter Outline

## Learning Objectives

Upon completing this chapter you will be able to:

1.  Place the human user of assistive technologies in the proper context relative to the activities and contexts of human performance
2.  Describe and apply an information processing model of the disabled human operator of assistive technologies
3.  Use basic human factors and neuroscience concepts to describe the interaction between persons with disabilities and assistive devices
4.  Describe how disabilities, learning (including experience), age, and changing conditions affect the human performance model and the interaction among the human, the activity, and the context
5.  Apply basic principles of human performance to specific application areas (activities) and contexts

## Key Terms

| | | |
|---|---|---|
| Abandonment | Motivation | Range |
| Apraxia | Motor Control | Recall |
| Central Processing | Morphology | Recognition |
| Cognition | Muscle Tone | Reluctant Users |
| Development | Optimal Use | Resolution |
| Effectors | Paralysis | Semantics |
| Engram | Perception | Sensors |
| Growth | Phonology | Spasticity |
| Intrinsic Enablers | Pragmatics | Syntax |
| Learning | Primitive Reflexes | Visual Accommodation |
| Memory | Psychosocial Function | |

In the previous chapter we described the assistive technology system and the interrelationships among its component parts. In this chapter we focus on the human user of assistive technologies. It is assumed that the reader has a general knowledge of normal human physiology and of disabilities, and therefore our emphasis is on those characteristics of disability that influence the use of assistive technologies. The Disability Statistics Center at the University of California, San Francisco, has provided the following statistics based on the National Health Interview Survey (NHIS), a continuing national household survey consisting of 49,401 household interviews with 128,412 people in 1992 (www.dsc.ucsf.edu). Data collected include information regarding basic personal assistance needs (i.e., whether people need help with such activities of daily living [ADL] as bathing, eating, dressing, or getting around inside) and routine personal assistance needs (i.e., whether people need help with such instrumental activities of daily living [IADL] as household chores, doing necessary business, shopping, or getting around for other purposes) as a result of chronic health conditions.

* Approximately 15% (37.7 million) of the United States'

population have a limitation that affects a major life activity such as working or going to school. These individuals report 1.6 conditions per person on average, for a total of 61 million limiting conditions.
* More than 19 million individuals ages 18 to 69 have physical or mental conditions that keep them from working, attending school, or maintaining a household. Females report a higher number of activity-limiting conditions than males.
* Minorities, the elderly, and those in lower socioeconomic populations have a greater incidence of disabilities and need greater assistance in both ADLs (52% over age 65) and IADLs (58% over age 65).
* A newborn can be expected to experience 13 years of limited activity out of a 75-year life expectancy.
* National disability-related costs are more than $170 billion annually.

These statistics indicate that activity-limiting disabilities are widespread, unevenly distributed across the general population, and expensive. Assistive technologies, if appropriately applied, can help to overcome the activity limitations imposed by disabilities. This requires a thorough understanding of human abilities and skills, especially in the presence of a disability.

In designing assistive technology systems, we build on the skills of the user and provide assistive devices that augment or replace functional limitations. Because our goal is to increase functional independence for individuals with disabilities, it is important to focus on remaining function, rather than on lost function. In this chapter we develop a description of the human user of assistive technologies.

## AN INFORMATION PROCESSING MODEL OF THE ASSISTIVE TECHNOLOGY SYSTEM USER

Human factors engineers and psychologists have developed the model shown in Figure 3-1 to describe the human component of a human-machine interaction (Bailey, 1989). This model is useful for describing the human operator of an assistive technology system. The individual blocks shown in Figure 3-1 delineate functional rather than structural components, and they are used to help identify the important considerations in human-machine interaction. Bailey (1989) lists three things that a system designer must know about the user: (1) what can be done (skills), (2) what cannot be done (limitations), and (3) what will be done (motivation). Motivation is directly related to the person's goals and needs and how well the assistive technology system meets them.

When designing assistive technology systems, we look at skills and limitations in the three component areas shown in Figure 3-1. Taken together, these components constitute the **intrinsic enablers** for the human. Input from **sensors** is necessary for obtaining data from the environment, and limitations can arise in both the sensitivity (minimum detectable levels of light, sound, or pressure) and range (allowable variation in size, amplitude, or magnitude of the sensory input). When assistive technology system use is being considered, the visual, auditory, tactile, proprioceptive, kinesthetic, and vestibular sensory systems all play important

roles. Sensory data produced by each of these systems are important for the successful use of assistive technologies. Some assistive technologies specifically address sensory loss. For example, reading and mobility systems for the visually impaired and hearing aids for individuals with auditory impairment are designed to compensate for these specific losses (Chapter 12). However, sensory function affects virtually all areas of assistive technology application, and it is important to consider sensory function as an integral part of the overall human capabilities required for the successful operation of an assistive technology system.

We shall use the term **effectors** to describe the neural, muscular, and skeletal elements of the human body that provide movement or motor output. The result of the movement of the effectors is motor output. These elements work together to allow movement under the control of central processing and in response to sensory input. Limitations can arise from impairments in any element or combinations of them. Effectors provide the motor outputs that can be used for the control of assistive technology systems. Often, assistive technology systems are controlled by hand movements. For example, powered wheelchairs typically employ joystick control activated by hand movements, and computers and augmentative communication systems utilize hand and finger movements for keyboard use. However, other anatomical sites may be used for control, and the components of postural control and reflexes also contribute to the generation of motor output.

Interposed between the sensors and effectors are the **central processing** functions of perception, cognition, neuromuscular control (including motor planning), and psychological factors. **Perception** is the interpretation and assignment of meaning to data received from the sensors, and it involves an interaction between information derived from sensed data and information stored in memory based on previous sensory experiences (Bailey, 1989). As Dunn (1991) points out, sensory and perceptual function provide the mechanisms by which an individual interacts with the environment. It is the combination and interpretation of data from all our sensory systems that provide a meaningful picture of the environment and our interaction with it.

We use the term **cognition** to refer to attention, memory, problem solving, decision making, learning, language, and other related tasks. As pointed out by Duchek (1991), virtually all aspects of performance are based on cognitive function. This applies to performance that utilizes assistive technology systems and to human performance in general. For example, the use of a powered wheelchair requires several types of cognitive function. The human operator must visually scan the environment, process the sensory data, make decisions as to the direction of movement desired, and activate the corresponding effector to cause the motion of the wheelchair in the desired direction.

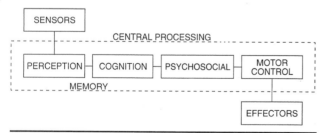

**Figure 3-1** An information processing model of the human operator of assistive technologies. Each block represents a group of functions related to the use of technology. Taken together, these components constitute the intrinsic enablers for the human.

Once in motion, the user must attend to the environment to avoid obstacles and hazards and make instantaneous decisions regarding speed and direction. The user may also be required to engage in problem solving to negotiate a tight space or recover from an error. Cognitive processes involved in this example include attention, decision making, problem solving, language (e.g., spatial concepts such as left, right, forward, back), and memory. Without these capabilities, it would be difficult to control a powered wheelchair effectively.

It is also sometimes difficult to separate cognitive performance from sensory or motor performance. For example, an individual using an electric feeding device (see Chapter 11) requires sensory input to locate food on a plate; decision making to select the desired food item to be eaten; sufficient motor skills to activate a control interface that directs the spoon to the plate to pick up food and move it to the mouth; and monitoring of the path of the spoon as it travels. Because this is a complex set of tasks, it is difficult to determine whether failure to complete them successfully is caused by a sensory or perceptual problem (e.g., difficulty in separating the food from the background of the plate), a cognitive problem (e.g., forgetting what the sequence of tasks is or inability to attend long enough to complete the task), or a motor limitation (e.g., inability to activate the control interface or inability to physically remove the food from the spoon because of lack of oral-motor control).

**Motor control** is the result of the integration of sensory, perceptual, and cognitive components into a motor pattern that is executed by the effectors. This process involves many degrees of feedback and feed-forward control, and there are many current theories relating to the precise mechanisms involved (see Burgess, 1989, for example). We use the term *motor control* to refer to the central processing components of effector regulation. These components may be in the brain or spinal cord, and smooth, precise movements are possible only through integration of information from the sensors, other central nervous system (CNS) components (e.g., perception, decision making), and feedback from the effectors.

*Motor planning* is used to describe the process by which purposeful movements are executed to accomplish a purposeful task (Warren, 1991). This is a central processing activity that requires the highest level of motor control. For example, the tasks of writing, eating, using a hand tool, and typing all require motor planning for successful completion. *Motor learning* occurs as we practice a task over and over, and many tasks become automatic with practice (i.e., we are not aware of the individual steps in the task). During the learning process, we must concentrate on each step in order to learn the task. However, even though the task may become automatic or subconscious, motor planning is still involved; an individual who has suffered CNS damage may

lose this ability. Thus motor output involves sensory data collection (from internal and external sensors), interpretation and integration of these data (perception), conscious planning of a movement (not always necessary), development of a movement pattern that is responsive to the plan and consistent with the sensory data (motor control), and execution of the movement (effectors). Motor control is discussed in detail later in this chapter.

**Psychosocial function** consists of identity, self-protection, and motivation. These factors are related to the acceptance of a disability, the approach a person takes to the assistive technology, and how effective the technology can be for the person. Concepts from self-identity and self-protection are used to describe how a person with a disability might interact with assistive technologies and how successful he is likely to be in using them. Motivation greatly influences how much an individual works to develop skill in using an assistive technology and the degree to which they are successful in that use.

Limitations in function can occur in any of these areas as a result of trauma, disease, or a congenital condition. A major goal of assessment for the purpose of designing assistive technology systems is to identify the disabled person's skills in the areas of sensory function, central processing, and motor output and control.

## ■ SENSORY FUNCTION AS RELATED TO ASSISTIVE TECHNOLOGY USE

In this section the major sensory systems that are involved in assistive technology system use are described. The emphasis is on human sensory performance and how it affects use of assistive technologies to compensate for sensory limitations. These compensatory technologies are discussed in succeeding chapters.

### Visual Function

Visual function is important (but not essential) for the effective use of assistive technology systems, especially regarding access systems. For example, in using augmentative communication systems, individual items must be found in arrays of vocabulary elements, scanning cursors must be tracked, and visual feedback is often used to signify successful message generation. Likewise, in order to use a powered wheelchair, visual scanning of the environment must be present and there must be adequate acuity and visual field to guide the chair around obstacles effectively, safely, and efficiently. For individuals who have visual impairments, reading print material or computer displays can be difficult or impossible, and assistive technologies can be of help.

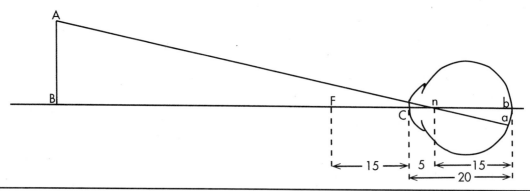

**Figure 3-2**   The visual angle is the angle just in front of the cornea, *C,* formed by object *AB.* (From Ruch TC, Patton HD: *Physiology and biophysics,* ed 19, Philadelphia, 1966, WB Saunders.)

When an individual's primary disability is visual, it is obvious that the assistive technology must accommodate needs in this area. We must often use other modalities, typically auditory or tactile senses; general purpose visual substitution systems for mobility and reading are discussed in Chapter 12. However, as Cress et al (1981) point out, the incidence of visual impairment in individuals with severe physical disabilities may be as high as 75% to 90%. Often these visual difficulties are not identified or treated. Because assistive technology application is so dependent on the use of visual input, we need to carefully evaluate visual function (see Chapter 4), and we need to specify and design systems such that we account for special visual requirements. Several types of measurements are typically employed to assess visual capability. These include visual acuity (target size), visual range or field size, visual tracking (following a target), and visual scanning (finding a specific visual target in a field of several targets). Each of these is important in the use of assistive technology systems; we describe how they are measured in Chapter 4.

**Visual acuity.**  We use the term *visual acuity* to refer to all those aspects of the visual system that are related to focusing an image on the retina and extracting sensory data from that image. Three factors are important in this process: (1) size of the object, (2) contrast between the object and the background, and (3) spacing between the object and surrounding background objects. One way to measure the size of an object is to determine the visual angle formed by that object when it is viewed at a known distance. Figure 3-2 illustrates the concept of visual angle. Visual angles of common objects include 13 minutes of arc for pica-typed letters, 2 minutes for a quarter held at arm's length, and 1 second for a quarter at 3 miles (Bailey, 1989). The minimal visual angle threshold for the eye is approximately 1 second of arc; however, the recommended visual angle for ease of viewing in normal light is 15 minutes of arc (21 minutes in reduced light) (Bailey, 1989).

*Visual angle* describes only the size of an object that is detectable. Contrast between the object and the background is equally important, and the visual threshold of interest is brightness. The minimal detectable brightness for normal human vision is a single candle seen at 30 miles on a dark, clear night (Bailey, 1989). This translates into measurable units of $10^{-6}$ millilamberts. For comparison, a tungsten filament light bulb emits 1 million millilamberts, and white paper has a brightness of 10 millilamberts in good reading light. The absolute value of the emission or reflection of light from an object is not as important as the degree to which the object differs from the background. The visual system functions best when contrast is high (Dunn, 1991). Busy visual fields have too many competing objects for the visual system to extract important visual data. In later chapters we discuss how assistive technology system assessment and design are affected by these considerations.

The eye is sensitive to colors in the visual spectrum (from violet to red), but it is not equally sensitive to all colors in this range. Also, different areas on the retina are sensitive to different colors (Bailey, 1989). If the eye is fixed and not allowed to rotate, the limits of color vision are 60 degrees to each side of the midline. Within this range, the response of the retina to colors is not equal for all wavelengths (colors). Figure 3-3 illustrates that blue objects are visible over the entire 60-degree range, whereas yellow, red, and green are recognizable only at points closer to the fixed (center) point of vision. This has implications for our design of systems for individuals who rely on peripheral vision or who have difficulty moving their eyes to track objects. If we use green or red, we may limit the person's ability to see the object; we can increase visibility by using blue or yellow. We can also effect contrast by using different colors for foreground and background.

**Visual field.**  With the head and eyes fixed on a central point, the normal range of peripheral vision in the right eye

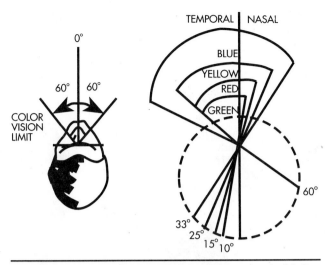

**Figure 3-3**  Color response of the eye differs with visual angle. (Modified from Woodson W, Conover D: *Human engineering guide for equipment designers,* Berkeley, 1964, University of California Press.)

is 70 degrees to the left and 104 degrees to the right (Bailey, 1989). If the eyes are allowed to rotate but the head remains fixed, the range is 166 degrees to each side of the central point.

This typical visual field may be altered in several ways by disease or injury to the eyes, visual pathways, or brain. The most common types of visual field deficits are shown in Figure 3-4. Visual loss may occur in one or more of the quadrants of the left or right field. Dunn (1991) discusses the major causes of these losses. These types of losses are common in persons with disabilities such as cerebral palsy, traumatic brain injury, and diseases affecting the eyes and visual system. When we specify and design assistive technology systems, we must be careful to take into account the size and nature of the individual's visual field.

**Visual tracking and scanning.**  Visual tracking is the ability to follow a moving object. This skill is necessary for many assistive technology tasks. Visual scanning differs from visual tracking in that the object does not move; instead the eyes are moved to image different parts of a scene in order to find a specific object or location within the scene. Oculomotor function is required for normal vision and for assistive technology applications in which the eyes are used as an effector (see the section on motor control in this chapter). Conjunctive eye movements are those in which the eyes move together (e.g., saccades, vestibuloocular reflexes, optokinetic reflexes, and smooth-slow pursuit). In disjunctive eye movements the eyes do not track together as in vergence during refocusing. These motor behaviors all need appropriate alignment of the eye muscles in addition to the intact motor system, and this is often not the case in persons with disabilities.

Eye movements are typically classified into two sets of systems: those which stabilize the retinal image and those which transfer gaze to a new target. The optokinetic (OKR) and vestibuloocular (VOR) reflexes are in the first category. All head movements serve as adequate stimuli for these reflexes; that is, the head movement serves as the input that generates the reflex. This is important because many individuals with disabilities have difficulty maintaining stable head or trunk position. Smooth pursuit eye movements also serve to stabilize the retinal image. Transfer of gaze is accomplished by saccades, vergence, and head movements.

**Visual accommodation.**  In the normal eye at rest, distant objects are focused on the retina. As the object is brought closer, the image falls in front of the retina unless the curvature of the lens is changed. The process by which the ciliary muscles change the curvature of the lens and hence the focal point of the eye is called **visual accommodation.** Accommodation is quantified by determining the change in the power of the lens of the eye as objects are brought closer. The power is calculated as the reciprocal of the focal distance of the eye, and it is measured in diopters (D). The closest point at which an object can still be focused is called the near point. For a person under 20 years of age with normal visual accommodation, the near point is approximately 10 cm and the accommodation is approximately 12 D. As we age, our accommodative ability decreases. For example, at age 50 the near point is at approximately 30 cm and the accommodation is reduced to less than 2 D; this leads to the prescription of reading glasses. Many types of disabilities affect accommodation; limitations in accommodation are referred to as *accommodative insufficiency.* When using assistive technologies, this can be a significant factor. For example, if a person is using a keyboard device with a visual display, the separation of these two system components may require constant accommodation as visual gaze is directed at the keyboard and then at the display and back to the keyboard. Appropriate placement of the keyboard and visual display can reduce the amount of accommodation that is required, and it can result in significantly improved overall system performance.

**Common visual deficits.**  Visual limitations are common in many types of disabilities. We have included two studies in this section to illustrate how these limitations can affect our design of assistive technology systems. We have chosen one example of a congenital disability (cerebral palsy) and one example of an adventitious disability (traumatic brain injury).

Duckman (1979) studied ocular function in a population of 25 children with cerebral palsy. He found that 92% of the children had ocular motor dysfunction of some type; 40% had significant refractive errors, 56% had strabismus, 100%

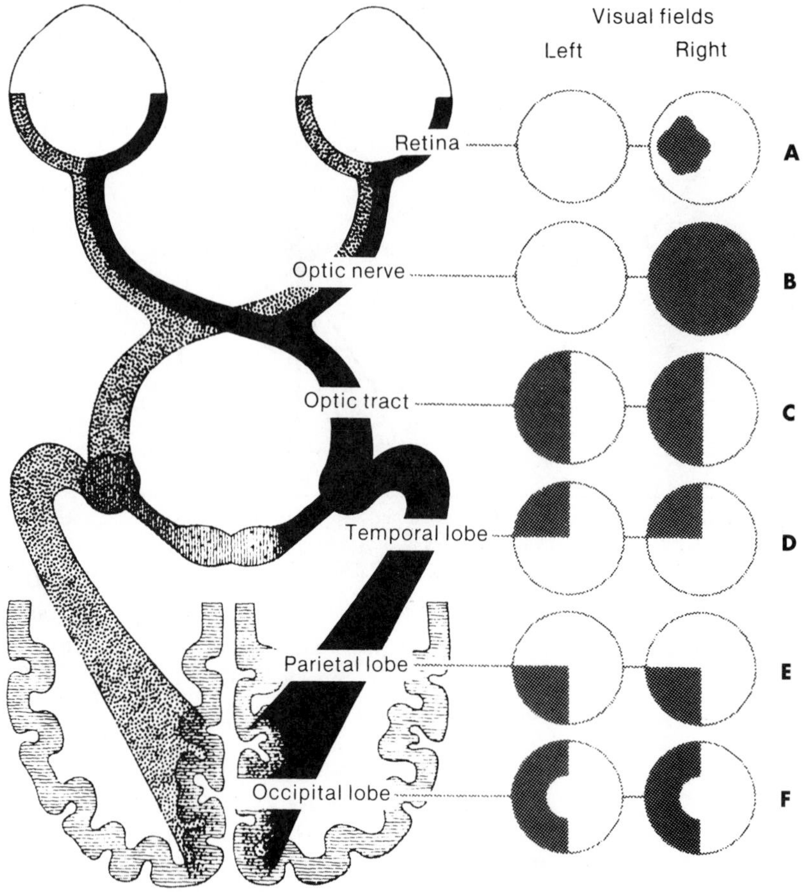

Figure 3-4 Types of visual field deficits. **A,** Retinal lesion: blind spot in the affected eye. **B,** Optic nerve lesion: partial or complete blindness in that eye. **C,** Optic tract or lateral geniculate lesion: blindness in the opposite half of both visual fields. **D,** Temporal lobe lesion: blindness in the upper quadrants of both visual fields on the side opposite the lesion. **E,** Parietal lobe lesion: contralateral blindness in the corresponding lower quadrants of both eyes. **F,** Occipital lobe lesion: contralateral blindness in the corresponding half of each visual field, but with macular sparing. (From Umphred DA: *Neurological rehabilitation,* ed 2, St Louis, 1990, Mosby, p 721. Courtesy Smith Kline & French Laboratories, Philadelphia.)

had accommodative insufficiency, 100% had poor directional concepts, and 78% had visual perception dysfunction. These results parallel other reports in the literature, and they indicate that the visual system is far from normal in this population. Duckman states that the poor directional concepts were so severe that "most children did not even have a concept of direction on their own bodies" (p. 1015).

The high degree of accommodative insufficiency was unexpected by Duckman, and he stated that "these children almost demonstrated 'paralyses' of accommodation" (p. 1015). Most of the children were unable to make shifts of as little as 0.25 D in their accommodative systems. This finding has direct bearing on tasks that require frequent redirection of gaze, such as looking at a keyboard to find the desired character and then looking at a display or screen to monitor the selections. It also helps explain the success of systems in which eye gaze is used in one (vertical) plane only rather than requiring movement horizontally and vertically (e.g., Goosens and Crain, 1987).

These considerations dictate that great care must be exercised when asking persons with disabilities to perform visual tasks. For example, communication systems using eye gaze as a method of indicating choices typically rely on printed targets (e.g., "yes" or "no") to which the eyes must

be directed (Goosens and Crain, 1987). Given the slow movements, tracking asymmetries, and difficulties with accommodation, it is not surprising that the use of these approaches is difficult for severely disabled persons and that development of these skills can take many hours of practice (see Light, Beesley, and Collier, 1988, for example).

Tychsen and Lisberger (1986) have shown that flaws in the visuomotor systems underlie deficits in the processing of visual motion. They note that the misalignment of the eye muscles (strabismus) in early life results in a permanent misalignment of the horizontal axes for both eyes, even after surgical correction of the muscle defect. Further, their tests demonstrate (1) a nasal-temporal asymmetry in the rate of smooth pursuit eye movement, given a horizontally moving target; and (2) a vertical asymmetry in smooth pursuit, given a vertically moving target. Psychophysical judgments by their subjects revealed that targets were seen to move more rapidly in one direction than in the other when the targets were traveling at the same speed.

Padula (1988) describes a similar situation for individuals suffering traumatic brain injuries. He describes a posttrauma vision syndrome with characteristics of exotropia, exophoria, accommodative dysfunction, convergence insufficiency, low blink rate (related to attention level), spatial disorienta-

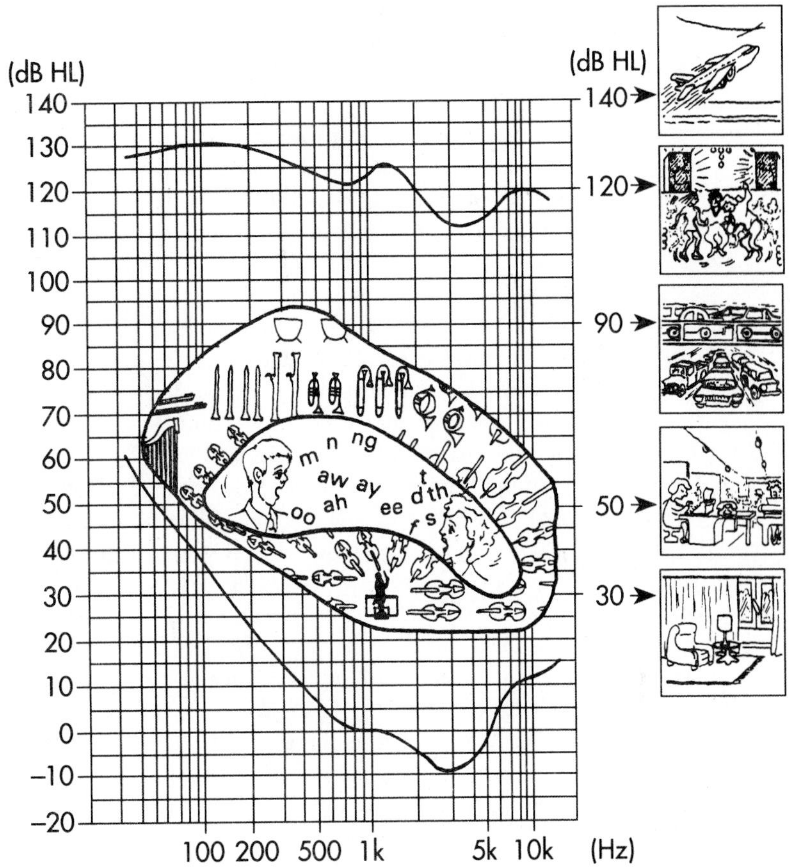

**Figure 3-5** The sensitivity of the human ear to frequency is shown on the plot. This curve is normalized to 0 dB at 1000 Hz. The reference pressure is 0.0002 dynes/cm². Along each side and in the center of the plot are shown frequencies and intensities of common sounds and speech. (From Ballantyne D: *Handbook of audiological techniques*, London, 1990, Butterworth-Heinemann.)

tion, and balance and posture difficulties. Individuals with this syndrome typically experience diplopia (double vision), movement of objects located in the periphery, visual memory problems, poor tracking ability, and poor concentration and attention. Padula also describes remarkable improvement in functional ability when prism lens glasses are utilized with these individuals. These characteristics and symptoms are similar to those described by Duckman (1979) for cerebral palsy.

## Auditory Function

Several types of auditory function are important for the use of assistive technology systems. *Auditory thresholds* include both the *amplitude* and *frequency* of audible sounds. The amplitude of sound is measured in decibels (dB). This unit is the logarithm of the ratio of the sound pressure being heard to the smallest sound pressure detectable by the ear (20 micropascals). This minimal threshold is equivalent to the ticking of a watch under quiet conditions at 20 feet away. Because of the logarithmic calculation of decibels, a doubling of the sound pressure level in decibels is a tenfold increase in the amplitude of the sound. Figure 3-5 shows sound pressure levels for a variety of typical sounds (Bailey, 1989).

The concept of sound pressure level and the values

shown in Figure 3-5 are particularly important in our consideration of the context for assistive technology use. One example of the application of these principles is Carolyn's use of an augmentative communication device that has voice synthesis output. She frequently goes shopping at a large mall (70-dB background noise) and goes out to dinner often. For dinner, her choice of restaurant may be a noisy fast food place (70 to 80 dB) or a quiet, elegant restaurant (50 to 60 dB). Because normal conversational levels are approximately 60 dB (see Figure 3-5), the quiet restaurant is more amenable to this function. Having these data, we can now evaluate different voice output communication devices to see whether they will meet Carolyn's needs. For example, assume that the specification for system one is a maximum of 50 dB and for system two it is 75 dB; the greater output of system two generally results in a heavier and larger device because the speaker and the batteries must both be larger to allow greater volume output. If we know some other things about Carolyn, such as whether she is able to walk or uses a wheelchair and how stable she is when walking, we can trade off the extra size and weight against the greater output amplitude capability.

Impairment of auditory function has two major effects: loss of input information and inability to monitor speech output. The latter can result in significant difficulties in oral communication. There are several assistive technology approaches to providing oral communication assistance to persons who have an auditory impairment. One approach is to provide feedback, either visually or tactually, that represents the person's speech patterns and relates them to typical speech. A second approach is to provide alternatives to oral communication, such as visual displays that are read by the listener. These and other approaches are discussed in Chapter 12.

**Auditory thresholds.** The typical range of frequencies that can be heard by the human ear is 20 to 20,000 hertz (Hz) (Bailey, 1989). The ear does not respond equally to all frequencies in this range, however, and Figure 3-5 shows the response curve of a normal ear. The vertical axis of Figure 3-5 is the sound pressure measured in decibels. The horizontal axis shows the frequencies of sound applied. The curve in this figure is the minimal threshold for detecting the sound for each frequency. The tone presented at 1000 Hz requires an intensity of 6.5 dB to sound as loud as a tone presented at 250 Hz with an intensity of 24.5 dB. This curve illustrates why alarms and other audible indicators usually have a frequency near 1000 Hz.

There are several types of tests that audiologists use in assessing hearing. Pure tone audiometry presents pure (one-frequency) tones to each ear and determines the threshold of hearing for that person. The intensity of the tone is raised in 5-dB increments until it is heard; then it is lowered in 5-dB increments until it is no longer heard. The threshold is the intensity at which the person indicates that he or she hears the tone 50% of the time. A typical audiogram is shown in Figure 3-6. On the curve shown in Figure 3-6, all values are displayed as hearing loss, and the "normal" level is shown as 0-dB loss. The curve of Figure 3-5 is incorporated into the plot of Figure 3-6. Thus for 125 Hz, a tone of 90.5 dB was

heard 50% of the time in the right ear (45.5-dB threshold from Figure 3-5 added to 45-dB loss from Figure 3-6). At 1000 Hz the threshold presented was 36.5 dB. This test gives the audiologist information regarding the range of frequencies over which the person can hear.

Even though the frequencies presented in the pure tone test are in the range of speech (125 to 8000 Hz), this test alone does not indicate the person's ability to understand speech. To evaluate this function the audiologist uses a speech recognition threshold test (SRT). In this evaluation, speech is presented, either live or recorded, at varying intensity levels, and the person's ability to understand it is determined. The person is asked to repeat either words or sentences presented at these varying intensities.

**Hearing loss.** Based on these and other tests, the audiologist determines both the degree of hearing loss and the type of loss. Four types of hearing loss are typically defined (Mann, 1974). These are (1) conductive loss associated with pathological defects of the middle ear, (2) sensorineural loss associated with defects in the cochlea or auditory nerve, (3) centrally induced damage to the auditory cortex of the brain, and (4) functional deafness resulting from perceptual deficits rather than physiological pathology. Auditory impairment is considered slight if the loss is between 20 and 30 dB, mild if from 30 to 45 dB, moderate if from 60 to 75 dB, profound if from 75 to 90 db, and extreme if from 90 to 110 dB (Stach, 1998). Selection of hearing aids for these types and magnitudes of loss is discussed in Chapter 12.

## Somatosensory Function

Somatosensory function plays an essential role in the design and selection of assistive technology systems. One view of the role of the somatosensory system is to provide information regarding "where the body ends and where the world begins" (Dunn, 1991, p. 239). As the major interface for many assistive devices, the somatosensory system plays a critical role in determining the effectiveness of assistive technology interventions. The close relationship between the motor and sensory systems is also evident in the decreased control capability exhibited in the presence of somatosensory impairment. For example, persons who have Hansen's disease (leprosy) lose peripheral sensation. This results in a loss of feedback to the motor system, and fine motor abilities are significantly compromised. This can result in significantly compromised capabilities relative to the control of assistive technologies. Somatosensory input is received from receptors in the periphery and includes pressure, hot-cold, tactile, and kinesthetic responses.

When sensation is lost, as in spinal cord injury, this input is absent and tissue damage can result from externally applied pressures such as those generated in sitting. This is especially important in the design of seating systems and

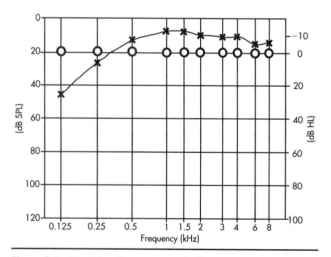

**Figure 3-6**　Typical audiogram test results for pure-tone testing. *SPL,* Sound pressure level. (From Ballantyne D: *Handbook of audiological techniques,* London, 1990, Butterworth-Heinemann.)

cushions (see Chapter 6). This leads to another role for assistive technologies, that of providing pressure relief and alternative means of sensory input when the somatosensory input is absent or inaccurate.

## Control of Posture and Position

The adequate control of posture and position in space are fundamental to successful use of assistive technologies. Movement of the limbs or head requires adjustment by the internal sensory and motor control systems to maintain a functional posture. Accommodation to external forces such as gravity or movement also require constant adjustment. This control of posture and body position in space is an integrative function of the visual, vestibular, proprioceptive, and kinesthetic senses and motor components of the trunk, pelvis, and extremities. As we discuss in Chapter 6, a fundamental requirement for the effective use of assistive technologies is that the user be positioned appropriately.

The vestibular system provides information regarding how the body is interacting with the environment (Dunn, 1991). This information is integrated with other sensory data to effect control of body position and to accommodate changes brought about by movement or changing environmental data. The sensory data provided by the vestibular system are used to relate internal sensory and motor maps to the external world. Humans constantly change their position in space to achieve greater functional control (e.g., compensating for upper extremity movement or changes in balance when picking up an object) or greater comfort or to move from place to place. When sensory or motor impairments are present, assistive technologies can be used to help compensate for postural deficits. Likewise, when postural deficits are present, the design of assistive technology systems must take them into account.

When changes in body position occur because of internal forces (e.g., reaching for a keyboard) or external factors (e.g., increasing the load on the arm by lifting an object), a sophisticated control system provides the necessary compensatory mechanical, neural, and sensory changes (Lee, 1989). This control system features both feedback (sensory data affects motor output) and feed-forward (internal commands alter the motor system, with sensory changes following) components. For individuals who lack the motor or sensory system function adequate for postural control, we can design seating and positioning systems that help stabilize the person and facilitate functional tasks (see Chapter 6). However, many of these systems are static, providing only one fixed position for the individual. As Kangas (1991) points out, this is inconsistent with normal posture, which is dynamic and varies widely with different functional tasks. Kangas also defines a functional position, which allows movement but which also stabilizes the individual to facilitate function (see Chapter 6).

As discussed earlier, Padula (1988) describes the use of prism glasses, which allow the individual to place visual and vestibular data in proper relationship to each other. In some cases we can use assistive technologies to alter sensory perception and affect motor performance. In one case an individual had continual neck flexion and only lifted his head for short periods. When he was fitted with prism lenses, he immediately lifted his head and brought it in line with his torso. Similarly, individuals who demonstrate a consistent left- or right-leaning posture have been brought to midline by the use of horizontally oriented prism lens. In motor-disabled children and adults with disabilities such as traumatic brain injury, these lenses have resulted in postural corrections independent of any additional technological intervention such as seating systems.

The visual-vestibular coupling also can be exploited in other ways. Vestibular and visual function are closely related. The degree of this coupling is directly connected to the degree of self-produced locomotion (Campos and Bertenthal, 1987). Self-produced locomotion allows much greater correlation of visual and vestibular feedback. This has obvious implications for dependent versus independent mobility using assistive technologies. Sensory input provided by the vestibular system (in concert with visual and proprioceptive data) is significantly different when an individual is in control of her own movement than when she is a passive "passenger." A common example of this phenomenon is the observation that the driver of a car on a winding road rarely gets carsick, whereas passengers often do. Likewise, when a person with a disability is pushed in a wheelchair, he receives different vestibular input than when management of the chair is under his control. This is important when considering the transition from a dependent manual mobility system to an independent powered system.

A recurring theme in this chapter is that prior experiences of the human user of assistive technology systems play a major role in both the specification and design of the system and in its success. A classic study done with newborn kittens illustrates this point for the postural control system (Held and Hein, 1963). Kittens and their mothers were reared in total darkness from birth to the initiation of visual exposure at 8 to 12 weeks of age. A special carousel was used to provide equivalent movement experiences for each kitten. Two littermates were used in each set of experiments. One kitten was allowed to move on its own; the other was moved passively by the motion of the first kitten. Only the kittens that had active movement showed fear of heights, whereas the passively moved kittens did not. These results indicate that development involving movement depends in large measure on the degree to which that movement is self-generated. An example of an assistive technology application in which these concepts are important is dependent mobility (e.g., the person is pushed by an attendant) compared with independent powered mobility.

The importance of postural and position control has other implications for the application of assistive technologies. Given that self-generated movement provides different information than passive movement, it is not surprising that children who are given access to a powered mobility system often initially spend a great deal of time turning in circles. If we attempt to "correct" this behavior, we may be depriving the child of important vestibular, visual, and kinesthetic development. If, however, we allow the child to experiment with the powered wheelchair and obtain the new sensory experiences associated with self-propelled locomotion, we will have greater success in getting the child to be accurate and safe with the wheelchair.

## ■ PERCEPTUAL FUNCTION AS RELATED TO ASSISTIVE TECHNOLOGY USE

Perception adds meaning to sensory data. Human interpretation of sensory events is based on both physiological function and prior sensory and perceptual experience. Assistive technologies can affect perceptual experience in many ways, some positive and some negative. Because the use of these technologies is often a new experience, a novice user who has a disability is likely to have significantly different perceptions of events and device interactions than do either more experienced users or nondisabled assistive technology practitioners (ATPs). In this section we shall explore the implications of perceptual function and assistive technologies.

All sensory systems have both physical and perceptual thresholds. We use the term *threshold* to describe the minimal level of input that results in an output from a sensory system. For example, the auditory system can be described in terms of the amplitude and frequency of the input information. These are physical parameters that describe the thresholds associated with sensory function. Auditory perceptual thresholds are described as loudness (related to amplitude) and pitch (related to frequency). The perceived loudness and pitch differ from individual to individual and are typical of perceptual thresholds that are often referred to as *psychophysical parameters*. Sensitivity to sound varies from person to person, and an acceptable sound for one person (e.g., a teenager listening to a rock band) may be perceived as uncomfortably loud by another person (e.g., a parent listening to the same rock music).

A major perceptual task is separating information about one portion of an image from the rest of the image, for example, picking one person out of a crowd or identifying one object in a picture when there are many objects present. This type of task is referred to as *figure-ground* discrimination because the desired object (figure) is extracted from the background (ground). Good figure-ground skill is important for many assistive technology-related activities, such as selecting one symbol out of an array of symbols on a communication device. Many disabilities interfere with the ability to make figure-ground discriminations.

*Auditory localization* refers to the ability to identify the spatial origin of a sound; it is based on a comparison of sound from the two ears. Separation of one source of sound from others in a noisy environment is also important for successful task completion and for the effective use of assistive technology devices in varying contexts. For example, a user of a powered wheelchair must be able to identify the location (e.g., street noise, a person approaching, a voice calling to her) of a sound if she is to respond to it. This ability is also what allows us to focus on one speaker at a party in which many conversations are going on simultaneously. Dunn (1991) uses the term *auditory figure-ground discrimination* to describe this capability.

Making discriminations of physical parameters is a perceptual task. Our estimates of length, distance, and time are examples of such discriminations. Time estimates are an important part of assistive technology use, especially when single-switch scanning is used. Accurate estimates of time require active participation in the task (Bailey, 1989). An active person generally overestimates time (i.e., thinks time has passed faster), and a passive person underestimates time (i.e., thinks it has passed slower). This is a formal recognition of the old saying "time flies when you're having fun." It also underscores the importance of making the human user of assistive technologies an active participant in the training process. For example, we often use computer-based games to develop switch skills. In this approach, the disabled child is required to activate a switch in order to obtain interesting graphic or auditory results. Using this approach, the child may activate the switch many times in a session in order to obtain new results, and a training session of 30 minutes may pass very quickly. Conversely, if we connect the switch to less interesting results, such as a single light or tone, and ask the child to practice hitting it, the training session time may drag for both the child and the teacher.

One of the major accomplishments of early childhood development is independent mobility, and early perceptual development is directly related to the acquisition of this skill. In children with motor disabilities, independent mobility is often dependent on the use of assistive technologies. Campos and Bertenthal (1987) studied the relationship between independent locomotion and perceptual development. They point out the importance of considering both growth and learning as important aspects of development. Campos and Bertenthal used an experimental paradigm that measured fear of heights (as determined by heart rate increases) in children who had developed locomotion and in those who were prelocomotor. They found that height wariness was greater in children who were independently mobile than in those who were not. They also found that the height wariness of prelocomotor infants (less than 12 months old) who had used walkers was higher than that of those who had not. In a related experiment, they studied a motorically disabled infant who had a cast and brace preventing independent mobility. When the cast and brace were removed, they found that the infant's wariness of heights increased. These and other studies demonstrate the relationship between motor experience and perceptual development and the role of assistive technologies in each. Kermoian (1998) describes evidence relating early mobility to cognitive development in young children as they actively engage in their environment. Typically developing children use creeping, crawling, and walking to obtain environmental interaction beyond their arm's reach. This interaction fosters cognitive and language development. Children who have mobility limitations can achieve similar benefits from the early use of assistive technologies for mobility (see Chapter 10).

Assistive technologies can also provide erroneous sensory data—that is, data that are not consistent with other environmental information available to the person. A classic example of this phenomenon is the use of prism glasses that reverse the image on the eye, creating a mirror image of the environment (Bailey, 1989). When these glasses are first put on, the world is reversed and the person becomes disoriented. However, as the glasses are worn for longer periods, the sensory perception is brought into conformance with the sensory data and the person begins to function as if the visual image was not reversed. When the glasses are removed, the person is initially disoriented, and a period of adjustment is required to bring sensory perception into line with the new, "normal" data.

Bailey (1989) describes another study in which subjects who wore prism glasses that displaced the visual image several inches to the left or right were asked to reach for a target. Once again, they adjusted the sensory perception to match the data, and they were able to access the targets accurately after a few minutes of practice. The most interesting result of this experiment, however, came when the glasses were removed. The subjects consistently missed the targets in the opposite direction from the original displacement provided by the glasses. Analysis of these results revealed that it was *kinesthetic* perception rather than *visual* perception that was altered, and the effect persisted for a much longer time than the original visual disorientation had. It was also determined that if one hand was observed doing a task during the wearing of the glasses and the other was not, only the hand that was observed with altered visual input was affected.

These experiments have profound implications for the application of assistive technologies. Because individuals with disabilities often have significantly different sensory experiences and sensory maps of the world than do able-bodied persons, it is difficult to predict the perceptual experience that an assistive technology system will provide to the person. Perceptual differences may result from the sensory input, as in the prism glasses experiment. For example, a person with an altered visual field may not receive visual data that provide a complete picture of the environment. If that person acts on the limited sensory data, he may make errors in using an assistive device. Because these errors will be reflected in motor performance, it is difficult to identify them as perceptual rather than motor. An individual who has a motor disability may have difficulty keeping her head aligned with the horizon (i.e., have a tilt of the head to the left or right); this affects her sensory input. If she then attempts to use a computer input system that requires horizontal and vertical movement (relative to the horizon) to move a cursor on the screen, she may have difficulty because the sensory data provided regarding the external world are not consistent with the way in which the cursor moves on the screen. In order to improve performance, we must bring the sensory (visual and kinesthetic) data into conformance with the perceptual information. This can be accomplished in several ways, such as orienting the screen to the same angle as the head or providing learning time that allows the person to adapt the perception of the computer task to the task of head movement.

## ■ COGNITIVE FUNCTION AND DEVELOPMENT AS RELATED TO ASSISTIVE TECHNOLOGY USE

Cognitive performance plays an important role in the use of assistive technologies. In this section we describe those aspects of cognitive performance that most often affect the design and implementation of assistive technology systems. There are several problems associated with adequately assessing the cognitive abilities necessary for the control of assistive technology systems. The most important of these is that the assistive technology often provides a function for which the person has no experience base. In the use of a powered wheelchair, the disabled human operator may have never been responsible for his or her own mobility and may not have experience in making the required decisions. A second difficulty is that there are many cases of effective technology use that would not have been expected given the measurable cognitive function of the user. For example, Richard, a young boy seen in our facility, was described as autistic and unable to spell. He was provided with an augmentative communication system that allowed him to use pictorial icons or spelling for choosing vocabulary (see Chapter 9). He was quite successful using this system for communicative interaction, but he was restricted to those stored utterances for which he had an iconic representation. One evening his family was deciding what game to play, and Richard was very interested in one particular game. He did not have an iconic representation of this game, so he typed in "I want to play [name of game]." His family was amazed, since this was the first indication that Richard was capable of spelling. Needless to say, he got his choice of game that night, and his school program was expanded to include spelling.

## Cognitive Development

In order to specify and design assistive technology systems for children, it is important to understand some fundamental concepts of cognitive development and to relate these to the use of assistive technologies by children. With the passage of federal legislation relating to early intervention and special education, services are being provided to very young (birth to 3 years) children (see Chapter 1). Many children in this age group have special needs that can be aided by assistive technologies. Although many of the principles that we have discussed can be applied directly to this population, there are unique characteristics that must also be considered. We discuss these in this section.

Changes that occur in a child arise from both environmental influences (experience) and biological maturation (Santrock, 1997). **Growth** can be defined as change arising from physical development of the CNS. We use the term **learning** to refer to changes that occur because of contact with some environmental influence. **Development** is a function of both growth and learning. A careful consideration of development, both current status and developmental change, is crucial to the successful application of assistive technology systems.

Although there are many theories of cognitive development, the work of Jean Piaget (see Brainerd, 1978, for example) is particularly useful because of its emphasis on object manipulation in the early years and the consideration of alternative methods of problem solving as the child grows into an adult. The major stages of development proposed by Piaget are shown in Table 3-1. Although there is some controversy regarding the details of Piaget's theory, the four basic stages shown in Table 3-1 provide a useful framework for us to consider in applying assistive technologies to solve problems of children with disabilities. One of the major factors illustrated in Table 3-1 is the change in problem-solving approaches and abilities as a child develops. The very young child does not approach problems in the same way as the adult, and we must consider this in our design of assistive technology systems.

One of the major controversies regarding Piaget's theory is the age at which symbolic representation emerges. This skill, necessary for cognitive functions such as problem solving, was believed by Piaget to begin with the preoperational stage (Stage II in Table 3-1). However, recent work has shown that infants as young as 6 months develop symbolic representation (Mandler, 1990). These skills are acquired by observation, as well as by direct manipulation of

| TABLE 3-1 | | Piaget's Stages of Human Development | |
|---|---|---|---|
| Stage | Age Range (yr) | Title | Characteristics |
| I | Birth to 2 | Sensorimotor | Child organizes physical action schemes for dealing with the immediate world |
| II | 2-7 | Preoperational | Child begins to use symbols and internal images; problem solving is unsystematic and illogical |
| III | 7-11 | Concrete operations | Child develops the operations to think logically but only with reference to concrete objects and activities |
| IV | 11 to adult | Formal operations | Individual develops capacity to think systematically and abstractly solve problems |

objects. For example, 9-month-old infants have been shown to be capable of imitating actions that they have observed but not practiced. Infants are also able to remember, after a short delay, where objects have been placed. These and other similar results indicate that very young children (less than 9 months old) are capable of forming symbolic representations of objects and manipulating these representations to carry out tasks.

Goldenberg (1979) applies the idea of observational learning to the case of children whose motor abilities are severely limited and who have limited capability for further motor development. He proposes two hypothetical situations: (1) a child whose only motor response is eye movement, and (2) a child whose only response is raising an eyebrow. The first child may engage the environment through movements of the eyes that cause an image to move on the retina. This motor action may or may not lead to interaction, depending on whether someone in the child's environment interprets the eye movements as meaningful and uses them as a basis for communication. In the second case, the child's action does not manipulate the environment for the child, but again its interpretation by another person may allow interaction with the environment. In each of these cases the provision of an assistive device that is sensitive to the motor actions of the child may enable development. However, in each case the importance of observational learning prevents us from saying that development is not occurring.

From the point of view of assistive technology systems, the early manipulation of objects and the use of tools are of particular importance. Table 3-2 summarizes some of the early skills in these areas. It is clear from Table 3-2 that at a

| TABLE 3-2 | Early Object Manipulation and Tool Use in Normal Children During the Sensorimotor Period of Development (Birth to 2 Years) |
|---|---|

| Developmental Age (mo) | Actions |
|---|---|
| 5 | Reinitiates familiar game during pause |
| 6 | Finds object hidden behind or under screen |
| 6 | Imitates novel body movement |
| 6-8 | Transfers object hand-to-hand |
| 7 | Leans forward to look for a dropped object |
| 8-10 | Anticipates circular trajectory of an object |
| 8 | Drops one object to reach for another |
| 8-9 | Moves to obtain object out of reach |
| 8-10 | Pulls support to obtain object without demonstration |
| 9 | Uses one object as a container for another |
| 12 | Pulls string to obtain object without demonstration |
| 12-14 | Retrieves object by pouring if container is too small for hand |
| 12-15 | Holds mechanical toy that another person has started |
| 13-15 | Uses string to obtain object against gravity |
| 15 | Moves around barrier to obtain object |
| 15-18 | Uses tool as extension of body to obtain object |
| 15-18 | Finds object where last seen or usually kept |
| 15-19 | Opens box to obtain object without demonstration or seeing object placed in box |
| 18-20 | Imitates two action combinations |
| 19-20 | Anticipates result of actions and adjusts behavior accordingly to situations and problems |
| 21 | Attempts to activate mechanical toy without demonstration |
| 22 | Anticipates means/end and result of applied means |

very early age the normally developing child can and does interact with objects and use an object as a tool to achieve a desired result; thus it is not surprising that assistive technologies have been used successfully with very young children. Brinker and Lewis (1982a) used the concept of co-occurrences, the provision of a contingent result when the child carries out a purposeful action, to foster the development of interaction skills in infants and very young children. They used a microcomputer to arrange events so that they could be consistently controlled by an infant's behaviors; therefore the infant was led to believe that the world was controllable (Brinker and Lewis, 1982b). The infant used switch activation to control graphics, toys, and tape recordings of songs or voices. Data on the number of switch activations and observable behaviors (e.g., facial expressions, reaching for a toy) of the infant showed that children as young as 3 months would develop purposeful movements to cause the contingent result. Given the skills shown in Table 3-2, these results are not surprising.

The direct manipulation of objects via robotic systems controlled by the child is an attractive contingent result in a computer-controlled and switch-activated system for very young children. Cook, Liu, and Hoseit (1990) developed a system that allowed a very young child to interact with a small robotic arm by a single-switch activation. They investigated whether both nondisabled and disabled children would use the robotic arm as a tool. Cook and co-workers used a continuous playback mode in which a movement was played back sequentially as long as the switch was depressed and the arm stopped when the switch was released. Typical tasks used were bringing a cracker within reach of the child and tipping a cup to reveal its contents. If a child was attempting to retrieve an object using the robotic arm, it was concluded that he was using it as a tool if the switch was pressed to bring the object closer (in the continuous mode) and then the object was reached for, and if still out of reach the switch was pressed again. Repeated use of this sequence of actions indicated the use of the robotic arm as a tool to retrieve the object. Fifty percent of the disabled children (all those with a standardized cognitive age level score of 7 to 9 months or greater) and 100% of the nondisabled children did interact with the arm and use it as a tool to obtain objects out of reach. Gross and fine motor skill levels were less related to success in using the robotic arm than were the levels in cognitive and language areas. This study illustrates the careful application of assistive technology to match the developmental level.

As children grow and develop, they are able to deal with objects and schemes of action more symbolically. These emerging skills affect the way in which we specify and design assistive technology systems for children who are between 2 and 6 years of age (in the second stage shown in Table 3-1). For example, augmentative communication systems that require the use of symbols can be designed and the vocabulary included can be expanded over that of the Stage I child. We can also include more complicated operational features such as two-sequence and three-sequence tasks. As concepts of time begin to develop, sequential selection of objects, such as that required in scanning, can be used. For the preoperational child, it is also important for us to consider other characteristics (Brainerd, 1978). For example, children in this age range typically exhibit centration, focusing on only one aspect of an object. Often this is a surface feature such as color or flashing lights; thus we need to design assistive technology systems carefully so that the most striking features are also the most important to their use. Children in this stage also exhibit animism, attributing life and consciousness to inanimate objects. We can exploit this characteristic by making devices fun to use and giving them names. A final example is the failure of children in this stage to separate play and reality; they apply the same ground rules to each situation. If we take this into consideration, we will, for example, allow a communication device to be used to create strange sounds (e.g., a belch) and we won't insist on always saying things properly. This approach can help the child develop skills in an interesting way and then apply them to other situations, such as moving to a given destination. Examples of characteristics of the preoperational child and their implications for assistive technology use are shown in Table 3-3.

Assistive technologies can play a role in cognitive development for children in this stage as well. Verburg (1987) studied 10 children ages 2 to 5 years who were provided with a miniature powered vehicle. The changes in scores on a developmental profile over the course of learning to use the powered vehicle were used to determine the effect of the device on cognitive development. Changes in scores were calculated in months, and those that exceeded the number of months of the training period were taken to indicate cognitive growth. For example, if a study lasted 3 months and the child's difference in beginning and ending scores was 5 months, it was decided that development had occurred as a result of the experiment. Five categories of development were used: physical, self-help, social, academic, and communication. The major effects of the use of the vehicle were in the social and academic categories, with 7 of the 10 children showing gains greater than the length of the study. Communication (three children), self-help (two children), and physical (one child) showed smaller gains. This study illustrates the importance of assistive technologies in enabling learning and associated development. An added benefit of Verburg's study was that parental protectiveness decreased as the children became more independently mobile.

The older child (Stage III in Table 3-1) has significantly more ways of using assistive technologies (Brainerd, 1978), and we can take advantage of these in our specification and design process. For example, decentration is now common, and we can include "optional" features that are secondary but useful without the concern that they will distract the

child from successful use of the device. For instance, a powered wheelchair controller with a high-speed and low-speed feature will be more understandable by a child in Stage III than it was for the child in Stage II. A major advance for children in this stage is the ability to apply logical operations to concrete (real and observable) problems. The emergence of these skills has a direct influence on our design of augmentative communication systems to be used for writing in school. We can begin to include features of word processors that allow editing of text, and the child can be expected to learn to use features such as printing and saving text. It is important, however, that our design of training materials for the use of assistive technology systems be based on concrete, real situations rather than more abstract concepts. Operational principles should also be concrete. This means not that they must be "simple," but that they rely on a logical problem-solving approach that focuses on real properties of objects and situations. Among the skills of children in this stage are the ability to carry out complex tasks consisting of several steps and recognizing that the processes are reversible, categorizing objects, combining classes of objects and extracting their common properties, recognizing that problems may be solved in more than one way, and reasoning deductively. Our success in specifying and designing assistive technology systems for children in this stage of development is directly related to how carefully we consider these and other characteristics of this age group.

The adolescent (Stage IV) is in transition between deductive, concrete problem solving and the inductive, systematic reasoning characteristic of adults. A key change in this stage is that problem solving and reasoning are systematic rather than random as in previous stages. Our design of assistive technology systems for individuals in the early part of this age range (11 to 15 years) must include consideration of the transition from concrete to formal operations, since most individuals alternate between these two during this period. The problem solving and decision making required for the use of systems can be more inductive, but we must also allow for basic operation that is concrete.

In summary, the specification and design of assistive technology systems for children are not just a matter of simplifying the features of adult systems. Instead there are specific characteristics of children in various age groups that must be taken into account to ensure the effectiveness of systems selected for them. By taking into account the nature of childhood and its unique "lifestyle," we can make assistive technologies fun, as well as useful. This increases the likelihood that they will be effective. Finally, we must remember that not only is the human component different in the case of children but there are activities and contexts that are unique to childhood. By incorporating the unique features of these other two components of our total system, we can further improve its efficacy.

**TABLE 3-3    Characteristics of the Preoperational Child That Influence Assistive Technology Use**

| Characteristic | Assistive Technology Implications |
|---|---|
| Symbolic Representation | Augmentative communication, use of language concepts in control of devices |
| Sequencing | Multiple symbol communication, multistep control of systems |
| Centration | Child may focus on color, size, or shape rather than function of assistive device |
| Animism | Give assistive devices a personality with names, etc. |
| Play equals reality | Make use of play routines to accomplish functional goals |

## Developmental Disabilities and Cognitive Deficits

When considering developmental delay or cognitive impairment caused by trauma (e.g., traumatic brain injury), it is tempting to relate an individual's functional capability to the stages of development such as those presented in Table 3-1. From the point of view of assistive technology use, this is undesirable for several reasons. First, the individual who has a disability has a significantly different nervous system than the nondisabled person for whom the developmental sequences have been established. The developmental delay or cognitive impairment is the result of other factors, and these must be taken into account when evaluating the level of cognitive functioning. Second, it is often true that an individual with cognitive impairment exhibits significant skill in one area but has severe deficits in others, even though all the functional skills are considered to occur concurrently in a nondisabled individual (Kauffman and Payne, 1975). Development in the presence of an abnormal nervous system is best considered as divergent from the path considered to be normal. This is in contrast to the view that development is proceeding along the same "normal" path but is delayed. Assistive technology application is most effective when individual skills are determined through assessment (see Chapter 4) and the system characteristics emerge from this assessment.

Individuals with congenital or adventitious cognitive impairments may have difficulties in attention, memory, problem solving, language, and other areas. When designing assistive technology systems for these individuals, it is important to give careful attention to the cognitive demands that use of the device places on the person and to include learning and operational aids within the total system. It is generally not our goal to make things *simpler* for someone with a cognitive deficit, but to make them *different*. For example, individuals who have a learning disability may benefit from alternative modes of information presentation. Often auditory information is more easily assimilated than visual information. Examples of approaches for individuals with memory loss and problem-solving limitations are described next.

## Memory

**Memory** is important for effective use of assistive technologies. When specifying and designing assistive technology systems, we need to be aware of the role of human memory in successful use. Human memory is often considered to have three components: (1) sensory memory, (2) short-term memory, and (3) long-term memory (Bailey, 1989). Each type of memory plays a role in the use of assistive technologies. Sensory memory describes the storage of sensory data for a very brief time following the removal of the stimulus. For our purposes, the most important types of sensory memory are visual and auditory. The afterimage that traces the path of a moving sparkler in the dark is an example of

sensory memory. Visual sensory memory is typically in the form of an image and lasts for about 250 millisecond (one-quarter of a second) (Bailey, 1989). Some assistive devices make use of this type of memory in their design. One example is the Pathfinder* augmentative communication system. In this device a set of 128 lights is arranged in a matrix 16 lights wide by 8 lights high. A detector is placed on the user's head, and when it is aimed at one of the lights, the Pathfinder detects this and the choice labeled by that light is activated. The device turns on the lights one at a time from the upper left corner to the lower right corner, row by row. However, even though only one light is turned on at a time, the user actually sees all the lights as being dimly lit. This effect results in part from sensory memory, and without it this input method would not be feasible. Auditory sensory memory is often in the form of an echo of the original input data, and it lasts for up to 5 seconds (Bailey, 1989).

Short-term memory is sometimes referred to as working memory (Bailey, 1989). Its duration is generally up to about 20 to 30 seconds, and we use it for temporary storage of information necessary to complete a task. This allows us to carry out many tasks associated with assistive technologies. In assistive technologies, short-term memory is employed for seldom-used device operational sequences that are looked up in a manual when needed (e.g., how to replace batteries in a hearing aid) or for remembering a piece of information briefly (e.g., a telephone number to be dialed). Because the capacity of short-term memory is approximately seven items, it is important to restrict the amount of information required to be stored in short-term memory. Individuals have difficulty remembering more than seven items if they do not have the opportunity to rehearse and transfer the information to long-term memory. Information stored in short-term memory arises from both external and internal sources. For example, when reading this sentence you are using stored information regarding letters and their combination into words, together with visual input from the page. Information in short-term memory is generally believed to be stored in an encoded form. The code may be a form that makes use of longer-term stored information or one that is more easily recalled than the original form of the information. There is evidence that some visual information, such as words, is actually stored in auditory form, by memory of their sounds rather than what they look like. This has implications for individuals who are unable to use oral language or who have not heard oral language because of a congenital hearing impairment, and we must take this into account when designing assistive technology systems for them. In general, the use of codes that take advantage of both internal and external data are the most effective.

When designing systems, we can take several steps to

---

*Prentke Romich Co., Wooster, OH.

help the human operator maximize his or her use of short-term memory. One way to do this is to group information into short sequences and to use patterns that are related to stored information. For example, an assistive device for writing may have several functions, such as entering text, storing text, and printing. If we design the system so that each of these tasks follows a similar, consistent sequence of actions, then the use of the system will be more easily learned. Bailey (1989) also discusses the use of rehearsal and patterns in codes as aids to users of systems. Rehearsal is the repeating of a new piece of information (e.g., a phone number) to ensure that it is not forgotten. There are several types of patterns. One approach is to group number or letter sequences into short (three- or four-character) groups and to include similar patterns in the groups. Examples of useful patterns for numbers are groups that end in the same number; for letters the groups may spell short words or be remembered as acronyms.

Long-term memory is where we store information that has lasting value. Whereas short-term memory consists of "throwaway" information we use only once, long-term memory is important for things we need to use often. Examples of the use of long-term memory in assistive technologies include recalling codes used for storage of information, remembering how to turn on a device and use its features, and remembering where we want to go and how to get there using a powered wheelchair. Long-term memory differs from the other two types primarily in the duration of the stored information. This type of memory is permanent even though we forget. There is evidence indicating that loss of information from long-term memory is a problem of access rather than actual loss of stored information (Bailey, 1989). As designers of assistive technology systems, we need to be aware of several memory processes related to remembering and forgetting: (1) encoding, (2) storage, and (3) retrieval. Each of these plays a major role in the design and use of assistive technology systems.

Encoding is the way in which we organize information to be stored, and it is important in retrieval of the stored information. As system designers we can help with this process by relating steps, tasks, or information to be remembered to the person's experience. Because each person has unique, and sometimes limited, experiences, careful attention must be paid to assessing the best ways to encode information for easy retrieval. For example, with speed dialing, in which one digit is used as a code for a stored phone number, it may be easier if phone numbers for certain people are recalled by letters instead of by the digit. Mom's number could be stored under *M*, sister Tammy under *T*, work under *W*, and so on. This method of encoding helps with recall because there is a relationship between the stored number and the code.

There are many theories regarding how and why we forget. From a systems design point of view, these are important, especially in relation to training individuals to use assistive technologies. One of the most important factors affecting forgetting is what the person does between the time the information is learned and the time that it is used (Bailey, 1989). The term *interference* is used to describe the process of forgetting. Bailey discusses two types of interference: proactive and retroactive. Proactive interference occurs when information acquired before the learning of new material interferes with the use of the new material in performance. This type of interference often occurs in assistive technology system use. For example, let's assume that Tom has learned to use one type of mechanical feeder, which requires that a switch be pushed to the right to rotate the plate and to the left to raise the spoon to mouth level. The spoon action is automatic once the switch has been activated. A new feeder is introduced that gives Tom more control because the second switch must be continuously pressed to scoop the food and raise the spoon and it can be stopped at any point and restarted. This can make eating more efficient, since if the spoon misses the food, it is not necessary to go through an entire cycle before trying again to get food. We would say that Tom has *proactive interference* if he persists in pushing the second switch only once, since this was a previously learned strategy, rather than maintaining switch activation until the food reaches mouth level. Even if Tom is able to adapt to the new strategy, he may revert to the old strategy if he is tired or stressed.

*Retroactive interference* occurs when a person learns to do task A, then learns task B, and finally is asked to perform task A. She may forget how to do task A because of concentrating on task B. This situation can occur when training a person to use an assistive technology system that has multiple functions or tasks. We can avoid this type of problem by allowing enough practice and use time for task A before we introduce task B. For example, assume that we are training a person with a visual impairment to use a screen reader. This is a device that provides speech output instead of visual output. The person has learned how to scan through the text by using the arrow keys on the keyboard (task A). Now we train him to save a file and retrieve it (task B). When he goes back to task A, he may have forgotten how to do it or forgotten details of this task. If so, we call this retroactive interference.

It is important for us to distinguish between **recall** and **recognition**. The task of recalling information relies exclusively on the person's abilities, with no assistance from the system. Recognition requires the person to identify the proper or desired item from a list presented by the device. This difference is evident in two types of computer user displays, which are discussed in Chapter 8. In one type of interface, called the command line interface (CLI), the computer screen merely displays a "prompt" and the user must type in the information desired, such as the name of a file to be retrieved or a program to be run. The second type of user interface is called a graphical user interface (GUI). In this approach the user is presented with a series of icons on the screen and a selection is made by moving a pointer to the desired icon and pressing a button. This then produces a list of items from which the user can choose by pointing at the desired item and pressing a button. The CLI approach depends on recall, and the GUI makes use of recognition. Because recognition is easier than recall, it should be included in assistive technology system design whenever possible.

Human memory includes information from all the senses. For example, somatosensory long-term memory plays a role in many aspects of assistive technology application. The feel of a switch or joystick is remembered, and a new, improved control may not be as effective because it is unfamiliar. Tactile memory is also important in seating and positioning systems. Often persons who have had one seating system for a long time are not comfortable in a new seating system even though it is more functional. The tactile memory of the old system is present, and the new system must be introduced gradually to ensure acceptance.

When an individual has memory deficits, it is necessary for us to alter the way in which we design assistive technology systems. Batt and Lounsbury (1990) present a case study in which they describe the development of computer use by an individual who had suffered memory deficits as a result of a cerebral vascular accident (CVA). He and his wife were both concerned that he had no activities other than

watching television, and they wished to make use of his personal computer for writing and correspondence. This activity was limited because he could not remember any verbal commands, and his cognitive deficits prevented him from using the owner's manual supplied with his computer. The word processing program that he wanted to use featured a menu approach with eight options, which perplexed the user because of his impaired memory. A simple color-coded flow chart was designed to break the complex list of options down into a manageable form (Figure 3-7). This chart allowed the user to progress through his choices without having to remember the previous selections or having more than one option for the next choice. By using the flow chart and a training program, the user was able to learn to write letters and his own memoirs. Writing his memoirs helped him deal emotionally with his disability, and it led to an increase in his self-esteem and a perception on his part that his memory and cognitive processing had improved.

## Language

A language is any system of arbitrary symbols that are organized according to a set of rules agreed to by the speaker and listener (Miller, 1981). This set of symbols may be the familiar alphabetic written language (referred to as *traditional orthography*) or it may be a set of pictographic symbols conveying meaning (such as hieroglyphics or other special

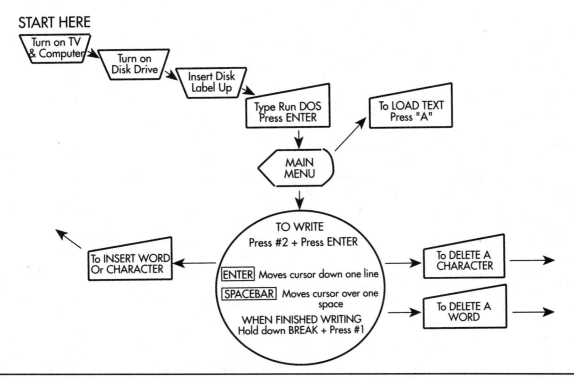

**Figure 3-7**   A flowchart used to assist a person with memory deficits to use a word processing program. (From Batt RC, Lounsbury PA: Teaching the patient with cognitive deficits to use a computer, *Am J Occup Ther* 44:366, 1990.)

symbols) or a set of hand movements (sign language) or gestures. Speech is the oral expression of language.

Language consists of five basic elements: (1) phonology, (2) morphology, (3) syntax, (4) semantics, and (5) pragmatics. **Phonology** describes the sounds used in any particular language and the rules for their organization. The smallest group of language sounds that can be considered unique is called a *phoneme*. To produce English speech using an electronic speech synthesizer requires approximately 60 phonemes (Fons and Gargagliano, 1981). However, different synthesizers or analysis methods may use a larger or smaller number. Phonemes and letters do not have a one-to-one relationship because phonemes represent spoken language and letters portray written language. There are, however, computer programs that convert written text to spoken language (Allen, 1981). Because there is not a one-to-one correspondence between phonemes and letters, all these programs require both a set of rules and a large number of exceptions in order to convert from text (letters) to speech output. (Voice synthesis is discussed in Chapter 9.) Words often have fewer phonemes than they do letters. For example, the word "night" has three phonemes: (1) *n*, (2) *igh*, and (3) *t*. We refer to the generation of language by the selection of phonemes as the *segmental* characteristic of spoken language. Some electronic speech synthesizers use allophones (combinations of phonemes) rather than phonemes. In this case it may take up to 130 allophones to generate an unlimited vocabulary in English (Smith and Crook, 1981). Prosodic or suprasegmental features such as pitch, duration, and amplitude give richness and add meaning to spoken language (Miller, 1981). These features convert a statement into a question by raising the pitch at the end of a sentence or increasing the amplitude and duration of a word to stress it in a sentence.

**Morphology** describes the rules for organizing the smallest meaningful units of language, which are called morphemes. *Free morphemes* are complete words that may stand alone (e.g., *run*); *bound morphemes* must be coupled to another morpheme (e.g., *-ing*) in order to form a complete word. *Words* are articulated sounds or series of sounds that are used alone as units of language and symbolize, communicate, and have meaning. **Syntax** refers to the rules for organizing words into meaningful utterances. Taken together, morphology and syntax constitute grammar, which is the set of rules for speaking and writing a language. Various grammatical rules are used by linguists to describe language usage (Miller, 1981) and by designers of augmentative communication systems to enhance communicative ability.

**Semantics** describes the relationship between words and their meaning. This is the "definition" of a word. The *lexicon* of a language is a list of all the words in that language. Semantics describes the meaning of the words. There are approximately 100 concepts that have a word in every language (Miller, 1981). The relationships between a word and its meaning can be complex. For example, the word *gold* may mean the color, the metal, or the concept of wealth (e.g., "good as gold"). This flexibility is what makes natural languages (as opposed to computer languages, music, etc.) powerful. They allow us to talk about anything, even without precise definitions.

**Pragmatics** is the relationship between language and language users. By understanding the rules of pragmatics, a user of a language is able to observe social conventions. No matter how many words a person knows, they are not functional unless he or she knows when and how to use them to convey ideas. This use of language is fundamental to effective communication, but the rules are not intuitive. This is especially important when a person obtains an augmentative communication system for the first time. She may not understand how effective language is used, and extensive training may be required just to develop adequate strategies of use.

Both semantics and pragmatics are important in applying assistive technology systems. Barnes (1991) uses the term "motoric language" to describe the language necessary to drive a powered wheelchair. She describes two categories of vocabulary that apply to wheelchair use: relational and substantive. *Relational vocabulary* refers to concepts such as *in, on, between, under,* or *over; substantive vocabulary* refers to the appropriate use of nouns, verbs, and adjectives. Interestingly, Barnes and her colleagues have found that a good substantive vocabulary is more predictive of success in powered mobility than is a good relational vocabulary. Because mobility involves the use of spatial concepts, relational concepts would be expected to be more important. However, the relational concepts are generally more complex and difficult to understand, so they may develop later.

## Language Development

The development of language begins very early in a child's life. At 1 or 2 months of age an infant can distinguish between speech and nonspeech sounds, and there is an inherent predisposition to be interested in communication (Miller, 1981). It is generally believed that skill in language use is developed primarily through practice. Children who are unable to speak because of a disability still develop language. First words are typically tied to gestures such as the direction of eye gaze. The direction of gaze leads to arm or other limb movement in the direction of the object, and this leads to vocalizing (e.g., whining) until the object is given to him and he can manipulate the object. The linguistic functions of requesting and asserting that are performed at this early age by gestures are those later performed by oral language. Table 3-4 lists several important stages in the development of early language (Chapman, 1981; Santrock, 1997).

**TABLE 3-4**  **Early Development of Language**

| Approximate Age (mo) | Language Use |
|---|---|
| 8-10 | Communicative intent via gestures |
| 3-6 | Babbling sounds (e.g., "goo-goo," "ga-ga") |
| 9-15 | Utterances expressing communicative intent |
| 16-22 | Utterances with discourse function (see Table 3-5) |
| 24+ | Utterances with symbolic function (symbolic play, evoking absent objects or events, etc.) |

**TABLE 3-5**  **Early Communicative Intents with Discourse Functions**

| Intent | Example |
|---|---|
| Instrumental | "I want" |
| Regulatory | "Do as I tell you" |
| Interactional | "Me and you" |
| Personal | "Here I come!" |
| Heuristic | "Tell me why" |
| Imaginative | "Let's pretend" |
| Informative | "I've got something to tell you" |

**BOX 3-1**  **Categories of Language Use**

**DORE'S PRIMITIVE SPEECH ACTS**
- Labeling
- Repeating
- Answering
- Requesting action
- Requesting object
- Calling
- Greeting
- Protesting
- Practicing

**CONVERSATIONAL ACTS**
- Requests (for information, action, acknowledgment)
- Responses to requests
- Descriptions of past and present events
- Statements (of facts, rules, attitudes, feelings, beliefs)
- Acknowledgments
- Organizational devices (regulate content and conversation, e.g., "By the way. . .")
- Performatives (accomplish task by being said, e.g., "Stop," "That's mine," "I'm first")
- Miscellaneous

From Chapman RS: Exploring children's communicative interests. In Miller JF, editor: *Assessing language production in children,* Baltimore, 1981, University Park Press.

Infants show an interest in sounds and respond to voices between 3 and 6 months of age. Babbling (producing sounds such as "goo-goo" and "ga-ga") follows during the next 3 to 6 months. Babbling is thought to be a result of biological maturation and not hearing, caregiver interaction, or reinforcement (Santrock, 1997). The purpose of this early communication is to attract the attention of parents and others. An infant's receptive vocabulary, or the ability to understand words, begins to develop in the second half of the first year and increases dramatically in the second year.

The first vocalizations begin to appear at 10 to 15 months. Typically, communicative competence (e.g., requesting, asserting, protesting) develops before linguistic competence (e.g., the use of symbolic representations such as words). Vocalizations during the first year are generally more in a play than a communication context, and the child develops a greater variety of sounds than are needed in adult speech. During the second year, vocalizations and communication begin to merge as the child learns to control the vocalizations sufficiently to communicate ideas and manipulate her world. Not surprisingly, the first words uttered by most children fall into one of two categories: (1) names for concrete objects, usually those that have been manipulated; and (2) words for social interactions, such as *move, up,* and *bye.* At 16 to 18 months, vocalizations have several communicative intents, as listed in Table 3-5 (Chapman, 1981). By 2 years of age the child has begun to develop imaginative

uses of language and to explore its manipulative potential. For children who have difficulty speaking, the design of augmentative communication systems must take into account these very early language skills. By providing means of achieving language skills that are alternatives to speech, assistive technologies can have a major impact on both functional competence and long-term development. For example, early communication systems should give the child the opportunity to carry out as many of the communicative intents shown in Table 3-5 as possible, even if the child is unable to speak.

As the child continues to develop, the conversational use of language increases and the categories of use are expanded. Box 3-1 lists two of several categorizations of speech acts (Chapman, 1981). These primitive speech acts and conversational uses of language are typically learned by the young child through practice. For the child who has difficulty with speech or motor control, the ability to perform these acts becomes a joint venture between the human and the augmentative communication device. In Chapter 9 we discuss the use of augmentative communication systems.

## Problem Solving and Decision Making

Problem solving is an important aspect of the use of assistive technologies. Bailey (1989) defines problem solving as "the combination of existing ideas to form a new combination of ideas" (p. 119). This definition emphasizes the importance of prior experience in developing a solution to a new problem. A problem is a situation for which the person has no ready response (Bailey, 1989). Decision making, on the other hand, is choosing between already defined alternatives. Assistive technology systems may require the use of problem solving, decision making, or both. Problem solving is the discovery of a correct solution in a new situation; decision making is the weighing of alternative responses in terms of desirability and the selecting of one alternative. When a novice is learning to use an assistive device, he or she employs problem-solving strategies. However, when an expert uses a system in daily life, he or she applies decision making more frequently than problem solving. Our recommendation and design of assistive technology systems must take into account the skills of the potential user in these two areas. Well-conceived and well-executed training programs can facilitate the development of both problem-solving and decision-making skills in the user. The emphasis of both problem solving and decision making on past events implies a dependence on memory skills.

Bailey (1989) discusses several steps in problem solving that can be aided by computers, and we can apply these to assistive technology system specification and design. These are (1) problem recognition, (2) problem definition, (3) goal definition, (4) strategy selection, (5) alternative generation, (6) alternative evaluation, and (7) alternative selection and execution. In order to alert the user to the fact that there is a problem (problem recognition), the system must provide information regarding only relevant changes. Assistive devices can facilitate problem recognition in several ways. The most common is through warnings that are displayed to the user. For example, some computer-based powered wheelchair controllers (see Chapter 10) have a visual output that displays a flashing light when there is something wrong (Figure 3-8). This alerts the user to the existence of a problem. The visual display also shows a code indicating the type of error (e.g., joystick disconnected, battery low). This is the problem definition stage, since the device has told the user what the problem is. Strategy selection is based on the first two steps—the recognition of a problem and the definition of the nature of the problem. In this example, a troubleshooting chart in which the error code is listed together with possible causes and solutions may aid strategy selection. This problem-solving aid can then be combined with the user's experience with similar problems to develop a strategy for solving the problem. The problem-solving strategy generally yields a set of alternatives (alternative generation) from which the most likely cause can be chosen (alternative evaluation). Finally, an alternative is chosen (e.g., disconnected joystick) and the error is corrected. This final stage is alternative selection and execution. If the alternative provides a solution to the problem, then all is well. If not, then additional alternatives must be evaluated and executed until the problem is solved. The problem-solving aids provided by the technology, in this case a warning display and code and a troubleshooting chart, help to convert a difficult problem into a series of decision-making steps. Whenever possible we should include aids for problem solving in our design of assistive technology systems.

It is possible to compensate for poor problem solving on the part of the user by incorporating some "intelligence" into the device. For example, in the design of an augmentative communication system for a person with aphasia, the combination of pictures or other symbols and categorization can help avoid the dependence on recalling a specific word. A "food" picture can be selected, which leads to the presentation of different types of food (e.g., fruits, meats) or eating situations (e.g., breakfast, lunch). Once a secondary category is selected, the choice can be more specific (e.g., pear, apple, banana). This approach converts a problem-solving or memory task (recalling the correct word or phrase) to a decision-making process (choosing one of

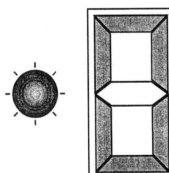
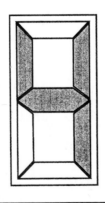

| Troubleshooting Chart | | |
|---|---|---|
| Code | Probable Cause | Correction |
| 01 | No power to motor | Check cable Check fuse |
| 02 | Weak battery | Recharge |
| 03 | Left motor cable disconnected | Reconnect cable |
| 04 | Joystick disconnected | Reconnect cable |
| • | | |
| • | | |
| • | | |

Figure 3-8  A display and troubleshooting chart used in diagnosing a malfunction in a powered wheelchair. The display is part of the wheelchair controller, and the chart is included in the user's manual.

several alternatives). By carefully designing the system to accommodate the possible number of choices and steps in a sequence of activities, the system can provide significant improvement in communicative performance.

## ■ PSYCHOSOCIAL FUNCTION AS RELATED TO ASSISTIVE TECHNOLOGY USE

How the human interacts with assistive technology involves more than the physical and cognitive components. Psychosocial factors have a significant influence on assistive technology usage as well. Psychosocial function is composed of both intrinsic and extrinsic factors. The intrinsic psychosocial characteristics of an individual are hard to separate from the influences of the person's social environment. In the human activity assistive technology (HAAT) model, these intrinsic psychosocial factors are discussed in relation to the human and the person's social environment is seen as a part of the context (see Chapter 2).

In an attempt to understand the psychosocial factors that influence human performance, Depoy and Kolodner (1991) organize the information into three major areas: self-definition or identity, self-protection or maintenance, and motivation for action. These areas can also be applied to assistive technology and can help us understand how psychosocial factors influence human performance related to assistive technology use.

### Identity and Self-protection

In terms of identity the main question that is asked is "Who am I?" The answer to this question involves notions such as self-concept, locus of control, well being, emotion, environment, and performance (Depoy and Kolodner, 1991). Of primary importance to the successful use of assistive technology is a clear self-concept on the part of the person with a disability. Robertson (1998) defines self-concept as "our definition of the goals, values, and beliefs that give direction and meaning to life" and states further that "knowing who we are unifies our actions, pulls the various parts of ourselves into a cohesive whole" (p. 452). The individual with a well-developed self-concept has clearly defined goals and expectations for the assistive technology system and is more likely to be successful in using the technology.

An individual's self-concept is closely linked to physical attributes. Any changes in physical skills and features as a result of illness or disability can have a profound effect on how an individual feels about himself. Individuals who acquire a disability go through various emotional stages of loss before accepting the disability. Different authors have identified these stages as shock, anxiety, denial, depression, internalized anger, externalized hostility, acknowledgment, and adjustment (Livneh and Antonak, 1990, 1991). The

sequence in which these stages are experienced and the duration of each stage vary depending on the individual (Livneh and Antonak, 1991). For example, a woman who sustains a stroke later in life will go through the stages in the process of adjusting to her disability. Her ultimate acceptance of the disability requires a balance between acknowledging her loss and appreciating her remaining abilities to participate in activities of daily life (Sabari, 1998). If she is in the stage of depression when it is time to select an assistive technology device, she may not be capable of exercising good judgment (Scherer, 1998). Furthermore, assistive technology that is recommended before acceptance of the disability may be seen as a reminder of the independence that she has lost and consequently may be avoided or abandoned altogether. On the other hand, a person who has grown up with a disability, such as cerebral palsy, does not go through this same type of process in accepting the loss. As Scherer (1993) points out, the person who is born with cerebral palsy is more likely to have adjusted to the disability. This individual is inclined to view assistive technology as opening up new opportunities.

A second critical psychosocial factor is self-protection. The fundamental purpose of the self is "to regulate behavior, to maintain mental health, and [to] maximize each person's productive contributions in valued roles in society" (Robertson, 1998, p. 452). To achieve stability and protect himself from internal and external psychological harm, the individual uses mechanisms of self-protection, such as defense mechanisms and adaptive strategies (Depoy and Kolodner, 1991).

Protecting oneself can factor into assistive technology use as well, particularly if a person does not feel comfortable using the device. For example, there are individuals with spinal cord injuries who may have lived more in their body than in their mind before their injury (Scherer, 1993). As a result, these individuals may have had limited exposure to computer technology and now are being asked to use it for functional activities. If a person is uncomfortable using an assistive technology device, this can be anxiety producing. To protect herself and reduce the anxiety, this person may avoid or abandon the device.

### Motivation

Bailey (1989) defines **motivation** as "any influence that gives rise to performance" (p. 154). In the context of assistive technology systems, motivation may result from the human, activity, context, or assistive technology components of the system. Lack of motivation by the consumer to use the device or perform the task is one of the principal reasons an assistive technology device is abandoned (Scherer and Galvin, 1996). We can define both internal motivating factors and external factors. Internal factors include desire to succeed, and external factors include praise and task-related effects such as feedback generated by the task. Feedback that results from the performance of a task can serve three purposes: (1) provision of knowledge regarding performance; (2) motivation to continue, which is the present state and does not equal the ultimate goal; and (3) reinforcement. A *reinforcer* is a stimulus whose occurrence tends to strengthen the response via a close temporal relationship.

Assistive technologies can provide motivation in many ways. It is often useful to couple social interaction with the occurrence of a desired result. For example, Mary Lou was particularly passive, and her use of a switch to activate graphics, toys, and sounds was inconsistent and slow (in some cases minutes). Mary Lou was especially fond of her father, and this was used to motivate her motor performance. A computer and voice synthesizer were used to allow her to generate a spoken phrase by activating a switch. The phrase used was "Come here, Dad." Her father was asked to leave the room, and Mary Lou used her switch to activate the stored phrase and request that her father return to the room. She found this to be a highly motivating task, and her response times were rapid. The social reward facilitated by the technology provided the necessary motivation for her to activate a switch, a difficult motor act for her. In this case all three of the purposes of feedback were accomplished, and each played an important role in her success. First, the provision of external feedback provided Mary Lou with the knowledge that she could summon her father. Second, she was motivated to act by the social reward of interacting with her father. Finally, the spoken phrase activated by her switch provided reinforcement for the accomplishment of the motor act, and she was motivated to repeat the action to repeat the social reward.

Because motivation is so important to the effective use of assistive technologies, we must carefully define the goals of the potential user and choose devices that meet these goals in a manner that is meaningful and motivating to the person. Depoy and Kolodner (1991) provide an overview of the major psychological theories relating to motivation. They define six factors that determine motivation for action: (1) elicitors of behavior, (2) symbols, (3) beliefs and perceptions, (4) cultural norms and expectations, (5) intrinsic motivation, and (6) history of experience (p. 313). Although the major schools of psychological thought view each of these factors somewhat differently, we can use them as a basis for discussing motivation as it applies to assistive technologies.

As we have discussed, elicitors of behavior can be either *intrinsic* (e.g., the desire to please) or *extrinsic* (e.g., synthetic speech feedback), and they are the forces that cause or trigger behavior. In assistive technology systems, external elicitors of behavior may include those resulting from social outcomes (the context) or successful completion of an activity. Examples of social results include conversational interaction, achieving a goal (e.g., moving a wheelchair to a given location), and reinforcement (e.g., getting a high grade). These social effects result because the individual completes an activity such as conversational communication, mobility, or studying for an examination.

From a psychological point of view, *symbols* are abstract representations of reality. Many actions in daily tasks are symbolic, and they are carried out to conform to expectations. For example, a major goal of communication is social politeness, in which the content of the communication is less important than the conformance to social norms (Light, 1988). In order for a person whose goal is social politeness to be motivated to use an augmentative communication system, the device must be capable of providing rapid and simple output that facilitates social interaction. This differs from the use of a system for making requests, in which the user's motivation is to receive a specific result. As Depoy and Kolodner (1991) point out, the degree to which the symbols are shared between the user of the assistive technology system and his or her communication partner has a major impact on the effectiveness of an interaction.

*Beliefs* have a strong effect on motivation. In our consideration of assistive technologies, we must specify or design a system that is consistent with the person's belief system in order for the person to be motivated to use it. Among the most highly valued beliefs is acceptance by others, and assistive technology systems can either facilitate or impede acceptance. A simple example is the choice of color in a wheelchair for a child. If the child is allowed to have a wheelchair whose frame is in his favorite color, he may be more accepted by his peers than if the wheelchair is the standard "hospital chrome." A more significant problem in acceptance was (and still is to a large extent) presented by the limited availability of female synthetic voices used in augmentative communication systems. Females have often acquired but not used communication systems with male voices, and this is at least partially related to the social acceptance of the total assistive technology system, which has a disparity between the person's characteristics and the quality and gender of her voice.

As we have emphasized throughout this chapter, *experience* plays a major role in the successful utilization of assistive technologies. The ways in which we perceive these experiences can also have a large impact on motivation. Our perceptions give us an understanding of events and also provide the basis by which we ascribe meaning to them. These perceptions can be motivating in several ways. Negative experiences can lead to avoidance of events, tasks, or actions. For example, a child who is introduced to a powered wheelchair without adequate preparation and training may have difficulty using the system and may be frightened by errant movements or collisions. This experience can dissuade the child from attempting to use the system. Alternatively, a child who has a positive experience in her first attempt at powered mobility will be highly motivated to repeat her actions.

The final factor underlying motivation is adherence to *cultural norms and expectations*. Assistive technology systems must foster such adherence if they are to be motivating and useful. Depoy and Kolodner (1991) describe cultural norms and expectations as "shared, common environmental elements that underpin behavior" (p. 317). Many individuals who have disabilities live in segregated group homes and spend the majority of their time in "special" educational or adult programs. This culture differs significantly from the world in which the majority of us live, and these two cultures may have widely different norms and expectations. One of the major goals of assistive technology application is to normalize the performance of an individual with a disability in order to facilitate greater independence and broader exposure to the world at large. In approaching this goal we must carefully consider the impact of cultural norms and expectations on motivation for performance using the assistive device. In some cultures—Asian, for example—if an elderly person becomes disabled as a result of a stroke, his continued independence is not viewed as being important. The extended family now perceives their role as taking care of that person. In this situation, outside intervention, including that provided by assistive technology, may not be seen as necessary. As another example, consider devices intended for self-feeding (see Chapter 11). These devices are imperfect, and a severely disabled person who uses one may achieve independence at a cost of neatness. It may be more "acceptable," in a public place such as a restaurant, for the disabled person to be fed by a human attendant, resulting in less mess. The person may choose to sacrifice independence, as obtained using the mechanical feeder, to achieve cultural acceptance. Alternatively, in her group home setting, she may choose independence (the use of the mechanical feeder) over neatness because her peers are more accepting than strangers in the restaurant. Another person may be less influenced by cultural acceptance and choose to use the mechanical feeder in both locations. Because no assistive device will be used effectively if the person is not motivated, these factors are important.

In her book *Living in the State of Stuck: How Technology Impacts the Lives of People with Disabilities*, Scherer (1993) presents the milieu personality technology model, which describes personality characteristics as one aspect influencing an individual's use of assistive technology. The three factors described earlier (identity, self-protection, and motivation) are all incorporated into these personality characteristics. **Optimal use** of the technology occurs when the individual is proud to use the device, motivated, cooperative, optimistic, has good coping skills, and has the skills to use the device. It is predicted that those individuals who are

unmotivated; intimidated by technology; embarrassed to use the device; impatient or impulsive; or have low self-esteem, unrealistic expectations, or limitations in the skills needed may become partial or **reluctant users.** Nonuse of the assistive technology occurs when the individual either avoids it altogether or abandons it after initial use. Characteristics of the person who avoids using a device may include someone who does not have the skills to use the device and someone who is depressed, unmotivated, embarrassed to use the device, uncooperative, withdrawn, or intimidated by technology. The personality characteristics related to the **abandonment** of a device can be attributed to an individual who is depressed, angry, embarrassed to use the device, withdrawn, or resistant; has low self-esteem or poor socialization and coping skills; or lacks the skills and or training to use the device. Being aware of the psychological factors that affect assistive technology use can facilitate the matching process for the ATP and optimize use of assistive technology systems.

## Assistive Technology Use Over the Lifespan

The person's developmental stage at the time that assistive technology is being considered influences the decision-making process and use of the device. We discussed child development and its implications for assistive technology use earlier in this chapter. In this section we consider factors that change over the lifespan and their implications for assistive technology use.

King (1999) characterizes how learners across the lifespan approach technology. Children from birth to 3 to 4 years of age are eager to explore and play. They will be motivated to engage in assistive technology by this need to explore. It is for this reason that very young children who are being introduced to powered mobility be encouraged to explore with the mobility device rather than asked to follow instructions for a particular protocol (Janeschild, 1997). Children of this age may have some fear of sounds or movement, but they have little or no fear of failure and embarrassment (King, 1999). At this age, they will use any and all parts of their body to interact with devices. As children age and their motor skills become more refined, so does their ability to control a device. The fingers and hands are then more likely used as control sites.

From the childhood to the early teenage years, children remain eager to explore and are interested in trying out control interfaces (King, 1999). As children approach adolescence, they become more motivated by the desire to be competent than by the need to explore (Early, 1993). Consequently, persons at this age will practice over and over even when they fail. They are not embarrassed about making mistakes or worried about the time involved in developing their skills. Their desire to learn how to interact with technology drives them to seek and accept instruction from adults and older or more skilled children.

The next age span described by King (1999) is the young adult to middle-aged adult, which encompasses roughly age 20 to ages 65 to 70. Individuals in this phase of the life cycle are typically engaged in job pursuits and are motivated by the need to achieve (Early, 1993). The young adults in this group (ages 20 to 30) have grown up with technology and in general are not intimidated by it. They remain eager to explore technologies and are fairly confident in their approach. The middle-aged adults in this group (ages 30 to 70) did not grow up with computer or video games. However, through their work they have most likely been exposed to some type of technology, and in most cases keeping their job depends on their ability to use technology. Those middle-aged adults who use technology are comfortable with it and not intimidated to use it. However, those who are not familiar with technology are uncomfortable using it and can find it threatening. These individuals prefer to learn about the technology and practice it in private, without being observed or supervised while gaining the needed skills.

Older adults (ages 65 to 70 and older) have similar characteristics as the group just described (King, 1999). They may have had little exposure to new technologies and tend to use devices and tools that they are familiar with. When it comes to using a new tool or device, they may be extremely fearful. Part of this fear is related to the belief that they may do something to the technology that will damage it or result in costly repairs. Given one-on-one training, encouragement, and practice, these individuals have the potential to become highly skilled in the use of new technologies. As these individuals age, however, they are likely to have sensory, motor, and cognitive deficits that affect the learning and use of technology. Older adults are motivated by a need to explore the past, review life accomplishments, and investigate present capabilities through leisure activities (Kielhofner, 1980). Someone who is otherwise fearful of using a computer may be motivated to overcome that fear if given the task of writing his life story or utilizing it for genealogy research.

To maximize the use of assistive technology, the ATP must take into consideration the learning characteristics of each stage in the human lifespan and be able to select technologies and interventions that match the individual's age group.

## ■ MOTOR CONTROL AS RELATED TO ASSISTIVE TECHNOLOGY USE

As we have stated, *motor control* refers to all the central processing functions that lead to planned, coordinated motor outputs. Many aspects of motor control are important in the use of assistive technologies. In order to perform a control task, the human operator must be able to locate a target, plan a movement to that target, and produce a desired action once the target is reached. This process involves both sensory and motor components. Sensation is involved in both the scanning of the environment to locate the target and in the regulation of the movement via sensory feedback during the task. For example, one of the tasks involved in writing is to pick up a pencil. The pencil is the target, and the steps in picking it up follow the sequence described above. These motor actions to targets are called *aimed movements*.

As we repeat a movement many times, *motor learning* takes place, and both the speed and accuracy of our movement improve. Another effect of motor learning is changes that occur in the variability of the path of movement or trajectory. Initially the path we use to move to the target varies widely from trial to trial. As we learn the movement, the trajectory becomes much more uniform and consistent from trial to trial. This motor learning is made possible by the formation of **engrams,** which are preprogrammed patterns of centrally represented muscular activity (Pedretti, 1996). They develop when there are many repetitions of a specific movement or activity. With repeated, consistent movements, the conscious effort of the person is reduced and the movements become more automatic.

For the sensory and motor components of these movements to be integrated, there must be maps of both the person's own internal neuromuscular system and the external worlds. These maps also consist of engrams, and they are constructed as we encounter the environment through experience.

In this section we consider the role of motor control in the use of assistive technology systems and the effects abnormalities may have. Our emphasis is on those aspects of motor control that are most important for the successful application of assistive technology systems.

### Aimed Movements to Targets

Control of assistive devices is achieved through aimed movements carried out by the user. This control requires the successful completion of a number of sensorimotor tasks. A set of targets *(selection set)* must be visually or auditorily scanned; the desired element chosen; and the element selected, activated, or manipulated through a motor act. This process applies equally to the use of devices in which several choices are to be made (e.g., a wheelchair joystick with four directions or a television remote control with a group of buttons, in which the targets are physical locations) and to objects to be manipulated (e.g., fork, washcloth). It also applies to systems in which the targets are on a screen (graphic) or spoken (auditory) and are presented one at a time for the user to select. The movement to and activation or manipulation of targets may be via any of the effectors discussed in the next section.

**Speed and accuracy of movements.** Human factors engineers often use speed and accuracy to measure motor performance in moving to targets (Bailey, 1989). In general, these two parameters are inversely related: as speed increases, accuracy decreases. The level of experience the person has also affects this relationship between speed and accuracy. For a novice, the inverse relationship generally holds. However, for experienced users of systems, increasing speed does not necessarily result in decreased accuracy. For example, Klemmer and Lockhead (1962) found that the fastest (and most experienced) keypunch operators were twice as fast as the slowest (and least experienced) operators. Surprisingly, the fastest operators were also 10 times as accurate as their slower colleagues. Thus we must not assume that because a task is completed faster it is necessarily less accurate.

Fitts (1954) found that the time to move to a target decreases for closer or larger targets and increases for more distant or smaller targets. This relationship, called Fitts's Law, "appears to hold under a wide variety of circumstances involving different types of aimed movements, body parts, manipulanda [types of controls], target arrangements, and physical environments" (Meyer, Smith, and Wright, 1982, p. 451). Jagacinski and Monk (1985) found that Fitts's Law was a good predictor of the speed/accuracy tradeoff for control of two-dimensional cursor movements on a video screen. This relationship held for both a helmet-mounted control and a hand-controlled joystick.

Using Fitts's Law, Radwin, Vanderheiden, and Lin (1990) evaluated both mouse movement and a head-mounted pointer for computer entry. They found that mouse input was faster and generally required less movement than the head pointer for able-bodied subjects. For disabled subjects they found that the speed and accuracy of head control were both dramatically affected by proper trunk stability provided through a seating system. Figure 3-9 is a plot of movement time (the distance from the origin radially outward) versus the direction of cursor movement on a computer screen. Both the dotted and solid lines are for the same subject, who had cerebral palsy. The solid curve represents the speed of head movements when the subject had inadequate thoracic support; the dotted curve shows that movement times were much faster and more symmetrical from left to right when adequate support was provided for the subject. This type of study underscores the importance of providing a stable position as a base of support for control tasks.

**Reaction time.** Although the inverse speed-versus-accuracy relationship holds for movement time to a target, it does not generally apply to reaction times. Reaction time can be broken down into contributions from the major information processing stages, as shown in Table 3-6 (Bailey, 1989). From this table, we can see that the majority of the reaction time is taken up by "cognitive processing," with

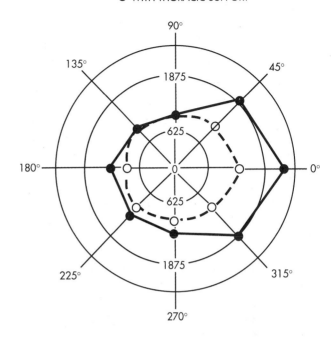

MOVEMENT TIME (ms) vs. DIRECTION (degrees)

**Figure 3-9**  A plot of movement time, from the origin radially outward, versus the direction of cursor movement, shown in degrees, for a head pointer controlled cursor on a computer screen (Reprinted with permission from *Human Factors*, Vol. 32, No. 4, 1990: "A Method for Evaluating Head-Controlled Computer Input Devices Using Fitts' Law" by R. G. Radwin et al. Copyright 1990 by The Human Factors and Ergonomics Society. All rights reserved.)

| TABLE 3-6 | Reaction Times Related to Stages of Human Processing |
|---|---|
| Delay | Typical times (msec) |
| Sensory receptor | 1-38 |
| Neural transmission to CNS | 2-100 |
| Cognitive processing delays (CNS) | 70-300 |
| Neural transmission to muscle | 10-30 |
| Muscle latency and activation time | 30-70 |
| Total delay | 113-528 |

From Bailey RW: *Human performance engineering,* Englewood Cliffs, NJ, 1989, Prentice Hall, p 43.

much smaller contributions from sensors, neural conduction, and effectors (muscles). Central processing is largely perception and motor control in our stage processing model (see Figure 3-1). The ranges shown in Table 3-6 indicate differences based on the type of sensory input. For example, reaction to an auditory stimulus is faster than that to a visual or tactile stimulus. Fastest reaction times occur when multiple sensory stimuli are available simultaneously.

The values in Table 3-6 are for nondisabled subjects; the presence of a disability can dramatically affect the results. For example, individuals who have sustained a stroke or head injury or who have cerebral palsy often exhibit **apraxia,** a motor planning deficit in which the peripheral components necessary to execute the motion are generally intact (Trombly and Scott, 1977). In these cases, reaction time can be significantly increased, and it is often difficult to separate central causes (e.g., apraxia) from peripheral (e.g., sensory or effector) factors. The use of assistive devices that depend on reaction time must take these factors into account. For example, some individuals with motor disabilities find it easier to release a switch than to activate it when asked to choose from sequentially presented choices. Alternatively, a step approach in which the user hits the switch repeatedly to move through the choices works better for some persons because it does not depend on their reactions being rapid. This brings the operation of the device under the control of the user to a greater degree, and it can result in improved performance. This type of selection method also allows the user to get into a motor pattern that is more automatic. These topics are discussed further in Chapter 7.

## Development of Movement Patterns through Motor Learning

Movement trajectories provide important information regarding motor control and motor learning. Although there are a large number of potential trajectories in an aimed movement task, only a few are actually used (Georgopoulos, Kalaska, and Massey, 1981). To understand this, place a pencil or pen on the table. Now think about all the different paths that your arm can take as you reach for the pencil. Even though all these paths or trajectories are possible, there are only a few that you would ever actually use. As the movement is practiced over and over, the variability of path trajectory decreases; that is, fewer of the possible trajectories are actually used in accomplishing the movement. Georgopoulos and co-workers also found that reaction times increased as the number of targets increased, but the change in reaction time was smaller than the change in the number of targets. This means that use of a keyboard with many targets results in slower reaction times than a single target presented by one switch. This helps to explain why, with some types of disabilities, it is easier for the individual to select from a group of targets once he is positioned near them (e.g., his hand is over the keyboard) than it is to move to the array of targets from a rest position (e.g., his hand is in his lap).

In a similar study, Flash and Hogan (1985) examined the configuration of the arm and hand in space during two-dimensional arm movements. They also found that, with practice, only a few of the many trajectories from a rest position to a target are actually used and variability decreases with practice in nondisabled subjects. If similar relationships exist in disabled persons, then our assessment and training of consumers to use devices that require aimed movements should include tasks designed to identify and emphasize trajectories for which motor performance is optimized.

An individual seen at our center presents a striking example of the application of these concepts to augmentative communication system use. At the time of assessment, Doug was a very proficient user of the HandiVoice 120.* His overall communication rate, determined during an interview, was 26 words per minute. He used whole words and phrases (selected with a single three-digit code) approximately 65% of the time and individual phonemes 35% of the time. Because of his cerebral palsy, he had some difficulty in hitting the keys, and our initial naive assumption was that providing the equivalent of the three-digit codes on individual keys and therefore reducing the number of keystrokes could dramatically increase his overall rate. This was addressed by placing the individual phoneme and word or phrase labels on the keys of a computer, with the corresponding words or phrases of the phonemes being spoken upon key activation. To our surprise, he was unable to use these labels; they were no longer meaningful to him. We then substituted the three-digit codes for the word or phoneme labels. Once again, Doug was unable to access the vocabulary with which he had demonstrated such facility when using the HandiVoice directly. At Doug's suggestion, we placed the HandiVoice next to the computer keyboard, and he looked at the keyboard, visualized the movement required, and then entered the correct word or phoneme codes to generate his message. He had, in fact, developed a set of motor patterns or engrams that he used with the HandiVoice, and he no longer made use of either the phoneme or word labels or their corresponding codes; his motor learning associated with the use of the HandiVoice had progressed to the stage of maximizing motor performance in the absence of cognitive attention to target locations. This skill had developed over long periods of practice with a carefully designed training program using the HandiVoice. This outcome, in retrospect, was predictable based on the concepts of aimed movements and reduction in hand path variability with practice described by Georgopoulis and co-workers (1981) and Flash and Hogan (1985). It is also consistent with the common experience of not being able to recall a phone number but being able to dial it once the motor pattern is begun.

Some assistive technology systems involve uncertainty in target locations, and in order to use them effectively, this must be taken into account. An example is augmentative communication systems with dynamic displays in which the selection set on the touch screen changes with each selection. Each time the user makes a choice, she is confronted

---

*Phonic Ear, Inc., Mill Valley, Calif.

with a totally new set of choices on the display. If the choices are totally random, then motor learning relative to movement to the targets will not occur. However, if the choices are *predictable*, even though they change from screen to screen, then motor patterns can develop and speed and accuracy can both improve with practice.

## The Relationship between a Stimulus and the Resulting Movement

In the use of assistive technologies, there are many situations in which a device generates an output that requires a response by the user. We can think of this output as a *stimulus* and the user's resulting movement as a *response*. For example, most computers now use a graphical user interface that displays a set of small pictures (icons) depicting the action to be taken. There are icons for loading a file, running a program, erasing a file, and many others. An icon is selected by moving an on-screen pointer using a mouse—an aimed movement to a target. The relationship between the stimulus (in this example, an icon) and the response (movement of the cursor with the mouse) is important. Fitts and Deininger (1954) used the term *stimulus-response (S-R) compatibility* to describe improvements in motor performance that resulted from a close relationship between the stimulus and the response. Fitts and Deininger used the task of a radial movement from the center of a circle to one of eight targets located around the circle to study S-R compatibility. The subject was asked to move to one of the eight locations as quickly as possible following a stimulus that represented one of the eight locations. Four stimulus sets were used in this experiment: (1) eight lights arranged in a pattern around a circle, corresponding to one of the eight target locations (spatial two-dimensional set); (2) numbers corresponding to locations around a clock face (1:30, 9:00, etc.) (symbolic two-dimensional set); (3) a horizontal string of eight lights (one-dimensional stimulus set); and (4) eight three-letter first names, each assigned to one of the eight locations (symbolic nonspatial set). Fitts and Deininger recorded reaction time and number of errors for each stimulus set to determine whether any of them led to increased performance (faster times and fewer errors). The fastest response times and fewest errors were obtained with the spatial two-dimensional stimulus set (clock face). This set was familiar to the subjects. The symbolic two-dimensional set (common three-letter names) was second best, followed by the one-dimensional and symbolic nonspatial sets. Therefore the sets with the least similarity to the task were the slowest and least accurate.

The implication for the design and use of assistive technologies is that motor performance can be improved if the correspondence between the stimulus and required response is high. For example, in a GUI a stored file can have a picture of a file folder and the data file system can be portrayed as a filing cabinet. Because of the limited motor experiences of many disabled persons, S-R compatibility may be considerably different from that of normal subjects (e.g., manipulation of objects may have been limited and file folders may be meaningless). As motor experience increases, the number of available motor responses may increase, and this creates more options for stimuli that match desired responses.

## ■ EFFECTOR FUNCTION RELATED TO ASSISTIVE TECHNOLOGY USE

The human operator controls the assistive technology through his various effectors, and they enable manipulation of the environment in a variety of ways. The presence of disability dramatically alters the use of effectors. Several factors are important to keep in mind when considering effector use for the purpose of controlling assistive technologies. First, there are a variety of ways of accomplishing the same task. For example, people type using fingers, toes, head wands, mouthsticks, and many other methods. This diversity in accomplishing tasks opens up many options that we would not consider if we restricted ourselves to the common ways of doing things. Second, we cannot interpret effector function from the point of view of a nondisabled person. We must attempt to obtain the perspective of the person with a disability; this underscores the importance of including this person in the process of service delivery.

### Description of Effectors

Effectors provide the motor outputs that underlie both stabilization and control. The large muscles of the trunk and pelvis provide strength for stabilization of the body. This stabilization is required for manipulation, or control. Control effectors include hand or finger, arm, head, eye (oculomotor control), leg, foot, and respiration and phonation. In this section we describe these effectors, and in Chapter 4 we discuss the process by which we assess an individual person's capabilities in the use of these effectors.

Figure 3-10 shows the body sites that can be used to control a device. We refer to these as *control sites*. Each control site is capable of performing a variety of movements. The mouth can be used in a number of ways, depending on the individual's capabilities. The flow of air can be used as a control signal. This regulation of airflow requires chest muscles and diaphragm control; in order to use airflow as a control signal, the individual must be able to control her *respiration*. Respiratory flow can be detected by sip (inhaling) or puff (exhaling) switches. If the airflow also includes sound production by the vocal folds, we refer to it as *phonation*. Phonation may produce sounds (including

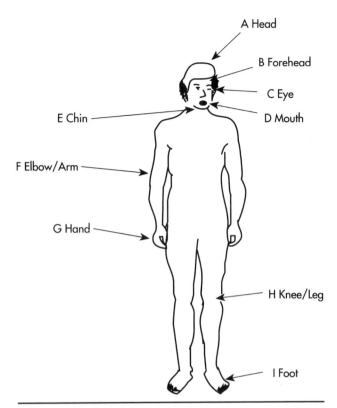

A Head
B Forehead
C Eye
D Mouth
E Chin
F Elbow/Arm
G Hand
H Knee/Leg
I Foot

Figure 3-10  Anatomical sites commonly used for control of assistive technologies. (From Webster JW, Cook AM, Tompkins WJ, Vanderheiden GC: *Electronic devices for rehabilitation*, New York, 1985, John Wiley and Sons, p. 207.)

whistling) or speech. Sounds can also be detected by various control interfaces. If the individual is able to use speech, we can use *speech recognition* as a control interface. Tongue movements can also be used for control.

For many persons with severe disabilities, eye gaze techniques are the first that are used as control signals in augmentative communication systems, and this method of communicative output can be developed to a high degree of competence (Goossens and Crain, 1987; Nolan, 1987). Often the first communication after a major injury (such as a traumatic brain injury) is yes/no questions answered by eye blinks or eye movement. The eyes can also be used in the control of assistive devices by using control interfaces that detect eye movements. For these reasons, we include oculomotor function with other effectors. Erhardt (1987) uses the following terms, which emphasize the role of the oculomotor system as an effector: *visual approach* (localization), *visual grasp* (fixation), *visual manipulation* (ocular pursuit), and *visual release* (gaze shift). By considering the role of the oculomotor system in these terms, its role as a control site is clear. For example, identification, selection, and indication of vocabulary elements in augmentative communication systems involves all these oculomotor tasks. To employ eye

movements to access an assistive device, we must detect the eye movement and use it as a signal for communication or control. Often eye movements are observed by another person, and the control or communication is carried out by that person (see Goossens and Crain, 1987, for example). However, there are also electronic systems that can measure eye position and use it as a control signal. Control interfaces for all these effectors are described in Chapter 7.

The head can be used as a control site in a number of ways. Movements of the head include tilting side to side, vertical movement, horizontal rotation, and linear forward and backward movement. Very few functional movements are purely horizontal or vertical or purely rotational with no tilt; most movements of the head are combinations of these components. Upper extremity sites include the movements of the shoulder, elbow, forearm, and hand and finger. Shoulder movements include elevation, flexion, extension, abduction (away from the body), and adduction (toward the body). The movements of the elbow are flexion and extension. The movements of the forearm consist of pronation (turning the palm down) and supination (turning the palm up). The wrist can flex or extend or move from side to side (radial deviation or ulnar deviation). The fingers can individually flex and extend or, together, perform a grasp and release movement. The thumb can flex and extend, abduct and adduct, and oppose each of the fingers. Control movements used in the lower extremities include raising and lowering of the leg at the hip (e.g., hip flexion and extension), knee flexion and extension or knee abduction and adduction, foot plantar flexion (toes point down) or dorsiflexion (toes point up), and foot inversion or eversion (side to side).

When the interaction between a person with a disability and an assistive device involves relatively fine control, the hand and fingers are the preferred control site because they are typically used for manipulative tasks. Even if hand control is limited, it may still be possible to enhance the existing function using assistive technologies, which makes it possible to use hand movements for control. If the hand is not controllable, then the use of the head as an interface site is preferred. With pointers of various types as control enhancers (e.g., a head pointer), it is possible to obtain relatively precise control using the head. Oculomotor control is most often used for indicating choices in augmentative communication when no other control site is available for pointing. Eye-controlled switches can be used for gross control using the eyes. Voice allows for relatively fine control with many possible control signals. Simple airflow with no speech is generally more gross and restricted to a few signals. For some individuals, fine control of the foot is possible. For fine manipulative tasks, the foot is less desirable than the hand or head because visual monitoring can be difficult and the foot is generally not as finely controlled as the hand. The use of the arm or leg is less desirable for precise tasks because these represent naturally gross movements controlled by large muscle groups. For this reason, they are the least desirable for manipulative functions.

Although we generally use an individual's "best" available control site, in some cases, more than one control site must be identified. This most often occurs when one person uses several types of assistive technologies. For example, head control may be used for augmentative communication and foot control for a powered wheelchair. In other cases, such as with some neuromuscular disabilities (e.g., amyotrophic lateral sclerosis), multiple sites need to be identified because of progressive paralysis. The course of this progression can vary from months to years. The variation in ability to use effectors over the course of the disease makes it necessary to find flexible control interfaces that can be used with multiple control sites or to find separate control interfaces for several sites initially (see Chapters 4 and 7).

## Factors Underlying the Use of Effectors

Two primary factors underlying the use of effectors are automatic movements and muscle tone. The former consists of primitive reflexes, righting reactions, and equilibrium reactions (Hopkins and Smith, 1993).

**Primitive reflexes** are characterized by immediate and automatic movement performed at a subconscious level (Hopkins and Smith, 1993). They are usually initiated by sensory stimulation. Present at birth or shortly thereafter, these reflexes are inhibited or (more often) integrated into volitional movements in order to control posture and perform basic movement patterns as the infant develops. Neurological damage before or at birth may affect the degree to which the infant is able to integrate or inhibit these reflex patterns, resulting in delayed motor development and impaired motor control (Fiorentino, 1978). Neurological damage later in life can also reduce the individual's ability to inhibit some of these primitive reflexes, resulting in impaired postural control and movement patterns.

Hopkins and Smith (1993) tabulate 17 primitive reflexes, including their initiation, stimulus, response, and adaptation in later life. The primitive reflexes that most commonly influence effector use are the asymmetrical tonic neck reflex (ATNR) and the tonic labyrinthine reflex (TLR) (Trefler, 1984). The ATNR occurs when the head is turned to one side, the arm on that side is extended, and the opposite arm is flexed. This reflex makes it difficult for the person to hold his trunk and head in midline, prevents use of both hands together, and contributes to scoliosis (Trefler, 1984). The tonic labyrinthine reflex is displayed by increased extensor tone in the supine position and increased flexor tone in the prone position. When sitting,

the result is increased extensor tone in the lower limbs, trunk, and neck, causing the person to slide forward in the chair (Davies, 1985).

Righting reactions and equilibrium reactions respond to more global stimuli, and they persist throughout life (Hopkins and Smith, 1993). *Righting reactions* support the vertical position of the head, alignment of the head and trunk, and alignment of the trunk and pelvis. These reactions are essential for the effective control of assistive technologies. Hopkins and Smith also list nine righting reactions. One reaction that can interfere with assistive technology use is the *positive supporting reaction*, which is elicited by pressure on the toe pads or ball of the foot. The pressure from the footrest of a wheelchair, for example, can elicit this reaction. Increased extensor tone of the lower extremities follows simultaneously with contraction of the flexor muscles. The result is strong extension of the legs, which affects upright posture.

*Equilibrium reactions* provide balance when the center of gravity is disturbed, such as by leaning to one side. As the nervous system matures, equilibrium reactions serve to regain balance. These reactions include the counterrotation of the head and trunk away from the direction of a displacement of gravity (e.g., by leaning) and the use of the extremities to gain balance by abduction. Hopkins and Smith (1993) describe 12 equilibrium reactions.

**Muscle tone** is defined as the resistance to stretch provided by neural activity, viscoelastic properties of muscle and joints, and sensory feedback to the CNS (Brooks, 1986). Normal muscle tone is high enough so that the individual can resist gravity and low enough to allow for movement (Bobath, 1978). Tone varies with age, level of activity, stress, and other factors. Muscle tone in infants is generally decreased, or *hypotonic,* and they begin to develop more normal tone as their nervous system develops. As we age, the amount of tone generally decreases for many reasons, including changes in muscle fibers, sensory receptors, and CNS function (Farber, 1991).

Disabilities can also lead to changes in muscle tone. Depending on the level of damage to the nervous system, impaired muscle tone can include flaccidity, spasticity, and rigidity. A reduction in normal muscle tone is referred to as *flaccidity* or *hypotonicity.* When muscle tone is increased it is referred to as *hypertonicity* or **spasticity.** Several types of disorders can result in spasticity. Increased muscle tone is often accompanied by exaggerated reflexes and imbalances between the antagonistic muscle pairs controlling joints. With *rigidity* there is an increase of muscle tone in both the antagonist and agonist muscles at the same time, resulting in resistance to passive range of motion throughout the range and in any direction (Undzis, Zoltan, Pedretti, 1996). It is possible for a person to exhibit a mixture of types of muscle tone and for her tone to fluctuate throughout the

| TABLE 3-7 | Effector Characteristics | | | |
|-----------|------------|----------|----------|-------------|
| Effector | Resolution | Range | Strength | Versatility |
| Fingers | High | Small | Low | Very high |
| Hand | Moderate | Moderate | Moderate | Moderate |
| Arm | Low | Large | Large | Low |
| Head | Moderate | Moderate | Moderate | High |
| Leg | Low | Moderate | High | Low |
| Foot | Moderate | Large | High | Low |
| Eyes | High | Small | N/A | Moderate |

*N/A,* not applicable.

course of a day. This fluctuation has a direct consequence on effector use and therefore on the control of assistive technologies.

Trauma or disease to the central nervous system that results in abnormal muscle tone, the presence of primitive reflexes, or abnormal righting or equilibrium reactions affect the individual's ability to maintain a stable upright posture and perform smooth, coordinated movements. When an individual does not have the ability to stabilize his body, assistive technologies can be used externally to obtain balance and functional positioning. (We discuss these assistive technologies in Chapter 6.) Lack of coordinated volitional movements may dictate the use of specialized controls that are enlarged or positioned in locations of maximal control (see Chapter 7).

## Characterization of Effector Movements

The movements of effectors can be characterized in several ways, as listed in Table 3-7. By defining the resolution, range, strength, and flexibility for an anatomical site, we can relate these to the skills required for the use of control interfaces.

**Resolution.** **Resolution** is used to define the degree of fine control, and it describes the smallest separation between two objects that the effector can reliably control. For example, the spacing of individual keys on a keyboard requires relatively fine motor control and an effector with good resolution. Alternatively, a 6-inch diameter single switch used to turn on a toy requires much lower resolution on the part of the effector. All the components of effector use that we have described contribute to the generation of high-resolution fine movements.

**Range.** We describe the maximal extent of movement possible as **range.** Some tasks require large range and others require small range. For example, the use of push rims on a manual wheelchair requires a relatively large range of movement, whereas the use of a computer mouse requires a relatively small range. The combination of resolution and

range allows us to define the workspace of the effectors. These are both affected by disease or injury. For example, *contractures* may occur as a result of increased tone. This is a shortening of the muscles and tendons that limits joint range of motion.

**Strength.** Another measure of effector performance is *strength* of movement. As designers of assistive technology systems, we must take into account the strength of the effector that we are considering for control of the system. In general the upper extremities function best when precision and control are required, and the lower extremities are best suited for power and strength. Control of assistive technology systems may require that a minimal level of strength, as reflected by the force required to activate a control interface, be available. Even if the necessary resolution and range are available, there may be insufficient strength to activate the control.

In some disabilities, strength is significantly reduced (or absent). For example, **paralysis** resulting from a spinal cord injury prevents the use of certain effectors, depending on the level of the injury (Table 3-8). In this case the major goal is to find an effector that is not paralyzed; head or chin control may be required, rather than a control interface activated by hand function. Partial paralysis or *paresis* is a muscle weakness that makes it difficult to move but does not prevent movement as paralysis does. In this case we must modify our assistive technology control interfaces to accommodate for reduced effector capabilities. For example, an adapted door handle could be used to require less force to be applied in order to turn the doorknob. In diseases such as muscular dystrophy, fine control is often available but muscle weakness results in very low levels of strength. This may lead to restricted movement over large distances, but fine movements such as those required for a contracted keyboard or a short-throw joystick may be possible.

It is also possible that strength is too great for adequate control. This often occurs when the foot is used for fine control such as typing on a keyboard. However, excessive strength is not restricted to the lower extremities. Spastic movements are poorly controlled, and they often lead to force in excess of that required for control. Because many control interfaces, such as joysticks, are designed for normal upper extremity levels of force, the excessive forces generated by spastic movements can result in damage to the assistive technology system, as well as poor performance.

**Endurance.** We are also interested in the ability of an individual to sustain a force. In contrast to strength, which is an indicator of the maximal force that can be exerted by an effector, *endurance* refers to the ability to sustain a force and to repeat the application of a force over time. In other neuromuscular disabilities, such as myasthenia gravis, the problem is one of *fatigue,* and initial strength may be within a

| TABLE 3-8 | Motions and Functions Available at Different Levels of Spinal Cord Injury | |
|---|---|---|
| Level of Injury | Active Motion Available* | Possible Functions |
| C3 | Neck motion | Unable to perform personal care |
| | Chin control | Directs others in transfers, personal care |
| | | Uses mouth or chin control for assistive technologies, ventilator on wheelchair |
| C4 | Neck motion | Same as C3 except: |
| | Shrugs shoulder | 1. No ventilator |
| | | 2. Shoulder switch available |
| C5 | Some shoulder motions | Assistance for bathing/dressing, bladder/bowel care, transfer |
| | | Uses mobile arm support for feeding, hygiene, grooming, writing, telephone (must be set up by attendant) |
| | Flex elbow, no extension | Uses chin or mouth control for assistive technologies |
| | | Can propel manual wheelchair short distances with hand rim projections |
| C6 | Wrist extension | Independent transfer, dressing, personal hygiene |
| | Forearm pronation | |
| | Full shoulder motions | Manual wheelchair possible with adapted rims, hand splints for writing, feeding, hygiene, grooming, telephone, typing |
| C7 | Wrist, elbow, shoulder motions; no finger grasp | Independent sitting |
| | | Drive with adapted controls; uses hand splints for manipulation |
| C8 | No intrinsic hand muscles; limited sensation in the fingers | Limited hand grasp with splints |
| T1 | Paralysis of intrinsic hand muscles; limited flexibility of hand | Weak unaided grasp |
| T2-T12 | Full use of upper extremities; increasing lower extremity function at lower levels; increasing trunk control at lower levels | Manual wheelchair; may use reachers; trunk supports required for higher levels |

Modified from Adler C: Spinal cord injury. In Pedretti LW, editor: *Occupational therapy: practice skills for physical dysfunction,* St Louis, 1996, Mosby.
*At each lower level, all the functions of higher levels are available plus those listed for the given level.

normal range. However, as the individual repeats a movement, there is a continual decrease in performance until total fatigue occurs. We can provide for this in several ways. First, the interface between the human and the device can be designed to minimize the amount of fatigue by requiring low energy expenditure. We can also design the device so it is flexible and reduces the amount of effort as the person tires. An example of the first approach is a joystick for a wheelchair, which requires very little travel and small force. An example of adaptation to fatigue is a variable scanning rate so that when the user is fresh, the scanning is rapid (and selections can be made quickly), but when the person tires, the scan rate slows down to accommodate. The slowdown could be automatically triggered by erroneous entries or manually selected by the user or an attendant. These approaches may be necessary in order to allow continued functional performance in the presence of fatigue. The careful consideration of the strength and endurance available to move an effector is crucial to the successful application of assistive technology systems.

**Versatility.** Some effectors are capable of being used for a variety of tasks and in a variety of different ways for the same task. We refer to this characteristic as *versatility*. For example, both the hand (fingers) and foot (toes) can be used to press a key or switch. However, the hand can also be used to grasp a handle (e.g., a joystick). Thus the hand is more versatile than the foot. The higher the versatility, the more options provided for the use of the effector to control an assistive device. This is directly reflected in our choice of control interfaces (see Chapter 7) and in the overall design of the human/technology interface.

## ■ SUMMARY

The emphasis of this chapter has been on the human operator of assistive technologies. The use of the basic information processing model shown in Figure 3-1 has allowed us to describe the many components that underlie human performance. This model is also utilized in succeeding chapters as we discuss specific assistive technology systems. In the next chapter we explore the assessment of these areas of performance for the purpose of matching assistive technologies to the skills and needs of persons with disabilities.

## Study Questions

1. Distinguish between sensation and perception.
2. Assume that you determine the total reaction time for an upper-arm reaching task. Referring to Table 3-6, how would you expect the various components of this total to change (i.e., increase or decrease) given the following conditions: (a) muscular dystrophy, (b) spinal cord injury at the T2 level, (c) traumatic brain injury, (d) cerebral palsy, (e) Hansen's disease (loss of peripheral sensation)?
3. What is the difference between visual tracking and visual scanning? How do the oculomotor mechanisms that underlie them differ?
4. What is visual accommodation, and how can it affect assistive technology use?
5. What are the three major characteristics that can be changed to increase visual input?
6. If you knew that a person with whom you were working had a severe peripheral visual loss, what color of stimulus would you use to try to maximize visibility (refer to Figure 3-3)?
7. If a person is reported as having a 40-dB hearing loss at 2000 Hz, what was the actual intensity of sound applied to the ear (refer to Figure 3-6)?
8. How is the degree of self-produced locomotion related to integration of visual and vestibular sensory function? Relate this to dependent and independent wheeled mobility.
9. Explain why prism glasses experiments produce the results they do, including the effects on kinesthetic perception.
10. Assume that you are trying to develop a word processing program for use as an augmentative writing system. How would your design differ for a preoperational, concrete operational, and formal operations person? Focus on the user interface (screen commands, loading files, etc.) to the system and special features that you would or would not include. Also include the method you would use to introduce the program to each group.
11. Is motor capability necessary for the development of cognitive skills? If yes, how much capability is required? Explain and justify your answer.
12. What are the major notions involved in self-concept?
13. How is self-concept related to the physical abilities and attributes of the assistive technology user?
14. List and describe the stages of loss typically experienced by a person who has sustained an injury or disease resulting in permanent disability.
15. How is the concept of self-protection related to the acquisition and use of assistive technologies?
16. How can difficulties in self-concept or self-protection lead to abandonment of assistive technologies?
17. What are the six factors that affect motivation? How can each of these be incorporated into an assistive technology system? Give an example for each factor.
18. What are the three types of memory distinguished on the basis of time?
19. What is the difference between recognition and recall? How does each apply to assistive technology device use?
20. What are the five basic elements of language? Distinguish between speech and language.
21. What is the difference between problem solving and decision making?
22. Design a flow chart similar to Figure 3-7 for a program of your choice. Assume that the user has short-term memory deficits that make it difficult to follow a sequence of steps.
23. Explain the meaning of the solid and dashed curves in Figure 3-9. What type of curves would you expect if the individual lacked good trunk support to each side?
24. What are the implications of a decrease in motor path variability on assistive technology use?
25. Distinguish between range and resolution for an effector system.
26. How does the age at which an individual is introduced to assistive technology influence acceptance and successful use of assistive technologies?
27. How does the age at which an individual is introduced to assistive technologies relate to the possibility of abandonment of those technologies?

## References

Allen J: Linguistic-based algorithms offer practical text-to-speech systems, *Speech Technol* 1(1):12-16, 1981.

Bailey RW: *Human performance engineering*, ed 2, Englewood Cliffs, NJ, 1989, Prentice Hall.

Barnes KH: Training young children for powered mobility beyond the standard joystick, *Developmental Disabilities Special Interest Section Newsletter, American Occupational Therapy Association* 14(2):1-2, 1991.

Batt RC, Lounsbury PA: Teaching the patient with cognitive deficits to use a computer, *Am J Occup Ther* 44:364-367, 1990.

Bobath B: *Adult hemiplegia: evaluation and treatment*, ed 2, London, 1978, William Heinemann Medical Books.

Brainerd CJ: *Piaget's theory of cognitive development*, Englewood Cliffs, NJ, 1978, Prentice Hall.

Brinker RP, Lewis M: Discovering the competent infant: a process approach to assessment and intervention, *Top Early Child Ed* 2(2):1-16, 1982a.

Brinker RP, Lewis M: Making the world work with microcomputers: A learning prosthesis for handicapped infants, *Except Child* 49(2):163-170, 1982b.

Brooks VB: *The neural basis of motor control*, New York, 1986, Oxford University Press.

Burgess MK: Motor control and the role of occupational therapy: past, present and future, *Am J Occup Ther* 43:345-348, 1989.

Campos JJ, Bertenthal BI: Locomotion and psychological development in infancy. In Jaffe KM, editor: *Childhood powered mobility: developmental, technical and clinical perspectives*, Washington, DC, 1987, RESNA Press.

Chapman RS: Exploring children's communicative intents. In Miller JF, editor: *Assessing language production in children*, Baltimore, 1981, University Park Press.

Cook AM, Liu KM, Hoseit P: Robotic arm use by very young children, *Assist Technol* 2(2):41-57, 1990.

Cress PJ et al: Vision screening for persons with severe handicaps, *TASH J* 6(Fall):41-49, 1981.

Davies PM: *Steps to follow: a guide to the treatment of adult hemiplegia*, New York, 1985, Springer-Verlag.

Depoy E, Kolodner EL: Psychological performance factors. In Christiansen C, Baum C, editors: *Occupational therapy*, Thoroughfare, NJ, 1991, Slack.

Duckek J: Cognitive dimensions of performance. In Christiansen C, Baum C, editors: *Occupational therapy*, Thoroughfare, NJ, 1991, Slack.

Duckman R: Incidence of visual anomalies in a population of cerebral palsied children, *J Am Optom Assn* 50:607-614, 1979.

Dunn W: Sensory dimensions in performance. In Christiansen C, Baum C, editors: *Occupational therapy*, Thoroughfare, NJ, 1991, Slack.

Early MB: *Mental health concepts and techniques for the occupational therapy assistant*, ed 2, Raven Press, New York, 1993.

Erhardt RP: Sequential levels in the visual motor development of a child with cerebral palsy, *Am J Occup Ther* 41(1):43-49, 1987.

Farber SD: Neuromotor dimensions of performance. In Christiansen C, Baum C, editors: *Occupational therapy*, Thoroughfare, NJ, 1991, Slack.

Fiorentino MR: *Normal and abnormal development: the influence of primitive reflexes on motor development*. Springfield, Ill, 1978, Charles C Thomas.

Fitts PM: The information capacity of the human motor system in controlling the amplitude of movement, *J Exp Psychol* 47:381-391, 1954.

Fitts PM, Deininger RL: S-R compatibility; correspondence among paired elements within stimulus and response codes, *J Exp Psychol* 48:483-492, 1954.

Flash T, Hogan N: The coordination of arm movements: an experimentally confirmed mathematical model, *J Neurosci* 5:1688-1703, 1985.

Fons K, Gargagliano TA: Articulate automata: an overview of voice synthesis Gelfan, *Byte* 6(2):164-187, 1981.

Georgopoulos AP, Kalaska JF, Massey JT: Spatial trajectories and reaction times of aimed movements: effects of practice, uncertainty, and change in target location, *J Neurophysiol* 46:725-743, 1981.

Goldenberg EP: *Special technology for special children*, Baltimore, 1979, University Park Press.

Goosens CA, Crain SS: Overview of non-electronic eye-gaze communication, *Augment Altern Commun* 3:77-89, 1987.

Held R, Hein A: Movement-produced stimulation in the development of visually-guided behavior, *J Comp Physiol Psychol* 81:394-398, 1963.

Hopkins HL, Smith HD, editors: *Willard and Spackman's occupational therapy*, ed 8, Philadelphia, 1993, JB Lippincott.

Jagacinski RJ, Monk DL: Fitts' law in two dimensions with hand and head movements, *J Mot Behav* 17:77-95, 1985.

Janeschild M: Early power mobility: evaluation and training guidelines. In Furumasu J, editor: *Pediatric powered mobility: developmental perspectives, technical issues, clinical approaches*, Arlington, Va, 1997, RESNA Press.

Kangas KM: Seating, positioning and physical access, *Developmental Disabilities Special Interest Section Newsletter, American Occupational Therapy Association* 14(2):4, 1991.

Kauffman JM, Payne JS, editors: *Mental retardation*, Columbus, Ohio, 1975, Charles E Merrill.

Kermoian R: Locomotor experience facilitates psychological functioning. In Gray DB, Quantrano LA, Lieberman ML, editors: *Designing and using assistive technology*, Baltimore, 1988, Paul H Brookes Publishing.

Kielhofner G: A model of human occupation. 2: Ontogenesis from the perspective of temporal adaptation, *Am J Occup Ther* 34:657-663, 1980.

King TW: *Assistive technology: essential human factors*, Needham Heights, Mass, 1999, Allyn & Bacon.

Klemmer ET, Lockhead GR: Productivity errors in two keying tasks: A field study, *J Appl Psychol* 46:401-408, 1962.

Lee WA: A control system framework for understanding normal and abnormal posture, *Am J Occup Ther* 43:291-301, 1989.

Light J: Interaction involving individuals using augmentative and alternative communication systems: state of the art and future directions, *Augment Altern Commun* 4(2):66-82, 1988.

Light J, Beesley M, Collier B: Transition through multiple augmentative and alternative communication systems: a three-year case study of a head injured adolescent, *Augment Altern Commun* 4(1):2-14, 1988.

Livneh H, Antonak R: Reactions to disability: an empirical investigation of their nature and structure, *J Appl Rehabil Counsel* 21:12-21, 1990.

Livneh H, Antonak R: Temporal structure of adaptation to disability, *Rehabil Counsel Bull* 34:298-319, 1991.

Mandler JM: A new perspective on cognitive development in infancy, *Am Sci* 78(3):236-243, 1990.

Mann RW: Technology and human rehabilitation: prostheses for sensory rehabilitation and sensory substitution. In Brown JHU, Dickson JF, editors: *Advances in biomedical engineering*, New York, 1974, Academic Press.

Meyer DE, Smith KJ, Wright CE: Models for the speed and accuracy of aimed movements, *Psychol Rev* 89:449-482, 1982.

Miller GA: *Language and speech*, San Francisco, 1981, Freeman.

Nolan C: *Under the eye of the clock*, New York, 1987, St. Martin's Press.

Padula WV: *A behavioral vision approach for persons with physical disabilities*, Santa Ana, Calif., 1988, Optometric Extension Program Foundation.

Pedretti LW: *Occupational therapy: practice skills for physical dysfunction*, 4th ed, St Louis, 1996, Mosby.

Radwin RG, Vanderheiden GC, Lin ML: A method for evaluating head-controlled computer input devices using Fitts' law, *Hum Factors* 32:423-431, 1990.

Robertson SC: Treatments for psychosocial components: intervention for mental health. In Neistadt ME, Crepeau EB, editors: *Willard and Spackman's occupational therapy*, ed 9, Philadelphia, 1998, Lippincott-Raven.

Sabari JS: Occupational therapy after stroke: are we providing the right services at the right time? *Am J Occup Ther* 52:299-302, 1998.

Santrock JW: *Life-span development*, Madison, Wis, 1997, Brown and Benchmark.

Scherer MJ: *Living in the state of stuck: how technology impacts the lives of people with disabilities*, Cambridge, Mass, 1993, Brookline Books.

Scherer MJ: The impact of assistive technology on the lives of people with disabilities. In Gray DB, Quatrano LA, Lieberman ML, editors: *Designing and using assistive technology: the human perspective*, Baltimore, 1998, Paul H Brookes Publishing.

Scherer MJ and Galvin JC: An outcomes perspective of quality pathways to the most appropriate technology. In Galvin JC, Scherer MJ, editors: *Evaluating, selecting and using appropriate assistive technology*, Gaithersburg, Md, 1996, Aspen Publishers.

Stach BA: *Clinical audiology*, San Diego, 1998, Singular Publishing Group.

Smith W, Crook SB: Phonemes, allophones, and LPC team to synthesize speech, *Electron Des* 25:121-127, 1981.

Trefler E: *Seating for children with cerebral palsy*, Memphis, 1984, University of Tennessee Press.

Trombly CA, Scott AD: *Occupational therapy for physical dysfunction*, Baltimore, 1977, Williams and Wilkins.

Tychsen L, Lisberger SG: Maldevelopment of visual motion processing in humans who had strabismus with onset in infancy, *J Neurosci* 6:2495-2508, 1986.

Undzis MF, Zoltan B, Pedretti LW: Evaluation of motor control. In Pedretti LW, editor: *Occupational therapy: practice skills for physical dysfunction*, St Louis, 1996, Mosby.

Verburg G: Predictors of successful powered mobility control. In Jaffe KM, editor: *Childhood powered mobility: developmental, technical and clinical perspectives*, Washington, DC, 1987, RESNA Press.

Warren M: Strategies for sensory and neuromotor remediation. In Christiansen C, Baum C, editors: *Occupational therapy*, Thoroughfare, NJ, 1991, Slack.

# PART 2

# Service Delivery in Assistive Technologies

# Delivering Assistive Technology Services to the Consumer

---

## Chapter Outline

## Learning Objectives

Upon completing this chapter you will be able to:

1. Describe principles related to assessment and intervention in assistive technology service delivery
2. Describe the methods used to gather and analyze information during assistive technology assessment and intervention
3. Understand the relationship between the consumer's life roles and performance areas and his or her needs for assistive technology
4. Identify and describe each of the steps in assistive technology service delivery
5. Discuss the matching of device characteristics to consumer needs and skills
6. Understand the need for training and how to develop effective programs
7. Define outcomes as related to assistive technology
8. Understand why outcomes in assistive technology need to be measured
9. Discuss the principles of outcome measurement and their relationship to service delivery and system effectiveness
10. Understand how measurement of outcomes in related disciplines can contribute to knowledge and development of assistive technology outcome measurements
11. Understand the unique outcomes measurement needs of the field of assistive technology
12. Describe the primary outcome measurement tools developed for outcome assessment in assistive technology service delivery programs

## Key Terms

Assessment
Criteria for Service
Criterion-Referenced Measurement
Device Characteristics
Expert Systems
Functional Performance Measures
Follow-along
Follow-up

Health-Related Quality of Life
Implementation Phase
Needs Identification
Norm-Referenced Measurements
Outcome Measures
Operational Competence
Performance Aid
Quantitative Measurement

Qualitative Measurement
Quality of Life Measures
Referral and Intake
Strategic Competence
Technology Abandonment
User Satisfaction Measures
User Satisfaction

Service delivery is the provision of hard and soft assistive technologies to the consumer. In Chapter 1 we delineated the components of the assistive technology industry, which has at its core the consumer and service delivery programs. This chapter describes the process by which the consumer obtains assistive technology devices and services. Chapter 2 described a model that is used as the basis for assistive technology assessment and intervention (Human Activity Assistive Technology [HAAT] model) and discussed the principles of assistive technology system design. This chapter builds on the HAAT model by delineating systematic methods of assessment and intervention that help the assistive technology provider (ATP) define the components of the model and integrate them into an effective assistive technology system for each individual consumer. The intrinsic enablers of the human and his or her relationship to the use of assistive technologies, as discussed in Chapter 3, provide the foundation for the discussion of evaluation of consumer skills in this chapter.

To effectively provide these services to the consumer, the ATP should be knowledgeable in the following areas:

1. The principles related to assessment and intervention and methods of gathering and interpreting information
2. The service delivery practices used to determine the consumer's needs, evaluate his skills, recommend a system, and implement the system
3. The measurement of outcomes of the assistive technology system that indicate whether the identified goals have been achieved
4. The identification and attainment of funding for services and equipment

In this chapter and in Chapter 5 we present general principles and practices related to each of these areas.

## ■ PRINCIPLES OF ASSISTIVE TECHNOLOGY ASSESSMENT AND INTERVENTION

The assistive technology intervention begins with an **assessment** of the consumer. Through this assessment, information about the consumer is gathered and analyzed so that appropriate assistive technologies (hard and soft) can be recommended and a plan for intervention developed. Information is gathered regarding the skills and abilities of the individual, what activities she would like to perform, and the contexts in which she will be performing these activities. The assessment also yields information regarding the consumer's ability to use assistive technologies. Based on the assessment results, a plan for intervention is developed. This plan includes implementation of the system, follow-up, and follow-along. Basic principles that underlie assessment and intervention in assistive technology service delivery are listed in Box 4-1.

---

**BOX 4-1**   **Principles of Assessment and Intervention in Assistive Technology**

- Assistive technology assessment and intervention should consider all components of the HAAT model: the human, the activity, the assistive technology and the context.
- The purpose of assistive technology intervention is not to rehabilitate an individual or remediate impairment, but to provide assistive technologies that *enable* an individual to perform functional activities.
- Assistive technology assessment is ongoing and deliberate.
- Assistive technology assessment and intervention require collaboration.
- Assistive technology assessment and intervention require an understanding of how to gather and interpret data.

---

## Assistive Technology Assessment and Intervention Should Consider All Components of the HAAT Model: Human, Activity, Assistive Technology, and Context

Often AT assessment focuses on the assistive technology only. This can lead to later rejection or abandonment of the technology. One way to reduce the probability of this is to systematically consider all four parts of the HAAT model. Needs and goals are often defined by a careful consideration of the activities to be performed by the individual. However, it is rare that the activity will be performed in only one context, so it is important to identify all the possible contexts in which the activities will be performed. This includes the setting and social context. More global considerations that can lead to success or failure are cultural and physical contexts (see Chapter 2). Thus the careful evaluation of the activities to be performed and the contextual factors under which that performance will occur are key to success. Once the goals have been identified, an assessment of the skills and abilities of the human operator (the consumer) must be identified. Only after consideration of these three components (activity, context, and human) can a clear picture emerge of the assistive technology requirements and characteristics. The assessment process must also include an assessment of the degree to which these characteristics match the consumer's needs. Chances of success in implementation of an assistive technology system are enhanced by attention to all four parts of the HAAT model during the service delivery process.

### Assistive Technology Intervention Is Enabling

The *primary* purpose of assistive technology intervention is not remediation or rehabilitation of an impairment, but provision of hard and soft technologies that *enable* an individual with a disability to be functional in activities of daily living. This principle places the focus on functional outcomes. Through the application of the HAAT model we can develop goals for the assistive technology intervention, and these goals ultimately are used to measure the functional outcomes of the intervention. Approaching intervention from this perspective requires that the ATP determine the individual's strengths and capitalize on them instead of focusing on deficits or impairments. For example, consider the functional activity of typing. If we were to use a rehabilitation approach, the goal would be to improve hand and finger control sufficiently to allow for typing, with the intervention focusing on exercises and activities for the fingers and hands. From an assistive technology perspective, however, the objective becomes enabling the person to perform the functional activity of typing regardless of how it is done. The impairment in the hands and fingers that causes the disability is not necessarily addressed. The disability of being unable to type is what is addressed in the assistive technology approach. Through the use of assistive technology, alternative approaches to using the fingers for typing are considered, such as using a mouthstick, head pointer, or a speech recognition system instead of the hands.

This focus on function does not mean an individual's potential for improvement is ignored. The *parallel interventions model* (Angelo and Smith, 1989; Smith, 1991) demonstrates how technology can be used to promote the dual objectives of enabling function and improving an individual's skill level. In one track, assistive technologies are provided that are based on the consumer's current skills and needs and maximize his function. Simultaneously, a second track provides intervention that focuses on improving his skill level so as to minimize his reliance on technology. Some individuals who have a severe physical disability may never have had the opportunity to develop their motor skills, and training to develop these skills can take months or years (Cook, 1991). A common example of this is an individual whose evaluation shows that she is able to use her head to activate a single switch to make simple choices on a computer. With training and a period of experience in using this switch, her head control may improve to the point where she can use a light beam positioned on her head to make direct choices with a dedicated communication device. The latter means of control would more quickly provide access to choices on a device and would be much less demanding cognitively. Although we have used an example related to physical access, the model could also be applied to developing cognitive and language skills. Careful decisions must be made in these situations in terms of funding, because often third-party funding sources allow the purchase of only one system for an individual.

## Assistive Technology Assessment Is Ongoing and Deliberate

Although assessment is typically considered a discrete event in the direct service delivery process, it is actually an ongoing process. Assistive technology assessment entails a series of activities linked together and undertaken over time. The activities that occur and the decisions that are made during the intervention are deliberate rather than haphazard. Information is gathered and decisions are made from the moment of the initial intake referral through follow-along.

The ATP reevaluates progress toward the goals of the intervention plan and makes necessary revisions. For example, during training, observation may reveal that the consumer can access the control interface more effectively if it is positioned at an angle instead of flat. As our decisions are implemented, we continuously assess their impact and make revisions to the intervention. Schon (1983) defines this as *reflection-in-action*. Schon also describes a reflective contract

between the consumer and the practitioner in which the practitioner gives up a claim to authority and their interaction becomes one of shared control. This type of interaction allows the consumer to question the ATP and the ATP to reflect openly on his knowledge base and on the meaning and results of his advice. This coincides with our earlier discussion in Chapter 1 in which we describe the consumer as a co-developer in the design of the assistive technology system.

Assessment is ongoing not only while the consumer is actively involved in the service delivery process but also potentially throughout the consumer's life. Because many individuals have lifelong disabilities, they will be in need of assistive technology throughout their lives. It is important not only to recommend assistive technology that enables the individual today but also to predict the technology that will be necessary to enable the individual in the future. The components of the HAAT model change over each individual's lifetime. Changes may occur in the individual's skills and abilities, life roles, and goals; the capabilities of technology; and the context in which the assistive technologies are used. Using the HAAT model as a framework, the ATP can predict some of these changes and plan for the consumer's future technology needs.

## Assistive Technology Assessment and Intervention Require Collaboration and a Consumer-Centered Approach

Given the nature of assistive technology and its impact on the consumer's activities of daily living, it is essential that the assessment and intervention be a collaborative process. McNaughton (1993) defines a collaborator as "one who works with another toward a common goal" (p. 8). Furthermore, she states that collaboration requires that (1) all participants be equal partners; (2) a problem-solving attitude be shared by all participants; (3) there be mutual respect for each other's knowledge and the contributions each person can make, as opposed to the titles he or she holds; and (4) each participant have available the information necessary to carry out his or her role (McNaughton, 1993).

Frequently, assistive technology services are provided via consultation, in which the ATP is called into a situation on a limited basis to specifically address the assistive technology needs of the consumer. There may be several people already involved with the consumer, including family members, teachers, vocational counselors, employers, therapists, and representatives from the funding source. The assistive technology assessment and intervention is more successful when these significant others are identified and involved at the beginning of the process.

There is a delicate balance between the opinion and "expertise" of the ATP (based on technical knowledge and experience with a variety of people) and the opinion and "expertise" of the consumer and family relating to the specific needs and goals of the person. The role of the ATP is to educate the consumer of the choices available to her so that she can make decisions related to the assistive technology in an informed manner. The challenge for the ATP is to do this without unduly influencing her choice. The value of this approach is that the consumer and the ATP inform each other throughout the process and develop a shared responsibility for the outcome. This approach has been referred to as the "educational model" of intervention (as opposed to the "expert" and "consumer-driven" models, which take one extreme position or the other). Lysack and Kaufert (1999) describe this process and its benefits.

The ATP should initiate the collaborative process by identifying significant others as a part of the intake referral phase. For example, Jerry, who has a developmental disability, lives in a small group home. During the intake, the ATP discovers there are several key people who need to be involved in the assistive technology intervention for Jerry: staff at his home; staff at the day program he attends; an occupational therapist, who consults with his residential program; his caseworker at the department of developmental services; and his parents, who live out of town. Each of these individuals is invited to participate in the initial assessment and decision-making process. Different participants will be working with the consumer to accomplish different goals. Communication among the collaborators regarding their respective goals for the consumer is critical. It is important to identify the ways in which the goals of the assistive technology intervention can be accomplished without interfering with other goals. Sometimes compromises need to be reached. For example, two professionals working with the consumer may be focusing on different goals, and compromises may need to be made by all parties in working toward these interdependent goals. One therapist may be working with a child on improving the strength in her neck muscles to improve head control, whereas the ATP's goal may be to support and position the head in an upright position to prevent deformity and allow optimal position for functional activities. The two professionals may need to set up a schedule to allow time when the child uses the supports so that functional activities can be performed and time when strengthening of the muscles is worked on without the supports. The success of the assistive technology system depends on coordination and teamwork among all the individuals involved with the consumer.

Beukleman and Mirenda (1998) discuss the importance of building consensus among the user, family members, and other team members. Negative consequences, such as a lack of vital information for intervention; lack of "ownership" of the intervention, resulting in poor follow-through with the recommendations; and distrust of the service provider, may result if the process of consensus building is not begun during the initial assessment. Initiating this process early on helps to avoid problems in the future with regard to the acceptance and utilization of a device.

## Assistive Technology Assessment and Intervention Require an Understanding of How to Gather and Interpret Data

In Chapter 2 we define human performance as "the result of a pattern of actions carried out to satisfy an objective according to some standard" (Bailey, 1989). It is both possible and desirable to measure human performance, and much of what we describe in this chapter is directed toward that end. When making measurements, we use clinical standards as guidelines for evaluating performance and making decisions. In assistive technology service delivery we need to be careful that we know what we are measuring. In some cases, as when we are determining the effectiveness of our service delivery process and outcomes, we want to measure the performance of the entire assistive technology system. Because we have defined this system to be the four components of the HAAT model (human, activity, context, and assistive technology), we must develop measurements and standards that apply to the entire system. In other cases (e.g., during an initial assessment) we want to measure *human performance* rather than system performance. Measuring human performance can be general or task specific (Sprigle and Abdelhamied, 1998). An individual's *general abilities* are measured when we evaluate separate components of the sensory, perceptual, physical, and cognitive systems, such as range of motion, sensation, strength, tone, or memory. Task-specific measurement involves the evaluation of the individual's *functional skills*. The ability of the person to complete a functional task, such as entering text into a computer document, requires a level of skill that combines physical, sensory, and cognitive abilities. In this case we must establish clear objectives for each task, develop a clinical standard to be applied, and then develop measures that evaluate the performance.

In this section we focus on the principles associated with measurement in assistive technology service delivery. These include the purposes, types, standards, and methods of measurement.

**Quantitative and qualitative measurement.** Information gathered by the ATP throughout the assistive technology intervention can be by either **quantitative measurement** or **qualitative measurement**. A *quality* is "an intelligible feature by which a thing may be identified"; to qualify is "to characterize by naming an attribute" (*Webster's Ninth New Collegiate Dictionary*, 1984, p. 963). A *quantity* is "an indefinite amount or number" (*Webster's Ninth New Collegiate Dictionary*, 1984, p. 963). Measurement of user satisfaction is an example that helps to illustrate the difference between these two types of measurements. We can quantify this measurement by developing a scale that rates the consumer's satisfaction from 1 (unsatisfied) to 5 (satisfied). Alternatively, we can qualitatively describe the user's satisfaction based on observations of his behavior (e.g., the user appears to be less depressed since beginning to use the device).

There is a need in all areas of rehabilitation and education for the development and use of tools that allow professionals to quantify assessment information more objectively. As Kondraske (1990) points out, in rehabilitation the purpose of these tools is primarily to document the degree of disability or impairment. In the field of assistive technologies there is a need to develop tools that can provide quantitative measures to aid in the prescription, design, and determination of the outcomes of assistive technology (Enders and Hall, 1990; Kondraske, 1990).

Although there is a need for quantitative measures, it is not always practical or possible to capture all the necessary information in a quantitative measure. Qualitative measures can be just as valuable. It is important that qualitative measures be reliable and consistent. We describe methods that can be used to help the ATP gather reliable and consistent qualitative information. Whether the measures are qualitative or quantitative, it is essential that the ATP document the person's needs, skills, and abilities related to assistive device use.

### Norm-referenced and criterion-referenced measurements.

Two commonly used standards are employed for measuring performance (for both the human and the total system): norm referenced and criterion referenced. In **norm-referenced measurements** the performance of the individual or system is ranked according to a sample of scores others have achieved on the task. Norm-referenced measures usually produce a percentile rank, a standardized score, or a grade equivalent that indicates where the individual stands relative to others in the representative sample (Witt and Cavell, 1986). Most norm-referenced measures are based on a sample of nondisabled persons. This can be a limitation in assistive technology assessment where the consumers have disabilities. The norm-referenced test results cannot be applied to a person who lacks skills necessary for success in the test. For example, a person who is unable to speak cannot be expected to achieve an age-appropriate score on a test whose answers require verbal responses. Likewise, a person with limitations in fine motor control cannot be expected to achieve an average score on a normalized manual dexterity test. For these reasons, norm-referenced measures are generally not used in assessment for assistive technologies.

An alternative way to assess human or system performance is to rate the performance according to a specified criterion or level of mastery. This is referred to as **criterion-referenced measurement,** and the person's own skill level in using the system is used as the standard. As an example of this approach, Jagacinski and Monk (1985) evaluated joystick and head pointer use by young adult nondisabled subjects. They found that skill in using these devices is acquired with some difficulty over many trials. The criterion used was whether the individual's performance (time to move to target) did not change by more than 3% over a period of 4 consecutive days. This is illustrated in Figure 4-1. In this figure, the horizontal axis represents the elapsed practice time and the vertical axis represents how quickly the person has been able to use the joystick or head pointer to move to a target. The horizontal dotted line is the final level of performance and serves as the criterion of performance. Using this criterion, they found that joystick use required 6 to 18 days and head pointer use required 7 to 29 days of practice to reach the criterion level of performance. When we use this approach to measurement, we accomplish two desirable goals. First, we base our assessment of progress on the person's unique set of skills and do not attempt to relate this performance to a normalized standard. In this example, we can compare the two alternative ways of accomplishing the same task (joystick and head pointer) and determine which method is likely to result in a higher skill level. The second goal we accomplish by using the person's own performance as a standard is that we have a way of measuring progress. This is extremely important in assessing the efficacy and cost effectiveness of assistive technology intervention. If no progress is made, or if the progress does not lead to a satisfactory level of performance, then we need to change the technology (e.g., use a different control interface) or the training approach or both.

### Methods for gathering and interpreting information.

There are several methods used to gather and interpret quantitative and qualitative information about the consumer: (1) collection of the initial database, (2) interview procedures, (3) clinical assessment, and (4) formal assessment procedures (Dunn, 1991). Each of these is used at one time or another during the service delivery process. Often more than one method is used to gather information about the same aspect of a consumer's skills, the context, the activity, or the use of assistive technology. For example, information on an individual's hand function can be collected through each of these methods. We will illustrate this with Sam, a 22-year-old man with quadriplegia secondary to complete C6 lesion of the spinal cord, who is being evaluated for his ability to access a computer.

Information collected for the *initial database* may include the reason for referral, medical diagnosis, and educational and vocational background information. This information is collected during the referral and intake phase of the service delivery process; its purpose is to provide preliminary data for planning the assessment. Sam's medical diagnosis is complete quadriplegia at the C6 level. If we refer to a text describing the effects of spinal cord injury at the C6 level on arm function (see Table 3-8), we expect Sam to have scapular movements, shoulder flexion, elbow flexion, and wrist extension but to lack finger flexion and extension. Most medical histories do not provide information on the consumer's assets and functional abilities. In some cases we may unintentionally limit the consumer's potential if we fail to look beyond the expectations we have acquired based on the medical diagnosis. As Christiansen (1991) points out, a medical diagnosis may provide guidelines for the assessment and expectations regarding the nature of the consumer's impairments, but it is inadequate for planning intervention.

The *interview* is another way to collect information and can occur at different points in the service delivery process. Typically an initial interview takes place during the needs identification phase as a means of gathering information regarding the consumer and her needs. It is important that the consumer, family members, rehabilitation or education professionals, and other care providers be interviewed. In Sam's case, during the initial interview we can find out what his goals are and determine his particular needs related to using a computer. We can also learn which tasks he has difficulty performing. Finding out whether Sam currently uses any adaptive equipment, or has in the past, to complete functional tasks also provides us with valuable information about his hand function. For example, we may learn that Sam is able to sign his name using an adapted splint to assist with grasping the pen, but that it is difficult for him to write

and he tires quickly. This difficulty has led him to pursue the use of a computer to facilitate taking notes at school and completing homework assignments. Another stage in which the interview is important is follow-up. At this stage, interviewing the consumer or caregivers provides valuable information on whether the device is being used and how. It is important that the ATP develop the ability to conduct interviews so that useful information is gathered.

*Formal assessment procedures* are administered in a pre-scribed way and have set methods of scoring and interpreta-tion. Therefore they can be duplicated and analyzed. They may or may not be standardized. Through formal assess-ment procedures, Sam's arm and hand abilities can be quantified. For example, we can evaluate Sam's muscle strength in his upper extremities by performing a manual muscle test (Daniels and Worthingham, 1986). During this test, the therapist follows certain procedures for isolating specific muscles and asks the individual to move that particular body part to the best of his ability under condi-tions of gravity eliminated, gravity, and gravity plus resis-tance. The result is graded by giving a score ranging from 0 to 5 for each movement according to the ability of the consumer to complete it. The problem with this type of measurement is that it only provides us with information regarding a specific muscle group and does not provide us with information on Sam's ability to functionally use his upper extremity. For a measurement that is more specifically related to assistive technology use, we can measure Sam's

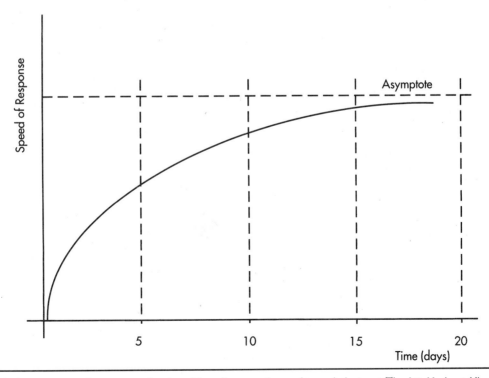

Figure 4-1    Speed of response to reach a target as a function of days of training. The *horizontal axis* is days of training. The *vertical axis* represents the speed to reach the target. The *dotted horizontal line* is the speed as performance levels off. This is used as the criterion for performance.

hand function as it applies to typing speed and accuracy. There are many software programs that teach typing using the computer and also include typing tests. By giving Sam a typing test we can gather information on reaction time, speed of typing, the number of errors made, and the types of errors made. However, it still does not tell us specifically how Sam has completed this task; for example, his posture in the wheelchair and whether he has used any strategies to stabilize himself are important. That type of information can be garnered only from skilled observation.

*Clinical assessment techniques* involve skilled observation of the consumer and are used throughout the assessment and intervention process. The ATP may structure these techniques so that a series of steps is followed to determine specific skills or they may be intentionally left unstructured to see what takes place. Observation can be done during a simulated task in a clinic setting or in a context familiar to the consumer (e.g., classroom or workplace). Through skilled observation during the structured task of a series of typing tests, we may observe that Sam's typing speed and accuracy improve when he stabilizes himself with his left forearm and types with his right hand. Data from the formal manual muscle test as described above do not give us this information, nor do the scores on the typing test. Given the limitations of existing methods of quantitatively evaluating human performance for the use of assistive technology, it is vital that the ATP be skilled in observation and qualitative appraisal of performance, as well as in quantitative evaluation methods.

All these considerations lead to one very important conclusion: In the application of assistive technology systems, success is largely the result of the combined efforts of knowledgeable and competent clinicians who, in collaboration with informed consumers and caregivers, make decisions based on both specific knowledge and experience. This is exactly the situation that exists in any other field of rehabilitation or special education. The complexity of the total system, including the diversity of the individual and of disabilities, technologies, and contexts of use, dictates that when designing an assistive technology device, best practice is often a matter of using clinical reasoning rather than precise measurements.

## ◾ OVERVIEW OF SERVICE DELIVERY IN ASSISTIVE TECHNOLOGY

Regardless of the type of service delivery model (see Chapter 1), there is a basic process by which delivery of services to the consumer occurs. Figure 4-2 illustrates the steps involved in this intervention process. The first step is **referral and intake.** At this point, the consumer, or someone close to her, has identified a need for which assistive technology intervention may be indicated and contacts an ATP to make

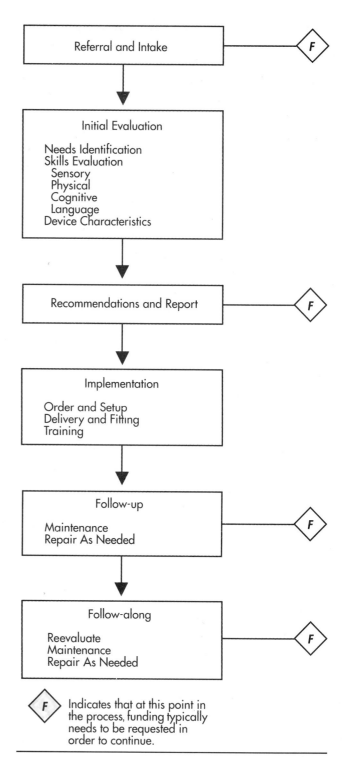

Figure 4-2   Steps in the service delivery process.

a referral. The service provider gathers basic information and determines whether there is a match between the type of services he provides and the identified needs of the consumer. Funding for the services to be provided is also identified and secured at this stage. Once the criteria for intake have been met, the *evaluation phase* begins. A more detailed specification of the consumer's assistive technology needs is the first step in this phase; this is referred to as *needs identification*. Following a thorough identification of the consumer's needs, the consumer's sensory, physical, and central processing skills are evaluated. Technologies that match the needs and skills of the consumer are identified, and a trial evaluation of these technologies takes place. The evaluation results are summarized and *recommendations* for technologies are made based on consensus among those involved. These findings are summarized in a written *report*, which is used to justify funding for the purchase of the assistive technology system.

When funding is secured, the consumer proceeds with the intervention in the **implementation phase.** At this phase, the equipment that has been recommended is ordered, modified, and fabricated as necessary; is set up; and is delivered to the consumer. Initial training on the basic operation of the device and ongoing training of strategies for using the device also take place during this phase.

Once the device has been delivered and training has been completed, we need to know whether the system as a whole is functioning effectively. This normally occurs during the follow-up phase, in which we determine whether the consumer is satisfied with the system and whether the goals that have been identified are being met. The follow-along phase actually closes the loop by putting in place a mechanism by which regular contact is made with the consumer to see whether further assistive technology services are indicated. If so, this brings the consumer back to the referral and intake phase and the process (wholly or partially) is repeated. Building this final phase into the service delivery process ensures that the consumer's needs are considered throughout her lifespan. Now let's take a more in-depth look at each of these steps.

## Referral and Intake

The service delivery process is usually initiated by a phone referral to the ATP. The purpose of the referral and intake phase is to (1) gather preliminary information on the consumer, (2) determine whether there is a match between the needs of the consumer and the services that can be provided by the ATP, and (3) tentatively identify services to be provided (Gaster, 1992).

The consumer, or the person making the referral on the consumer's behalf, recognizes a need for assistive technology services or devices, and this triggers the referral to the ATP. These identified needs are called **criteria for service,** and they define the objectives for the intervention. If there is a third party involved in the referral, such as a state vocational rehabilitation agency, they will have a set of policies and procedures that governs who is eligible to seek assistive technology intervention and what devices and services they

cover. For example, it is the policy of vocational rehabilitation agencies that the assistive technology helps the individual obtain or maintain employment. Langton and Hughes (1992) describe a framework for inclusion of assistive technology in the vocational rehabilitation case management process called "tech points." They identify key points during the consumer's vocational rehabilitation at which technology should be considered. This approach is valuable because it includes a mechanism through which the vocational case manager can monitor whether a criterion for assistive technology services exists for individuals in his caseload. Langton and Hughes also present a case study that illustrates the application of the tech point framework.

Depending on the policies of the ATP, referrals are accepted from a variety of sources. These sources include the consumer, a family member or care provider, a rehabilitation or educational professional, or a physician. At this time, information regarding the consumer's background and perceived assistive technology needs is gathered for the initial database. This includes personal information (e.g., age, place of residence), medical diagnosis and health information, and educational or vocational background. Information related to the individual's medical diagnosis and health information that may guide the assessment include the stability of the individual's condition (e.g., cerebral palsy), expected improvement (e.g., a person in rehabilitation after a head injury), or expected deterioration (e.g., amyotrophic lateral sclerosis).

The appropriateness of the referral is viewed from the perspective of both the ATP and the referral or funding source. When exchanging information about the consumer's needs and the services provided by the ATP, each party can determine whether there is a match. One outcome is that the needs of the consumer do not match the services provided by the ATP. For the consumer's benefit, this should be acknowledged and the consumer referred to another source that can more appropriately address her needs. The assistive technology provider should have, within the organization's mission statement, a policy that establishes what services are provided and who is eligible to receive services. For example, some assistive technology service providers specialize in certain disabilities (e.g., visual impairment), and others focus on specific technologies (e.g., seating technologies). Professional codes of ethics and standards of practice (see Chapter 1) require that ATPs practice within their specialization and not try to provide services outside of this realm.

The other outcome is that there is a match between the needs of the consumer and the services provided by the ATP. In this case, funding is sought and plans are made to move forward with the initial evaluation, starting with a thorough identification of the consumer's needs. From the information provided, the ATP also determines the level of service that would be most beneficial to the consumer.

There are a number of scenarios. First is the individual who has never used or been evaluated for assistive technologies. This could be an individual who is newly disabled or someone with a long-standing disability. An individual with a long-standing disability who may not have previously been a candidate for assistive technology services may now be able to access assistive devices because of recent advances in technologies. In this situation an in-depth assessment is warranted. Referrals may also be received from consumers who have used technology for some time and would like to evaluate current commercially available technologies. If this person's functional status has remained stable, it may not be necessary to conduct a complete evaluation. In some cases the assistive technology is not working or has been abandoned by the consumer and he is seeking a referral to see if modifications to the system can aid in making it more functional. Sometimes the consumer may only require further training or reevaluation of how she is using her current system to see whether training in new strategies would be beneficial. Similarly, there may be a new care provider who needs training or technical assistance.

## Initial Evaluation

Through a systematic evaluation, the ATP gathers information and facilitates decisions related to eventual device use. Because of the cost of the assistive technology to the consumer (or third-party funding source), it is essential that the ATP be able to assist the consumer in making informed decisions in the selection of a device. Current knowledge of the available technology and use of a systematic process facilitate the ATP's ability to make such decisions. This section focuses on the type of information gathered and the procedures used during the evaluation. Examples of assessment forms that capture most of the data discussed here are included in Appendices 4-1A and 4-1B.

## Needs Identification

Through the **needs identification** process we determine the individual's needs and goals, which provide the basis for the assistive technology intervention. Identifying the needs of the consumer is the most critical component of the service delivery process and is completed at the onset of evaluation. The information collected during needs identification is the cornerstone for measuring the effectiveness of the final outcome. Therefore it is important to take this step seriously and ensure that there is a consensus among those involved as to the nature and scope of the problem to be addressed by the assistive technology intervention and the goals identified to target these problem areas.

Information gathered during needs identification is also used by the ATP to justify purchase of services and equipment. Third-party payers who fund services and equipment want to know what the problem or need is and how the equipment is going to address the need. Finally, the needs identification process results in the development of a plan for completing the remainder of the evaluation. This includes composition of the evaluation team, determination of needed evaluation tools and devices, and identification of further information to gather (either through evaluation of the consumer or by request from outside sources).

Figure 4-3 provides a model for gathering and analyzing information regarding the person's life roles, performance areas, related activities, and tasks. The consumer's life role at the time influences his needs and goals. Is the individual a child or an adult? What are his life roles? Life roles include student, parent, employee, volunteer, and so on. It is important to note that as the individual's life roles change over time, so may the technology that is needed. Changing life roles, and therefore technology needs, is one of the reasons that consumers may return after a time to be reevaluated.

In relation to the consumer's life roles, there are performance areas (self-care, work, school, play, leisure) in which activities are accomplished. Identifying these performance areas helps the ATP to define the activities for which the consumer needs assistance. For example, play (performance area) is very important for a young child (life role), and a child with a disability may be precluded from manipulating toys (activity). Identifying the context in which the consumer will perform these activities is also critical. In Figure 4-3 we show needs identification for a student who is attending college. A major activity for this student is reading the material assigned from the textbook. The major part of this activity will take place at home for him, but he will also need to do some reading at school.

A task analysis of the skills required to complete the activity is conducted. The consumer and others identify to the best of their ability which tasks the consumer can likely perform himself and which tasks may need to be assisted with technology. This may be unknown in some cases, and the evaluation can determine which tasks the individual needs assistance with. In our example the activity of reading is broken down further into small tasks. If the student has a physical inability to hold the book and turn the pages, resulting in the need for manipulation of reading material, we identify this as a need in the third column. Another student may have difficulty with the activity of reading because of a visual impairment and require different technologies to meet this need.

The consumer's prior history with technology should also be discussed as part of the needs identification. Useful information can be gathered from the consumer's previous success or failure with using assistive technology. Has he had experience in using technology before, and if so, what technology was used and was the experience successful? If not, why? In our example the student had attempted to turn

| Life Roles/ Performance Areas | Activities | Difficult Tasks to Perform | Contexts | Prior Technology History |
|---|---|---|---|---|
| 1. College student education | 1. Reading class assignments in textbook | 1a. Holding the book<br>1b. Turning the pages | 1a. Home<br>1b. Library | 1. Has used mouthstick and bookholders in the past; encountered problems positioning book and mouth becoming tired from holding mouthstick |

| Intervention Goals: | Directions: |
|---|---|
| 1. Evaluate alternatives for holding reading material and turning pages in order to increase Joe's independence in reading. | 1. Identify consumer's life roles and performance areas.<br>2. Identify activities consumer is interested in performing.<br>3. Identify the specific tasks the individual has difficulty performing.<br>4. Identify the contexts in which these activities are carried out.<br>5. Determine if consumer has used technology in the past for the activity and what the outcomes were. |

Figure 4-3    Identifying consumer needs using the HAAT model.

the pages of different books with the use of a mouthstick, which turned out to be unsuccessful. It is important to identify and discuss reasons why the mouthstick did not work out for the individual. Perhaps the mouthstick was cumbersome and uncomfortable to use for any extended period, or perhaps he could physically perform the task with the mouthstick but didn't like the aesthetics of it.

Beukelmen and Mirenda (1998) discuss the need to identify actual or potential "opportunity barriers" and "access barriers" for the consumer. Although their model specifically targets consumers with augmentative communication needs, it also holds true for other areas of assistive technology. *Opportunity barriers* are imposed by individuals or situations that are not under the consumer's control. Generally the provision of assistive technology does not result in the elimination of these barriers. Beukelman and Mirenda (1998) identify five types of opportunity barriers: policy barriers, practice barriers, attitude barriers, knowledge barriers, and skill barriers. Policy barriers are legislative, regulative, or agency policies that govern situations in which consumers find themselves. For example, there are regulations in some school districts that restrict the use of school-purchased assistive technology to use in the school, preventing it from being taken home. Practice barriers refer to routine activities that are not dictated by policy but that constrain the use of assistive technologies. If the school's policy doesn't *require* that the device stay in the school, but the local teacher or principal has the practice of keeping the

devices in the school, the result is the same as if it were a policy. Attitude, knowledge, and skill barriers all apply to those individuals with whom the consumer interacts and on whom the effective use of the device depends. If the consumer's job supervisor has a negative attitude regarding the use of automatic speech recognition because it is distracting to other workers, it is an attitude barrier that prevents the consumer's participation in that job. Alternatively, the supervisor may have insufficient knowledge or skill regarding automatic speech recognition to ensure that it is effectively installed and made available to the consumer. The approach taken by the ATP to overcome opportunity barriers is very different depending on the type of barrier. It may involve training (for skills or knowledge), lobbying (for policy, attitude, or practice barriers), or a combination of the two.

*Access barriers* are barriers related to the abilities, attitudes, and resource limitations of the consumer or her support system (Beukelmen and Mirenda, 1998). During the needs assessment before an augmentative communication evaluation, for example, all the consumer's current ways of communicating can be identified. Known constraints related to user and family preferences and the attitudes of communication partners are other access barriers that should be identified. A potential barrier to accessing technology, one commonly seen during augmentative communication assessments, is resistance on the part of parents to pursue an augmentative communication device because they are worried that the use of such a device will inhibit the child's development of natural speech. As we discuss later in this chapter, the ability to find funding for assistive technology systems and services may also pose a barrier. Identifying potential and actual barriers (both opportunity and access) during needs assessment will help the ATP formulate strategies for assessment and intervention.

The information for the needs assessment can be derived from an interview or through a written questionnaire completed by the consumer or his representative. In Appendix 4-1A we provide one example of a questionnaire. Instruments such as the Matching Person and Technology Assessments (Scherer, 1998) can also be used by the ATP to identify the areas of the individual's needs and his predisposition to use assistive technology. If the information is gathered through a written questionnaire before actually meeting the consumer, it should be reviewed at the time of the first meeting with the consumer. The purpose of reviewing this material at the first meeting is to ensure that all the necessary information has been provided and to analyze the information to develop the goals. The total team should also be present at this meeting, and everyone's input regarding the needs and goals of the consumer can be discussed and a consensus reached.

## Skills Evaluation: Sensory

As discussed in Chapter 3, auditory, tactile, and visual senses all play a role in the use of assistive technology. In recommending assistive technologies, the ATP needs to be aware of the consumer's sensory abilities and limitations. The ATP is not expected to diagnose sensory impairments such as hearing loss or visual impairments. Consumers who have sensory impairments have usually undergone evaluation by a specialist (e.g., audiologist, ophthalmologist, or optometrist), and are able to provide the ATP with a report that details the degree of their impairment. If this testing has not occurred, the ATP should make a referral to an appropriate source before proceeding.

The ATP needs to be able to identify sensory functions that are available for using assistive technologies. If the primary disability is sensory, an alternative sensory pathway may need to be used and we need to know what the consumer's sensory capabilities are. For example, in the case of a consumer who is blind and who needs to read, the ATP must evaluate tactile and auditory skills that can substitute for vision during reading. This is discussed further in Chapter 12.

In other cases a consumer may have a sensory disability secondary to either a physical or cognitive limitation. For example, if a consumer is hard of hearing, the ATP needs to know how this will effect interaction with technology. This includes everything from hearing warning beeps when a computer error is made to understanding voice synthesis on a communication device.

**Evaluation of functional vision.** The most critical visual skills needed for assistive technology use are sufficient acuity to see the symbols used in the system of choice or to identify small objects in the environment; adequate visual field to allow input of information from a display (e.g., the keyboard or the monitor) or the environment; and sufficient visual tracking ability (e.g., for reading or tracking a moving cursor). During the initial interview, known visual problems should have been identified, but a visual screening may also identify previously undetected deficits. The ATP can evaluate the effect of these deficits related to the use of technologies.

Identifying any *visual field deficits* a consumer may have is extremely important in the application of assistive technology. Visual field is commonly assessed by having the consumer look straight ahead and then indicate when she first sees a moving stimulus appear in her peripheral visual field. The stimulus is held approximately 18 inches away and moved in an arc toward the consumer's midline. This is typically done for the right and left peripheral fields and the upper and lower fields. Peripheral field vision is considered intact if the stimulus is seen when it is parallel to the person's cheek and impaired if the individual does not indicate that she sees the object as it approaches the center of her face (Dunn, 1991).

We can often compensate for visual field limitations by carefully considering the placement of displays and controls to ensure that they fall within the visual field and by restricting the visual range (field size) required by the user of the assistive device. To help the user identify the visual field during scanning, a visual cue such as a colored piece of tape can be placed to the left of each row to be scanned. We can also use compensatory strategies. For example, a user of a powered wheelchair who has a restricted visual field can be taught to rotate his head from side to side to ensure that the entire field is visualized.

In some cases it is difficult to identify the effects of visual field limitations on assistive technology use. For example, individuals with a visual field deficit may make errors in typing because they do not see the whole keyboard. If we are not careful, we may interpret this as a physical limitation instead of identifying the visual field deficit. If we had assumed motor limitations, we might have made the keys larger so that the consumer could hit them more easily, an expensive and unnecessary step.

*Visual tracking* is the ability to follow a moving object. This skill is necessary for many assistive technology tasks, such as following a moving cursor on a screen, following the rotation of a plate with food in a feeder, or following objects in the environment while driving a wheelchair. Visual tracking is usually tested by having the consumer follow a moving object with her eyes. The object is held approximately 18 inches in front of the consumer and moved horizontally, vertically, and diagonally. The ATP notes whether the two eyes track together, whether the eye pursuits are smooth or jerky, whether there is a delay in the tracking, and whether the eyes can track without head movement.

Limitations in visual tracking ability may significantly reduce the options that we have for specifying and designing an assistive technology system. In particular these results have implications for the use of scanning augmentative communication systems in which the cursor moves left, right, up, and down (four-way directional scanning). It may be that an individual with a disability is able to track more easily to the right and down than to the left and up. In this case, two-way directional scanning, right and down, is preferable to using all four directions. When the cursor gets to the extreme right of the display, it automatically wraps around and begins from the left side again. Similarly, when it gets to the bottom, it wraps around to the top.

*Visual scanning* differs from visual tracking in that the object does not move; instead the eyes are moved to image different parts of a scene in order to find a desired object or location. This skill is used, for example, to locate obstacles during mobility and to scan a keyboard to find a specific key. The eye movements used in visual scanning are the same as those used in tracking. We often assess this capability by presenting arrays of pictures, symbols, words, or letters and asking the consumer to choose one item from the array. If the individual has difficulty visually scanning, then the number of items in the array should be limited. This often happens in the use of augmentative communication systems, where we begin with only two or three vocabulary choices and gradually expand the system to include more when the individual's visual scanning skills increase.

In Chapter 3 we described *visual accommodation* as the ability of the eyes to adjust to objects near and far. This is impaired in many persons with disabilities, and it is important to be aware of possible accommodative insufficiency during the assessment process. If an individual has problems accommodating, this may be observed by changing the visual focus between a monitor and keyboard. If the monitor and keyboard are far apart, the person may have more difficulty than if they are visually close. If a consumer appears to require much effort to copy letters on the screen, consider repositioning the keyboard or other input system so that the change of gaze is not too great.

An individual's ability to see objects (visual acuity) is affected by (1) the size of the object, (2) the contrast between the object and the background, and (3) the spacing between the object and surrounding background objects. These three considerations apply to symbols, as well as to objects. For testing of visual acuity, actual objects, photographs, line drawings, orthographic symbols, letters, and words are used. It is helpful to have a set of materials that includes objects of 3 to 4 inches high; large letters, pictures, and symbols 1 to 2 inches high; and letters and words down to the size of standard typewritten letters (an eighth of an inch) (Cook, 1988). Information gathered from the initial interview can guide the ATP as to the type and size of symbol to start with. The goal is to find the smallest size of symbol that can be seen well by the consumer and that results in accurate selections. This is tested by presenting two items of the selected size and symbol type at a time to the consumer. The individual is asked to identify one of the two items using the manner in which he usually indicates a choice (e.g., eye gaze, pointing, yes/no). Three trials of each size and symbol are completed before proceeding to the next smaller size, until the individual is no longer able to identify the item successfully. It is desirable for the consumer to be able to see a small size for a number of reasons. First, the smaller the size, the larger a given array of symbols can be. Second, this allows greater options in hardware and software, including standard keyboards and software that have been developed for the nondisabled population.

If the consumer is able to read but appears to have difficulty seeing words, the effects of various foreground-background combinations (to improve contrast) and letter spacing can be assessed using computer displays and software designed for this purpose (see Chapter 8). For example, most word processing software allows alteration in the background and foreground (letters) colors. Special software designed for persons with visual impairments also adds size variation to these capabilities. For computer applications, these features can improve performance.

We can improve visual performance by using enlarged graphics or text and by designing control panels with dark backgrounds and light lettering or controls. Identifying switches or keys with colors more distinguishable to the individual may be helpful. Switches can be light colored and placed on a dark background to improve recognition, and language board arrays can have bold dark letters or pictures on a white background, or vice versa. Likewise, video screens and the input array need to be carefully planned so that the amount of information presented is not cluttered.

**Evaluation of visual perception.** As we discussed in Chapter 3, visual perception is the process of giving meaning to visual information. Visual perceptual skills that need to be considered during the assessment include depth perception, spatial relationships, form recognition or constancy, and figure-ground discrimination. Formal testing of the consumer's visual perception may have been completed before the assistive technology assessment, and results of this can be gathered during the initial interview. It is necessary to observe the consumer during functional tasks and note any apparent perceptual problems. If there is still some concern regarding the exact nature of the problems, a formal evaluation such as the Motor Free Visual Perception Test (Colarusso and Hammill, 1972) or the Test of Visual Perception can be used. These tests and other visual perceptual evaluations are described by Dunn (1991).

If an individual has difficulties with visual perception, adaptations can be made. For example, if the person has difficulty finding an item in an array, decreasing the number of items in the field or creating more contrast between the foreground and background may help. Likewise, if icons are to be used with an individual who has perceptual problems, it may be helpful to select simple line drawings. Sometimes perceptual problems may be so severe that they preclude the use of assistive technologies such as powered wheelchairs because of safety concerns.

**Evaluation of tactile function.** There are three particular circumstances in which attention needs to be paid to the evaluation of tactile sensation. These occur during seating and positioning assessments, when evaluating tactile input for the use of control interfaces, and when considering the use of tactile alternatives to vision or hearing.

Somatosensory input is necessary for detecting forces or pressures exerted on the surface of the skin. Individuals who lack sensation may sit for prolonged periods without shifting position, and this can result in skin breakdown. The ATP needs to be aware of an individual's sensory status in these situations and be able to evaluate pressure on the sitting surface. Dunn (1991) presents a specific testing protocol for tactile response. Additionally, observation and monitoring of the skin surface is necessary. In Chapter 6 we discuss sitting pressure problems and relief activities in more detail.

Somatosensory function is responsible for providing information regarding the location of a control interface, the movements required to activate it, and whether it is successfully activated. Lack of ability to receive appropriate sensory input (e.g., because of Hansen's disease, nerve injuries, or sensory loss from aging) can severely limit the effective use of control interfaces. The initial interview generally reveals whether somatosensory deficits are present. During functional tasks, the ATP's skilled observation can identify limitations caused by sensory deficits. Dunn's (1991) sensory testing protocol can also be applied in this situation. In the case of decreased tactile sensation, the control interface needs to provide adequate feedback so that it compensates for the loss of sensory function (see Chapter 7). For example, it is possible to adapt computer keyboards to provide an audible beep whenever a key is pressed. This simple adaptation may be sufficient to compensate for an individual's tactile loss.

When visual or auditory function is inadequate for the input of information, we often use tactile substitutes (see Chapter 12). To determine whether this alternative sensory input is viable for an individual, we must evaluate tactile function. In particular, the skin response on one or more fingers is evaluated using two-point discrimination and similar tests. This evaluation is necessary because certain

---

**BOX 4-2**    **Steps in the Physical Skills Evaluation**

1. Obtain Functional Position
2. Identify Potential Anatomical Sites
   a. Evaluate functional movement skills
   b. Measure range
   c. Measure resolution
3. Select Candidate Interfaces
4. Perform Comparative Testing of Interfaces
   a. Non-computer-aided
   b. Computer-aided

---

diseases (e.g., diabetes) that result in loss of vision also cause reduced tactile sensation.

**Evaluation of auditory function.** The ATP, through the initial interview and observation during functional tasks, should be aware of any significant auditory impairments that may affect device use. In cases of suspected hearing loss, a formal evaluation by an audiologist should be requested. Basic information sought by the ATP should include whether the individual responds to auditory stimuli, is distracted by some or all sounds, recognizes specific auditory stimuli (e.g., someone calling her name), and responds appropriately to auditory stimuli (Dunn, 1991). For example, many augmentative communication devices emit a beep when a selection is made. For some individuals, this cueing is helpful; however, for others the beep may produce a startle reflex that interferes with the succeeding motor movement. The individual may eventually habituate to the beep, but it is important to consider a device that has the option of disabling it.

## Skills Evaluation: Physical

The overall goal of the *physical skills evaluation* is to determine the most functional position for the individual and evaluate his ability to access a device physically. Box 4-2 lists the steps involved in completing this process.

**Evaluation of seating and positioning needs.** Regardless of whether problems related to seating and positioning have been identified during the initial interview, the individual's seated position needs to be considered first during the physical evaluation. Careful observation of the individual's posture, reflex patterns, and muscle tone while at rest and while performing tasks is necessary. Changes in body position and their effects on the consumer's ability to control a device should be noted.

The individual needs to be in a position that optimizes her ability to operate an assistive device. Stabilization of the pelvis and trunk maximizes function in the extremities. If the individual does not have the ability to stabilize herself, external support provided by a seating system may be required. Individuals require varying degrees of support, and determining the appropriate amount of support needed is critical. As Kangas (1991) points out, there is a difference between stabilization or support and restraint, and for individuals to be successful in using assistive technologies, we need to offer support instead of restraint. This was the situation with Steven, who has cerebral palsy and was evaluated for an augmentative communication system. Based on this evaluation, an augmentative communication device was recommended. It was several months before funding was authorized and the device was ordered and prepared for delivery to Steven. By the time Steven returned for the delivery of his communication device, he had received a new wheelchair and seating system. The seating system supported him in all directions, including blocks at his knees. Unfortunately, even though Steven "looked good" in his new wheelchair, he was now so restricted he was unable to use his typical movement patterns to select the keys on his device. Steven's ability to operate his communication device improved once the knee blocks were removed and some of the other supports were adjusted to be less restraining. This example also illustrates the need for the ATP to know whether the consumer intends to have revisions made in his wheelchair or seating system in the near future. Sometimes it is advantageous to postpone evaluating an individual's ability to access a control interface and operate a device until these revisions have been made. In Chapter 6 we discuss in detail principles related to seating and positioning for various needs and technologies that are available to meet these needs.

### Identifying potential anatomical sites for control.

In Chapter 3 we identify the control sites that can potentially be used by the consumer to operate a device (see Figure 3-10) and describe the various movements each control site is capable of performing.

In evaluating individuals with physical disabilities, it helps to keep in mind the movement capabilities of each of these anatomical sites and the hierarchy in which these sites are considered. The hands and the fingers are the preferred control sites because they are naturally used during manipulation tasks and finer resolution can be achieved. If the hands are not an option for control, the head and mouth are considered next. With the use of mouthsticks, head pointers, or light beams, it is possible to achieve the fine resolution and range needed to control a device. The next option to consider is the foot. Some individuals are able to develop fine control of the foot for typing (Figure 4-4); however, problems with positioning the device so that it can be seen by the user make this site less desirable than the hands or the head. The least desirable sites are the legs or

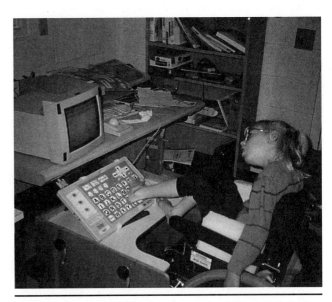

**Figure 4-4**   Child using her foot to control an expanded keyboard.

the arms because they are controlled by larger muscle groups, so the movements of these sites are gross in nature compared with the fine movements of smaller muscles (Cook, 1988).

Simulation of functional tasks is used to evaluate the types and quality of movement an individual possesses. Functional tasks are chosen for evaluation because they are often more meaningful to the consumer than physical performance components such as strength and joint range of motion. They also provide the ATP with an opportunity to gather qualitative information regarding the consumer's movements, and results of such tasks are more likely to reflect the consumer's true abilities.

We present a model based on clinical experience to determine the best anatomical site for accessing a control interface. The hands, being the control site of choice, are the first to be assessed. Basic hand function can be observed and rated using a "grasp module" (Figure 4-5), which includes a total of seven functional grasp patterns. The consumer's ability to complete each grasp pattern is rated (unable, poor, fair, or good). Notations are also made regarding how the consumer completed the movement and the factors that made it successful or not. For example: Did the object need to be positioned in a particular way for the consumer to grasp it? Was there a delay in initiating the movement? Did the consumer have difficulty releasing the object? Was the movement pattern isolated or synergistic in nature? Did the consumer appear to have problems with depth perception when reaching for the object?

If the consumer has the potential for hand use, it is then necessary to determine the minimal and maximal arm range within a workspace and the resolution in hitting a target. A range and resolution board, as shown in Figure 4-6, can be

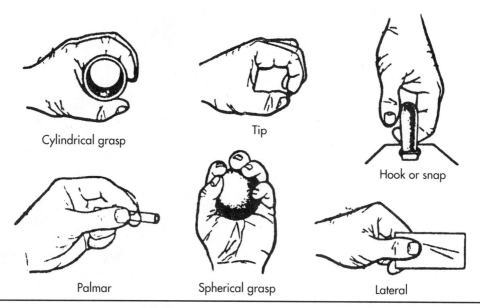

Cylindrical grasp          Tip                    Hook or snap

Palmar          Spherical grasp          Lateral

Figure 4-5   Functional grasp patterns for evaluating hand use.

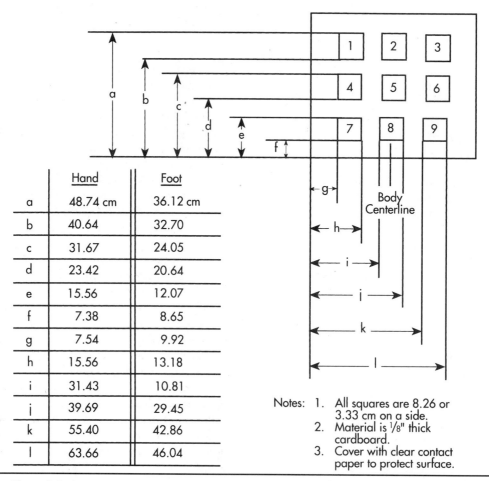

| | Hand | Foot |
|---|---|---|
| a | 48.74 cm | 36.12 cm |
| b | 40.64 | 32.70 |
| c | 31.67 | 24.05 |
| d | 23.42 | 20.64 |
| e | 15.56 | 12.07 |
| f | 7.38 | 8.65 |
| g | 7.54 | 9.92 |
| h | 15.56 | 13.18 |
| i | 31.43 | 10.81 |
| j | 39.69 | 29.45 |
| k | 55.40 | 42.86 |
| l | 63.66 | 46.04 |

Notes: 1. All squares are 8.26 or 3.33 cm on a side.
2. Material is ⅛" thick cardboard.
3. Cover with clear contact paper to protect surface.

Figure 4-6   Range and resolution board used for evaluating the ability to hit a target using a given control site.

used to measure both of these. If possible, the consumer is asked to use her thumb or a finger to point to each corner of each numbered square. If the consumer is unable to point to the corners, she is asked to touch each square with her whole hand. This provides information regarding the approximate size of the workspace and the best locations for a control interface, as well as a rough measure of accuracy of movement. Both arms are evaluated as appropriate.

If the hands are eliminated as a control site, other anatomical sites must be considered. For example, we can also measure range and resolution for the foot and head. With a range and resolution board of smaller dimensions, the same task can be used to evaluate foot range and targeting skills, as well as the consumer's range and resolution using a mouthstick, light pointer, or head pointer. Appendix 4-1B shows a sample assessment form for documenting the information gathered during the physical skills evaluation. After completion of this component of the skills evaluation, the ATP should have a good idea of the user's physical skills and the anatomical sites that can best be used to control an interface.

**Selecting candidate control interfaces.** Once the ATP has identified anatomical sites that the consumer can potentially use, the next step in the process is to select control interfaces that have potential to be used successfully by the consumer. In Chapter 7 we present a set of control interface characteristics that are useful in selecting interfaces that most closely match the consumer's available anatomical sites.

**Comparative testing of candidate control interfaces.** Having chosen potential anatomical sites and candidate control interfaces, we next measure the consumer's ability to use these interfaces. Comparative testing provides the ATP with data on the consumer's speed and accuracy in using particular control interfaces. These data can be used to compare different interfaces operated with a given site. If a control enhancer (e.g., mouthstick, head pointer) or modification (e.g., keyguard) is being considered, its use should also be evaluated (Chapter 7). This is one area where gathering quantitative information on the person's ability to use the control interface is extremely valuable and can assist the ATP in making decisions regarding the selection of a control site and interface. It is also important to note the consumer's preferences during this process.

During the assessment process, speed of response is often used to compare control interfaces. *Speed of response* is a temporal (time-based) measurement that can be quantified. Because these measurements are typically made in the controlled setting of the clinic, they must be carefully applied to contexts outside the clinic. Another measure used to compare control interfaces is *accuracy of response*. This is often based on moving to the correct position, and it is therefore a spatial measurement, rather than a temporal

(time-based) measure. Measurement of accuracy requires a standard of performance. This is usually the number of correct responses out of the total number of trials. Speed of response and accuracy are generally inversely proportional to each other for novice users.

Having defined these two basic parameters, we can now describe methods for measuring them. The selected control interface is first placed in a position where the consumer can activate it. It may be necessary to try different locations for the control interface before finding the position at which the consumer has the greatest control. The consumer's time to move from a rest position to target the control interface can be measured using a stopwatch.

Computer-assisted assessment provides several useful features. First, data collection and analysis can be automated, relieving the clinician of tedious record keeping. Performance measures for each possible control site/interface pair can be obtained. The effects of different positions for the control interface or the use of control enhancers and modifications can also be measured. Because several different control site/interface combinations can be evaluated, this data collection process can facilitate the choice of interfaces based on measured results. Second, the computer can provide a variety of contingent results (including graphics, sound, and speech) when the control interface is activated. This variety of results not only makes the task more interesting, but it also can allow assessment of visual and auditory capabilities.

## Skills Evaluation: Cognitive

In Chapter 3 we described the major cognitive skills associated with assistive technology use. Although there are standardized test batteries that are used for cognitive assessment (Duchek, 1991), in general we do not use them for evaluating consumer's cognitive skills related to assistive technologies. Instead, clinical observation is the major strategy utilized for the collection of information regarding a consumer's cognitive function. Clinical observation yields information that is often not provided by standard tests. For example, when observing a consumer using a switch-activated program on the computer, we can obtain an indication of his level of attention, understanding of cause and effect, degree of motivation, and ability to follow directions.

All three types of memory discussed in Chapter 3 (sensory, short term, and long term) are important for the use of assistive technologies. We can evaluate memory tasks related to assistive technology by using structured clinical observations. For example, we can have the consumer memorize a group of codes and then note the consumer's ability to remember these codes during an encoding task.

Problem solving can also be measured during functional tasks. For example, when using an electric feeder, it is necessary to rotate the plate in order to position the food so the spoon can pick it up. This requires a high degree of problem-solving skills. If the person lacks these skills, use of the device becomes frustrating and an alternative should be considered. The value of this type of cognitive assessment is that it occurs during completion of a functional task, which may be predictive of assistive technology system use.

## Skills Evaluation: Language

The evaluation of language skills required for the use of assistive technology devices focuses on both expressive and receptive abilities. In addition, the abilities to sequence items, use symbol systems, combine language elements into complex thoughts, and use codes are important in operating various types of assistive technologies. Whereas the most extensive language evaluation is carried out for augmentative communication system recommendations (see Chapter 9), language skills and use are also important in employing other assistive devices such as mobility systems (see Chapter 10) or systems for manipulation (see Chapter 11). Also, language and hearing are closely coupled, and assistive technologies intended for persons with hearing impairments must address language, as well as auditory skills (see Chapter 12).

Specific areas that are evaluated include categorization, sequencing, matching, social communicative skills (e.g., degree of interaction), receptive language skills (e.g., recognition of words or symbols, understanding of simple commands), motor speech skills, and pragmatic language skills. Advanced language capabilities (e.g., syntax and semantics) are also evaluated when possible. The evaluation of these skills for augmentative communication device use is discussed in Chapter 9.

## Matching Device Characteristics to the User's Needs and Skills

The assessment process we have described to this point provides the basis by which the ATP and the rest of the assistive technology service delivery team carefully define the goals to be accomplished and determine the skills the consumer has available for assistive technology system use. It is necessary to systematically transform these goals and skills into characteristics of assistive technology devices. We use the term **device characteristics** to refer to general properties of the technology. A *feature* is a particular implementation of a characteristic. Characteristics of automobiles include, for example, engine, color, size, performance (acceleration, gas mileage), and doors. Features for these same characteristics might include four-cylinder engine, blue color, compact size, 35 miles per gallon, and two doors. As consumers, we have certain needs, and we match those needs to general characteristics to select specific features of

interest to us. We also have skills that apply to our selection. For example, we may not be able to use a standard manual transmission and choose only automatic transmission cars for consideration. Life roles also play a part in our selection decision. For instance, parents with small children may choose a minivan rather than a compact car.

In assistive technology service delivery, we can use a similar matching process to choose features that match the consumer's needs and skills. This systematic approach is superior to using trial and error with all the possible devices that *may* work and then trying to pick one. To use this approach, however, we must first define a set of characteristics to be considered. A generic set of assistive technology device characteristics is listed in Box 4-3. The categories in this box parallel those used in Figure 2-7 to describe the components of the assistive technology portion of the HAAT model. In the following chapters we consider more specific characteristics for certain areas of assistive technologies: seating systems, control interfaces, computer adaptations, augmentative communication systems, mobility devices, manipulation devices, and sensory aids.

**The human/technology interface.** The human/technology interface is the portion of the device with which the consumer directly interacts. The most general human/technology characteristics, applying to all devices, are the physical properties. These include the force exerted by the

---

### BOX 4-3    Assistive Device Characteristics

**HUMAN/TECHNOLOGY INTERFACE**
Physical properties
Mountability
User feedback
Number of inputs
Selection methods
Selection set

**PROCESSOR**
Commands
Control parameters
Data or information processing

**ACTIVITY OUTPUT**
Magnitude
Precision
Flexibility

**ENVIRONMENTAL SENSOR**
Range
Threshold

**PHYSICAL CONSTRUCTION**
Mountability
Portability
Packaging

human/technology interface on the person and the force exerted by the person on the interface, the size and weight of the interface, and its texture and hardness. A seating system may be too hard or soft to be effective, and this feature can be related to the needs of the individual consumer. All human/technology interfaces must be attached either to the person, to a wheelchair, or to a stable work surface. Consideration of this "mountablilty" characteristic can often mean the difference between success and failure of the human/technology interface. For example, if a consumer has very limited range of arm movement, a switch must be positioned within this range.

Just as the human user exerts forces on the human/technology interface, the human/technology interface provides feedback to the user. This may be as a direct consequence of the interface. For example, a seat cushion exerts a certain force, depending on its materials, design, and construction. In other cases the user feedback is a separate component, such as a flashing light indicator on a television control or a tactile display on a reading device for a person with total visual impairment. We can describe human/technology user feedback sources in terms of the characteristics of magnitude, type, and origin and match them to the consumer's needs. For example, the *magnitude* of a visual display is the brightness of the light. The *types* of human/technology interface feedback are other characteristics and include visual, auditory, and tactile varieties. Each of these can be matched to the corresponding user skill. The *origin* refers to the source of the feedback, such as that provided by a seat cushion or the voice output provided from the screen reader.

The next three characteristics listed in Box 4-3 apply to human/technology interfaces used with electronic assistive devices (including power mobility). The *number of inputs* required to operate any device is a characteristic. We refer to this characteristic as the *size of the input domain* (see Chapter 7). There are many types of control interfaces available, with varying numbers of inputs and requiring different physical skills for activation. The most appropriate control interface for any given consumer is largely determined by the physical and interface assessments that are described here and in Chapter 7.

Depending on the size of the input domain related to the consumer's needs and skills, a *selection method* can be chosen. In Chapter 7 we describe two basic selection methods: direct and indirect. In direct selection, all the choices are presented to the user at one time and the user has the physical ability to choose any one element directly. With indirect selection, there are intermediate steps required for the user to make a selection. If the number of input signals required (based on needs) is greater than the number the consumer can control (based on physical skills), then some form of indirect selection must be used. Individual devices may have both these methods or they may be restricted to

only one method. Direct selection requires greater physical skill than indirect selection; however, indirect selection requires greater cognitive, visual, perceptual, and possibly auditory abilities. The consumer's skills must be taken into account when picking specific device features.

Selections are made from a *selection set* consisting of the choices available to the consumer. Features of this set include size, number of choices, format (e.g., print, tactile), and type of symbol (real objects, pictures, computer icons, line drawings, traditional orthography, or symbols used to represent an idea). The type of symbol system that is most appropriate to a given individual is determined during the language assessment. The question of symbol system type is obviously essential for augmentative communication devices, but it is also important in other applications. For example, in electronic aids to daily living (EADL), the devices to be controlled must be labeled, and often we use symbols rather than words to make the systems available to persons who have difficulty in reading. Speech labels, generated by synthetic speech, are also used in the selection set for individuals who have either visual or cognitive limitations. Along with determining the type of symbols used in the selection set, the size of the selection set is also determined. The number of choices required is often dictated by the consumer's needs, as well as other factors such as how many will fit on a display given the consumer's visual acuity. The choice of these features for a consumer is based on her skills in several areas, including sensory, cognitive, and language.

**The processor.** Recall that the processor is the element of our assistive technology device that relates the human/technology interface to the other components. Sometimes this is simply a mechanical linkage (e.g., in a reacher), and in such cases there are not many choices in characteristics. However, processors for electronic devices have several characteristics that must be carefully matched to the consumer's needs and skills. The first of these is the basic set of *commands* that are necessary to operate the device. It is important to ensure that the consumer can use these so that the system will be functional for him. For example, in a powered wheelchair system the basic commands are forward, backward, left, and right. In a communication device, some basic commands include printing a document and speaking. In an EADL the commands may include lights on and off, TV channel selection, and telephone dialing. These are essential for operation. The greater the number of commands, the more flexible the system is to the user. For example, an EADL that can control the television with three functions (power, volume, and channel), turn three appliances on and off (lights, drapes, and door lock), dial a telephone (three commands), and access an emergency message machine has 10 functions. The more commands included, the more confusing the system can become. The consumer, family, care providers, and ATP need to evaluate the effect of a specific command size during the assessment.

A second characteristic of the processor is the *control parameters*. In contrast to commands, control parameters allow adjustments to be made to the system; they are nice to have but not always essential. Control parameters include such things as variable speed for forward and reverse, or indoor and outdoor speed levels in a powered wheelchair. In an augmentative communication device, control parameters adjust the voice synthesizer pitch, voice type, and rate to affect the way the speech output sounds. A control parameter also provides the ability to switch between different applications for multiple activity outputs. For example, it is possible to operate an EADL, communication device, and computer access system from a powered wheelchair controller. Individual control parameters need to be presented to the consumer for the systems being considered, and both the consumer and the ATP need to evaluate their effectiveness.

The final general processor characteristic is *data or information processing*. In this case the device is internally processing information rather than dealing with commands or control signals. One example, used in augmentative communication systems and screen readers for the blind, is the generation of spoken output from text using software programs. By listening to several speech systems, the consumer can determine the intelligibility of each and identify which one is preferred.

Another type of information processing is word prediction, in which the software program guesses at the desired word based on the entries the consumer makes. This type of application can also adapt to the user by learning her most frequently used words. Encoding involves the use of a symbol (e.g., number, letter, mnemonic, color) to represent a vocabulary item or a command (e.g., TV ON in an EADL). The user selects the code instead of directly selecting the element, which can increase the user's rate of data entry. Encoding schemes can be cognitively difficult, and the consumer should try them during the assessment. The consumer may indicate a preference of one encoding method over another after having a chance to try several.

Information processing is also used in sensory systems to convert the input from the environmental sensor to a form that can be presented to the user. For example, a hearing aid uses a microphone to detect voices, amplifies them (data processing), and presents the amplified signal to the ear (see Chapter 12). Different hearing aids have different data processing, and this characteristic can be evaluated by the consumer.

**The environmental interface.** As we discuss in Chapters 2 and 12, the environmental interface is that portion of the assistive technology system that is used to take in information from the external world for use in a sensory substitution system. For example, when the person has a visual limitation, we use a camera, and when a person has an auditory impairment, we use a microphone. Characteristics that apply to this element include the *range* of the input signal (i.e., how big or small the signal can be and still be detected). The smallest signal that can be discerned from background noise is the *threshold*. As an example of how these characteristics can be applied, consider the two problems of reading and mobility for persons with severe visual impairments. For reading, the device needs very little range because only one letter or line of text needs to be viewed at a time. However, for mobility the environmental sensor needs to take in a variety of sizes (e.g., from a dish to a tree). For reading, the threshold is low (a letter in fine print), but for mobility the threshold can be much higher.

**Activity output.** The activity output is what the system accomplishes for the consumer (e.g., communication, mobility, manipulation). The first characteristic that describes the activity output is its *magnitude*. This includes the volume for a speech synthesis system, the force or torque generated by a powered wheelchair, and the brightness of a video screen display. *Precision* is a measure of how accurately the system performs the functions and how exactly it accomplishes its task. For example, a reacher may be able to pick up a cup but not a button. If the consumer needs to pick up the button, then this particular reacher has insufficient precision to accomplish the task. If an output can be used in different contexts or can be used to accomplish different goals for the consumer, we would say that it is *flexible*. Flexibility can be an important factor when the consumer has many tasks that he wishes to perform. Careful consideration of context must also be included in choosing specific activity output features.

**Physical construction.** The final category of characteristics is physical construction. No matter how well a system works in an assessment session, it will not be effective in everyday use unless the person has access to it at all times. This is determined primarily by the *mountability* of the system. Special consideration must be given to both the mounting of the system (or placement on a desk) and the attachment of any components to a wheelchair if necessary. For example, mounting of a communication system to a wheelchair must be considered during the assessment to ensure that the chosen system is compatible with the consumer's wheelchair.

*Portability* is a measure of the degree to which the device can be moved from place to place. This characteristic includes a consideration of size, weight, and power source. For electronic devices, portability often requires that the device be battery operated and that it be small and lightweight enough to be carried or attached to a wheelchair. If the person is ambulatory, her ability to carry the device needs to be assessed. There are differences in batteries (e.g., life may be a few hours or a few days between charges) and size and weight. For mobility devices, the ability to transport the wheelchair in the trunk of a car may need to be considered. Some wheelchairs fold so that they can be transported in a car trunk, whereas others, such as powered wheelchairs, do not typically fold.

We generally leave consideration of the characteristics of color, shape, and overall design to the last when developing a recommendation of assistive technologies for a consumer. We refer to these as *packaging* characteristics. Consideration of the consumer's preferences in this area can contribute to motivation to use the system, as well as overall user satisfaction. However, the consumer's packaging preferences cannot always be integrated into the system (e.g., the wheelchair may not come in bright orange). All these features should be discussed with the consumer and others to ensure that the device selected will meet the consumer's needs.

**Evaluating the match between characteristics and the consumer's skills and needs.** It is our premise that a large part of the assessment up to this point is best completed without the introduction of specific devices. The reason for this is to keep the focus of the assessment on the functional results to be achieved by the technology instead of secondary features of technology, such as color, size, and design. Once the basic functional characteristics have been defined and agreed on, differences in the secondary factors of size, weight, color, and overall design become important, and they may be the basis for a final decision. After the assessment phases described earlier, one or more devices that have the potential to meet the consumer's skills and needs are identified for the consumer to evaluate. There are two primary ways in which the ATP can evaluate specific technologies for use by the consumer: (1) trial using the actual device and (2) simulation of device characteristics.

Ideally the consumer will have the opportunity to try the devices being considered and evaluate their usefulness before a recommendation is made. However, because of the expense, it is not always possible for the ATP to have access to every available device, nor is it a prerequisite for conducting a skilled assessment. It is desirable that the ATP have available a set of devices that represents a broad range of characteristics. A service delivery program can carefully choose equipment to be used for evaluations, making it possible to address the major characteristics of devices during consumer assessment. In some cases a local manufacturer's representative might loan a device to the ATP for a consumer trial. If these devices are available, it is helpful to demonstrate the various features to the consumer and have the consumer try them. There may be two or three devices being considered, and, if possible, each device should be tried and evaluated by the consumer. Sometimes a short trial

during a one-time assessment is not adequate and it is necessary to have the consumer use the device for an extended period. Some manufacturers and service delivery programs lease devices for this purpose. At the end of the lease, the effectiveness of the device can be evaluated and a decision can be made regarding purchase.

In lieu of having the actual device available, the ATP can simulate device characteristics. This requires that the ATP be knowledgeable about the characteristics and features available for specific assistive technologies. For computer-based products, the assistive technology adaptations are often software based, and demonstration disks can be obtained from manufacturers or downloaded from a manufacturer's Web site. These demonstration programs illustrate the essential features of the software, but they are not fully functional.

To position a control interface for simulation during assessment, universal mounting systems that can be adjusted and placed in various positions can be used. This is important to ensure that the control interface is in a functional position for the consumer and remains stable during the assessment.

**Decision making.** To propose a set of candidate assistive technology devices for a consumer, it is necessary to choose characteristics of these systems that will meet the needs and be consistent with the skills possessed by the consumer. The most important principle in this process is the relationship between the tasks the assistive technology device must accomplish for a person (embodied in the consumer's goals) and the characteristics that must be contained in the device for those tasks to be accomplished. This does not imply a one-to-one relationship between each device characteristic and goal, but that each goal may be accomplished only if a set of essential characteristics is included in the assistive technology system. For example, the goal may be mobility, and the characteristics of the type of cushion, wheelchair type, and color all contribute to the accomplishment of this goal.

Many characteristic-goal relationships are subtler, however, and generic characteristics of devices are not always equivalent to specific features of commercially available assistive technologies. For example, a generic characteristic of all EADLs is turning lights on and off. However, different manufacturers of EADLs may accomplish this function in different ways. Developing recommendations and a plan for implementation should be based on the consideration of device characteristics that have been evaluated by the consumer.

Computer-based **expert systems** that assist in the decision-making process for assistive technologies are being developed. Depending on the expert system, collection and interpretation of data are incorporated. Expert systems use artificial intelligence to guide the ATP through the assessment and decision-making process. Expert systems attempt to mimic the skills of an ATP using software programs that are capable of making decisions much like humans do. In assistive technologies, several preliminary systems have been developed. Garrett et al (1990) have developed an expert system called VOCAselect for use in selecting augmentative communication systems for specific consumers. Their system is based on 17 features that are determined during the assessment process. In addition to features related to consumer performance (e.g., input method, vocabulary size), they include physical construction (e.g., portability) and information regarding available support services (e.g., price range acceptable, training availability). These factors are then related to specific features of each available communication device. The expert system matches the specific requirements of the user, based on goals and needs, as well as on assessment of skills, to appropriate devices. By including the weight of factors (e.g., characteristic A is twice as important as characteristic B) and a scale of responses (e.g., priority for speech output is 9 out of 10), this type of expert system can focus on specific options even more closely. Garrett et al report that preliminary trials indicate exact agreement in device selection between the expert system and a speech-language pathologist.

Stapelton and Garrett (1995) carried out an evaluation of this system. Respondents to a survey indicated strongly (greater than 79%) that this system would be of value in making recommendations for augmentative communication systems. They also present an example of the use of this program for a specific case. Stapelton et al (1995) extended the VOCAselect concept to the selection of computer adaptations (see Chapter 8). This computer program is similar to VOCAselect, but it is built on characteristics of devices and software used to make computers accessible to individuals who cannot use a keyboard or mouse for entry or use the standard screen for output. In operation this software is functionally identical to VOCAselect. Stapelton et al (1995) present a example of the use of this system.

An expert system for seating and mobility systems is available to clinicians at www.rehabcentral.com. Using this approach, clinicians enter evaluation data for a specific client, and product alternatives that best fit the client's needs are suggested. Each product that is suggested is linked to its respective Web site, where the ATP can find further information. Each product also is linked to any related messages that may have been posted on the rehabcentral message boards.

Whether an expert system is used or not, the process we have described is highly effective in defining the features of a recommended system. It is important to recognize that the features that are most limiting must be considered first, followed by those that are less restrictive. For example, in an augmentative communication system, the type of symbol system is often the most limiting characteristic. If a consumer requires pictures as a symbol, many devices are eliminated immediately. In contrast, spoken output as a characteristic is not as limiting, since most devices use similar speech synthesizers. For each type of assistive technology, it is important for the ATP to identify a set of general characteristics that fit within the categories of Box 4-3. We present these in later chapters. If the characteristics are generic, then specific features can be selected in sequence to define the final assistive technology system. The major advantage of the assessment methods described here is that they are based on a consideration of the consumer's goals and skills first and a consideration of assistive technology system characteristics second. Thus the system is matched to the consumer (within the limits of current technology) rather than the consumer being forced to adapt to the system. Without a structured approach like the one presented here, however, it is very difficult to meet consumer's goals.

It is clear that many characteristics of devices should be considered, and the features (and their costs) will differ from one system to the next. In addition to specific features of the device, other important factors include the contexts of use, the amount of training required before the device can be used effectively, cost, availability of a family member or caregiver to support and facilitate the training and implementation of the device, and ease of use of the device.

## Recommendations and Report

The recommendations summarize the information gathered during the evaluation and suggest a design for the assistive technology system. At the conclusion of the assessment, everyone involved should sit down to review it and come to a consensus regarding the final recommendation. A written report is prepared that details the assessment and recommendations for an assistive technology system. The written report synthesizes the assessment process and starts out by defining the needs and goals that have been addressed. A summary of the consumer's skills applicable to device use is provided, with a description of generic characteristics to be incorporated into a device. This is followed by specific recommendations for equipment, including descriptions, part numbers if applicable, manufacturer's name, any modifications that need to be made, and cost. Recommendations for soft technologies are also included in the written report. These may include recommendations for developing skills that are necessary before purchase of a device, training once the device has been purchased, and strategies for incorporating the technology into the individual's context. Finally, a plan for implementation of the recommendations is provided. This includes logistics such as seeking funding from the appropriate sources and who will take responsibility for implementing the recommendations.

Often the written report is aimed at various individuals, thus presenting a unique challenge for the ATP writing it.

The report, first of all, needs to be geared toward the consumer, who may not be familiar with medical or technical jargon. Rehabilitation or educational professionals working with the consumer may also be receiving the report and its recommendations. These professionals typically need information on what the consumer's skills have been in using the technology and what skill areas they may need to address to facilitate the use of the device. Some of these professionals may be very knowledgeable in assistive technology, but for others this may be their first experience with it. The contact person for the funding source will also be reading the report, and his or her interest is typically in the "bottom line," or what it is going to cost. This person wants evidence that the system recommended is going to meet the consumer's needs at the lowest possible cost. In the section on funding in this chapter, we describe how to write a report to a third-party payer in order to justify the purchase of an assistive technology system.

## ■ IMPLEMENTATION

Once the recommendations have been made and funding is obtained, the implementation phase begins. This aspect of the delivery process consists of ordering specified equipment, obtaining commercially available equipment or fabricating custom equipment, making needed modifications, assembling or setting up equipment, thoroughly checking it as a system, fitting the device to the consumer, and training the consumer and caregivers in its use.

### Ordering and Setup

Many recommended interventions have components from several manufacturers, and these must be integrated into a total system. Some of these may be standard commercially available components and others may be commercial assistive technologies. These devices are ordered from the manufacturer or equipment supplier and may take up to 6 weeks to be received after ordering. The recommendation may have also included a custom device or devices that require an adaptation. Examples of custom modifications include mounting a switch to a wheelchair or table, making a cable for connecting two devices together (e.g., a communication device and an EADL), programming a device for unique vocabulary, and adapting a battery-powered toy so it can be controlled with one switch. The design and fabrication of these system components can occur during the waiting time for the delivery of the commercially available technologies. Once all the individual devices and adaptations are available, it is necessary to assemble them into a total package. For example, a wheelchair obtained from one source and a seating system from another will need to be interfaced to each other. The complexity of this assembly process varies

widely, and some systems require much more effort than others.

### Delivery and Fitting

Once the equipment is obtained, modified, or adapted as necessary and integrated into a system, the system is ready to be delivered to the consumer. This may occur in a clinic setting, in a school or at a job site, or in the consumer's living setting. The choice of locations depends on the nature of the equipment, the ease of transport of the consumer, and the complexity of the system (i.e., what support services of technicians and tools are required). We refer to all system deliveries as a "fitting" because we are interfacing the human (consumer) with the rest of the system. In some cases, such as custom seating systems, the process resembles a fitting for an orthotic or prosthetic device. In other cases the fitting focuses on installation of the system, mounting the control interface and the device to a wheelchair, and interconnection of the various components. The fitting phase may also include some amount of assessment as adjustments are made to optimize the consumer's ability to utilize the system. An example of this is the use of head switches to control a powered wheelchair. The head switches must be attached to the wheelchair and wired into the controller unit. This is done before the fitting, and during the fitting, the location of the head switches (e.g., how close they are to the consumer's head) is adjusted to maximize performance.

The complexity of many assistive technology systems may require more than one session to obtain all the proper adjustments, mountings, and fittings. The ATP must be prepared to continue making adjustments and adaptations in the system until the consumer's goals and needs are met. This phase of the delivery process often involves some reassessment, but its success is directly related to the quality of the initial assessment and recommendations, and difficulties experienced at this time can often be traced to incomplete or inaccurate assessments.

### Facilitating Assistive Technology System Performance

A major concern of everyone involved in the delivery of assistive technology services is whether the device recommended is going to meet the stated goals. It *cannot* be assumed that intervention ends with the delivery of the device. Most users of technology, even those with previous technology experience, require assistance in facilitating their performance with the device. The ATP, as the designer of the system, is responsible for providing the means to facilitate human performance. This is where the soft technology components discussed in Chapter 1 come in.

Bailey (1989) identifies three methods that facilitate human performance: written instructions, performance aids, and training. He describes the major difference between each of these facilitators as being "the time that elapses between when information is presented and when the performance takes place" (Bailey, 1989, p. 325). A performance aid is used immediately, written instructions are read and also used fairly quickly, but information presented during a training session may not be used until months later. In designing performance facilitators for individual users, the ATP should keep this difference in mind. The ATP also needs to know how to provide a balance among these facilitators. For example, many manufacturers of augmentative communication devices develop an abundance of written instructions. Even if the user were to read all this information, most of it would be stored away in memory and forgotten. It has been found that when workers on a job site need information that can be found in similar documents, they either take a guess at the solution or ask someone else (Bailey, 1989). The same thing happens with assistive technology users. An example of this is a person who is hard of hearing and obtains a hearing aid. It may work fine for a relatively long period; then the batteries are discharged and need to be replaced. Often the user merely puts the hearing aid in a drawer because it "doesn't work anymore" instead of replacing the batteries. If the user does replace the batteries, it is generally because he asked someone else what to do or was instructed in the process when the aid was sold to him, not because he looked it up in the user's manual. Bailey admits that there are few guidelines to help the ATP determine when to use performance aids, written instructions, or training but emphasizes that "the best decisions are made when as much as possible is known about the potential users, the activity to be performed, and the context in which the performance will take place" (p. 326). As applicable, each of the following chapters has a section on specific training ideas.

**Training.**  Bailey (1989) defines training as "the acquisition of skills, knowledge, and attitudes that will lead to an acceptable level of human performance on a specific activity in a given context" (p. 387). This is referred to as *performance-based training*. In the field of assistive technology, prior authorization from the funding source to conduct training is usually required. For a funding source to authorize training, an estimate of the amount of time that will be needed is typically required. The ATP is then required to abide by this estimate, and unfortunately the training of individuals to use the assistive technology becomes *time based* rather than performance based. Time-based training is completed within a specified period, whether or not the user achieves a level of skill. The ATP's time estimate is based on previous training experiences with particular types of assistive technology, consumers with similar skills and limits, and similar environmental conditions and support. The experienced ATP is able to accurately estimate the amount of training a particular individual will need with the recommended system.

For an individual to become a proficient assistive technology user, training over time is required. Without adequate training, there is an increased likelihood that the device will be abandoned. The training process is facilitated if the ATP starts out by developing a set of well-defined, measurable objectives for training. This will help focus the training sessions and will serve as an indicator for termination of training. It is also important that there be one person affiliated with the consumer who takes on the role of the facilitator and learns the operation of the device and basic concepts so that she can assist with the use of the device as needed.

Training oriented toward establishing **operational competence** is initiated at the delivery and fitting (Pallin, 1991). This phase of training is intended to make it possible for the user of the technology, his care providers and family, and any other support person to begin using the assistive technology system. Examples of considerations included in training for operational competency for the consumer are (1) how to turn an electronic device on and off, (2) making adjustments in operational parameters (e.g., adjusting a scanning rate), (3) loading an initial vocabulary in an augmentative communication system, (4) explaining basic maintenance (e.g., battery charging, cleaning), (5) introducing basic functions and how they work (e.g., choosing what to say on a communication device, using an adapted telephone dialer), and (6) basic troubleshooting so that the consumer and others have some strategies to use if problems develop with the system. It is important to present information in small doses to avoid overwhelming the consumer and others. This is especially key for complicated computer-based devices, which may have many features, options, and operational modes. At the initial fitting session it is only necessary to present enough information so that the consumer can begin to use the system. Subsequent training addresses the acquisition of the necessary skills for more advanced operations.

In addition to basic operational competence, it is necessary for the consumer to develop strategies that maximize the effectiveness of the system. To facilitate this, the ATP provides training for **strategic competence**. The training focuses on the *application* of the system, rather than basic operation. As this phase of training progresses, the consumer begins to develop her own set of strategies. For example, the person using a manual wheelchair will develop strategies for navigating curbs or inclines and the user of an AAC device will develop strategies for communicating in a noisy restaurant. These strategies can then be shared with other consumers by the ATP.

**Performance aids.**  A document or device containing information that an individual uses to assist in the comple-

---

## CASE STUDY 4-1

### TRAINING

Marilyn is a 45-year-old woman who sustained a brain-stem stroke. Her only available control site is very slight movement of her right thumb. She will use this movement to control a computer that provides both verbal and written augmentative communication (see Chapter 9) and EADL (see Chapter 11). She resides in a skilled nursing facility where she has daily visits from family and church members. One session a week for 4 weeks will be carried out. Her training program will include the following:

**Session One:**
**Basic operational competence:** Instruction in how to connect the switch to the AAC system and to mount the switch for independent access; discussion of setup of software parameters for scanning; presentation of an overview of system features; instruction in charging of batteries and the use of the swing-away mounting systems for the computer and the switches.
**Basic linguistic competence:** Instruction in how to use commands in the word processor to load, save, edit, print, use pictures and use different fonts; instruction in how to retrieve and use vocabulary; and selection of preliminary vocabulary.
**Basic strategic competence:** Discussion of when to use features to maximize effectiveness of the AAC device.
**Basic social competence:** Discussion of how augmented communication differs from speech.

**Session Two:**
**Intermediate operational competence:** Instruction in storage and retrieval of vocabulary in the electronic AAC device.
**Intermediate linguistic competence:** Instruction in how to use advanced features of the word processor and how to add vocabulary to the system.

**Intermediate social competence:** Discussion of how to be a good communicator.

**Session Three:**
**Advanced operational competence:** Instruction in how to load and use new vocabulary files and how to print. Instruction in how to use the AAC menu to select and control the EADL; demonstration of how to connect devices to remote control receivers and how to make phone calls using the AAC device.
**Intermediate strategic competence:** Discussion of how to use strategies for conversations with visitors. Development of strategies for conversations with nursing staff.

**Session Four:**
**Advanced linguistic competence:** Practice with word processor for writing. Instruction in how to use special features to enhance speech output.
**Advanced strategic competence:** Discussion of when to use different system features. Development and use of conversational repair strategies, and effective use of commenting (see Chapter 9).
**Advanced social competence:** Instruction in how to vary conversational vocabulary and moods for differing categories of interaction and partners, and how to select vocabulary and modes for differing social situations.

Marilyn, her husband, and the staff of the long-term care facility in which she is currently living will devote the period between the sessions to practice. Before the start of each session, information from the prior session will be reviewed to see if Marilyn has any questions. At the fourth session Marilyn will be evaluated to see how she is doing in using the device and to determine if she has further training needs.

---

tion of an activity is called a **performance aid.** By decreasing the amount of information to be remembered, the performance aid reduces the amount of cognitive processing required to complete an activity. With a performance aid, the user does not have to rely as much on long-term memory. This results in reduced errors, increased speed for certain tasks, and a reduced amount of training required. Performance aids do not necessarily have to be written; picture symbols can also be effective for individuals who cannot read. Bailey (1989) describes five quality standards for performance aids: (1) accessibility, (2) accuracy, (3) clarity, (4) completeness and conciseness, and (5) legibility.

Performance aids are commonly used with individuals

who have memory deficits as a result of damage to the brain. One type of performance aid is simple step-by-step instructions that assist the user in carrying out a sequence of tasks. For example, Tim is a young man who has sustained a head injury. He uses a computer to complete school assignments but has problems remembering the sequence of steps to get into his computer word processing program. The steps to do this have been simply written and are posted next to his computer. Because Tim also has visual acuity problems, the instructions are printed in large, bold letters. For Tim, this simple performance aid has meant the difference between success and failure in using his computer.

Another type of performance aid assists in remembering

several items of information. An example of this type of aid is a printed list of codes with their meanings, which an individual may have stored in her augmentative communication system. Often a list such as this is attached to the side of the device so the user can view it easily as needed. Sometimes codes and their meanings are built into software programs and presented on the screen each time the user selects a letter. This is referred to as *word prediction software* and is discussed further in Chapter 9.

**Written instructions.** Written instructions should be considered an integral part of the system and be available to the user at the time of the system delivery. Instructions are helpful when step-by-step directions with detailed information are required or when graphic information needs to be presented. Written instructions may be compiled and presented in the form of user manuals, handbooks, or computer software. The ATP must not assume that the instructions provided by the manufacturer are going to be adequate. Written instructions provided by the manufacturer of the system may include too little or too much information or they may be difficult to follow by the user. It is recommended that instructions from the manufacturer be reviewed and supplemented as needed. When the manufacturer's documentation is overwhelming, the ATP can review the documentation and condense it into a quick reference sheet that provides simplified and frequently used information.

Bailey (1989) provides detailed guidelines for developing the various types of written documents, including software documentation. For our purposes, it is important to remember to keep our audience in mind and write the instructions for the people who will use them. For example, if the primary person facilitating the performance is the parent, the instructions may be different from those generated if the facilitator is a teacher. In the field of assistive technology this may mean a new or revised set of instructions for each individual consumer, even for use of the same device.

## ■ FOLLOW-UP AND FOLLOW-ALONG

Once the system has been implemented, it is tempting to think that the intervention has been completed. This perception, however, is totally false; the delivery of the system marks the beginning of the time of use, and it therefore signals the beginning of the evaluation of system effectiveness. We use the term **follow-up** to refer to activities that occur during the period immediately following delivery of an assistive technology system and that address the effectiveness of the device, training, and user strategies. The term **follow-along** is used to describe those activities that take place over a longer period. This phase addresses factors such as changes in needs or goals, availability of new devices, and other concerns.

We include a formal follow-up phase in our delivery process for several reasons: (1) assistive devices can seldom be used right out of the box without ever needing to be adjusted; (2) electronic devices are not 100% reliable, and a significant portion of them require repair during the first year of use; (3) training programs seldom proceed flawlessly, and questions arise during the initial period of use; and (4) perceived device failures are often the result of operator error caused by a lack of device understanding. A carefully developed follow-up program will identify these problems easily and address them quickly.

Repair and maintenance are often conducted during the follow-up phase. *Repair* refers to action taken to correct a problem in a system. *Maintenance,* on the other hand, is a systematic set of procedures that is aimed at keeping the device in working order. Examples of maintenance functions are proper battery charging, cleaning, tightening mounting hardware, and lubrication of moving mechanical parts. A regular schedule will ensure that necessary maintenance takes place. Assistive technology system failures result in a major disruption of the consumer's life. For example, a consumer depends on his powered wheelchair for mobility. If it fails, he may have a manual wheelchair as a backup, but his independence may be significantly reduced. Repair of assistive technologies is most often carried out either through manufacturer's representatives or directly through the manufacturer. In the latter case the device must be returned to the factory for repair, and the consumer may be without it for several days or even longer. Prompt attention to repair needs of consumers is an important part of follow-up.

As part of a formal follow-up program, contacts with the consumer (via telephone, on the job site, in the home, or in the clinic) are scheduled on a regular basis, such as at 1, 3, 6, and 12 months after delivery. These contacts occur whether there is a perceived problem or not, and they are in addition to other activities such as training or repair. This regularly scheduled contact is important because there may be unnoticed problems, or more often there are underutilized features that are discovered during the follow-up sessions. Mortola, Kohn, and LeBlanc (1992) found in a follow-up study that 63% of 196 assistive devices delivered by their center were not being used for mechanical reasons. In most of these cases the consumer had not informed the ATP of the device failure.

As we have defined it, follow-along has a much longer time frame than follow-up. Whereas follow-up typically covers the first year of operation of an assistive technology system, follow-along is carried out over the individual's lifetime. Consumers may return for service after a period of years for several reasons. They may have found that the device is not working as they would like and is not meeting their functional goals. Another reason is to obtain information about advances in technology since they obtained their device. In other cases the consumer may have changed in significant ways. This change is often seen in children who have grown significantly and need a revision in their seating system. Change can also be the result of a degenerative condition such as amyotrophic lateral sclerosis, and in these cases the device may need to be altered to accommodate decreased physical function. In other cases the change in consumer condition is a result of the development of new skills that make it possible to consider new device features. For example, a consumer who has suffered a traumatic brain injury (TBI) may initially receive a communication device that is based on very simple replay of sentences. As she recovers, her ability to spell effectively may improve and a device with this capability should be considered.

There are other reasons for follow-along. One of the most important of these is a change in the life roles and context of the consumer. For example, Martin, who has severe cerebral palsy and has used an augmentative and alternative communication (AAC) device for several years, decides to move into an apartment on his own. The success of this transition could depend heavily on the availability of assistive technologies. An EADL would allow him to control lights and appliances; answer and dial the telephone; and control the television, VCR, and other entertainment devices. This reevaluation is dictated not by changes in his condition, but by changes in his life roles and the context in which he will be using his technology.

As opposed to follow-up, follow-along is often initiated by the consumer rather than the ATP. This is because the ATP is not aware of the changing physical, sensory, and cognitive conditions in the consumer. On the other hand, the consumer cannot possibly be aware of changes in technology. For this reason, it is important that the ATP develop a mechanism to maintain contact with her consumers to inform them of changes in technology. This mechanism should empower each consumer to take personal responsibility for his long-term assistive technology needs. One frequently used method for doing this is a regular newsletter that is sent to consumers by the ATP.

Another reason for both follow-up and follow-along is to evaluate the effectiveness of the assistive technology system by measuring outcomes. This provides a measure of how well the system meets the original needs identified during the assessment. In the next section we describe the measurement of outcomes.

## ■ EVALUATING THE EFFECTIVENESS OF ASSISTIVE TECHNOLOGY SERVICES AND SYSTEMS

Measuring the outcomes of the assistive technology services we provide is a primary focus in the industry today and will continue to be in the forefront of assistive technology service delivery. Consumers want measures that reflect their needs for improved function and quality of life. Payers seek efficient provisions of services using the fewest possible resources, and as providers, we seek information on how to deliver efficient and effective assistive technology services.

When we consider outcome measures for assistive technology systems, we need to develop measures and standards of performance that allow a careful determination of the effectiveness of such systems. For instance, a child who is evaluated for a powered wheelchair (see Chapter 10) will have a level of accuracy, speed, and reliability that we can measure. Speed of response and accuracy are both employed to assess powered wheelchair performance. The speed of response is important in describing how quickly a disabled consumer reacts to obstacles, and accuracy is a measure of how well the consumer can navigate a specific course. If we use this as the baseline performance, we can determine progress over time by comparing performance with this baseline. In a clinic or laboratory setting, these measures can be used to select a control interface (see Chapter 7) and to determine such things as the feasibility of safe powered mobility. However, to determine the success of the desired functional outcome (independent mobility), measures must be made in the intended context. This raises several additional questions. For example: What is the standard for accuracy of powered wheelchair use in a shopping mall? Is it a minimal number of collisions with people and objects? If so, how many are acceptable? Is it being able to successfully negotiate a crowded store? If so, what is being measured to assess success (e.g., minimal breakage, no collisions, how fast the user gets to the door)? Obviously, measuring and assessing assistive technology system performance in the real world is not an easy task. In the remainder of this chapter we focus primarily on the measurement of outcomes of the use of assistive technology devices and the provision of services.

### Overview

The effectiveness of assistive technology systems in meeting the needs of consumers is related to many factors. Sackett (1980) identifies four types of evaluation to consider: effectiveness, efficacy, availability, and efficiency. These can each be related to different questions and to different assessment instruments. For evaluating *effectiveness* we ask the question, Does it work? Effectiveness is measured in terms of the impact of the product on the consumer's life and needs. Therefore the outcome measurements that we collect must begin with and focus on the consumer and the results of the assistive technology intervention. These outcomes allow us to determine the *efficacy* of the service delivery structure and process. Efficacy is the ability to produce a desired result or effect; the question to be asked is, Can it work? This is what is measured when we evaluate a service delivery structure and process. It provides us with useful information on how we are delivering services so that necessary revisions can be made.

The entire assistive technology industry is evaluated by the success of service delivery and assistive technology system utilization by the consumer. As we have described, the consumer and the delivery of assistive technology services are at the core of the assistive technology industry (see Figure 1-2). Gathering information on outcomes should be included as a regular part of the service delivery process so this information can be utilized as feedback to the rest of the industry. For example, a manufacturer could be determined to have good manufacturing practices and meet all industry standards; however, the most meaningful standard is the effectiveness of the equipment for consumers. Likewise, the effectiveness of the equipment is only as good as the service provider who delivers it. If, as a whole, there are problems with consumer utilization of assistive technology, all of the industry will be affected. This is related to evaluation of *availability,* which asks the question, Is it reaching those who need it? (Sackett, 1980).

Finally, the question, Is it worth doing? needs to be answered. This addresses the relative importance of the service being provided by comparing it with other programs that could be purchased with the same resources. This evaluation measure is referred to as *efficiency.* Third-party payers want to know that the assistive technology services and devices are worth paying for. It is the ATP's responsibility to provide this justification.

A wide range of outcome data needs to be collected, and determinations need to be made regarding what measures will be used, how many measures are needed, and how focused the measures need to be (Smith, 1996). When developing outcome measures for assistive technology devices and services, it is important to be clear about who the stakeholders are in this process (DeRuyter, 1995). This is not as obvious a question as it first seems. If outcome measures are used to inform funding sources, are these funding sources consumers of the outcome results or stakeholders in the process? Likewise, providers may be considered either consumers or stakeholders, depending on the type of outcome measure used and the implications for its

implementation. If user satisfaction is to be used as an outcome measure, is that a measure that relates to the provider, the funding source, or the user? Certainly the user of the technology is a consumer, but not all outcome measures are user centered. In the remainder of this section we focus on those measures that are have been demonstrated to have reliability and validity in the measurement of outcomes at several levels.

We can distinguish among structure, process, and outcome measures in assistive technology delivery. The *structure* of the delivery system refers to aspects such as the staffing, staff expertise, equipment on hand, budget, and range of services provided. The *process* of assistive technology delivery includes the stages of assessment and intervention that we have described in this chapter. Process measures ascertain whether these stages have occurred and whether the procedures meet an acceptable standard. **Outcome measures** evaluate the end result of the assistive technology intervention. Figure 4-7 illustrates the interrelationship among the assistive technology system, the service delivery process, and their outcomes.

There are a number of different levels at which we can evaluate the effectiveness of both devices and services by measuring outcomes. Traditionally at the clinical level the question being asked is, Did the intervention remediate the individual's impairment? This is the impairment level of the ICF classification of the World Health Organization (see Chapter 1). In the provision of assistive technologies, this level is seldom the major focus, but it is important because assistive technologies can lead to improvement in impairment and thus in function. The *parallel interventions model* (Angelo and Smith, 1989; Smith, 1991), described earlier in this chapter, illustrates how intervention to affect the level of impairment is related to the use of assistive technologies. The next level is the functional level, when the question is, Can the individual accomplish tasks that she could not do without the assistive technology? This is the activity level of the ICF classification of the World Health Organization. In this case, **functional perfor-**

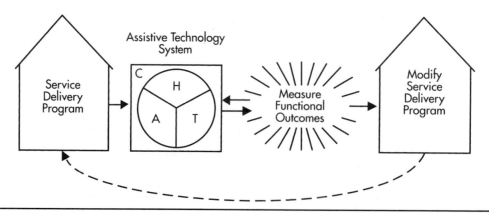

**Figure 4-7**    Interrelationship among the assistive technology system, the service delivery process and structure, and their outcomes. *H,* Human; *A,* activity; *C,* context; *T,* assistive technology.

**mance measures** are typically employed to determine effectiveness.

When services were primarily clinical and delivered in institutional settings, measures of impairment and functional measures were the focus of outcome evaluation. However, there has been a move toward community-based services in rehabilitation over the past decade. This has been driven by rising costs of institutional care and is being addressed by shortening stays and transferring more care to the community. As we have described in this chapter, many services, including most of assistive technology services, are more appropriately delivered in the community where they will be used.

Community-based services are also being driven by an emerging alliance between the largely institution-based rehabilitation establishment and the largely community-based disability community. This alliance has implications for responsibility for care, including responsibility for choices of assistive technology devices and services (Lysack and Kaufert, 1999). As we described in Chapter 1 and this chapter, consumers play a larger role in decision making regarding what they receive and the evaluation of the quality of both the devices and services. The question being asked by the consumer at this level is, Do the assistive technology services and devices provided meet my needs? In order to answer this question, **user satisfaction measures** related to assistive technology services and devices have been developed.

As we discussed in Chapter 1, the classification of disability over the past 20 years has begun to focus on its social dimensions (Fougeyrollas and Gray, 1998). This social model, now incorporated into the World Health Organization (WHO) ICF classification (WHO, 2001), provides a richer and more complete view of both disability and the role of assistive technologies in the lives of people who have disabilities. It is no longer important to achieve success only in the clinic or laboratory. The real test is in daily community use of the technologies. The question being asked at this level is, What is the impact of this assistive technology device or service on my quality of life? The primary outcome measures used for assessing the effectiveness of assistive technology devices and services in this broader social context are **quality of life measures**.

Each of these primary types of measurement of assistive technology device and service outcomes is discussed in the following sections.

## Measuring Clinical and Functional Outcomes

In the past, health care and rehabilitation quality of service was measured by looking at factors such as timeliness and the completeness of the services provided (e.g., whether a discharge summary was completed for the consumer within 1 week of discharge). These are actually process measures, and they do not reflect outcomes of the assistive technology

intervention. Within the past decade or so, rehabilitation service providers have begun to focus more on the functional outcomes achieved by the consumer as a result of intervention. Because the focus of assistive technology practitioners is on reducing disability and maximizing an individual's functional status, it is only natural that one of the factors to measure is functional outcome related to assistive device use.

There are a number of tools that have been developed and studied that measure functional outcomes of individuals who have been through the rehabilitation process. Examples of functional outcome measures include the Barthel Index (Mahoney and Barthel, 1965), the Klein-Bell ADL Scale (Klein and Bell, 1979) and the Functional Independence Measure (UDS, 1997).

Unfortunately, many of these traditional tools used in the field of rehabilitation do not document the efficacy of technological intervention (Christiansen, Schwartz, and Barnes, 1988; Smith, 1996). As Smith (1996) points out, many instruments are limited in their scope in three ways: (1) they tend to be developed for a particular population, such as individuals who have sustained a stroke; (2) many instruments are developed for a particular health care setting, such as long-term care or acute rehabilitation settings; and (3) they frequently focus on a specific functional area, such as hand function or self-care.

**The Functional Independence Measure.** The Functional Independence Measure (FIM) is an example of one functional outcome measure. We have chosen the FIM as an example because it is widely used in assessing the outcomes of rehabilitation interventions. The FIM is based on a medical model of assessment, which places importance on cure (Smith, 1996). The FIM measures the individual's performance on 18 items under the categories of self-care, bowel and bladder management, transfers, locomotion, communication, and cognition (UDS, 1997). The scoring of the FIM is on a 7-point scale. The individual only obtains the full 7 points if he does not require any assistance or assistive device to perform a function. Thus the FIM is not directly applicable to assistive device outcome measurement because its maximal score in any category can only be obtained if the person does not use any technology. Use of technology automatically implies that the person is not totally functionally independent. This appraisal of functional independence is inconsistent with the current view that an individual is independent if she can manage her own life (Smith, 1996). Another concern regarding the FIM and other tools that measure function is that they do not impart information regarding the impact of assistive devices on the quality of life of the user (Jutai et al, 1996).

**The Occupational Therapy Functional Assessment Compilation Tool.** The Occupational Therapy Functional Assessment Compilation Tool (OT FACT) (Smith, 1990) was designed to address some of the limitations identified earlier by providing a means to assess an individual's overall performance. OT FACT takes into consideration environmental factors and any devices or adaptations that contribute to this performance. With OT FACT, the summary of the data is presented in a graphical form that shows the effectiveness of technology (e.g., a mouth wand) on the individual's performance (Figure 4-8). A major advantage of OT FACT is its use of a trichotomous scale (Smith, 1996). This approach uses a branching scale that assigns a score of 2 if there is no deficit, 1 for partial deficit, and 0 for total deficit. OT FACT uses software branching to focus the description of functional ability. The score drives the branching to new questions. If a 2 (no deficit) or 0 (total deficit) is entered, no further questions are asked in that functional area. If a 1 (partial deficit) is entered, additional questions are asked via software-directed branching. In this way the individual's functional ability is explored more fully for the given skill area.

## User Satisfaction As an Outcome Measure

Any discussion of assistive technology effectiveness must consider the recommended system and how well it meets the consumer's needs. Therefore the measures we use must be consumer oriented. This means that the factors we use to evaluate the effectiveness of assistive technology systems must be based on criteria that are important to the consumer. **User satisfaction** is the consumer's perception of the degree to which the assistive technology system achieves the

desired goal. This is a multidimensional phenomenon that requires qualitative measures (Demers, Weiss-Lambrou, and Ska, 1996). In addition, general user satisfaction scales are global, and they do not take into account various factors that affect a person's use or nonuse of assistive technologies. In assistive technology applications, on the other hand, rating scales that address specific aspects of use are employed (see Brooks, 1990, for example). For a large sample of users, these surveys can be statistically analyzed to determine the most important factors in achieving user satisfaction. These group statistics may indicate a significant lack of satisfaction, and this information can be used to make changes in the service delivery structure and process to improve user satisfaction. For any individual assistive technology system, satisfaction is one parameter to be evaluated during the follow-up and follow-along processes. One limitation with satisfaction survey instruments is that they often "top out"; that is, individuals use either the highest or lowest score, and the range of a scale is lost. For example, assume a 5-point scale is used, with levels of "very dissatisfied," "dissatisfied," "neutral," "satisfied," and "very satisfied." Most individuals will reduce this to a 3-point scale, using the two ends and "neutral." This is especially true if several parameters are measured with the same scale. Also, user satisfaction scales are one-dimensional, measuring only satisfaction. Multidimensional scales can be more informative (Jutai, 2001).

**Canadian Occupational Performance Measure.** The Canadian Occupational Performance Measure (COPM)

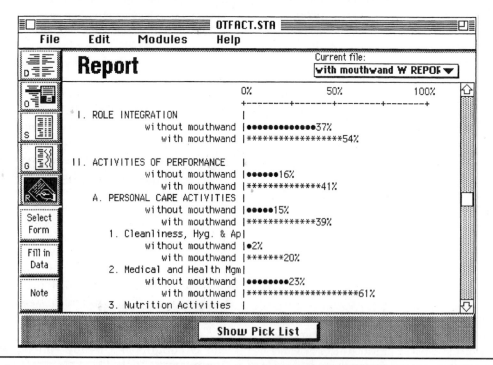

**Figure 4-8** Sample consumer functional profile generated by OT FACT, showing the effectiveness of technology on the individual's performance. (From Smith RO: *OT fact*, Rockville, Md, 1990, American Occupational Therapy Association.)

assesses the perspective of the individual with a disability (Smith, 1996). This is a general evaluation instrument that includes domains such as "functional mobility (e.g., transfers, indoor, outdoor)" and "quiet recreation (e.g., hobbies, crafts, reading)." Only questions that are relevant to the individual are included in the administration of the COPM. When using the COPM, the person being assessed helps to identify the areas of importance. A unique feature of this instrument is that it includes both the functional performance of the individual and personal preference and personal satisfaction in the scoring. When used in this way, the COPM becomes a user satisfaction measure. This mix of quantitative and qualitative data provides a valuable perspective that is useful for assistive technology outcomes assessment (Smith, 1996).

**Quebec User Evaluation of Satisfaction with Assistive Technology.** Five criteria were used in the development of the Quebec User Evaluation of Satisfaction with Assistive Technology (QUEST) (Demers, Weiss-Lambrou, and Ska, 1996). The first is the recognition that user satisfaction is a multidimensional phenomenon that includes a broad range of variables, each of which can affect the user's satisfaction with assistive technology. The second criterion relates to the inclusion of three types of variables: those involving the environment (context in the HAAT model), pertinent features of the person's personality (the human), and the characteristics of the assistive technology itself. The third criterion is the recognition that the user himself should determine the relative importance of the satisfaction variable. This reflects the highly subjective nature of the user satisfaction measure. The fourth criterion provides for the user to express her opinion freely within the constraints of an interview context. Finally, the QUEST was designed to be simple to understand and easy to use by ATPs when evaluating satisfaction. The QUEST requires approximately 30 minutes to administer and is guided by a three-part form.

The first part of the instrument is the general information questionnaire. This form is designed to determine the context in which the user's satisfaction or dissatisfaction developed. It consists of 18 open-ended questions designed to include the three domains of environment (context; e.g., living arrangements, social supports, funding considerations), user characteristics (human; e.g., gender, age, nature of disability, types of functional problems), and assistive technology characteristics (e.g., when the device was acquired, frequency and patterns of use or nonuse, number and types of assistive technologies used).

The second part of the QUEST instrument is an assessment of satisfaction. This includes a set of 27 variables that represent the factors most likely to affect user satisfaction with assistive technologies. Each of the variables represents a specific category, but they are randomly ordered in the presentation to the user. This ensures that the user's answers are not artificially influenced by the category of the question. Three tasks are used in this part of the evaluation. In the first task, the person is asked the degree of importance that he attributes to each variable. Each of the variables is printed on a card. There is a board for classifying the variable from very important (a score of 3) to no importance (0). The evaluator asks the user where he would like each card placed and then circles the response on the form. After completing the 27 variables, the user is given an opportunity to add other satisfaction variables that he feels are important. This task personalizes the assessment in terms of the individual's preferences. The second task requires that the evaluator reorganize the variable according to the three categories, and only the variables selected as being quite or very important (scores of 2 or 3) are included. For this task, a 6-point scale (0 [very dissatisfied] to 5 [very satisfied]) portrayed on a semicircular dial is used. For each of the variables included from Task 1, the user is asked to indicate his satisfaction by moving the dial or instructing the evaluator where to place it. The evaluator then circles the result on the summary form. Finally, the user is asked to express a global satisfaction score for the device. This task, as in Task 1, personalizes the assessment to the individual user. The third and final part of the QUEST requires that the evaluator reorganize the results from Part 2 into the three global categories (environment, person, and assistive technology). Only the values for those variables rated as quite or very important in Task 1 are included. The summary sheet then serves to facilitate the interpretation and utilization of the data in assessing satisfaction and addressing those areas in which satisfaction is low.

Weiss-Lambrou et al (1999) utilized the QUEST to determine satisfaction of consumers with seating aids. They describe the application of QUEST to this situation with a group of 24 subjects who used modular type seating aids (see Chapter 6). They found that the most important variable (user comfort) was also rated as the least satisfying. This study illustrates the value and importance of a consumer-driven measure of user satisfaction. Weiss-Lambrou et al describe the application of QUEST in this context in detail.

**Assistive technology abandonment.** One of the most tangible indicators of lack of consumer satisfaction is when the consumer stops using a device even though the need for which the device was obtained still exists. We call this situation **technology abandonment,** and it is useful to look at some of the factors that lead to it. Phillips and Zhao (1993) surveyed more than 200 users of assistive technologies and identified four factors that were significantly related to the abandonment of assistive technologies: (1) failure of providers to take consumers' opinions into account, (2) easy device procurement, (3) poor device performance, and (4) changes in consumers' needs or priorities.

It is not surprising that consumers more often abandon devices when their opinion is not considered, and we have stressed the importance of consumer involvement in the assessment process. If the *structure* of the delivery system supports an effective *process,* then by defining the needs and the activity the goal will be identified. This will help to avoid unfulfilled expectations. If consumers continually have unmet expectations, then changes need to be made to the structure or process or both. On an individual consumer basis, the failure to meet goals may result from a variety of factors such as unrealistic expectations, inappropriate needs assessment, poor device selection, and changing needs over time.

The "easy device procurement" factor refers to the situation in which a consumer obtains a device from a supplier without an evaluation; the consumer just goes into a store and buys a device. This most often occurs with "low-tech" devices such as crutches, canes, or reachers. If the consumer obtains assistive technologies in this manner, then she assumes total responsibility for matching her needs, goals, and skills to the purchased technology.

Poor device performance may be the result of inaccurate or inappropriate expectations on the part of the user, a mismatch between consumer skills and device characteristics, or actual device failure. The overall lack of standards of performance for devices makes it difficult to ensure that a given level of expected performance will be achieved. Changes in needs or priorities can be accommodated by an assistive technology design approach that features flexible allocation of functions (see Chapter 2). However, it is significant that one of the largest groups of devices for which this factor was important in Phillips and Zhao's study were those intended for temporary use (e.g., crutches).

Technology abandonment studies such as that by Phillips and Zhao underscore the importance of considering the entire assistive technology system (as represented by the HAAT model) when designing a system for an individual consumer. The human operator must be a part of the decision making, as well as a part of the needs and skills assessment process. Likewise, the context of use must be carefully considered. Just because a system works well in a clinical setting does not mean that it will meet the user's needs in other settings. Careful definition of the activities to be performed can ensure that the system will allow the consumer the maximum possible participation and that the activities chosen will be those of greatest interest to the consumer. This will also allow both the ATP and the consumer to develop realistic expectations for assistive technology system performance and will lead to a higher probability of user satisfaction and reduced chance for abandonment. Finally, technology abandonment is not always a negative outcome. In many cases a consumer abandons a device because improvement in his physical condition means that he no longer needs it. The assistive technology may have served him very well and met his needs completely during its period of use. We need to develop ways of looking at abandonment that take into account temporary need or lack of use as a result of improvement. Success can be defined in terms of functional results, user satisfaction, timeliness, and cost effectiveness, and we must develop methods for measuring each of these parameters.

## Quality of Life As an Assistive Technology Outcome Measure

ATPs, assistive technology suppliers (ATSs), and assistive technology manufacturers often claim that their service or device "improves the quality of life" of the consumer. This is an appealing concept. Who wouldn't want to do this? There are, however, several difficulties with this concept when we attempt to actually measure it. In fact, the term *quality of life* is itself controversial and subject to misuse (Wolfensberger, 1994). Despite these limitations, it is tempting to want to measure quality of life. It is being applied with increasing frequency to outcomes measurement in medicine and in rehabilitation (Oldridge, 1996). In a medical service context, quality of life is often related to life expectancy and optimal life quality during the time a person is alive. In rehabilitation the concept of quality of life takes on a bit of a different meaning, since the goal is not "repair" or cure but rather maximizing function and independence for the individual. In both cases the concept of health is important. The World Health Organization defines health as "a state of complete physical, mental and social well-being, not merely the absence of disease" (WHO, 1948). Assistive technologies can certainly contribute to both quality of life and a healthy life. Measures designed to assess the degree to which this goal is achieved have begun to emerge over the past decade, and we are in a position to evaluate the assertion that a service or device actually does improve a consumer's quality of life. We discuss several measures of quality of life in this section.

**Health-Related Quality of Life.** The concept of **health-related quality of life** (HRQL) refers to the impact of health services on the overall quality of life of individuals, and it represents the functional effect of an illness and its consequent therapy on an individual as perceived by the person receiving the therapy (Oldridge, 1996). It measures one dimension of quality of life. Others are independence, income, adequate housing, and a safe environment. The definition of HRQL is "the value assigned to duration of life as modified by impairment, functional states, perceptions and social opportunities that are influenced by disease, injury, treatment or policy" (Patrick and Erickson, 1993; quoted by Oldridge, 1996). Rehabilitation in general, and assistive technologies in particular, addresses the long-term effects of disease and injury.

Therefore they affect HRQL as defined here. However, as Oldridge points out, there are many instruments that have been developed to measure HRQL. Many of these are medically oriented and unsuited to assistive technology outcomes measurement. However, the general concepts underlying HRQL do have relevance to assistive technology outcomes measurement, and there is a need to develop new instruments that are more sensitive to the impact of assistive technologies on HRQL. Oldridge (1996) describes the types of HRQL measurements, their application, and the underlying principles on which this construct is based.

**Psychosocial Impact of Assistive Devices Scale.** In order to address the need for quality of life-related measures in assessing assistive technology outcomes, Day and Jutai (1996) developed the Psychosocial Impact of Assistive Devices Scale (PIADS). The development of the PIADS was based on information obtained through focus groups on the experiences of users of assistive technology (Day and Jutai, 1996). The initial set of constructs was developed and evaluated by a set of users. The scales were modified to include both positive and negative impacts on quality of life of assistive technology users by defining a scale from −3 (maximal negative impact) to +3 (maximal positive impact). The final version of the PIADS is a 26-item self-rating scale intended to measure the impact of rehabilitative technologies and assistive devices on the quality of life of the users of these products. Three subscales are included in the PIADS. These are competence (the effects of a device on functional independence, performance, and productivity), adaptability (the enabling and liberating effects of a device), and self-esteem (the extent to which a device has affected self-confidence, self-esteem, and emotional well-being). This multidimensional aspect of the PIADS contributes to its reliability and validity as a measure of the psychosocial impact of assistive technologies on the consumer.

The PIADS has been applied to measurement of outcomes with a variety of assistive technologies. The original study focused on eyeglass and contact lens wearers (Day and Jutai, 1996). In subsequent studies it has been demonstrated that the subscales of the PIADS remain consistent over populations and types of disabilities (stroke, amyotrophic lateral sclerosis, cerebral palsy) or types of assistive technologies. For example, Jutai et al (2000) used the PIADS to evaluate the psychosocial impact of EADLs (see Chapter 11). The goal of this study was to determine the perceived benefit of EADLs to the consumer's quality of life. Two groups were included: users of EADLs and those for whom EADLs were appropriate but who had not yet received them. Users' perceptions were measured at two points 6 to 9 months apart to determine the stability of the perception of psychosocial impact. Jutai et al found that EADLs produced similar degrees of

positive impact on users and positive perceptions of anticipated impact on those without EADLs. The two measures of those using EADLs indicated that the psychosocial impact was stable over the time frame employed. This study demonstrated the utility of the PIADS as an instrument for quantifying the psychosocial impact of assistive technologies.

Jutai et al (1996) discuss the use of instruments like the PIADS to evaluate the outcomes of service provision in assistive technologies. The importance of quality of life outcome measures, in addition to clinical, functional, and user satisfaction assessments, is demonstrated through a series of case studies related to ease of implementation, clear definition of the desired outcomes, ethical considerations, and responsibility to the user of the assistive technology.

**Matching Person and Technology model.** The Matching Person and Technology (MPT) model and assessment instruments have been developed to allow consumers to prioritize their own outcomes in relation to measurable changes in the perceived quality of life as opposed to the absence of disease or sickness or functional ability (Galvin and Scherer, 1996). This instrument has much in common with the QUEST and PIADS. The developers of the QUEST used the MPT as one of the theoretical bases for their work (Demers, Weiss-Lambrou, and Ska, 1996). As in these other measures, the MPT is a multidimensional instrument that taps domains related to overall impact on quality of life. Three domains are included in the MPT (Galvin and Scherer, 1996). The *milieu* dimension assesses characteristics of the environment and psychosocial setting in which the assistive technology is to be used. The *personality* dimension focuses on the individual's personality, temperament, and preferences. Finally, the *technology* component addresses characteristics of the assistive technology itself. Like the QUEST and PIADS, the MPT is designed to be applied across a wide range of disabilities and assistive technology types. The multidimensional nature of the MPT makes it possible to separate influences of the technology, environment, and personal preferences. For example, a consumer may have characteristics (goals, skills, and abilities) typically associated with assistive technology nonuse as measured by the milieu/environment variable but appear to be an optimal user according to characteristics identified for personality and technology. In this case the milieu/environment influences may need to be addressed before the consumer can gain maximal benefit and satisfaction from the use of the assistive technology. Galvin and Scherer (1996) describe the MPT instrument and its application in detail. The MPT has been shown to have reliability and validity in determining the factors related to device abandonment and in assessing the impact on quality of life of assistive technology use.

## Relationship of Outcome Measures to the HAAT Model

The framework utilized throughout this text is the HAAT model. This framework is useful in placing the various outcome measures described in an overall structure. Each HAAT element can be related to outcome measures. The *activity* defines the consumer goals to be achieved based on a consideration of life roles, performance areas, and tasks. There may be several goals for one consumer because she has several different life roles (e.g., worker, mother, wife). Goals that are defined form the basis for a consumer-driven outcome assessment. Functional measures such as OT FACT and the COPM can be used to accurately determine the goals and the associated functional capabilities of the consumer. Important questions to be addressed in this domain include (1) Was the goal achieved? How well was it achieved? (outcome measures), and (2) Were the needs adequately addressed during the assessment to allow definition of goals? (process measure).

Constraints that are placed on the achievement of goals are defined by the HAAT context. This is directly related to the milieu of the MPT and the environment of the QUEST and the adaptability subscale of the PIADS. Outcome measures arising from the context include whether the system is able to function in the required contexts and how well. These may relate to the physical context (e.g., heat or cold, bright light, noisy environment), settings (e.g., home versus employment), or social factors. The inclusion of social factors links the process to society as a whole via cultural considerations (see Chapter 2). One aspect of culture is the funding priorities that are mandated by society's attitudes toward persons with disabilities. Society as a whole determines funding priorities. If the consumer obtains a system purchased though a particular source, he is obligated to comply with the mandate of that funding source. For example, vocational rehabilitation agencies fund services and devices if they are related to employment, and a consumer who receives a computer from this source is obligated to use it for employment rather than recreation. However, if the consumer uses her own money to buy the services or system, she can use them as she sees fit. Thus the funding source is linked to the assistive technology system through the social context. The area of funding is discussed further in Chapter 5.

The human component of the HAAT model is directly related to the personality dimension of the MPT, the self-esteem, and competence subscales of the PIADS, and the personality feature of the QUEST. Each of these instruments taps a slightly different perspective on the human element of the HAAT model and relates to the overall perception of consumer satisfaction and improvement in quality of life as a result of the acquisition of an assistive technology system.

The desired assistive technology characteristics, the final element of the HAAT model, are defined by the combination of consumer skills, goals, personality, and contextual constraints. The QUEST addresses these through its assistive technology characteristics criterion, the MPT through the technology dimension, and the PIADS through the adaptability subscale. These characteristics are based on the consumer tasks that must be accomplished; the personality, perceptual, and motivational characteristics; and the characteristics of the assistive technology relevant to device use or nonuse. Questions of importance that can be addressed by the various outcome instruments include (1) Were the skills accurately determined? (2) Were these characteristics able to accommodate for contextual constraints? (3) Were the characteristics and associated tasks consistent with the consumer's skills? and (4) If the identified tasks are successfully completed, is the goal achieved?

Process and structure can also be evaluated by determining how well the needs and goals; human skills, perceptions, and motivation; and contextual constraints described by the HAAT model are identified. The assessment determines the human skills available to meet the goals. One typical process measure is how accurately these skills were determined. An example outcome measure is the degree to which these skills apply to the use of assistive technologies. For example, assume that it is determined during the assessment that a consumer can use a standard keyboard (see Chapter 7). By evaluating his success in performing functional daily tasks with the keyboard, we can measure both the outcome and the process. If he is physically unable to use the keyboard, then we must review our assessment procedures to see whether the assessment process is sound. If the process is all right but an error in ATP judgment was made, then we need to alter the structure by providing more staff training to increase the likelihood that correct recommendations will be made. When considering the effectiveness of training, a process goal, such as the degree to which the consumer has moved from novice to expert status with a given system, can be measured. Alternatively, the consumer may be able to use the keyboard physically, but the total system may not meet her needs and she may be dissatisfied with the overall result. This outcome will have an impact on process and structure as well, but it also may require revision in the system to make it functional.

## Conclusions

The effectiveness of the assistive technology system and the efficacy of the ATP to provide services are both measured by their ability to meet the needs of the consumer. Obviously this is appropriate. However, it is easy to lose sight of this emphasis if a program is built from a perspective of "experts" providing a service for consumers, rather than collaborating with the consumer, family, and others to meet a goal. The collaborative approach releases the ATP from the burden of having all the answers and accepting total responsibility. Responsibility for successful outcomes is shared with the consumer and others. This avoids the paternalistic protection of the consumer and empowers him to take responsibility for the outcome. Each member of the team becomes 100% responsible for success. This encourages cooperation, communication, and interaction, all factors that are essential for effective utilization of the system. The most effective service is operated from the point of view of establishing desired outcomes and then developing the structure and process to realize them. Too often ATPs and other professionals tend to protect their service from scrutiny rather than welcoming evaluation and its implications for improvement.

The development of appropriate process and outcome measures for assistive technology service delivery is still at an early stage. Since the mid-1990s, however, a number of new tools have been developed and validated and are now available for the ATP to employ in evaluating the effectiveness of assistive technology systems. The outcome measures described in this chapter have been developed to allow determination of skills, abilities, and motivation; functional performance requirements and skill levels; consumer satisfaction with the recommended system; and overall impact on the quality of life of the consumer and significant others. Each of these measures has been developed and validated to focus on different aspects of assistive technology outcomes. As we have seen, several of these have common characteristics. Work is underway to relate three measures, the PIADS, QUEST, and MPT, to each other and to develop a common understanding of the important variables leading to successful assistive device application and use (Jutai, 2001). Continued research and development, particularly on the psychosocial aspects of assistive technology use and nonuse, will continue to inform our assessment of outcome measures and the development of assistive technologies that are more effective in meeting the needs of consumers.

## ■ SUMMARY

This chapter describes the principles of assessment and intervention and the service delivery process to the consumer. The steps in the process include referral intake, needs assessment, evaluation, recommendation, implementation, follow-up, and follow-along. The current state of outcome measurement in the field of assistive technology is also discussed.

## Study Questions

1. Describe the five principles for assistive technology assessment and intervention.
2. Distinguish between quantitative and qualitative assessment procedures.
3. What are the four methods of gathering assessment information?
4. What is the difference between clinical and formal assessment procedures?
5. What is the meaning of the term *criteria for service* as used in assistive technology referral?
6. List the steps involved in assistive technology service delivery, and write a brief description of each one. Which of these steps is the most important? Justify your choice.
7. Describe the difference between opportunity barriers and access barriers. Give an example of each.
8. List three types of opportunity barriers and how they can be addressed during the assessment process.
9. What consumer skills do we evaluate during the assistive technology skills assessment?
10. Describe the ideal relationship between the consumer and the ATP in the assessment and recommendation process for assistive technologies.
11. What visual functions do we measure during the sensory assessment, and how does each of these apply to the use of assistive technologies?
12. Describe the steps involved in the physical evaluation. What are the major outcomes of the physical skills evaluation?
13. What are the major areas that are assessed in the cognitive evaluation for assistive technologies? Why do you think these areas were chosen?
14. Why do we include a separate "device characteristics" section in the assessment? What are the outcomes of this portion of the evaluation?
15. Who are the audiences for the written assessment report? What challenges does this present?
16. Describe the major steps in implementation of an assistive technology system.
17. What are the major types of performance facilitators? When is each type used? What is the role played by each?
18. What are the major goals of a follow-up program, and how does this differ from follow-along?
19. What is the difference between repair and maintenance?
20. What are the three major domains in which outcome measures are employed in assistive technology service delivery?
21. How do the three measurement domains of Question 20 relate to an improvement in the service delivery process?

22. What is OT FACT and how does it narrow the description of a consumer's functional skills and needs?
23. What are the limitations in the use of the FIM for assessing the outcome of assistive technology intervention?
24. What are the strengths of the COPM in relation to determination of consumer needs and satisfaction?
25. Describe the major features of the QUEST and how it is employed to assess user satisfaction.
26. What are the most common reasons that consumers abandon technology?

27. What is the HRQL, and how is it related to assistive technology outcome measures?
28. What are the three subscales of the PIADS? Why does the inclusion of these three scales increase the usefulness and validity of the PIADS?
29. Describe the relationship of the four HAAT model components to the outcome measures described in this chapter.
30. What are the roles and responsibilities of the ATP in determining the effectiveness of assistive technology services and devices?

## References

Angelo J, Smith RO: The critical role of occupational therapy in augmentative communication. In American Occupational Therapy Association, editors: *Technology review '89: perspectives on occupational therapy practice,* Rockville, Md, 1989, American Occupational Therapy Association, pp 49-53.

Bailey RW: *Human performance engineering,* ed 2, Englewood Cliffs, NJ, 1989, Prentice Hall.

Beukelman DR, Mirenda P: *Augmentative and alternative communication, management of severe communication disorders in children and adults,* Baltimore, 1998, Paul H Brookes.

Brooks NA: User's perceptions of assistive devices. In Smith RV, Leslie JH, editors: *Rehabilitation engineering,* Boca Raton, Fla, 1990, CRC Press.

Christiansen C: Occupational therapy, intervention for life performance. In Christiansen C, Baum C, editors: *Occupational therapy,* Thorofare, NJ, 1991, Slack.

Christiansen CH, Schwartz RK, Barnes KJ: Self-care: evaluation and management. In DeLisa JA, editor: *Rehabilitation medicine principles and practice,* Philadelphia, 1988, JB Lippincott.

Colarusso RP, Hammill DD: *Motor free visual perception test manual,* Novato, Calif, 1972, Academic Therapy Publications.

Cook AM: Assessing physical and sensory skills necessary for augmentative communication. In Coleman CL, editor: *ACTion augmentative communication training modules,* Sacramento, Calif, 1988, Assistive Device Center.

Cook AM: Development of motor skills for switch use by person with severe disabilities, *Developmental Disabilities Special Interest Section Newsletter* 14(2), 1991.

Daniels L, Worthingham C: *Muscle testing: techniques of manual examination,* ed 5, Philadelphia, 1986, WB Saunders.

Day H, Jutai JW: Measuring the psychosocial impact of assistive devices: The PIADS, *Can J Rehabil* 9:159-168, 1996.

Demers L, Weiss-Lambrou R, Ska B: Development of the Quebec User Evaluation of Satisfaction with Assistive Technology (QUEST), *Assist Technol* 8(3):3-1, 1996.

DeRuyter F: Evaluating outcomes in assistive technology: do we understand the commitment? *Assist Technol* 7:3-16, 1995.

Duchek J: Assessing cognition. In Christiansen C, Baum C, editors: *Occupational therapy overcoming human performance deficits,* Thorofare, NJ, 1991, Slack.

Dunn W: Assessing sensory performance enablers. In Christiansen C, Baum C, editors: *Occupational therapy overcoming human performance deficits,* Thorofare, NJ, 1991, Slack.

Enders A, Hall M, editors: *Assistive technology sourcebook,* Washington, DC, 1990, RESNA Press.

Fougeyrollas P, Gray DB: Classification systems, environmental factors and social change: the importance of technology. In Gray DB, Quatrano LA, Lieberman, ML, editors: *Designing and using assistive technology: the human perspective,* Baltimore, 1998, Brookes Publishing.

Galvin JC, Scherer MJ: *Evaluating, selecting and using appropriate assistive technology,* Gaithersburg, Md, 1996, Aspen Publications.

Garrett R et al: Development of a computer-based expert system for the selection of assistive communication devices, *Proc RESNA 13th Ann Conf,* pp 348-349, June 1990.

Gaster LS: Continuous quality improvement in assistive technology. Presented at RESNA International Conference, June 1992, Toronto.

Jagacinski RJ, Monk DL: Fitts' law in two dimensions with hand and head movements, *J Motor Behav* 17:77-95, 1985.

Jutai J: Personal correspondence, April 2001.

Jutai J et al: Outcomes measurement of assistive technologies: an institutional case study, *Assist Technol* 8(2):110-120, 1996.

Jutai J et al: Psychosocial impact of electronic aids to daily living, *Assist Technol* 12(2):123-131, 2000.

Kangas KM: Seating, positioning and physical access, *Developmental Disabilities Special Interest Section Newsletter, Special Issue on Assistive Technology, Part 1* 14(2), 1991.

Klein RM, Bell B: *The Klein-Bell ADL Scale mannual,* Seattle, 1979, University of Washington Medical School, Health Sciences Resource Center/SB-56.

Kondraske GV: Quantitative measurement and assessment of function. In Smith RV, Leslie JH, editors: *Rehabilitation engineering*, Boca Raton, Fla, 1990, CRC Press.

Langton A, Hughes JK: Back to work, *Team Rehab Rep* 3(3):14-18, 1992.

Lysack C, Kaufert J: Disabled consumer leaders' perspectives on provision of community rehabilitation services, *Can J Rehabil* 12(3):157-166, 1999.

Mahoney RI, Barthel DW: *Functional evaluation: the Barthel Index, Maryland State Med J* 14:61-65, 1965.

McNaughton S: Connecting with consumers, *Assist Technol* 5(1):7-10, 1993.

Mortola PJ, Kohn J, LeBlanc M: Success through client follow-up, *Team Rehabil Rep* 3(8):49-51, 1992.

Oldridge NB: Outcomes measurement: health-related quality of life, *Assist Technol* 8:82-93, 1996.

Pallin M: Techniques for the successful use of augmentative communication systems. Presented at *Demystifying Technology Workshop*, Sacramento, Calif, 1991, Assistive Device Center.

Patrick D, Erickson P: *Health status and health policy. Quality of life in health care evaluation and resource allocation*, New York, 1993, Oxford University Press.

Phillips B, Zhao H: Predictors of assistive technology abandonment, *Assist Technol* 5:36-45, 1993.

Sackett DL: Evaluation of health services. In Last JM, editor: *Mosley-Rosenau's public health and preventive medicine*, ed 11, New York, 1980, Appleton-Century-Crofts.

Scherer M: *Matching Person and Technology: a series of assessments for evaluating predispositions to and outcomes of technology use in rehabilitation, education, the workplace and other settings*, Webster, NY, 1998, The Institute for Matching Person & Technology.

Schon DA: *The reflective practitioner: how professionals think in action*, New York, 1983, Basic Books.

Smith RO: *Administration and scoring manual: OT FACT*, Rockville, Md, 1990, American Occupational Therapy Association.

Smith RO: Measuring the outcomes of assistive technology: challenge and innovation, *Assist Technol* 8(2):71-81, 1996.

Smith RO: Technological approaches to performance enhancement. In Christiansen C, Baum C, editors: *Occupational therapy*, Thorofare, NJ, 1991, Slack.

Sprigle S, Abdelhamied A: The relationship between ability measures and assistive technology selection, design, and use. In Gray DB, Quatrano LA, Lieberman ML, editors: *Designing and using assistive technology: the human perspective*, Baltimore, 1998, Paul H Brookes.

Stapelton D, Garrett R: VOCAselect Version 1.0: an AAC device selection tool, *Proc Australian Conference of Technology for People with Disabilities*, 114-116, 1995.

Stapelton D et al: Computer access selector: a tool to assist in the selection of computer access devices, *Proc Aust Conf Technol People Disabil*, pp 129-131, 1995.

Uniform Data System for Medical Rehabilitation (UDS): Functional Independence Measure, version 5.1, Buffalo, NY, 1997, Buffalo General Hospital, State University of New York.

*Webster's ninth new collegiate dictionary*, Springfield, Mass, 1984, Merriam-Webster.

Weiss-Lambrou R: Wheelchair seating aids: how satisfied are consumers? *Assist Technol* 11:43-53, 1999.

Witt JC, Cavell TA: Psychological assessment. In Wodrich DL, Joy JE, editors: *Multi-disciplinary assessment of children with learning disabilities and mental retardation*, Baltimore, 1986, Paul H Brookes.

World Health Organization: *Constitution of the World Health Organization: basic documents*, Geneva, 1948, WHO.

World Health Organization: *International classification of functioning, disability and health: ICIDH-2*, Geneva, 2001, WHO.

Wolfensberger, W: "Lets hang up 'quality of life' as a hopeless term." In Goode D, editor: *Quality of life for persons with disabilities: international perspectives and issues*, Cambridge, Mass, 1994, Brookline Books.

# Sample of a Written Questionnaire

---

**BACKGROUND INFORMATION QUESTIONNAIRE**

This questionnaire will help us in providing the services that the client may need. Please answer all applicable questions and return the form as soon as possible so that an evaluation may be scheduled.

---

**General Information**

Form completed by: _____    Relationship to client: _____

Client's name: _____    Date: _____

Address: _____    Birth date: _____

City/State/Zip: _____    Phone: _____

Language(s) spoken: _____

Please mark the ethnic group that applies (optional):

☐ Asian          ☐ American Indian          ☐ African American

☐ Caucasian      ☐ Hispanic                 ☐ Other

Spouse/parent/guardian: _____    Phone: _____

Address: _____

City/State/Zip: _____

Residence:

☐ Home: ___ Alone    ___ With Family        ___ With Attendant        ☐ Group Home

☐ Skilled Nursing Home    ☐ Rehab Facility    ☐ Extended Care Facility    ☐ Other _____

---

**Referral Information**

Referred by: _____    Relationship to client: _____

Address: _____

_____

Phone: _____

How did you learn about our services?

☐ Professional        ☐ Friend        ☐ Conference        ☐ Yellow Pages        ☐ Other _____

Reason for Referral:

☐ Communication                    ☐ Computer Access            ☐ Ergonomics (Work Site)

☐ Postural Seating/Wheelchair      ☐ Environmental Control      ☐ Lease/Rent Device

☐ Pressure Management/Wheelchair   ☐ Powered Mobility           ☐ Repair Device

☐ Other _____

Goals/Expectations:

**Medical/Health Information**

| Primary Diagnosis | Other Condition | | Onset Dates | Specifics/Comments |
|---|---|---|---|---|
| ☐ | ☐ | Amyotrophic Lateral Sclerosis | _____ | _____ |
| ☐ | ☐ | Traumatic Brain Injury | _____ | _____ |
| ☐ | ☐ | Muscular Dystrophy | _____ | _____ |
| ☐ | ☐ | Multiple Sclerosis | _____ | _____ |
| ☐ | ☐ | Spinal Cord Injury | _____ | Level: _____ |
| ☐ | ☐ | Stroke | _____ | _____ |
| ☐ | ☐ | Cerebral Palsy | _____ | _____ |
| ☐ | ☐ | Developmental Delay | _____ | _____ |
| ☐ | ☐ | Emotional/Behavioral Disability | _____ | _____ |
| ☐ | ☐ | Learning Disabiltiy | _____ | _____ |
| ☐ | ☐ | Cognitive Impairment | _____ | _____ |
| ☐ | ☐ | Hearing Impairment | _____ | _____ |
| ☐ | ☐ | Seizures | _____ | _____ |
| ☐ | ☐ | Other | _____ | _____ |

Anticipated Course of Condition:     ☐ Stable        ☐ Improving        ☐ Deteriorating        ☐ Fluctuating

General Health Condition:        ☐ Excellent        ☐ Good        ☐ Fair        ☐ Poor

Medications: _____

List any joint dislocations, deformities, other orthopedic problems, and past or pending surgeries:

_____

_____

Services Currently Receiving:     ☐ OT        ☐ PT        ☐ Speech Therapy     ☐ Other _____

---

**Sensory/Perceptual Abilities**

Vision

| | | | |
|---|---|---|---|
| Visual deficits? | ☐ Yes | ☐ No | Comments: _____ |
| Wear glasses or corrective lenses? | ☐ Yes | ☐ No | Comments: _____ |
| Perceptual deficits? | ☐ Yes | ☐ No | Comments: _____ |
| Lighting affect vision? | ☐ Yes | ☐ No | Comments: _____ |
| Can fixate vision on stationary object? | ☐ Yes | ☐ No | Comments: _____ |
| Can follow a moving object? | ☐ Yes | ☐ No | Comments: _____ |
| Can look right/left without moving head? | ☐ Yes | ☐ No | Comments: _____ |
| Preference for placement of objects? | ☐ Yes | ☐ No | Where in visual field? _____ |

Hearing

| | | | |
|---|---|---|---|
| Known hearing loss? | ☐ Yes | ☐ No | If yes, include audiology results |
| Wears hearing aid? | ☐ Yes | ☐ No | Comments: _____ |
| Reacts to sounds? | ☐ Yes | ☐ No | Comments: _____ |
| Understands speech? | ☐ Yes | ☐ No | Comments: _____ |

**Activities of Daily Living**

☐ School: _____    Full Time _____    Part Time _____    Grade Level _____

☐ Day Program: _____    Days per Week _____

☐ Work: _____    Position _____

      Full Time _____    Part Time _____

☐ Other Program: _____

Please indicate how many hours per day are spent in the following:

| | Hrs. | | Hrs. | | Hrs. |
|---|---|---|---|---|---|
| a regular chair/couch | ___ | driving/riding in a car | ___ | a manual wheelchair | ___ |
| powered wheelchair | ___ | standing unsupported | ___ | standing frame | ___ |
| lying in bed | ___ | sitting on the floor/mat | ___ | sitting at a desk | ___ |
| other _____ | ___ | | | | |

---

**Social Interaction, Learning, and Behavior**

Choose one that best describes level of alertness:

    ☐ No interest in surroundings

    ☐ Little interest in surroundings

    ☐ Sometimes observant; sometimes sees humor in situations

    ☐ Very alert; observant; sees humor in situations

For children, choose one that best describes his/her social play:

    ☐ Unoccupied behavior    ☐ Play among others; little interaction

    ☐ Onlooker behavior    ☐ Interaction with other peers

    ☐ Solitary independent play

Can he/she:

| | | |
|---|---|---|
| Sit and concentrate on a task for appropriate amount of time? | ☐ Yes | ☐ No |
| Concentrate within a distracting environment? | ☐ Yes | ☐ No |
| Make eye contact with people and/or tasks? | ☐ Yes | ☐ No |
| Classify different objects into categories? | ☐ Yes | ☐ No |
| Carry out tasks of 2 or more steps? | ☐ Yes | ☐ No |
| Understand concept of direction? (i.e., up, down) | ☐ Yes | ☐ No |
| Know his/her actions can cause something else to happen? | ☐ Yes | ☐ No |
| Make choices when 2 objects or activities are presented? | ☐ Yes | ☐ No |
| Follow directions or commands given? | ☐ Yes | ☐ No |

List activities/objects/people that the client finds motivating or interesting.

_____

Comments about social behavior:

**Functional Abilities**

Feeding:  ☐ Independent  ☐ Assisted  ☐ Dependent  ☐ Tube Feed  ☐ Electric Feeder

Chewing/
Swallowing:  ☐ Independent  ☐ Assisted  ☐ Dependent

Dressing:  ☐ Independent  ☐ Assisted  ☐ Dependent

Transfers:  ☐ Independent  ☐ Assisted  ☐ Dependent

If assisted:  ☐ Two-Man Lift  ☐ Sliding Board  ☐ Stand-Pivot

**Motor Skills**

Does the client have motor control in the following:

| | | | | | |
|---|---|---|---|---|---|
| Eyes | ☐ Yes | ☐ No | Mouth | ☐ Yes | ☐ No |
| Neck/Head | ☐ Yes | ☐ No | Trunk | ☐ Yes | ☐ No |
| Right Arm | ☐ Yes | ☐ No | Left Arm | ☐ Yes | ☐ No |
| Right Hand | ☐ Yes | ☐ No | Left Hand | ☐ Yes | ☐ No |
| Right Leg | ☐ Yes | ☐ No | Left Leg | ☐ Yes | ☐ No |
| Right Foot | ☐ Yes | ☐ No | Left Foot | ☐ Yes | ☐ No |

Which part of the body is best controlled? _____

Are there any positions or supports that help control movement?  ☐ Yes  ☐ No

If yes, describe: _____

Please mark all capabilities below (and dominant side when applicable):

☐ Write with pen or pencil  ☐ R  ☐ L      ☐ Point with a finger  ☐ R  ☐ L
☐ Type with one digit  ☐ R  ☐ L      ☐ Type with more than one digit  ☐ R  ☐ L
☐ Grasp/release object  ☐ R  ☐ L      ☐ Hold objects  ☐ R  ☐ L
☐ Use both hands for a two-handed activity      ☐ Type with head or mouthstick
☐ Reach capabilities:  ☐ Forward  ☐ Sideways  ☐ Backward

Problems that may interfere with motor function:

☐ Incoordination/poor balance      ☐ Endurance/fatigue  ☐ Tremor
☐ Tone:  ☐ Too little  ☐ Too much  ☐ Reflexes  ☐ Joint contractures

**Mobility/Positioning**

Check all that apply:

☐ Sits independently in regular chair                ☐ Unable to sit upright
☐ Sits in wheelchair without support                 ☐ Walks independently
☐ Sits in wheelchair with support (describe below)   ☐ Walks with assistance
_____              ☐ Depends on wheelchair for mobility

☐ Manual Wheelchair:        (Used Where? _____ )

    Brand Name/Manufacturer: _____ Date Obtained: _____

    Model: _____

    Funding Source: _____

    How Propelled:          ☐ Hands          ☐ Feet          ☐ Assisted/Dependent

    Type/Description of Seating System: _____

    Accessories (e.g., Laptray): _____

    Problems with Wheelchair: _____

    _____

☐ Power Wheelchair:        (Used Where? _____ )

    Brand Name/Manufacturer: _____ Date Obtained: _____

    Model: _____

    Funding Source: _____

    Controlled By:    ☐ Joystick      ☐ Sip & Puff      ☐ Chin Switch      ☐ Switch Array

    Control Site:     ☐ Hand          ☐ Head            ☐ Foot             ☐ Other _____

    Type/Description of Seating System: _____

    Accessories (e.g., Laptray): _____

    Problems with Wheelchair: _____

    _____

Is there a history of pressure sores?    ☐ No    ☐ Yes    (Current?   ☐ No    ☐ Yes)

Please check all means of <u>transportation</u> that are used:

☐ Car                      ☐ Family van                  ☐ Day program's vehicle
☐ Van/bus for wheelchairs  ☐ Public transportation       ☐ Paratransit

**Communication Skills**

Select all methods used to communicate:

☐ Speech          ____ Sounds          ____ Single Words          ____ Phrases          ____ Whole Sentences

Intelligibility:          ____ To All Listeners          ____ Only to Familiar Listeners

☐ Gestures          ☐ Eye Gaze          ☐ Facial Expressions

☐ Sign Language

Type:          ____ ASL          ____ SEE          ____ Other _____
Number of signs used ____
List 5 most commonly used signs _____

☐ Pointing          (How? with finger? foot? eye gaze? _____)

☐ Handwriting          ☐ Drawing          ☐ Typing

☐ Communication Board or Notebook:          (Symbols Used:  ☐ Pictures          ☐ Words          ☐ Letters)
Number of symbols used ____ Approx. size of symbols _____

☐ Electronic Communication Device: _____

Symbols Used:          ☐ Pictures          ☐ Words          ☐ Letters          ☐ No. of Symbols ____
How long has this device been used?: _____
Is this successful/How successful has it been? _____

What is the client's means of indicating "YES": _____          "NO": _____

Can the client spell?          ☐ Yes          ☐ No          (Approx. grade level____ )

Is communication spontaneous?          ☐ Yes          ☐ No

To whom can the client reliably communicate the following:

|  | All | Friends | Family/Caregiver | No One | Method: |
|---|---|---|---|---|---|
| Attract attention | ☐ | ☐ | ☐ | ☐ | _____ |
| Pain/discomfort | ☐ | ☐ | ☐ | ☐ | _____ |
| Frustration/happiness | ☐ | ☐ | ☐ | ☐ | _____ |
| Hunger/thirst | ☐ | ☐ | ☐ | ☐ | _____ |
| Fatigue/boredom | ☐ | ☐ | ☐ | ☐ | _____ |
| Refusal | ☐ | ☐ | ☐ | ☐ | _____ |
| Choice of items | ☐ | ☐ | ☐ | ☐ | _____ |
| Convey new information | ☐ | ☐ | ☐ | ☐ | _____ |
| Discuss past/future events | ☐ | ☐ | ☐ | ☐ | _____ |

Can the client convey medical needs to professionals?          ☐ Yes          ☐ No

How would you like to see the client's communications skills improve? _____
_____

# Assessment Forms

### ■ INITIAL EVALUATION FORM ASSESSMENT SECTION

I. Motor
  A. Grasps
    1. Finger, hand, and wrist movement
      a. Check the following finger/hand movement functions for both the right (R) and left (L) hands. For numbers 1, 2 (or 2a) and 3, place the object on the table and ask the person to hand it to you. If the person cannot pick the object up, then hand it to him or her. For numbers 4, 5, and 6, hold the object in a comfortable location oriented as shown and ask the person to grasp it, move it from front to back and side to side, and release it. For number 7, place the push button on the table and ask the person to press it. Place a number in the box as follows: 1, poor; 2, fair; and 3, good.

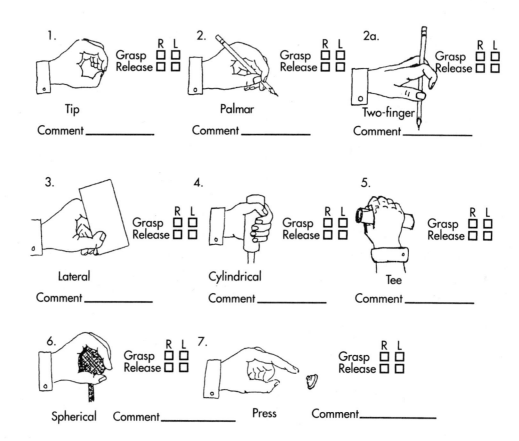

B. Range: Hand

Present hand range sheet. Locate the sheet with the client's midline centered on square #8.

The squares are numbered and each corner is lettered as shown. The targets are the corners. Use the sequence: touch the square then 1A/1B/1C/1D and repeat for all squares within the person's range. Circle locations reached. For children, it may be necessary to use the smaller (foot) range sheet.

Compare your impression of the time required to reach the square (tracking time) to the time required to move among the corners A, B, C, D (select time).

Use the distance table (see Figure 4-5) to fill in the following block.

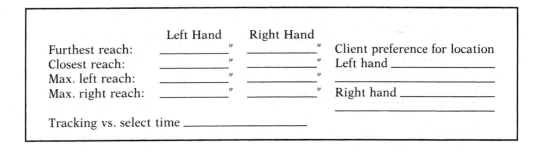

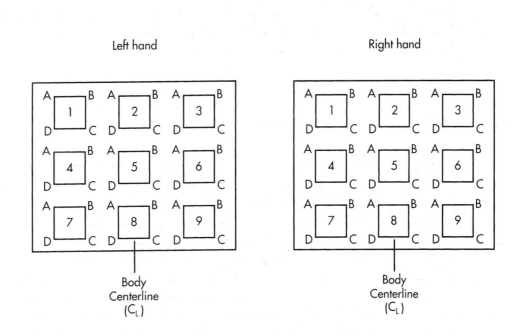

C. Body Part Movement and Control

For each movement requested place a + (present) or − (absent) in the appropriate column. Note whether required movement can be initiated (I), controlled (C), and terminated (T).

| | Left | | | Right | | | |
|---|---|---|---|---|---|---|---|
| **ARM** | I | C | T | I | C | T | COMMENTS |
| Tasks:  Tester places object (cup, toy, etc.) at person's midline 10″ from his or her body and instructs. Reposition if necessary and note new position. | | | | | | | |
| Lift 6″ | | | | | | | |
| Extend by reaching | | | | | | | |
| Rotate as if to pour (put object in cup to be poured) | | | | | | | |
| Rotate in the opposite direction | | | | | | | |
| Turn upright again | | | | | | | |
| Move 6″ to the left | | | | | | | |
| Move 6″ to the right | | | | | | | |
| Pull back | | | | | | | |

If adequate arm and hand movement are available, omit the following tasks:

| **KNEE** | I | C | T | I | C | T | COMMENTS |
|---|---|---|---|---|---|---|---|
| move knee to the left | | | | | | | |
| move knee to the right | | | | | | | |
| **JAW** | | | | | | | |
| open | | | | | | | |
| close | | | | | | | |
| **MOUTH** | | | | | | | |
| blow through a straw | | | | | | | |
| sip through a straw | | | | | | | |
| **VOICE** | | | | | | | |
| produce a sound | | | | | | | |
| produce a variety of words | | | | | | | |

D. Range: Foot

Present the foot range sheet unless the interview indicates there is no foot movement possible or hand movement is adequate. If foot control appears to be feasible, then repeat the same tasks that were done with the hand. Start by locating the heel of the foot at the site labeled "X." Allow the person to move the entire foot as necessary to complete the task.

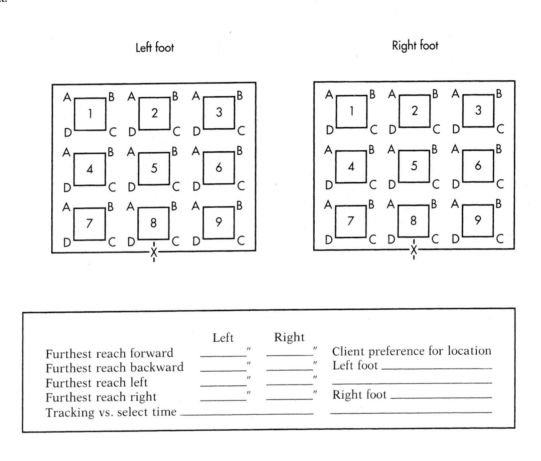

E. Head Control

Measure range of movement in the planes shown. Check the space representing the person's degree of movement to indicate if he or she has no movement, partial movement, or full range of movement.

Directions

| Movement plane | left | | | right | | | |
| --- | --- | --- | --- | --- | --- | --- | --- |
| | None | Partial | Full | None | Partial | Full | Comments |
| Horizontal | | | | | | | |
| | Up | | | Down | | | |
| Vertical | | | | | | | |
| | Left | | | Right | | | |
| Tilt | | | | | | | |

Is a headpointer used now? _____ If so, describe: _____

_____

If the client has used one before but doesn't now, explain why: _____

_____

Reflexive head movements noted: _____

_____

Restraints to head movement:

_____

_____

Sketch

Head

List those anatomical sites appearing to be most suitable for interfacing

Most suitable _____
Next most suitable _____
Third most suitable _____

II. Symbol Location, Type, and Size
  A. *Symbol Location Task*
    1. *Peripheral*
       Instruct the person to keep head and eyes fixed straight forward. Ask the person to indicate when he or she can see your finger or pointer without moving his/her eyes. If the person cannot keep his/her eyes fixed, provide an object to stare at. Start with your finger or pointer approximately 12 inches from the side of his/her head (at the ear) and move it around the head toward the face. Mark the areas in which the person can see your finger.

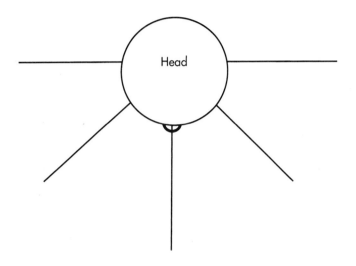

    2. *Tracking*
       Using your finger or pointer, have the person track horizontally at the level of the eyes. Begin at the nose and go left/right. To track vertically, begin at the nose and go up/down.

|  | Yes | Comments |
|---|---|---|
| Can the person track horizontally? | _____ | _____ |
| Can the person track vertically? | _____ | _____ |

  B. *Symbol Size Verification*
    1. *Instructions*
       Select the stimuli according to the information available. If information is lacking, begin with a more "basic" symbol system (e.g., select pictures over words or letters) and begin with the largest size set. Place the stimuli approximately 18 inches from the subject's eyes. Determine the method of selection and explain it to the consumer.

Present two stimuli to the consumer and say, for example, "Please point to (look at) the comb," or "Is this a comb?" Three trials should be run. If no errors are made, the size of the stimuli should be reduced, with three trials run at each size tested. A more advanced symbol system may then be tested if appropriate. If some errors are made, a more basic symbol system should be tested and the positioning of the stimuli should be reexamined.

2. *Data Sheet*

Use a plus mark in the choice column to designate a correct response and use a circle to designate an error. Be sure to note a symbol system and stimulus size for all trial groups.

| | | Trials<br>+      ◯ |
| Symbol System | Size | Correct/Incorrect |

a. _____ _____ 1. _____
                            2. _____
                            3. _____

b. _____ _____ 1. _____
                            2. _____
                            3. _____

c. _____ _____ 1. _____
                            2. _____
                            3. _____

d. _____ _____ 1. _____
                            2. _____
                            3. _____

Optimal symbol type: _____
Optimal size: _____

If you were not able to establish an optimal stimulus, explain why.

# CHAPTER 5

# Funding Assistive Technology Services and Systems

## Chapter Outline

PUBLIC SOURCES OF FUNDING
Medicare
Medicaid
Children's Medical Services
Programs for the Developmentally Disabled
CHAMPUS
Education
Vocational Rehabilitation
PASS
Veterans Administration

PRIVATE SOURCES OF FUNDING
Self-funding
Private Health Insurance
Worker's Compensation

OTHER SOURCES OF FUNDING

THE FUNDING PROCESS AND GUIDELINES FOR PROCURING FUNDING

IDENTIFYING THE FUNDING SOURCE

JUSTIFYING FUNDING FOR ASSISTIVE TECHNOLOGY SERVICES AND DEVICES

APPEALING THE FUNDING DENIAL

BILLING AND CODING FOR SERVICES

PAYMENT PRACTICES

SUMMARY

APPENDIX 5-1: SAMPLE FORMS FOR DOCUMENTING CONSUMERS' EQUIPMENT NEEDS

## Learning Objectives

Upon completing this chapter you will be able to:

1.  Identify the major categories of funding for assistive technology services and equipment
2.  Describe the types of assistive technology devices and services covered by each category of funding
3.  Distinguish between categories of funding as they relate to specific consumer characteristics
4.  Describe the process for procuring funding
5.  Describe the process by which funding decisions can be appealed

---

### Key Terms

| | | |
|---|---|---|
| Appeals Process | Managed Care | PASS |
| CHAMPUS | Medicaid | Procedure Codes |
| Diagnosis Codes | Medical Necessity | Public Funding Sources |
| Fee for Service | Medicare | Third-Party Payer |

---

Assistive technology services and devices are now more widely available to individuals with disabilities. Unfortunately, funding remains a major barrier for individuals trying to access assistive technology equipment and services. Evaluation, implementation, and ongoing maintenance and repair of assistive technologies can be costly, and most consumers do not have the financial resources available to purchase the necessary services and equipment. Therefore funding by third-party sources is necessary in order for individuals to procure assistive technology services and equipment. Acquiring this funding is an inherent part of the assistive technology practitioner's (ATP's) role as a service provider and is an ongoing challenge for both the consumer and the ATP.

In countries in which there is a national health or social service system (e.g., Australia and Canada), funding for assistive technology services and equipment is often provided by a central agency. In the United States funding is decentralized, meaning it is provided by numerous sources rather than by a system solely dedicated to the funding of assistive technology services and equipment. Funding for assistive technology is usually rendered through agencies that have been primarily developed for the provision of other types of services. Equipment and services may be funded solely through one source of funding or through a combination of sources. The various funding sources can be categorized as three general types: public, private, and other.

### ■ PUBLIC SOURCES OF FUNDING

**Public funding sources** include federal, state, and local government agencies; several public sources of funding are listed in Box 5-1. There are more than 30 programs established by the United States Congress that affect U.S. residents with disabilities and more than 12 agencies on the federal level that oversee these programs (Morris and Golinker, 1991). Typically, Congress authorizes funding through a specific piece of legislation, such as the 1986 Amendments to the Rehabilitation Act of 1973 (Public Law 99-506), which is discussed in Chapter 1, and designates a federal agency to determine the scope and criteria for the program. Within each state, an agency is designated to receive the federal funds and ensure compliance with the programs mandated by the federal government. The funds are then distributed to agencies or programs on a local level, which are responsible for providing the services to individuals with disabilities. Each program has a set of regulations that mandate the services to be provided.

### Medicare

**Medicare,** which was established by Congress in 1965, is the health insurance program operated by the federal government. It covers individuals age 65 and older and those adults under age 65 who are blind, are totally and permanently disabled, and have received Social Security Disability Insurance (SSDI) benefits or Adult Disabled Child benefits for at least 24 months. Medicare, which is administered by the Health Care Financing Administration (HCFA), has two types of coverage. Part A covers inpatient hospitalization, skilled nursing facility, home health care, and hospice care. Part B is a supplemental policy in which the individual pays a small premium to cover services such as outpatient therapies and durable medical equipment.

*Durable medical equipment* is defined by Medicare as equipment that is primarily and customarily used to serve a medical need, can withstand repeated use, and is generally not useful to a person in the absence of an injury and illness. Some assistive technology equipment, such as a wheelchair or seat cushion, are covered under Part B as durable medical equipment. Equipment purchased or rented under Part B must be used in the patient's home and deemed "necessary and reasonable" for the treatment of the injury or illness or for improving the function of an impaired body part. A physician's prescription is necessary to substantiate medical necessity for the device. This prescription indicates the individual's diagnosis and prognosis, the reason for the device, and the length of time the device will be needed. The provider must also substantiate the reasonableness of the device by indicating other alternatives that were considered and demonstrating that the one recommended is the least costly in terms of its expected therapeutic benefits. Reimbursement for the equipment is denied if the provider fails to prove reasonableness.

## BOX 5-1  Assistive Technology Financing Options

**PUBLIC PROGRAMS**

MEDICARE

MEDICAID

Required and Optional Services

Intermediate Care Facilities for Persons Who Are Mentally Retarded (ICFs/MR)

Early and Periodic Screening, Diagnosis and Treatment (EPSDT)

Home and Community-Based (HCB) Waivers

Community-supported Living Arrangements

MATERNAL AND CHILD HEALTH

Maternal and Child Health Block Grant to States

Children with Special Health Care Needs

Special Projects of Regional and National Significance (SPRANS)

EDUCATION

Individuals with Disabilities Education Act (IDEA) State Grants (Part B)

IDEA Programs for Infants and Toddlers with Disabilities and Their Families (Part H)

State-operated programs

Vocational education

Head Start

VOCATIONAL REHABILITATION

State grants

Supported Employment

Independent Living Parts A, B, and C

SOCIAL SECURITY BENEFITS

Title II: Social Security Disability Insurance (SSDI)

Title XVI: Supplemental Security Income (SSI)

Work incentive programs

DEVELOPMENTAL DISABILITY PROGRAMS

DEPARTMENT OF VETERANS AFFAIRS PROGRAMS

OLDER AMERICANS ACT PROGRAMS

**ALTERNATIVE FINANCING**

Revolving Loan Fund

Lending library

Discount program

Low-interest loans

Private foundations

Service clubs

Special state appropriations

State bond issues

Employee Accommodations Program

Equipment Loan Program

Corporate-sponsored loans

Charitable organizations

**U.S. TAX CODE**

Medical care expense deduction

Business deductions

Employee business deductions

Americans with Disabilities Act (ADA) credit for small business

Credit for architectural and transportation barrier removal

Targeted jobs tax credit

Charitable contributions deduction

**PRIVATE HEALTH INSURANCE**

Health insurance

Worker's Compensation

Casualty insurance

Disability insurance

**CIVIL RIGHTS**

The Americans with Disabilities Act

Rehabilitation Act, Section 504

**UNIVERSAL ACCESS**

Rehabilitation Act, Section 508

Decoder Circuitry Act

**TELECOMMUNICATIONS**

Telecommunications for the Disabled Act of 1982

Telecommunications Accessibility Enhancement Act of 1988

National Council on Disability: *Study on the financing of assistive technology devices and services for individuals with disabilities,* Washington, DC, 1993, The Council.

## Medicaid

**Medicaid** is the health insurance program, established in 1965 by Title XIX of the Social Security Act, for persons who are unable to pay the costs of their medical care; it is administered at the state level The federal government mandates certain services, eligibility, and benefits requirements. There are also optional services that states may elect to include as a part of their Medicaid program. Mandatory and optional Medicaid services are listed in Box 5-2. Each state modifies its program to accommodate its particular situation, and the scope of services provided by Medicaid varies widely from state to state. Assistive technology is not specified as one of the services mandated by the federal

government, nor is it found on the list of optional Medicaid services. However, assistive technology services and devices *are* within the scope of each state's Medicaid program (Golinker and Mistrett, 1997).

The federal definitions of the intent and scope of mandated and optional services should be used as a starting point to determine the basis of Medicaid funding for assistive technology. In order to receive federal funding for Medicaid, all states must comply with these definitions of services. Golinker and Mistrett (1997) identify eight services among the list of mandatory and optional Medicaid services under which funding for assistive technology and services may qualify. These services are early and periodic

---

**BOX 5-2    Mandatory and Optional Medicaid Services**

**MEDICAID SERVICES**
Title XIX of the Social Security Act requires that in order to receive federal matching funds, certain basic services must be offered to the categorically needy population in any state program:
- Inpatient hospital services
- Outpatient hospital services
- Physician services
- Medical and surgical dental services
- Nursing facility (NF) services for individuals aged 21 or older
- Home health care for persons eligible for nursing facility services
- Family planning services and supplies
- Rural health clinic services and any other ambulatory services offered by a rural health clinic that are otherwise covered under the state plan
- Laboratory and x-ray services
- Pediatric and family nurse practitioner services
- Federally qualified health center services and any other ambulatory services offered by a federally qualified health center that are otherwise covered under the state plan
- Nurse-midwife services (to the extent authorized under state law)
- EPSDT services for individuals under age 21

If a state chooses to include the medically needy population, the state plan must provide, as a minimum, the following services:
- Prenatal care and delivery services for pregnant women
- Ambulatory services to individuals under age 18 and individuals entitled to institutional services
- Home health services to individuals entitled to nursing facility services

If the state plan includes services either in institutions for mental diseases or in ICF/MRs, it must offer either of the following to each of the medically needy groups: the services contained in 42 Code of Federal Regulations (CFR) sections 440.10 through 440.50 and 440.165 (to the extent that nurse-midwives are authorized to practice under state law or regulations); or the services contained in any seven of the sections in 42 CFR 440.10 through 440.165.

States may also receive federal funding if they elect to provide other optional services. The most commonly covered optional services under the Medicaid program include the following:
- Clinic services
- Nursing facility services for persons under age 21
- ICF/MR services
- Occupational, physical, speech, hearing, and language therapy and other rehabilitative services
- Optometrist services and eyeglasses
- Prescribed drugs
- Tuberculosis-related services for infected persons
- Prosthetic devices
- Dental services

States may provide home and community-based care waiver services to certain individuals who are eligible for Medicaid. The services to be provided to these persons may include case management, personal care services, respite care services, adult day health services, homemaker/home health aide, habilitation, and other services requested by the state and approved by HCFA.

Modified from Health Care Financing Administration, Department of Health and Human Services: www.hcfa.gov/medicaid, 2001.

---

screening, diagnostic treatment services, home health care services, prosthetic devices, occupational therapy, physical therapy, rehabilitative services, skilled nursing facility, and services and intermediate care facility services for persons with mental retardation, developmental disabilities, and related conditions (ICF/MR-DD). Because assistive technology devices and services are not listed as such in the Medicaid vocabulary, it is recommended that use of these terms be avoided when applying for funding under Medicaid (Golinker and Mistrett, 1997). Instead, the device being requested should be identified by its specific name in all documentation and any descriptive terms used should match those in the definition of one of the Medicaid services listed above.

One of the general criteria for funding of all Medicaid services is that the requested equipment or service be considered a medical necessity. Another general criterion for funding of Medicaid services is that prior approval or prior authorization is required for nearly all services and equipment. Before commencing any services or purchasing any equipment for a Medicaid beneficiary, the ATP needs to request approval from Medicaid for the purchase of such

services or devices. In some states a certain amount of occupational and physical therapy services may be provided without prior authorization. Because the ATP may not know whether this threshold has already been reached, it is generally safer from a reimbursement standpoint to get prior approval for the services to be provided.

## Children's Medical Services

Medical and related services are provided to children under the age of 21 who have chronic disabling conditions and meet income limitations. This program is funded jointly by the federal and state governments. All children are eligible for medical diagnosis and evaluation. In some states, funding of assistive technologies is provided by Children's Medical Services (CMS).

## Programs for the Developmentally Disabled

Within each state, programs for the developmentally disabled provide a range of services, including case management, advocacy, community living, and purchase of other services. Assistive technology services and equipment may be funded from these programs.

## CHAMPUS

The Civilian Health and Medical Program of the Uniformed Services **(CHAMPUS)** is a federally funded program that provides medical benefits to dependents of active duty members of the armed forces and to retired members. CHAMPUS contracts with various health insurance companies to administer this program, which provides medically necessary equipment and assistive technology services.

## Education

As discussed in Chapter 1, the Education for All Handicapped Children Act of 1975, the Handicapped Infant and Toddlers Act of 1986, and the 1991 reauthorization of these through the Individuals with Disabilities Education Act (IDEA) are vehicles through which assistive technology and related services can be justified. Children from birth to 2 years of age must have an Individualized Family Service Plan (IFSP), and children 3 years to 21 years old must have a written Individual Education Plan (IEP) (see Chapter 1). Assistive technology must be considered in the development of the child's IEP. If assistive technology is identified as being necessary for a "free and appropriate public education" (FAPE), it must be included in the IEP and this service must be provided.

## Vocational Rehabilitation

The federal government provides states with funds to administer programs that help individuals with disabilities to enter, remain in, or return to employment. An Individual Written Rehabilitation Plan (IWRP) that outlines the individual's vocational objectives and services to be provided is required. Those who need assistive technology to complete training in a vocational rehabilitation program or obtain employment (competitive, supported, or sheltered) are eligible for funding of assistive technology equipment and services. In fact, of all federally funded programs, vocational rehabilitation programs are the only ones that require an evaluation for assistive technology as a part of determining eligibility for services (Morris and Golinker, 1991). With an increase in opportunities for supported and sheltered employment, the range of individuals who can be served by vocational rehabilitation programs is becoming larger. For example, individuals with more severe disabilities are now eligible for employment and vocational rehabilitation services. Staffs of vocational rehabilitation programs may not be aware of the benefits of assistive technology, and efforts by ATPs to provide ongoing training can increase their awareness regarding assistive technology.

## PASS

The Plan for Achieving Self-sufficiency **(PASS)** is a program that allows individuals to put aside income for equipment or services that will assist them in achieving a vocational objective. This includes assistive technology services and devices such as augmentative communication devices and adapted computer equipment. The Social Security Administration (SSA) oversees this program and must approve the PASS before it can go into effect. The SSA excludes the money earned to pay for the devices from earned income, which allows the consumer to continue to receive his applicable benefits. The consumer develops a written plan that identifies needs and feasible occupational goals, with a timetable for attaining these goals.

## Veterans Administration

The Veterans Administration (VA) directly provides assistive technology equipment and related services, as well as contracts with outside programs to provide these services. Individuals who have a service-connected disability are eligible for purchase of assistive technologies by the VA.

## ■ PRIVATE SOURCES OF FUNDING

In addition to federal funding sources, there are private sources of funding. These are identified in Box 5-1.

## Self-funding

Personal sources of funding include out-of-pocket cash paid by the consumer, private trust funds, and loans. Because of the cost of assistive technology equipment and services, paying cash could be a hardship on the consumer. Sometimes this is the only alternative, however. Some individuals have trust funds set up where money received from a legal settlement is kept to provide for the equipment and services they may need, including assistive technologies. Individuals who use personal funds to purchase assistive technology may be eligible for a deduction or credit on their taxes and should consult with a tax accountant.

Low-interest loans are also available for the purchase of assistive technology. In procuring a loan, the consumer shares the responsibility of paying for the equipment, which may increase the consumer's involvement in the process (Reeb, 1989). The Easter Seal Society has recently set up a national loan fund to help persons with disabilities purchase assistive technologies. The loan fund was made possible by a U.S. Department of Education grant. Up to 75% of the equipment costs can be financed. The maximal amount that can be financed is $3200.00. Some manufacturers and vendors also provide low-interest loans. A consumer in need of a loan should check with these sources as well.

## Private Health Insurance

The consumer may have private health insurance that will cover assistive technology equipment and related services. Insurance companies that provide health insurance plans have a variety of plans. The ATP should not assume the consumer has coverage based solely on the company name on the plan. Individuals who have private health insurance are provided with or can obtain the details of their plan, which stipulates whether any rehabilitative therapies are covered. One or more of these professionals may be involved in the evaluation, and their services may be covered under this provision. Rehabilitation engineering services usually are not provided for under any private health insurance plan. Some plans also cover a portion of the cost of durable medical equipment (DME). As in public health insurance, funding by private health insurance companies is based on a medical diagnosis and justification of medical necessity. Most private forms of health insurance require the use of Current Procedural Terminology (CPT) codes for billing (see section on billing and coding later in this chapter).

## Worker's Compensation

Expenses incurred as a result of work-related injuries are covered by Worker's Compensation benefits. Under certain conditions, equipment, home modifications, and services are covered. Worker's Compensation benefits are financed jointly by individual employers or groups of employers and state governments (Burton, 1996). A designated state agency or board develops the regulations for Worker's Compensation and private insurance companies typically administer the program.

## ■ OTHER SOURCES OF FUNDING

There are alternative sources for funding that do not fall under the categories of public or private agencies (see Box 5-1). These sources include service clubs, private foundations, and volunteer organizations. There are various community service clubs (e.g., Kiwanis, Rotary Club) that may be a source of funding for a local individual who has no other means of funding. Service clubs are more likely to provide funding if one of their goals is to help certain disability groups or if the consumer is a member of the club or personally knows someone who is a member.

There are foundations related to a specific disability group that directly supply equipment and services to individuals with that particular disability. Other disability-related foundations provide partial funding or assist the consumer in obtaining funding. The American Federation for the Blind provides low-interest loans, for example, to individuals who are visually impaired and need to purchase

equipment (Matheis et al, 1991). There are also a number of volunteer organizations (e.g., Telephone Pioneers of America) that may contribute by fabricating a custom device. Usually the labor is provided and the consumer pays for the cost of materials.

## ■ THE FUNDING PROCESS AND GUIDELINES FOR PROCURING FUNDING

Just as the assistive technology system is an ongoing process, so is the process of obtaining funding. It is not just the device that needs to be purchased; funding must be obtained for defining and implementing the total assistive technology system. There are several points during the process at which funding may need to be pursued (shown in Figure 4-2).

The first point at which funding is secured is after the intake referral, when the need for an evaluation has been identified. The second point at which funding is addressed is after the recommendations for the implementation of assistive technologies. At this point there needs to be justification that the equipment recommended is the most appropriate and cost effective for that particular individual. Resources for training of the consumer and care providers in the use of the device should also be requested at this stage. Some funding sources may not understand the need for training, in which case the ATP should advocate for these services and educate the funding sources regarding the importance of this component in the successful use of the device.

Finally, there is a critical need for funding during both the follow-up and follow-along phases. What happens when the device is dropped and the display is broken? Who pays for the repair? What happens when the individual moves to another care facility and the instruction manual and the charger for the device do not make it to the new facility? Who trains the staff at the new facility on the basic operation of the device? Who pays for these services? It is necessary that these issues be brought to the attention of the funding source at the onset of intervention so they can be considered as part of a total package in the delivery of the assistive technology system.

Earlier we described the various funding sources; in the next section we provide guidelines for navigating the complex process of obtaining funding.

## ■ IDENTIFYING THE FUNDING SOURCE

There are a number of problems that have been identified as a result of the decentralized funding system described earlier (Enders and Hall, 1990; National Council on Disability, 1993). It is not always obvious where to look for funding, and identifying the appropriate source for funding can be difficult for the consumer and the ATP. Each of the agencies that provides funding for assistive technologies may have a different standard of need, with little consistency among the various agencies. For example, educational agencies fund assistive technology that provides a student with access to education. Medicare and Medicaid typically only fund durable medical equipment that is medically necessary, such as wheelchairs and seat cushions. In state vocational rehabilitation agencies there is a standard that the assistive technology must significantly contribute to the individual's ability to be productive at work for it to be funded. This agency most likely will not fund assistive technologies that contribute to the individual's independence in self-care and home management skills.

Dealing with the multiple public or private agencies is a challenge. Procedures for obtaining funding for assistive technologies, levels of funding, and staff familiarity with the scope of and need for assistive technology and related services vary from agency to agency. For example, some funding agencies require that equipment and services be purchased from an approved list of vendors. Other funding agencies require approval for services and equipment before implementation. It is the responsibility of the consumer and the ATP to locate for each agency the regulations that apply to assistive technology and pursue funding based on those regulations. These regulations are often unclear and open to interpretation, making it difficult to initiate a request for funding. Commonly there is no coordination of services among agencies and many agencies see themselves as the payer of last resort; that is, they won't provide funding unless the consumer has received denial from other potential sources. All these issues can result in delays in the service delivery process.

It is not uncommon to seek funding for an assistive technology system from multiple sources, as shown in Case Study 5-1. The ATP may be working with a consumer on a variety of needs at the same time. It is also not unusual for a funding source to pay for an evaluation but not the equipment. The reverse is also true in cases where the funding source has not been educated about the value of a proper assessment before recommendation of a device or the need for training on strategies for using the equipment once it has been acquired by the consumer. Education of third-party payers is necessary in these situations.

To simplify the process of obtaining funding, it is recommended that a funding strategy be developed for each consumer. Beukleman and Mirenda (1998) identify five steps in developing such a strategy:

1. Survey the funding resources that are available to the individual.
2. Identify various funding sources for the various

## CASE STUDY 5-1

### FUNDING FOR MIRANDA

Miranda is 14 years old and a freshman in high school. She has cerebral palsy and uses a wheelchair for mobility. She is also nonverbal. Her teacher referred her to the Assistive Technology Center for an augmentative communication evaluation. During the needs assessment, it was discovered that Miranda was also in need of a new seating and mobility system. Her mother also expressed a desire for Miranda to be more independent at home and to be able to turn the TV and her stereo system off and on. Miranda has a range of assistive technology needs, and it became apparent to the ATP that funding for Miranda was going to have to come from multiple sources. Given the information that was shared during the needs assessment, the ATP completed a personal funding worksheet for Miranda. The ATP will seek funding from the state Medicaid system for the seating and mobility system, from the school system for an augmentative communication device, and from Miranda's personal resources for an electronic aid to daily living (EADL) to turn her TV, stereo, and appliances off and on. Her father is also involved in the local Rotary Club and that may be another source of funding for the EADL.

activities of an intervention (i.e., assessment, equipment, and training). The use of a personal funding worksheet such as the one shown in Box 5-3 is helpful.
3. Prepare a funding plan with the consumer and the family members.
4. Assign responsibility to specific individuals for pursuing funding for each aspect of the intervention.
5. Prepare necessary documentation for the funding request. Be sure to make all requests in writing so a written record is available if an appeal is necessary.

Keeping current on funding information is time consuming but absolutely essential for the ATP. Every state has a technology assistance project (see Chapter 1) that disseminates information on funding resources and strategies. For contact information refer to the Rehabilitation Engineering and Assistive Technology Society of North America (RESNA) Technical Assistance Project Web site (www.resna.org). *Assistive Technology: A Funding Workbook* (Morris and Golinker, 1991) also provides information on funding resources and strategies. Another source of funding information and advocacy are the independent living centers found in each state. Networking with other assistive

| BOX 5-3 | Personal Funding Worksheet |
|---------|---------------------------|

Client: _____

Type of Intervention (e.g., AAC, mobility): _____

| Funding Source | Assessment/ Recommendations | Equipment Purchase | Training | Follow-up and Follow-along |
|----------------|------------------------------|--------------------|----------|----------------------------|
| Medicare | | | | |
| Medicaid | | | | |
| Children's Medical Services | | | | |
| Developmental Services | | | | |
| CHAMPUS | | | | |
| School | | | | |
| Vocational Rehabilitation | | | | |
| PASS | | | | |
| Veterans Administration | | | | |
| Self-funding | | | | |
| Private Health Insurance | | | | |
| Worker's Compensation | | | | |
| Community Organizations | | | | |
| Other | | | | |

Modified from Beukelman DR, Mirenda P: *Augmentative and alternative communication, management of severe communication disorders in children and adults,* Baltimore, 1998, Paul H Brookes.

technology professionals at conferences, via listservs, and over the phone are other invaluable resources.

## JUSTIFYING FUNDING FOR ASSISTIVE TECHNOLOGY SERVICES AND DEVICES

**Third-party payers** will not fund assistive technology services or equipment without adequate documentation and proof of need. The essential question funding sources want answered is how this technology will improve the individual's functioning. Whether it is a medical, vocational, or educational need, there are essential components that should be included in any written justification. Golinker and Mistrett (1997) identify components to address when justifying a medical need for a device, but these elements can apply to other justifications as well. These components are summarized as follows:

1. A description of the specific functional limitation that the device and service addresses
2. A detailed description of the device, including features, accessories, and customization
3. A specific description of the effect of the device or service (e.g., how it will alleviate or ameliorate the functional limitation described in item 2)

4. A description of the evaluation process, how the recommendation was arrived at, and what other alternatives were considered
5. An explanation of why the device being recommended is the least costly solution
6. A description of the expertise of the ATP (or interdisciplinary team) recommending the services or equipment, including general professional experience and specific experience in assistive technology services

A specific criterion for funding under Medicare, Medicaid, and private health insurance is **medical necessity.** This requires that the justification include "identification of a medical diagnosis, or condition, that is specifically coupled to the functional impairment being addressed by the device" (Golinker and Mistrett, 1997, p 217). A physician's prescription is required for devices that are medically necessary. Appendix 5-1A provides an example of a form to use to justify funding for augmentative communication devices and Appendix 5-1B shows an example of a justification form for seating and wheeled mobility systems.

When funding is being pursued through a vocational rehabilitation agency, it is important that the written justification specify how the device will enhance the individual's ability to function in a work setting. For assistive technology services and equipment to be considered, they need to be part of the consumer's IWRP. Similarly, when funding is being pursued through special education, the justification needs to address how the equipment will give the child access to a free and appropriate education in the "least restrictive environment." All assistive technology services and equipment must address goals written in the child's IFSP for children from birth to 2 years old or the IEP for children ages 3 to 21. Medicaid and Medicare will not fund equipment and services that are education related, and educational agencies will not fund services that are medically necessary.

It is likely that the staff person reading the funding justification has never met the consumer and may not have had any experience with a person with a disability or with assistive technology. It is important that the justification be easily understood and clearly depict who this person is, what her needs are, and how the system can help. It may be helpful to include a picture or videotape of the consumer with the system being recommended.

## ■ APPEALING THE FUNDING DENIAL

At any point in the funding process, a denial for funding may be received. When requests for funding have been denied, it helps to be persistent and submit an appeal for the denial. It is through this persistence that funding sources may eventually include assistive technologies as a regular part of the support they provide.

Every funding agency has an **appeals process** whereby the ATP can appeal a funding denial. The first step taken by the ATP is to determine the procedure for an appeal. The next step, if possible, is to find out why the request was denied. By knowing the reason for denial, the ATP can be sure to submit an appeal that specifically addresses the reason and thus decrease the likelihood of the appeal being denied as well. Sometimes a request is denied because a piece of information was inadvertently omitted, such as a billing code, and resubmission of the request with the necessary information is all that is needed. The denial may have been made because the agency believes that the plan or policy does not include such a benefit, or it may be based on the fact that the provider does not think that the request meets the criteria for funding.

Mendelsohn (1996) discusses typical grounds for appeal and the format that appeals may take. The purpose of an appeal is to convince the funding agency that the denial was erroneous and have the decision reversed. The appeal should be made in writing to the funding source. It should explain why the denial for funding was inappropriate and provide any additional information that may have been omitted in the initial request (Golinker and Mistrett, 1997). During the appeals process it may be necessary to ask for assistance from a skilled advocacy layperson or an attorney.

## ■ BILLING AND CODING FOR SERVICES

Preparing the billing form correctly and using the proper codes on billing forms are necessary to ensure payment. Medical payers require that the provider use diagnosis codes and procedure codes when services are billed. **Diagnosis codes** are used to describe the person's condition or the medical reason for the services being requested; it is this condition that is the key to establishing medical necessity. The most widely used diagnosis-coding system in the United States is *The International Statistical Classification of Diseases and Related Health Problems,* tenth revision (ICD-10) (World Health Organization, 1992).

**Procedure codes** are used to describe the services that the provider carried out and that are being billed. The HCFA Common Procedure Coding System (HCPCS) is the most commonly used procedure-coding system. It has three levels: (1) the American Medical Association's Physician's CPT is referred to as Level I HCPCS; (2) Level II HCPCSs are the HCFA-developed alphanumeric codes, including codes for durable medical equipment, prosthetics, orthotics, and supplies (DMEPOS); and (3) Level III HCPCSs are local codes created as needed by Medicare and other carriers (Acquaviva, 1998).

The CPT codes are a set of five-digit codes that pertain to the medical service or procedure performed by physicians and other service providers. The CPT Editorial Panel of the American Medical Association establishes the CPT codes, which have become the industry standard for reporting, and updates them on an annual basis. There is a Physical Medicine and Rehabilitation section of the CPT codes under which occupational, physical, and speech therapy can bill for certain procedures that may encompass assistive technology intervention. The codes in this section are defined in 15-minute segments. For example, an occupational therapist who has instructed a consumer with a visual impairment on the use of sensory aids to increase independence in self-care can bill using CPT code 97535 ("Selfcare/Home management training, e.g., activities of daily living (ADLs) and compensatory training, meal preparation, safety procedures, and instruction in the use of adaptive equipment direct one-on-one contact by provider, each 15 minutes"). Practitioners may use codes in any section of the CPT as long as the service is within the scope of practice for the practitioner (Acquaviva, 1998). A new code specific to assistive technology has been drafted and is in the process of getting approved as an addition to the CPT codes.

## ■ PAYMENT PRACTICES

The traditional method of payment for health care has been **fee for service.** Under this method of payment, providers are paid a certain rate per unit of service and there is no incentive to limit procedures or look at alternative types of treatment at a lower cost (AOTA, 1996). As a result of skyrocketing health care costs in the United States, however, payment practices in the health care field have changed significantly over the last decade. **Managed care** has emerged as a means of controlling health care costs. The term *managed care* is used to describe "any method of health care delivery designed to reduce unnecessary utilization of services, and provide for cost containment while ensuring that high quality of care or performance is maintained" (Rognehaugh, 1998, p. 134). Managed care plans are now a major part of private health insurance offerings, as well as part of publicly funded insurance programs such as Medicare, Medicaid, Worker's Compensation programs, and CHAMPUS.

Several measures are used by managed care plans to limit either provider payments or enrollee use of services. The primary cost-cutting mechanism utilized in managed care is capitation. Negotiating with providers for a prepaid amount cuts costs. In this arrangement the managed care organization (MCO) agrees to pay the provider a set amount of money on a per-member, per-month basis in exchange for the provider's assuming responsibility for furnishing all or certain health services to a patient for a specified period of time (AOTA, 1996). The provider takes the risk that the capitation rate will be sufficient to cover all the costs of care for the members. An enrollee in the MCO's plan is restricted to using providers that have a contractual agreement with the MCO.

Other measures utilized by MCO's to control costs include precertification or preauthorization, mandatory second opinion, case management, and use of a third-party administrator (AOTA, 1996). For ATPs the implications of managed care are many. Primarily it makes it difficult or impossible to get paid for services if the ATP does not have a contract with an MCO or is not part of a group that contracts with an MCO. The ATP also should determine if the provider requires preauthorization or second opinions before carrying out any services with the consumer. Case

managers are being used more often, particularly in situations where the individual has had an injury or accident resulting in a long-term disability. Most case managers in the United States are nurses who may have limited experience with assistive technology. The case manager is a gatekeeper who controls access to the services that are provided to the individual, including assistive technology. One way for ATPs to learn more about case management and conversely to educate case managers about assistive technology is through the Case Management Society of America (CMSA) and its online forums, which can be accessed at the CMSA Web site (www.cmsa.org).

Consumers and ATPs need to continually be involved in educating funding sources and advocating for the inclusion of assistive technology equipment and services in agencies' policies. As we discuss in Chapter 4, ATPs need to expand their documentation of the benefits and outcomes of assistive technology. This documentation provides helpful information when advocating for increased allocation of funding by public and private agencies.

## ■ SUMMARY

The various sources of funding for assistive technology services and equipment are described in this chapter. Sources of funding for assistive technology are either public or private and include programs such Medicare, Medicaid, vocational rehabilitation, education, private health insurance, low-interest loans, and grants. The ATP should be knowledgeable about the different funding sources, as well as the process for successfully obtaining funding. This includes identifying the appropriate funding source for the consumer, writing a funding justification, billing and coding for assistive technology, and appealing denials as needed. Furthermore, it is important that the ATP advocate at the public policy level for increased coverage of assistive technology services and equipment.

## Study Questions

1. List the major steps in identifying a funding source for a particular assistive technology device or service.
2. What are the major categories of funding for assistive technology devices?
3. What are the major assistive technology funding sources typically available for a child who is in an educational program and needs an augmentative communication device?
4. What are the most likely funding sources for support of assistive technology devices and services for an adult who sustains a head injury at the age of 25?
5. Describe two distinct funding sources, and identify at

least one criterion that must be met by the consumer to be eligible for funding of assistive technology services from each source.
6. What are the types of personal funding?
7. What restrictions are typically placed on private insurance funding of assistive technology devices and services?
8. What is the source of the benefits available under Worker's Compensation?
9. What are the major challenges in identifying the most likely funding source for a given situation?
10. Define the term *medical necessity*.

11. When writing a medical justification for a device for a consumer, what elements should be included?
12. What are CPT codes, and how can they be used in securing funding for assistive technology services and devices?
13. List three types of alternative funding sources for assistive technology devices and services.
14. What are the five steps recommended for developing a funding strategy?
15. Describe the two types of billing codes commonly used in health care.

16. What is managed care, and how does it affect assistive technology service delivery?
17. What is meant by the term *capitation*? What are the implications of capitation for assistive technology service delivery?
18. What are the major steps taken to appeal a funding denial?
19. How can consumers and ATPs work together to inform funding sources of the needs for assistive technology services and devices?

## References

Acquaviva J, editor: *Effective documentation for occupational therapy*, ed 2, Bethesda, Md, 1998, American Occupational Therapy Association.

American Occupational Therapy Association Managed Care Project Team: *Managed care: an occupational therapy sourcebook*, Bethesda, Md, 1996, The Association.

Beukelman DR, Mirenda P: *Augmentative and alternative communication, management of severe communication disorders in children and adults*, Baltimore, 1998, Paul H Brookes.

Burton J: Worker's compensation, twenty-four-hour coverage, and managed care, *Work Comp Mon* 9(1):11-21, 1996.

Enders A, Hall M, editors: *Assistive technology sourcebook*, Washington, DC, 1990, RESNA Press.

Golinker L, Mistrett SG: Funding. In Angelo J: *Assistive technology for rehabilitation therapists*, Philadelphia, 1997, FA Davis.

Matheis D et al: *The buck starts here . . . a guide to assistive technology funding in Kentucky*, Frankfort, Ky, 1991, Department of the Blind.

Mendelsohn S: Funding assistive technology. In Galvin JC, Scherer MJ, editors: *Evaluating, selecting, and using appropriate assistive technology*, Gaithersburg, Md, 1996, Aspen Publishers.

Morris MW, Golinker LA: *Assistive technology: a funding workbook*, Arlington, Va, 1991, RESNA Press.

National Council on Disability: *Study on the financing of assistive technology devices and services for individuals with disabilities*, Washington, DC, 1993, National Council on Disability.

Reeb KG: *Assistive financing for assistive devices: loan guarantees for purchase of products by persons with disabilities*, Washington, DC, 1989, Electronic Industries Foundation.

Rognehaugh R: *The managed care health care dictionary*, ed 2, Gaithersburg, Md, 1998, Aspen Publishers.

World Health Organization. *The International statistical classification of diseases and related health problems*, rev 10 (ICD-10), Geneva, 1992, WHO.

# APPENDIX 5-1

# Sample Forms for Documenting Consumers' Equipment Needs

## ■ APPENDIX 5-1A

### Communication Prosthesis Payment Review Summary

### Instructions

#### 1. PATIENT INFORMATION
- Name—Patient's complete name
- Address—Patient's home address
- Birthdate—Month/day/year
- Health Insurance Number—Appropriate number for coverage
- Medial Diagnosis—Document medical diagnosis (ICD-9-CM) for the patient
- Speech-Language Diagnosis—Document speech-language diagnosis (ASHACS) for patient

#### 2. FACILITY INFORMATION
- Facility—Where the patient is receiving treatment
- Address/Phone Number—Facility address and phone (with area code)
- Physician/Specialty—Physician in charge of this case
- Speech-Language Pathologist—SLP working with patient

#### 3. DEVICE INFORMATION
- Item Description—General description of device being recommended
- Manufacturer—Maker of the device
- Distributor/Dealer—Local source of supply, including service and training

#### 4. PATIENT'S PHYSICAL STATUS
- Check the square that characterizes the patient's current physical condition per medical/clinical documentation or personal observation.
- Adequate/inadequate ratings related to physical parameters only as they apply to the use of the specific communication device selected.
- Nonessential indicates status is not related to the use of the device for this patient.

#### 5. PATIENT'S COGNITIVE PREREQUISITES
- Check the appropriate square that best describes the patient's current status.
- If applicable, provide the name of the testing instrument and the scores obtained.

#### 6. SELECTION OF AUGMENTATIVE COMMUNICATION DEVICE
- a. Current Means—Describe how this patient currently communicates and why it is not the best method of choice.
- b. Other Devices—List other devices considered for this patient and why they would not be applicable.
- c. Rationale—What characteristics of this device influence the determination that this was the best choice, e.g., portability, size, symbols, service, or training.
- d. Indicators—Has the patient had an opportunity to use the device? How long? Rental? What was observed, e.g., increased initiations or ADLs

#### 7. PROGNOSIS
- a. Communication Ability—Will the patient's ability to communicate basic needs, such as health and safety information, improve?
- b. Independence—Will the patient's independence increase with the use of the device?
- c. Placement—Will the community placement be affected? Example: group home vs. nursing home.
- d. Academic Ability—Will the patient's ability to learn and retain new information change?
- e. Vocational Training—Will the patient's ability to advance in vocational rehabilitation improve?

#### 8. COMMENTS—Give any comments unique to this device or what it will offer for this individual that would help in determining payment. Use space provided on the reverse side of the summary form.

PLEASE HAVE THE SUMMARY SIGNED AND DATED BY THE
PHYSICIAN AND THE SPEECH-LANGUAGE PATHOLOGIST.

---

**Communication Prosthesis Payment Review Summary**

**1. PATIENT INFORMATION**
Name _____
Address _____
City _____ State ____ Zip _____
Birthdate _____ Health Ins. # _____
Medical Diagnosis _____
Speech-Language Diagnosis _____

**2. FACILITY INFORMATION**
Facility _____
Address _____
City _____ State ____ Zip _____
Telephone _____
Physician _____
Specialty _____
Speech-Language Pathologist_____

**3. DEVICE INFORMATION**
Item Description_____
_____
Manufacturer _____
Distributor/Dealer _____

**4. PHYSICAL STATUS PER DOCUMENTATION**
   (Check Appropriate Square)

|  | Adequate | Inadequate | Nonessential |
|---|---|---|---|
| a. General medical status | ☐ | ☐ | ☐ |
| b. Respiratory | ☐ | ☐ | ☐ |
| c. Hearing | ☐ | ☐ | ☐ |
| d. Vision | ☐ | ☐ | ☐ |
| e. Head control | ☐ | ☐ | ☐ |
| f. Trunk stability | ☐ | ☐ | ☐ |
| g. Arm movement | ☐ | ☐ | ☐ |
| h. Ambulation | ☐ | ☐ | ☐ |
| i. Seating/positioning for use of device | ☐ | ☐ | ☐ |
| j. Ability to access the device (switches, etc.) | ☐ | ☐ | ☐ |

Summary _____
_____
_____
_____
_____

**5. COGNITIVE PREREQUISITES**
   (Check Appropriate Square)

|  | Present | Absent |
|---|---|---|
| a. Attempts to communicate with consistent response mode | ☐ | ☐ |
| b. Functional yes/no | ☐ | ☐ |
| c. Understands that communication will cause an action to occur | ☐ | ☐ |
| d. Understands that symbols (i.e., words, pictures, Bliss, sign) stand for verbal communication | ☐ | ☐ |

|  | Guarded | Poor | Absent |
|---|---|---|---|
| e. Prognosis to develop intelligible speech | ☐ | ☐ | ☐ |

|  | Present | Absent | Unknown |
|---|---|---|---|
| f. Demonstrates memory retention of verbal instruction | ☐ | ☐ | ☐ |

g. Names of standardized tests and scores (if applicable)
Spelling _____ _____
Reading _____ _____
Cognition _____ _____

**6. SELECTION OF DEVICE**
a. Patient's current means of communication: _____
_____
b. Other devices considered and rationale for elimination:
_____
_____
c. Rationale for selection of specific devices: _____
_____
d. Indicators for success with recommended devices: _____
_____

**7. PROGNOSIS**
a. Communication ability: _____
_____
b. Independence within environment: _____
_____
c. Placement in less restrictive environment: _____
_____
d. Academic ability: _____
_____
e. Vocational training/retraining: _____

Physician _____    Speech-Language Pathologist _____
          (Signature/Date)                                                      (Signature/Date)
                                                              1988 Specialized Product/Equipment Council (SPEC)

| Communication Prosthesis Payment Review Summary |
|---|
| **8. ADDITIONAL COMMENTS** |

**DEVELOPED BY
SPECIALIZED PRODUCT/EQUIPMENT
COUNCIL (SPEC) 1988**

## APPENDIX 5-1B

| **Funding Justification Letter for Seating and Mobility Systems** |
|---|

Date:

**To whom it may concern:**

Attached please find a detailed assessment, medical justification and equipment recommendation for

_____ (First Name) _____ (Last Name)

who was referred to us for _____

He/she presents as a _____ year old with a diagnosis of _____

He/she weighs _____ lbs., is _____ inches tall, and requires a wheelchair for

_____

_____

He/she presently uses _____, which is _____ years old.

**Observation of seated posture in this equipment shows:**

_____

_____

**The problems(s) with this equipment is (are):**

_____

_____

**Our assessment revealed:**

_____

_____

**He/she requires a:**       Seat height of: _____ inches

                             Frame depth of: _____ inches

                             Frame width of: _____ inches

**Our recommendation is that the following equipment be provided:**

_____

_____

**We expect the following outcomes**

1. _____

2. _____

3. _____

4. _____

**Other family members present:**

**Evaluator Name:** _____

Evaluator Title: _____

Facility: _____

**Physician Name:** _____

Physician Title: _____

Facility: _____

**RTS Name:** _____

RTS Title: _____

Company: _____

**If you have any additional questions, please feel free to call me at:** _____

Source: www.rehabcentral.com

---

**Justify Mobility/Seating**

**Mobility system and seating chosen and why:**

|        | **Mfg** | **Model** | **Size** |
|--------|---------|-----------|----------|
| Manual | _____ | _____ | _____ |
| Power  | _____ | _____ | _____ |

**Environment where equipment will be used:**

| Home | ◯ Full time | ◯ Part time | **School/Work** | ◯ Full time | ◯ Part time |
|------|-------------|-------------|-----------------|-------------|-------------|
| **Community** | ◯ Full time | ◯ Part time | **Institution** | ◯ Full time | ◯ Part time |

Other: _____

**Drive system for powered w/c:** _____

**Small turning radius needed for environmental access?**  ◯ Yes  ◯ No

**Narrow width needed for environmental access?**  ◯ Yes  ◯ No

**Mobility system:**  ☐ Folds side/side  ☐ Breaks apart  ☐ Back folds down onto seat only

☐ Doesn't fold at all  ☐ Has quick-release axles

**Available adjustment/growth:**

Frame depth: ____ inches    Seating depth: ____ inches

Frame width: ____ inches    Seating width: ____ inches

**Further growth achieved by:**

☐ Purchase of frame parts    ☐ Adjustment    ☐ Replacement of seating

---

**Mobility Base**

**Lighter weight required:**  ☐ To allow self-propulsion  ☐ To allow lifting  ☐ Family preference

Other: _____

**Heavy duty required for:**  ☐ User weight greater than 250 lbs.  ☐ Extreme tone problems

☐ Overactive user  ☐ Broken frame and/or components on previous chairs

☐ Multiple power seat functions

Other: _____

**Portability required for:**  ☐ Increased community access

Other: _____

**Seat height specified for:**

☐ Foot propulsion  ☐ Transfers  ☐ Accomodation of leg length  ☐ Table/desk access

Other: _____

**Variable wheel placement required for:**

☐ Improved hand access to wheels  ☐ Improved stability

☐ Changing angle in space for assistance with postural stability

☐ 1-arm drive access  ☐ Stability (amputee placement)

Other: _____

**Angle adjustable back:** _____ **degrees**

Required for:  ☐ Postural control  ☐ Control of spasticity  ☐ Accommodation of limited ROM

Other: _____

**Reclining back:** _____ **degrees**  ◯ **Manual**  ◯ **Power**

Required for:  ☐ Pressure relief  ☐ Transfers  ☐ Clothing or diaper changes, catheterization

☐ Head positioning  ☐ Repositioning  ☐ Relief from gravity

☐ Rest periods  ☐ Accommodation of limited ROM

Other: _____

**Backward tilt:** _____ **degrees**   ◯ **Manual**   ◯ **Power**

**Manufacturer:** _____

Required for: ☐ Facilitation of postural control   ☐ Repositioning   ☐ Pressure relief
☐ Head positioning   ☐ Management of spasticity   ☐ Transfers
☐ Relief from gravity   ☐ Rest periods   ☐ Control of lower extremity edema

Other: _____

**Foreward tilt:** _____ **degrees**   ◯ **Manual**   ◯ **Power**

Required for facilitation of:

☐ Head control   ☐ Trunk extension   ☐ Upper extremity movement/contol   ☐ Transfers

Other: _____

**Arm style:**  ☐ Fixed   ☐ Removable   ☐ Flip back   ☐ Fixed height
☐ Swing-away   ☐ Adj. height   ☐ Adj. angle   ☐ Desk length
☐ Full length   ☐ Special height   ☐ Custom length   ☐ Reinforced
☐ Flip back/locking   ☐ Reclining

Required for: ☐ Change of height/angles for variable activities   ☐ Durability
☐ Improved wheel access   ☐ Push-ups/transfers
☐ Upper extremity support   ☐ Support for UE support surface

Other: _____

**Foot/leg support:**  ☐ Elevating (Power)   ☐ Elevating (Manual)   ☐ Articulating   ☐ Angle adj. foot
☐ Swing-away   ☐ Fixed   ☐ Angle adj. knee   ☐ Lift off
☐ Depth adj. foot   ☐ Swing under   ☐ Heavy duty   ☐ Recessed calf panel
☐ Rotational hanger bracket(s)   ☐ Flip-up footplate

Required for: ☐ Comfort   ☐ Reduce swelling   ☐ Accommodation of ROM
☐ Durability   ☐ Transfers   ☐ Suppport
☐ Proper foot placement   ☐ Proper knee flexion angle   ☐ Proper leg placement

Other: _____

**Wheels:** _____

**Axle adjustment:** ◯ None   ◯ Semi adj.   ◯ Fully adj.

**Handrims:** _____

**Casters/forks:** _____

Required for: ☐ Durability   ☐ Access for propulsion
☐ For ease of maintenance (no flats)   ☐ Use over rough terrain
☐ Angle adjustment for postural control   ☐ Grasp
☐ Seat height adjustment   ☐ Decreased pair from road shocks
☐ Decreased spasms from road shocks

Other: _____

**Push handles:** _____

☐ Extended or angle adjustable
Required for: ☐ Caregiver access   ☐ Caregiver assist

Other: _____

**Brake extensions:** _____
Required for: ☐ Access   Other: _____

**Antitippers:** _____
Required for: ☐ Safety   Other: _____

**Bag & pouch:** _____
Required to hold: ☐ Medicines   ☐ Clothing changes   ☐ Diapers
☐ Orthotics   ☐ Special food   ☐ Catheters   ☐ Ostomy supplies

Other: _____

Required for: ☐ Safety          ☐ Long distance driving
☐ Operation of power seat functions
☐ Compliance with transportation
Other: _____

**Swingaway/retractable joystick:** _____

Required for: ☐ Allow table access     ☐ Allow special placement
Other: _____

**Base chosen accommodates:** _____

☐ Required seating     ☐ Needed joystick style/size
☐ Switches needed for driving or seat function
☐ Computer access     ☐ ECU capability     ☐ Communication device
☐ Add-on power tilt     ☐ Add-on power recline
☐ Add-on power elevating leg rests          ☐ Add-on power seat elevator
Other: _____

**Overall comments on mobility equipment:**

_____

_____

## Seating and Accessories

**Seat cushion:** _____

**Seat support:** _____

Required for: ☐ Comfort          ☐ Pressure relief
☐ Ease of use          ☐ Low maintenance
☐ Increased stability     ☐ Accommodation of ROM/asymmetries
☐ Control of posture/alignment
Other: _____

**Back cushion:** _____

**Back support:** _____

Required for: ☐ Accommodation of ROM/assymetries
☐ Comfort          ☐ Pressure relief          ☐ Support
☐ Improved swallowing/respiration          ☐ Control of posture/alignment
☐ Ease of use          ☐ Low maintenance          ☐ Increased stability
Other: _____

**Interfacing seat:** _____

**Interfacing back:** _____

Required for: ☐ Growth and/or angle adjustments
☐ Wheelchair folding          ☐ Disassembly for cleaning
Other: _____

**Head rest:** _____

Required for: ☐ Optimal positioning
☐ Support during tilt/recline          ☐ Improving vision
☐ Safety          ☐ Placement of switches
☐ Accommodation of ROM          ☐ Control of posture/alignment
☐ Improved feeding/swallowing/respiration
Other: _____

**Anterior chest support:** _____

Required for: ☐ Safety          ☐ Support          ☐ Stability          ☐ Alignment
☐ Accomodation of TLSO          ☐ Added abdominal support
☐ Assistance with head position/alignment
☐ Assistance with shoulder control/alignment
Other: _____

**Lateral trunk supports:** _____

- [ ] Swing-away for transfers                    [ ] Contoured for more support

Required for:
- [ ] Accommodation of asymmetries/decreased ROM
- [ ] Support          [ ] Alignment          [ ] Safety
- [ ] Improved head and UE function            [ ] Control spasticity

Other: _____

**Lateral hip support:** _____

- [ ] Removable for transfers

Required for:
- [ ] Support          [ ] Control of spasticity          [ ] Alignment          [ ] Safety
- [ ] Accommodation of asymmetry/ROM
- [ ] Contoured for more support

Other: _____

**Lateral knee support:** _____

- [ ] Removable for transfers

Required for:
- [ ] Accommodation of asymmetry/ROM
- [ ] Control          [ ] Alignment

Other: _____

**Medial and/or anterior knee support:** _____

- [ ] Removable/flip down for independence

Required for:
- [ ] Accommodation of asymmetry/ROM
- [ ] Alignment          [ ] Control of position
- [ ] Control of spasticity

Other: _____

**Foot positioners:** _____

Required for:
- [ ] Accommodation of asymmetry/ROM
- [ ] Alignment          [ ] Safety          [ ] Stability
- [ ] Control of position          [ ] Control of spasticity

Other: _____

**Pelvic belt/bar:** _____

- [ ] Pad for comfort/protection over bony prominences

Required for:
- [ ] Safety          [ ] Alignment          [ ] Independent use
- [ ] Maintainence of pelvic position
- [ ] Special pull angle to control rotation

Other: _____

**UE support surface:** _____

Required for:
- [ ] Support          [ ] Work surface          [ ] Control of upper extremity position
- [ ] Improves shoulder/head position
- [ ] Placement of communication aids
- [ ] Protection of flailing upper extremities

Other: _____

**Overall comments on seating equipment:** _____

_____
_____
_____
_____
_____
_____
_____
_____

# PART 3

# The Activities: General Purpose Assistive Technologies

## CHAPTER 6

# Seating Systems As Extrinsic Enablers for Assistive Technologies

*Elastomeric gels*
*Water filled*
*Viscous fluid filled*
Honeycomb
Foam Cushions
*Planar*
*Standard contoured*
*Custom contoured*
Alternating Pressure Cushions
Hybrid Cushions
Cushion Covers
Seating for Pressure Distribution and Postural Support

Pressure Relief Activities

PRINCIPLES AND TECHNOLOGIES OF SEATING FOR
  COMFORT
Technologies to Enhance Sitting Comfort for Wheelchair
  Users
Technologies That Increase Ease of Sitting for the Elderly
*Static lounge chairs*
*Self-propelled wheelchairs*
*Attendant-propelled wheelchairs*
Seating Individuals in the Workplace

SUMMARY

## Learning Objectives

Upon completing this chapter you will be able to:

1.    Identify the potential outcomes of seating for postural control, pressure management, and comfort
2.    Describe the evaluation for seating
3.    Describe key biomechanical principles related to the seated position and the application of seating technologies
4.    Delineate the principles of seating for postural control
5.    Characterize the major seating technologies for postural control
6.    Delineate the factors that contribute to the development of pressure ulcers
7.    Describe the hard and soft technologies for management of pressure ulcers
8.    Characterize the major principles and technical approaches used to improve comfort during seating

## Key Terms

| | | |
|---|---|---|
| Abductor | Fulcrum | Resilience |
| Center of Gravity | Functional Task Position | Scoliosis |
| Compression | Gravitational Line | Shearing |
| Dampening | Lever Arm | Stiffness |
| Density | Line of Application | Stress |
| Envelopment | Moment | Tension |
| Equilibrium | Pelvic Obliquity | Torque |
| Fixed Deformity | Pelvic Rotation | Translational |
| Flexible Deformity | Planar | Rotational |
| Force | Pressure | Windswept Hip Deformity |
| Frictional Forces | Pressure Ulcer | |

For a user of assistive technologies, a prerequisite to any interaction or activity is a physical position that is comfortable and promotes function. The primary purpose of seating devices is to maximize a person's ability to function in activities across all performance areas (self-care, work or school, play or leisure); for this reason, we consider them to be general-purpose extrinsic enablers.

In the first part of this chapter we describe the needs served by seating systems, evaluation of individuals for seating, and biomechanical principles related to seating. The remainder of the chapter provides in-depth information on each of the three categories of seating needs, including related principles and the technologies used for intervention. Seating components are typically interfaced with some type of mobility base. For purposes of this text, however, we have separated these two systems. We see mobility as a specific-purpose extrinsic enabler and discuss it in Chapter 10.

# OVERVIEW OF NEEDS SERVED BY SEATING

Seating, like other areas of assistive technology, has seen rapid growth and significant changes in the last 20 years. Assistive technology practitioners (ATPs) ought to be aware of the ramifications of seating (and lack thereof) and the technology that is available to address the varied seating needs of individuals with disabilities. Three distinct areas of seating intervention have emerged, with each area based on a particular consumer need served. These three categories of seating intervention, as suggested by Hobson (1990), are (1) seating for postural control and deformity management, (2) seating for pressure management, and (3) seating for comfort and postural accommodation.

The needs of children and adults with cerebral palsy have led to the development of seating interventions for postural control and deformity management. These individuals typically have abnormal muscle tone, muscle weakness, primitive reflexes, or uncoordinated movements that impair their ability to maintain an upright posture in a wheelchair. This affects their ability to participate in activities of daily living, can compromise their general health status, and can result in skeletal deformities.

Although individuals with cerebral palsy represent the largest group with seating needs for postural control and deformity management, individuals with other disabilities, such as muscular dystrophy and multiple sclerosis, often have needs in this area as well. Another more recent application of this technology is with individuals who are in the early stages of rehabilitation. For example, individuals who have an acquired brain injury are susceptible to postural deformities if not managed properly. The inherent challenge with this population is providing seating equipment that can be adapted as the person improves with rehabilitation. It is difficult to predict the extent to which a person will regain motor control, and it is important that postural deformities be prevented while control is regained so that the person can reach his or her fullest potential.

The primary population served by the category of seating interventions for pressure management is individuals with spinal cord injury. These individuals can have partial or complete paralysis and reduced or absent sensation below the level of their lesion. As a result, they are susceptible to breakdown of the tissue over bony prominences on weight-bearing surfaces. Also benefiting from technologies in this category are others who have limited mobility and therefore a reduced ability to relieve pressure from weight-bearing surfaces, such as individuals with multiple sclerosis, those with muscular dystrophy, and the elderly. An additional need in this category is to manage posture so as to distribute pressure more evenly and prevent deformities.

The third category of seating addresses the need to improve an individual's level of physical comfort through postural accommodation. Persons in this category may or may not be in a wheelchair and typically have normal or near normal sensation; however, any prolonged sitting causes them discomfort from which they are unable to obtain relief. Therefore they have unique needs and are not completely served by either category described above. Specialized seating can help to alleviate this chronic discomfort and maximize function.

Related to the categories described above are a number of potential outcomes that can be realized through appropriate seating intervention. The overall goal of every seating intervention is to maximize the individual's function. Specific outcomes that lead to increased function are listed in Box 6-1 (based on Bergen, Presperin, and Tallman, 1990). As a result of neurological damage, some individuals have abnormal muscle tone and reflexes and have difficulty voluntarily controlling their posture and movement. An appropriate positioning system can reduce the influence of the abnormal tone and reflexes (outcome 1) and facilitate normal movement components (outcome 2). Outcomes 3 and 4 are concerned with the prevention of skeletal deformity or tissue damage. Seating systems can provide external support so as to maintain skeletal alignment and prevent bony deformities and shortening of the muscles. In other cases the desired outcome of the seating system is to reduce the likelihood of the individual acquiring tissue damage. Distributing pressure across the weight-bearing surface with an appropriate seating system can reduce the occurrence of pressure ulcers.

The last five outcomes more directly relate to improved function as a result of the seating system. Providing a stable base of support and enhancing postural alignment often results in increased comfort and tolerance for sitting. External stabilization reduces the need for the individual to "fix"

---

**BOX 6-1    Potential Outcomes of Proper Seating and Positioning***

1. Normalization or decreased influence of abnormal tone and reflexes on the body
2. Facilitation of components of normal movement in a developmental sequence
3. Maintenance of neutral skeletal alignment and active and passive joint range of motion within normal limits; control or prevention of deformity or muscle contractures
4. Prevention of tissue breakdown
5. Increased comfort and tolerance of desired position
6. Decreased fatigue
7. Enhanced respiratory, oral-motor, and digestive function
8. Maximized stability to enhance function
9. Facilitation of care provision (e.g., therapy, nursing, education)

*Data from Bergen AF, Presperin J, and Tallman T: *Positioning for function: wheelchairs and other assistive technologies,* Valhalla, NY, 1990, Valhalla Rehabilitation Publications.

his body or prop himself up with his arms in order to maintain a position, thus lessening fatigue. An appropriate seating system can stabilize the person's trunk and pelvis so that manipulative tasks can be performed more easily and technology can be readily accessed (Nwaobi, Hobson, and Trefler, 1985; Nwaobi, 1987).

Improvement in the person's physiological functions, such as respiration, oral function, and digestion, can also be obtained by providing trunk and head support. In one study, vital capacity, forced expiratory volume, and expiratory time of children with spastic cerebral palsy (ages 5 to 12 years) were all greater when they were positioned in an adapted seating system than when they were seated in standard, sling-type wheelchairs (Nwaobi and Smith, 1986). In addition, children were found to have significant improvement in oral-motor skills and speech intelligibility following improved alignment of the head, neck, and trunk with the use of a postural support system (Hulme et al 1987; Hobson and Nwaobi, 1987).

Improvements in a person's seated position also facilitate educational and therapeutic goals and the caregiver's ability to provide care. Teachers' perceptions of a child were found to be more positive when the child was well positioned (good body alignment and head erect) with adaptive equipment (Brown, 1981). In particular, children who were poorly positioned were more likely to be rated as frustrated and weak than children who were well positioned.

## ■ EVALUATION FOR SEATING

The process of assessing individuals for the purpose of recommending seating technologies requires a systematic method that includes consideration of many factors. We describe in Chapter 4 some of the essential parts of assessment for assistive technologies. The purpose of this section is to provide a framework for evaluating consumers specifically for seating. Figure 6-1 outlines a framework to guide the ATP through the decision-making process and ultimate selection of seating and positioning technologies that match the needs and skills of the user.

As with other areas of assistive technology, the process of delivering seating services is a transdisciplinary effort involving the skills of several professionals. Occupational and physical therapists typically provide expertise in neuromotor function, human development, and knowledge of disabilities. A physician documents the medical status and prognosis of the consumer and medical justification for the seating system. The physician can also indicate whether surgery or other medical procedures are planned and what effects these procedures may have on the consumer's seating. Assistive technology suppliers often provide knowledge of available technologies and their application to meet specific goals. Sometimes a rehabilitation engineer provides this service. In

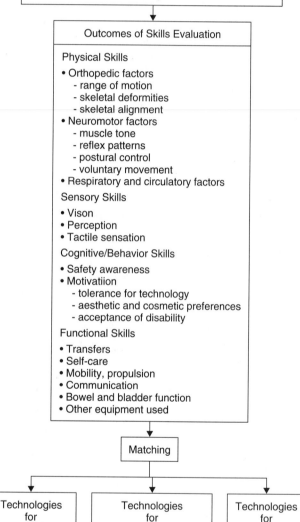

Figure 6-1    Framework for seating and positioning decision making.

cases where the consumer's need cannot be met by commercial products, the rehabilitation engineer can design a custom system. In addition to a solid knowledge base, it is important that all these professionals have prior clinical experience that has prepared them to engage in seating intervention. These professionals complement each other and together constitute a strong team for effective seating intervention.

## Needs Identification

Figure 6-1 lists the desired outcomes of the identification of needs. It is important to determine exactly what an individual's specific needs are regarding seating. From the identified needs, goals to be addressed by the seating intervention are developed. It is the ATP's responsibility to facilitate the identification of these goals, as well as the prioritization of them. It is not always possible to achieve every goal in all cases. In some cases, difficult as it may be, goals with lesser priority must be given up for goals with higher priority. For example, the goal of increasing comfort may require a reclined position that may be inconsistent with a desire to achieve a more upright position for increased function. Or a goal of correcting a flexible deformity in the spine may require such aggressive external positioning that it is not comfortable for the individual. The goal of correcting this deformity must then be compromised slightly so that a comfortable (and thus tolerable) position is achieved.

Discussion of the *contexts* in which the individual is to use the seating system contributes to determining the goals of the system and selecting the technology to be used. The contexts include physical factors such as heat, light, and sound; the setting in which the technology is to be used; and the social and cultural context. Certain factors present in the individual's contexts may have a bearing on which systems are considered for that individual.

Heat is the most important of the physical factors to be considered during seating intervention. The climate the person lives in can have an effect on the materials used in seating systems. If the system is to be used in extreme hot or cold temperatures, this should be taken into consideration when selecting materials. Exposure to light sources also may affect some materials and can be a concern for the eventual recommendation.

The settings in which the person will use the system also must be considered during the evaluation. Depending on the person's life roles, the system may be used at home, at school, at work, or in the community. The accessibility of the system in all settings in which it is to be used needs to be considered during the seating evaluation. A seat cushion that solves someone's needs for pressure relief but raises her up so high on the seat that she can no longer get under her desk at work is not practical. Recreational activities may require special seating requirements. In some cases more than one system is necessary. For example, one seating system may be required for a powered wheelchair that is used only at school and another system for a manual wheelchair that is used in other settings, or there may be a need for positioning outside of a wheeled base (e.g., in a side-lying position or in a standing position).

The type of residence the person lives in may affect the type of seating system recommended. For example, there are generally differences in the type of use and care a system gets between a group residential facility and an individual home. If the person lives in a group residential setting, many people will provide care over time and this needs to be taken into consideration. In many cases the caregiver is responsible for ensuring that the seating system is set up, maintained, and functioning properly. Therefore the caregiver's needs can be as important as the needs of the consumer. How the person is transported is another factor that affects the recommendation of a seating system. If the person uses the seating system during private or public transportation, the system needs to provide for safety in these situations. These and other accessibility issues that pertain to wheelchair mobility are addressed in Chapter 10.

### Physical Skills

The physical evaluation includes assessment of orthopedic, neuromotor, respiratory, and circulatory factors (see Figure 6-1). It is recommended that evaluation of physical skills take place with the person both in a sitting position and supine on a flat surface such as a mat.

**Orthopedic factors.** Orthopedic evaluation involves measurement of joint range of motion and assessment of skeletal deformities and skeletal alignment to determine optimal angles for sitting. Obtaining information regarding limitations in range of motion and deformities is necessary to determine whether the goal of the seating system will be to prevent deformities, correct deformities, or accommodate deformities that are present (Trefler, Hobson, and Taylor, 1993).

Starting with the consumer supine on the mat, mobility of the lumbar spine and pelvis are assessed, followed by *range of motion measurements* of the hips, knees, ankles, upper extremities, and neck. Joint angle and body measurements as shown in Figure 6-2 should also be made at this time. Next it is determined whether the individual's head, shoulders, and trunk can be aligned with the pelvis. Range of motion and skeletal alignment should also be assessed in a sitting position to determine how the body parts are affected by gravity. Bergen, Presperin, and Tallman (1990) describe in detail a process for measuring joint angles and assessing skeletal alignment.

Through the range of motion assessment, it is determined whether skeletal deformities are present and whether they are fixed or flexible. In **fixed deformities,** permanent changes have taken place in the bones, muscles, capsular ligaments, or tendons that restrict the normal range of motion of the particular joint. Fixed deformities affect the skeletal alignment of the other joints and typically require a seating system that is made to accommodate the deformity. Often, increased tone and muscle tightness cause persons to assume certain postures, and they may appear to have a deformity. With externally applied resistance (passive

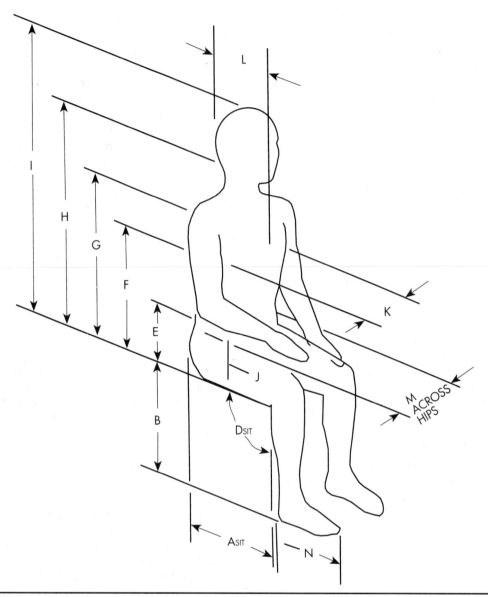

**Figure 6-2** Joint angle and body measurements taken during the evaluation. *A$_{SIT}$* (R & L), behind hips/popliteal fossa; *B* (R & L), popliteal fossa/heel; *D$_{SIT}$*, knee flexion angle; *E*, sitting surface/pelvic crest; *F*, sitting surface/axilla; *G*, sitting surface/shoulder; *H*, sitting surface/occiput; *I*, sitting surface/crown of head; *J*, sitting surface/hanging elbow; *K*, width across trunk; L, depth of trunk; *M*, width across hips; *N*, heel/toe. (From Bergen AF, Presperin J, Tallman T: *Positioning for function: wheelchairs and other assistive technologies.* Valhalla, NY, 1990, Valhalla Rehabilitation Publications.)

stretch) in the opposite direction, however, it is possible to move the joint and reduce the deformity. The person is then considered to have a **flexible deformity** at that joint. Depending on the situation, the seating system may be designed to correct a flexible deformity. Specific deformities and their effects on sitting posture are described in the section on seating principles for postural control.

Some individuals have had surgery to correct one or more deformities. The ATP should be aware of any past surgery the consumer may have undergone and be knowledgeable about the implications it has for seating intervention. In other cases the team may decide during the evaluation that surgical or orthotic intervention should be considered before seating intervention takes place. If this is the situation, referral to the appropriate medical professional is necessary. Letts (1991) examines surgical interventions related to the seated position.

**Neuromotor factors.** *Muscle tone* is evaluated to determine its effects on movement patterns and posture, particularly as related to seating and functional activities. To get an accurate picture of the individual's tone, changes should be noted in response to passive and active movement; alterations in body position (e.g., reclining the back of the wheelchair); external stimuli (e.g., noises, temperature); and internal stimuli (e.g., emotions such as happiness or disappointment) (Bergen, Presperin, and Tallman, 1990).

The ATP also needs to be aware of the presence of *primitive reflexes* and the effects they have on the person's sitting posture. The reflexes that most commonly affect sitting are the asymmetrical tonic neck reflex (ATNR), the symmetrical tonic neck reflex (STNR), the tonic labyrinthine reflex (TLR), and the positive supporting reaction (Trefler, Hobson, and Taylor, 1993); these are described in Chapter 3. By being aware of abnormal tone and primitive reflexes that affect the person's seated position, the ATP can design a seating system that optimally inhibits such pathological responses.

Tone and reflex patterns influence postural control and voluntary movement. Likewise, tone and reflex patterns are directly affected by posture. Therefore all these components should be evaluated simultaneously and general patterns described. It is important to establish how much internal control and movement the individual has so that the seating system provides adequate support beyond the person's volitional control but does not inhibit it. One measure of control is the degree to which the person can maintain an upright sitting posture. The amount of existing head and trunk control and that which is emerging should be measured through visual observation and hands-on evaluation of the individual (Bergen, Presperin, and Tallman, 1991).

**Respiratory and circulatory factors.** The person's *respiratory status* and *circulation* are other factors addressed during the evaluation. With skeletal deformities, pulmonary and cardiac function can be compromised. It is important to know whether certain positions enhance or limit respiration. Circulation, particularly in the lower limbs, needs to be considered as well. Some individuals may have a condition that predisposes them to circulatory problems; particularly for these consumers, positions that impair circulation should be avoided.

## Sensory and Perceptual Skills

*Vision and visual perception*, as discussed in Chapter 3, contribute to a person's balance and sitting posture, and deficits in these areas need to be considered during the evaluation. It is particularly important to be aware of what happens to the person's head when he looks around the environment. A person's awareness of body position *(proprioception)* in space also influences body posture. *Tactile sensation* is another factor to consider. Some individuals may react defensively to the touch of certain textures or positioning components on their body. Other individuals lack tactile sensation, which can contribute to skin breakdown. The

ATP should determine whether there is any known decrease in sensation, particularly in the buttock area, and whether there is a history of pressure ulcers. The condition of the person's skin on weight-bearing surfaces (including areas on the trunk that are braced by lateral supports) should be checked for evidence of skin breakdown, circulation, color, smoothness, sensation, and moisture (Tredwell and Roxborough, 1991).

## Cognitive Skills

Cognitive skills such as problem solving and motor planning are not as much of an issue in seating as in mobility. However, there are a few areas that require consideration. Individuals with poor safety judgment may not be aware of the need to keep a positioning belt fastened, and special considerations may be necessary. Knowing the individual's language and communication skills (see Chapter 9) will help determine how the ATP gathers information during the evaluation. For example, if a person relies on an augmentative communication device or on yes/no responses, these modes of communication should be utilized during the evaluation process. If it is known that the consumer is not reliable in her responses, then the ATP should seek assistance from a caregiver in interpreting the consumer's responses to the seating system.

## Psychosocial Skills

Motivation plays a significant role in the individual's acceptance of the technology. Some individuals may have had a bad experience with previous technology, may have a low tolerance for technology, or may not have fully accepted their disability, resulting in the rejection of seating technology. Additionally, because seating systems often are considered by the individual to be an extension of his or her body, aesthetics are a significant factor in acceptance or rejection of the system. Behavioral problems, such as a person who is agitated and throws himself against the back of the chair, can also present a safety problem that needs to be addressed. Working together with the consumer and the caregiver to address these concerns is essential.

## Functional Skills

Activities in which the individual is to participate from the seating system need to be identified and evaluated. These functional skills may include transfers to and from different surfaces (e.g., bed to wheelchair, car to wheelchair), self-care skills (e.g., feeding, dressing), wheelchair mobility, written and verbal communication, and bowel and bladder care. Additionally, equipment the person will use while in the seating system needs to be taken into consideration. For example, respiratory equipment and augmentative communication devices are frequently mounted on the wheelchair and need to be in a position that is functional for the user.

It is important that the individual's ability to perform functional activities be evaluated both in the existing system and in a simulation of the proposed system. By observing the consumer performing functional activities from her existing system, the ATP learns two things. First the ATP can determine the consumer's level of independence and areas where function is impeded. The ATP can also learn what strategies the individual currently uses to complete functional activities. Using the methods described below, the ATP can then simulate different positions with the consumer. The ATP can have the individual perform functional tasks while in these simulated positions. Changing the sitting position will affect the person's ability to perform certain activities. It is important to select a system that maximizes the person's function and does not interfere with the use of strategies that have proved to be beneficial. For example, a teenager who uses an abnormal ATNR to operate a single switch should not be prohibited from doing so unless another movement can be found that accomplishes this task. It will sometimes be necessary to trade an ideal seated posture for a posture that allows the individual to be more functional.

## Matching Device Characteristics to a Consumer's Needs and Skills

The information that has been gathered regarding needs and skills provides us with a profile of the user. We can then define which of the three categories in Figure 6-1 matches the consumer's profile. This allows us to identify potential technologies and evaluate their effectiveness in meeting the consumer's needs.

The next step is to actually simulate with the consumer one or more of the alternatives. By having the consumer try variations of the positioning system, the ATP can observe the effects of changes in body position and materials. Trial positioning is also helpful for assessing the person's ability to use control interfaces. Changes in position can be made to see whether there are beneficial or adverse effects on the person's ability to control a device or perform other functional skills. Finally, simulation makes it easier to document the need for and effectiveness of a particular system so that funding can be obtained.

There are various strategies and tools available that can help in this process. Simulation of a positioning system can be accomplished by templating, using equipment that is commercially available, or using equipment specifically designed for this purpose (Presperin, 1989; Bergen, Presperin, and Tallman, 1990). Templating is an inexpensive method of simulating a seating system that uses tri-wall (cardboard) to mock up the intended components. Plywood and foam

pieces can also be used in a simulation. Many centers that specialize in seating have an array of commercially available products on hand for the purpose of simulating positioning systems. In addition, manufacturers and local rehabilitation technology suppliers often have products available for demonstration or short-term loan. If specific cushions or positioning components are being considered for a consumer, it helps to have him try the actual product and determine whether he likes it. In some instances it may be desirable for the consumer to take the system home for a trial period. This allows the person to use the system over a longer period and in his natural environment.

There are also sophisticated simulation frames available that are adjustable to fit individuals of different sizes and with varying degrees of deformity. There are several commercially available simulators that are designed to accommodate different positioning components (e.g., head supports, foot supports) and support surfaces (e.g., planar, modular, custom contoured). Some of these simulators also allow custom contouring of a surface to the individual using the vacuum forming method discussed later in this chapter. The adjustments available on these simulators include seat depth, seat-to-back angle, back height, and system tilt in space. These simulators also can be attached to a powered mobility base so that the person can actually experience controlling the wheelchair while in the simulator. A photo of the individual positioned appropriately in the simulator can demonstrate the benefits of the seating system to the third-party funding source.

Simulation also allows the ATP to compare the pressure-relieving capabilities of various seating surfaces so that the most suitable system is selected for the individual. Besides palpating and visually examining the weight-bearing surfaces, there is technology available that can assist the ATP in obtaining objective pressure measurements of the consumer on various seating surfaces. These methods are described in detail later in this chapter in the section on hard and soft technologies for pressure management.

Another tool used by ATPs to assist them in matching the consumer's needs and skills to the appropriate technology is an expert system. Expert systems use a computer program that systematically leads the ATP through the decision-making process and results in the selection of the most suitable device. The development and use of expert systems is still in its infancy.

There are several critical questions that can help the ATP evaluate the effectiveness of the technologies that have been simulated and to select an appropriate seating system for the consumer. These questions summarize the needs evaluation, the skill assessment, and the simulation and are shown in Box 6-2. The primary concern is whether the simulated seating system meets the goals identified during the needs assessment. Providing a stable seating surface is important for safety and for optimal performance in functional activities. Whether the individual is able to perform functional activities successfully while seated in the system is considered. As we have said, care should be taken to select a system that does not hinder the person's ability to perform weight shifts and transfers or impede wheelchair mobility. Another factor is whether the consumer or caregiver needs to remove the cushion or seating system from the wheelchair, and if so, whether the weight and design of the system allow for this. Some consumers, for example, need to be able to remove the seat cushion from the wheelchair to fold up the chair for transportation. In other situations a complete seating system may need to be detached from the wheeled base and stored in a car for transportation. In these cases a caregiver is usually responsible, and the ATP must ensure that this person can handle the system. How comfortable the seating system feels to the user is another important consideration. In some cases this is the primary goal of the seating intervention, but in all cases, if the consumer does not find the system comfortable, she is not likely to use it.

The seating system should be reliable and durable enough to meet the needs of the user. Some systems require more maintenance (e.g., regulating amount of inflation, cleaning) than others and may not be an appropriate choice for a consumer who is not able to provide the needed maintenance. Other systems may be too susceptible to damage or deterioration to meet the consumer's needs adequately. Ultimately the cost of the seating system and the resources available for purchase need to be considered. The benefit the consumer is to receive from the recommended system needs to be justified, particularly when a costlier alternative is being recommended. We discuss funding of seating systems in Chapter 5. All the strategies and tools we have described make it easier and more efficient for the ATP to recommend a suitable seating system for the consumer.

## BIOMECHANICAL PRINCIPLES

To design and implement seating systems effectively for consumers with disabilities, it is important to understand how the laws of physics govern the actions and effects of the mechanical elements of the postural control system. These principles are embodied in *biomechanics,* the study of body position and movement. In this section we present the major concepts of biomechanics, which are fundamental to an understanding of seating and positioning systems for persons with disabilities.

### Kinematics: Study of Motion

When we design seating systems we need to consider the position of the consumer, the position of the seating system components, and their movements. The term *kinematics* describes movement. We use the term *displacement* to define the position of a body in space; a change in displacement results in a new position. For example, in a postural support system, one goal is to bring the trunk to a midline position. This may require a *displacement* from the rest position to midline by application of an external lateral trunk support. The rate of change in displacement is called *velocity.* It is also important to know how fast the velocity is changing (increasing or decreasing); we call this change *acceleration.* One of the most common accelerations is that of gravity. When we use the term *gravity* we are actually referring to the acceleration of an object toward the center of the earth. Acceleration of an object is directly related to the force generated by the object's movement.

There are two fundamental types of displacement: translational and rotational. When all parts of a body move in the same direction, at the same time, and for the same distance, we call the movement **translational** (Nwaobi, 1984). For example, a person walking generates translational movement. Displacements caused by external positioning components can also be translational. If the direction, distance, and time of the movement occur simultaneously, but the movement is through an angle instead of in a straight line, the movement is called **rotational**. Rotational movements occur around an axis called the **fulcrum**. The majority of body movements are rotational, such as hip or elbow flexion and shoulder flexion or extension. Some positioning components cause rotational displacements (e.g., reclining the back of a wheelchair causes rotation at the pelvis and hip).

### Kinetics: Forces

Force is a major element in biomechanics and seating for individuals with disabilities. **Force** is anything that acts on a body to *change* its rate of acceleration or alter its momentum. Forces always occur in equal and opposite action-reaction pairs between bodies, although it is often convenient to think of one body being in a force field. Forces can be applied to the body internally or externally. Internal forces are generated inside the body, such as muscle contractions that cause movement of the joints. Externally applied forces come from outside the body and act on it in some way, such as the forces applied by a support surface and components of a seating system such as lateral supports. The force resulting from the acceleration of gravity is another external and ever-present force that acts on the body and influences its posture and movement. This force on the body acts along a line called the **gravitational line,** and its effect is localized around a point in the body called the **center of gravity.** The force of the Earth's gravitational field tends to pull the body toward the center of the Earth, and this force must be accounted for in designing a seating system. The center of gravity changes as posture changes from standing to sitting and in different sitting positions.

Four properties of force, which ultimately determine its result, are magnitude, direction, line of application, and point of application. *Magnitude* is the amount or size of the force measured in newtons, pounds, or kilograms. Forces are applied in some *direction,* either pushing or pulling, and are applied along a particular **line of application.** The force acts at a particular point on the body, called the *point of application* (Nwaobi, 1984).

**Types of forces.** There are three different types of force. Each of these types produces different effects on the body, and it is important to understand these differences when designing seating and positioning systems. **Tension** forces act in the same line but away from each other (pulling apart), such as the force applied on the antagonist muscle during contraction of the agonist muscle. **Compression** occurs when forces act toward each other (pushing together), such as the force of the vertebrae on the disks in the spinal column. **Shearing** occurs when the forces are parallel to each other (sliding across the surfaces), such as the movement that occurs as the head of the femur moves across the acetabulum during hip movement. Each of these types of forces can also be applied externally to the body, such as the force exerted by a seating surface on the ischial tuberosities (compression), the force exerted by lateral supports to extend the trunk (tension), or the force exerted on the tissues in the buttocks when a seat back is reclined (shearing).

**Stress. Stress** is the resulting molecular change inside biological (e.g., soft tissue and bone) or nonbiological (e.g., metals, plastics, or foams) materials. Stress is caused by the same three types of forces—tension, compression, or shear—and can result in damage to the biological tissue or other material if prolonged. For example, a shear force applied to a foam seat cushion can result in tearing of the

foam. This is a change in the molecular structure of the foam caused by an externally applied force. Likewise, a piece of connective tissue that is subjected to severe or prolonged compression loading by sitting (e.g., under the ischial tuberosities) may be damaged by crushing of the tissue. This externally applied force results in compression inside the tissue, causing a change in the structure of the biological material.

**Pressure.** Every force is applied over a surface area. For example, with a postural support system, the force of each component is applied to an area of the body. It is important to determine the effect of each of these forces, and the concept of pressure is important. **Pressure** is defined as force per unit area. This means that a force applied over a very small area generates more pressure than the same force applied over a larger area. Imagine a 10-lb cat lying on a surface such as your stomach. The force generated by the cat is applied over the entire surface of its body and the pressure is uniform. Now imagine the same cat standing on your stomach. The force of the cat is the same, but the pressure at each of the cat's paws is much greater (and it hurts more) because the area of application (the paw) is much smaller than when the force is distributed over the whole surface area of the cat. This basic concept of distributing pressure by increasing the area of application is applied extensively in seating and positioning systems.

**Newton's laws of motion.** The English scientist Sir Isaac Newton formulated three laws relating to forces on bodies at rest and in motion. *Newton's first law* states that a body at rest tends to remain at rest and a body in motion in a straight line tends to remain in motion unless external forces act to change either of these states. This is often stated as the body's having *inertia,* and it is what we feel when a vehicle stops quickly and our bodies keep moving (or try to move against a seat belt). *Newton's second law* relates three parameters: the mass of a body, the change in velocity (acceleration), and the forces acting on that body. The force is equal to the mass (in kilograms) multiplied by the acceleration of the body (force = mass × acceleration). This means that the greater the force, the greater the acceleration, or conversely, the greater the mass for the same force, the smaller the acceleration. The force of gravity is the mass of the object multiplied by the acceleration of gravity. This force is commonly referred to as the *weight* of an object, and it is the reason that an object weighs less on the Moon, since the gravitational acceleration there is less than that on Earth.

*Newton's third law* is the one most applicable to seating and positioning systems. This law states that if one body exerts a force on another, there is an equal and opposite force, called a reaction, exerted on the first body by the second. For our purposes in this chapter, this means that every force exerted by the human body while sitting in a wheelchair or a seating system is balanced by an opposite force exerted by the sitting surface on the person. The force generated by the body is equal in magnitude and opposite in direction to the force generated by the seating system. This is often referred to as **equilibrium.** When a body is at rest and all internal and external forces are balanced, the body is in a state of *static equilibrium.* When forces are balanced around a body during movement, resulting in a constant velocity, we describe it as *dynamic equilibrium.* Both types of equilibrium are important in seating and positioning systems.

When rotational movements occur, the concept of point of application of the force becomes important. As stated earlier, a rotational movement occurs around a line, called the fulcrum, and the movement occurs in a plane perpendicular to that line (Nwaobi, 1984). Figure 6-3 shows the forces exerted on the femur by a pommel (a seating component that is placed between the thighs to position the legs away from midline; sometimes also called an abductor). The pommel acts at a location distal to the head of the femur (identified in the figure as *PF*). The product of the distance of the point of application of a force from the fulcrum (head of the femur in Figure 6-3) and the magnitude of the force is called **torque** or **moment.** The longer the distance from the fulcrum (sometimes called a **lever arm**), the greater the torque for the same force. When we apply Newton's third law to this type of situation, we balance torques rather than forces. So we must match the torque resulting from the muscle action on the femur (MD × MF) with the torque resulting from the pommel (PF × PD). Because the pommel is further from the fulcrum (i.e., PD > MD), the force applied by the pommel is less than that applied by the muscle (MF > PF). Let us hypothetically assume that the

muscle exerts a force of 3 newtons (N) (MF) and the point of application in which the force of the muscle is exerted is located 12 cm (MD) from the fulcrum. This results in a torque of 36 N-cm. When a pommel is located 36 cm (PD) from the fulcrum, the force exerted by the abductor is only 1 N-cm (PF). The fact that the pommel force is less than the muscle force is sometimes referred to as obtaining a "mechanical advantage" from the existence of the lever arm. We shall apply this concept further when we discuss postural control and deformity management.

**Friction.** Throughout this discussion, we have assumed that ideal circumstances exist. For example, a shear force applied to a body causes it to move across a surface, and ideally it encounters no resistance to movement from that surface. In reality, of course, this is not true, and we know that **frictional forces** exist between two bodies in contact moving in opposite directions. Two types of friction are defined: static friction and dynamic friction. *Static friction* is that force that must be overcome to start a body in motion. Static friction is proportional in magnitude to the perpendicular (compression) force holding the two bodies together. Static friction is independent of the area of contact between the two bodies. Once motion is initiated, the resistive force is generally smaller, and it takes less force to keep the bodies moving relative to each other than to start movement. Friction during movement is called *dynamic friction.* Both these frictional forces are affected by surface conditions such as moisture, heat, texture, and lubricants and both are important considerations in the recommendation and design of seating surfaces.

By employing these principles to support surfaces of a seating system, forces can be applied to prevent or retard the formation of bony deformities and to accommodate existing deformities (Nwaobi, 1984). Managing forces appropriately can also minimize tissue breakdown. Throughout this chapter we relate these principles to the management of seating pressures and control of posture.

## Postures and Center of Gravity

As mentioned earlier, gravity is an ever-present force acting on and influencing the body and its movements. The center of gravity is known to be important in governing balance and dynamic control. There is a direct relationship between how much muscle force is required to maintain a posture in the presence of gravity and the efficiency of that posture (Adrian and Cooper, 1989). For example, standing on one leg is less efficient than standing on two because the base of support has been reduced and more muscle forces and energy must be expended to maintain the position. Likewise, sitting with weight primarily on one ischial tuberosity requires more muscle activation and energy than if the weight is evenly placed on both sides.

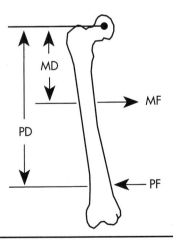

**Figure 6-3** Rotational equilibrium. *MD,* Muscle lever arm; *PF,* pommel lever arm; *MF,* muscle force; *PF,* pommel external force. (From Nwaobi OM: Biomechanics of seating. In Trefler E, editor: *Seating for children with cerebral palsy: a resource manual,* Memphis, 1984, University of Tennessee.)

There are several principles to keep in mind that relate the body and the supporting base to the efficiency of balance and control. For example, keeping the center of gravity over an area directly above the supporting base helps maintain balance. Also, the lower the center of gravity, the more stable the structure. Finally, the larger the base, the greater the range over which the body can move without becoming unstable.

**Standing posture.** In standing, the two feet provide the base of support. When the body is viewed from the front, the center of gravity from top to bottom is roughly located in the upper sacral region (Nwaobi, 1984). This varies among individuals, depending on body weight, gender, presence of a disability, and age. Zacharkow (1988, p. 3) summarizes the line of gravity (viewed laterally) in the "idealized erect standing posture" as passing through the mastoid processes of the jaw, a point just in front of the shoulder, a point just behind the center of the hip joints, a point just in front of the center of the knee joints, and approximately 5 to 6 cm in front of the ankle joints (Figure 6-4, *A*). In this posture the pelvis is in a neutral position and there is a natural lordosis of the lumbar spine (Nwaobi, 1984; Zacharkow, 1988).

**Sitting postures.** In sitting the center of gravity is lowered and the new base of support, consisting of the buttocks, the back of the thighs, and the feet, is larger. In spite of this, pelvic stability is greater in standing than in sitting. This is because of a passive locking mechanism at the hip joints provided by ligamentous support when the hips are fully extended during standing (Zacharkow, 1988). During sitting, the hips are flexed and this mechanism is lost. As shown in Figure 6-4, *B*, the pelvis also rotates backward during sitting, which causes the lumbar lordosis present during standing to convert to a kyphotic, or flexed, position. This is partially caused by tension of the hip extensors, particularly the hamstrings, when the hips are flexed. Posterior tilt of the pelvis increases further if the knee is extended in sitting. In this relaxed sitting posture the line of gravity is posterior to the ischial tuberosities and anterior to the lumbar spine.

There are unsupported sitting postures other than the relaxed sitting posture described above that can be obtained

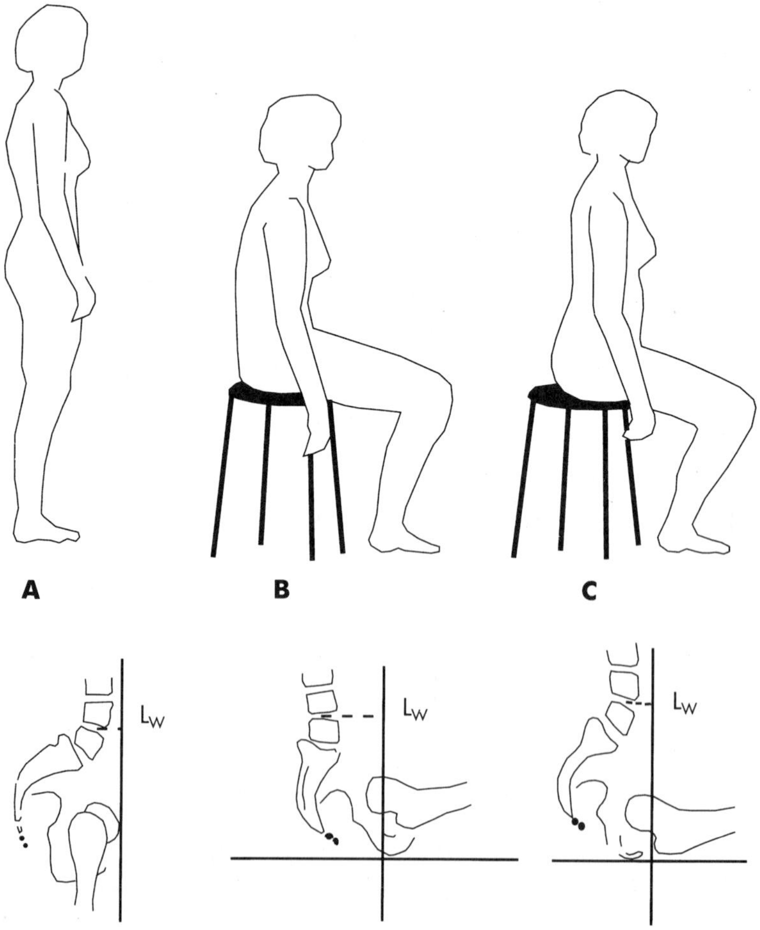

Figure 6-4    **A,** Line of gravity in erect upright standing. **B,** Relaxed unsupported sitting resulting in backward tilt of the pelvis and flattening of the lumbar lordosis. **C,** Erect sitting with reduction in backward pelvic tilt and increased lordosis. $L_w$ represents the lever arm. (From Frankel VH, Nordin M: *Basic biomechanics of the skeletal system,* Philadelphia, 1980, Lea and Febiger.)

(Zacharkow, 1988). The muscles of the spine can be activated to overcome the backward rotation of the pelvis and lumbar kyphosis and achieve an erect or lordotic sitting position (Figure 6-4, *C*). It can be seen in Figure 6-4, *C*, that the pelvis rotates forward and the line of gravity runs through the ischial tuberosities. Even though the line of gravity remains anterior to the lumbar spine, the distance between the two is shorter than in the posture described above.

A third position is a forward sitting posture in which the line of gravity runs just in front of the ischial tuberosities and then intersects the spine (Figure 6-5). This position can be obtained either with maximal flexion of the spine and little or no pelvic rotation or with a straighter spine and forward rotation of the pelvis (Zacharkow, 1988). A forward sitting posture such as this is referred to as a **functional task position** (Kangas, 1991) or *posture of readiness* (Adrian

and Cooper, 1989). In this position a person is usually getting ready to perform an activity and his center of gravity shifts toward the direction of activity. In sitting or in standing, an individual in a state of readiness flexes forward at the ankle and the trunk in anticipation of the activity. The arms and hands are naturally brought forward into the visual field and the feet shift behind the knees and bear more weight.

These sitting postures can be analyzed in terms of the biomechanical principles shown in Figure 6-6. The force of gravity *(W)* applies a rotational force (torque) to the body with the fulcrum of the rotation being the hip joint *(O)*. Each of the sitting postures has a different relationship between the line of gravity and the fulcrum. The distance between the line of gravity and the fulcrum is the lever or moment arm *(OA)*. This moment (force times the length of the lever arm: $W \times OA$) must be balanced by the moment on the other side of the fulcrum (muscle activity: $F \times OB$). If the line of gravity falls through the fulcrum, there is no lever arm ($OA = OB = 0$) and a condition of static equilibrium exists. As stated above, the line of gravity actually passes anterior to the pelvis as shown in Figure 6-6 and this creates a moment or torque. In the relaxed, unsupported sitting position (Figure 6-4, *B*), the length of the lever arm is increased because the line of gravity falls farther from the fulcrum. In this position the moment is increased, and the muscle force necessary to maintain equilibrium is increased as well. The lever arm is reduced in the erect sitting position shown in Figure 6-4, *C*. In the forward sitting position (see Figure 6-5), the line of gravity passes closer to the fulcrum (distance *OA* is reduced) and the moment ($W \times OA$) is also reduced. This reduces the amount of muscle force required to maintain static equilibrium. By analyzing these different

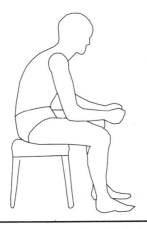

Figure 6-5    Forward sitting posture. (From Zacharkow D: *Posture: sitting, standing, chair design & exercise,* Springfield, Ill, 1988, Charles C Thomas.)

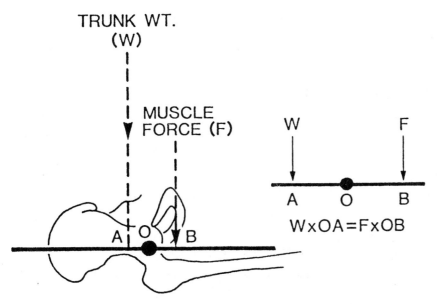

Figure 6-6    The moment resulting from the force of gravity must be balanced by a muscle force to achieve equilibrium. (From Nwaobi OM: Biomechanics of seating. In Trefler E, editor: *Seating for children with cerebral palsy: a resource manual,* Memphis, 1984, University of Tennessee.)

sitting postures, we can see how center of gravity (where the line of gravity falls) affects postural control.

For nondisabled individuals, the postural control system can adapt to a wide range of environmental conditions, including the force of gravity. However, individuals who have disturbances in one or more components of their postural control can be significantly affected by small changes in their center of gravity.

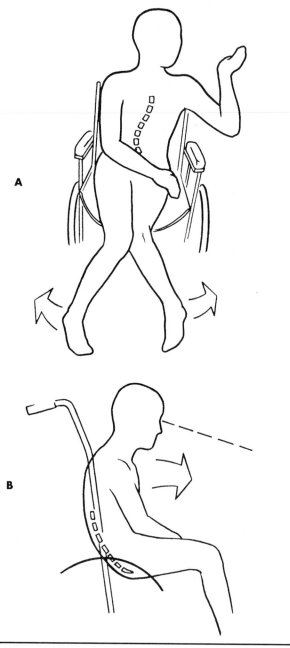

**Figure 6-7** **A,** Viewed from the frontal position: sitting in a sling seat causes internal rotation of the hips. **B,** Viewed from the side: sitting in wheelchair with sling seat and back results in an elongated C posture. (From Bergen AF, Presperin J, Tallman T: *Positioning for function: wheelchairs and other assistive technologies,* Valhalla, NY, 1990, Valhalla Rehabilitation Publications.)

**Sitting posture in a wheelchair.** Standard wheelchairs are made with a sling upholstery seat and back. The reason for this is that it is easily folded for transportation in an automobile. If you have ever sat in such a wheelchair or observed someone in one, you will have noted that what typically happens to the posture is that the hips slide forward and rotate inward, bringing the knees together (Figure 6-7, *A*). This causes the shoulders and trunk to collapse and round forward into an elongated C-type posture (Figure 6-7, *B*). This posture cannot possibly be comfortable for any length of time, and it does not allow an individual to use her hands to their maximal functional ability.

Sitting in a wheelchair with a sling seat without external stabilization has ramifications for pressure distribution, posture, and comfort. In this posture there is a posterior pelvic tilt and most of the weight is placed on the ischial tuberosities, the coccyx, and possibly the lower sacrum. The sling seat conforms to the forces generated by the individual instead of providing forces that resist and stabilize. This is an application of Newton's third law: each action (force) has an equal but opposite reaction. The internal forces of the body are not balanced by external forces from the sling seat. Thus the seat fails to support the alignment of the body, and the changes in posture cited above take place. An individual who uses a wheelchair likely has weakness and abnormal tone and may already have asymmetrical posture. Because the sling seat conforms to the forces generated by the individual, this asymmetry is further aggravated. It is important to understand the biomechanics of normal sitting so that these principles can be applied to seating for individuals with disabilities.

## ■ PRINCIPLES OF SEATING FOR POSTURAL CONTROL AND DEFORMITY MANAGEMENT

Children and adults who have irregular tone, muscle weakness, abnormal reflex patterns, shortening of a muscle group, or skeletal deformity are likely to require external positioning devices to control their posture and prevent deformities. Within this category, some individuals have mild impairment and require only minimal support, whereas other individuals have severe physical impairment and require extensive postural support. The components making up a seating system can provide support to the body that can align the body, normalize tone, prevent deformities, and enhance movement.

### Guidelines for Postural Control

The most important principle related to postural control is that proximal stabilization, near the center of the body, facilitates movement and control of the head and the extremities (e.g., function). During normal development, the infant achieves stability in the proximal joints before using the distal limbs for manipulation. For example, before a baby can successfully reach out and grab a toy while sitting, he must have mastered the ability to maintain a balanced sitting posture. Otherwise the hands must be used to maintain balance, which limits their use for manipulation. This is the basis of seating for postural control. For the individual who does not have the mechanisms to control body posture internally, external positioning components are used. Tredwell and Roxborough (1991) present a classification scheme (Box 6-3) that is useful in describing the amount of control a person exhibits in sitting. Each category is matched with a brief description of the recommended degree of support provided by the seating system.

When providing any type of external support, care needs to be taken so that the individual is not excessively positioned. We need to keep in mind that sitting is a *dynamic activity*. We often associate sitting with relaxation and lack of activity and movement, when in fact many activities are performed while sitting, such as writing, driving, talking on the phone, and typing. It is not uncommon to see individuals "properly" positioned to the point that they are no longer able to use the motor movements they have used in the past to complete functional tasks. The *fewest* restraints necessary to optimize function should be used (Bergen, Presperin, and Tallman, 1990).

In this section we present a set of general guidelines for proceeding with the development of a postural seating system for an individual. As in all applications of assistive technologies, the unique needs of each individual must be considered rather than applying a standard prescription. References such as Bergen, Presperin, and Tallman (1990), Trefler, Hobson, and Taylor (1993), and Letts (1991) are valuable resources that can assist the ATP in dealing with the intricacies of the application of these principles.

**Pelvis and lower extremities.** We have described the important role of the pelvis in relation to the center of gravity and sitting. The pelvis is a key point of control, and its position affects the posture of the rest of the body. Therefore alignment and stabilization of the pelvis is normally the first area addressed when positioning an individual. A position with the pelvis in neutral or in a slight anterior tilt is desired (Bergen, Presperin, and Tallman, 1990). The pelvis should be level and in midline.

A position with the hips flexed at approximately 90 degrees is recommended for most individuals (Bergen, Presperin, and Tallman, 1992; Taylor, 1987; Trefler, Hobson, and Taylor, 1993; Tredwell and Roxborough, 1991). This angle of hip flexion helps to inhibit extensor tone and reduces posterior tilt of the pelvis, thus keeping the individual positioned back in the seat. In some instances it is necessary to increase the amount of hip flexion (thus reducing the angle to less than 90 degrees) to further inhibit extensor tone. On the other hand, in some instances 90 degrees of hip flexion is not achievable (because of deformity) or is not the most appropriate position. A thorough evaluation will have provided the ATP with information regarding the amount of mobility in the pelvis, hips, and lower extremities; postures the individual tends to assume; and the degree to which these postures can be corrected. The degree of hip flexion found to be most appropriate subsequently determines the back-to-seat angle of the support surface.

Asymmetrical postures that may be present in the pelvis and hips include pelvic obliquity, pelvic rotation, pelvic tilt, and windswept hips. These postural asymmetries are often interrelated. They may be flexible postures or fixed bony deformities that restrict the mobility of the pelvis and prevent the attainment of the recommended pelvic position.

An individual with a **pelvic obliquity** has one side of the pelvis higher than the other when viewed in the frontal plane (Figure 6-8). The obliquity is named for the side that is lower; for example, with a left pelvic obliquity the left side is lower than the right. This is often accompanied by **pelvic**

---

| BOX 6-3 | Levels of Postural Control in Sitting |
|---|---|

**THE HANDS-FREE SITTER**
Can sit for prolonged periods without using the hands for support
Seating system is designed primarily for mobility, to provide a stable base of support, and to be comfortable

**THE HANDS-DEPENDENT SITTER**
One or both hands are used to maintain support while sitting
Seating system is designed to provide pelvic or trunk support to free up the person's hands for functional activities

**THE PROPPED SITTER**
Lacks any ability to support self in sitting
Seating system provides total body support

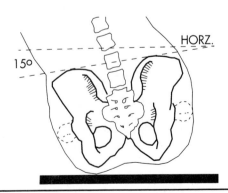

**Figure 6-8**  Pelvic obliquity viewed in the frontal plane. (From Siekman A: The biomechanics of seating: a consumer's guide, *Action Digest*, pp 8-9, March/April 1992.)

**rotation,** wherein one side of the pelvis is forward of the other side (Figure 6-9). **Windswept hip deformity** manifests itself with one hip adducted and the other hip abducted. This deformity has usually been found to be the end stage of a sequence that proceeds as follows: hip subluxation and dislocation, pelvic obliquity, scoliosis, windswept hip deformity. Therefore all these components are present in this deformity. The hip on the high side is typically dislocated, and the opposite hip may or may not be dislocated (Letts, 1991). When fixed deformities such as these are present, the seating system should be designed to accommodate them rather than to attempt to correct them (Taylor, 1987).

Support to the pelvis can be provided under, behind, in front of, or from the sides. At the very least, a firm seating surface for the individual to sit on will level and stabilize the pelvis. Individuals who are moderately to severely involved typically need more support for stabilization. This support can be provided by contours around the buttocks and up into the lumbar area. In cases where the individual has severe extensor tone, it may be necessary to reduce the seat-to-back angle. This can be accomplished by inclining the front of the seat or placing a wedge under the front of the seat. If it is desirable to keep a 90-degree angle of hip extension or greater, the back must also be reclined; this is called *orientation in space.* Finally, an antithrust seat can be used (Figure 6-10). With this approach, a depression is made in the cushion to accommodate the pelvis and stop forward movement. Supports to prevent lateral shifting of the pelvis or external rotation of the hips can be provided either by bolsters attached to the wheelchair or by blocks built into the seat surface.

To support the pelvis from the front, various types of pelvic positioning belts or knee blocks are used. The placement of the belt is important to effectively maintain pelvic position. Depending on the person's pelvic mobility, comfort, and positioning needs, the pelvic positioning belt is placed at an angle ranging from 45 to 90 degrees to the seating surface, as shown in Figure 6-11. In most cases a belt with an angle of pull at 45 degrees sufficiently maintains the pelvis in position. If there is excessive hip extension or a need for anterior pelvic mobility, positioning the belt at a 90-degree angle of pull is more effective. Pelvic positioning belts can be soft and flexible (e.g., webbing or padded vinyl)

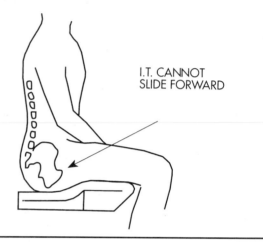

**Figure 6-10**    Antithrust seat. (From Bergen AF, Presperin J, Tallman T: *Positioning for function: wheelchairs and other assistive technologies,* Valhalla, NY, 1990, Valhalla Rehabilitation Publications.)

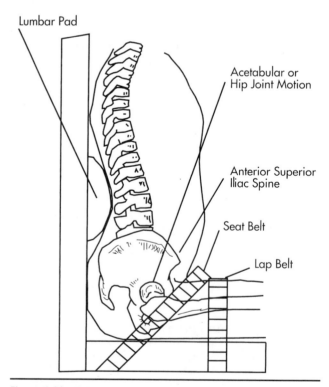

**Figure 6-11**    Pelvic positioning belts can be applied at 45 degrees (seat belt) or at 90 degrees (lap belt). (From Church G, Glennen S: *The handbook of assistive technology,* San Diego, 1992, Singular Publishing Group.)

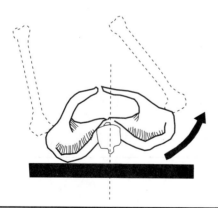

**Figure 6-9**    Pelvic rotation. (From Siekman A: The biomechanics of seating: a consumer's guide, *Action Digest,* pp 8-9, March/April 1992.)

or rigid when more support is required. A rigid pelvic positioning device, also called a subASIS bar (Figure 6-12), is typically a closely fitting, padded metal bar that is attached to the wheelchair frame or seat insert to position the pelvis below the individual's anterior superior iliac spines (ASIS). It is designed to be used in conjunction with a complete seat and back system for individuals who require greater control to maintain the neutral position of the pelvis and prevent pelvic rotation.

Adequately positioning the lower extremities helps to maintain the pelvic and hip positions. The positions of the legs and feet affect the position of the pelvis and therefore need to be addressed simultaneously. It is recommended that the legs be positioned in neutral abduction and with approximately 90 degrees of knee flexion. An **abductor** component (also referred to as pommel or medial knee support) can be used to keep the legs in a neutral abducted position, but unfortunately such components are frequently misused. One common misuse of an abductor is to place it in the groin area to prevent the individual from sliding forward in the seat. When correctly used, the abductor should be placed at the most distal point of the knee and extend approximately one third the distance of the thigh (Bergen, Presperin, and Tallman, 1990). Figure 6-13 shows an example of this type of component.

A frequently encountered problem in the lower extremi-

ties is hamstring tightness, which may or may not result in flexion contractures of the knees. Recall that these muscles are closely related to the position of the pelvis. Attempts to position the individual to stretch these muscles and reduce the flexion contracture only result in posterior pelvic tilt and a sliding forward in the chair into a sacral sitting position. Instead, it is best to accommodate this problem by modifying the seating surface (shortening the seat depth or undercutting the front edge) so the legs are allowed to flex under the seating surface. This maintains the correct pelvic position. If there is fixed knee extension, the lower leg must be completely supported with pads or troughs that match the range of motion in the knee.

Support for the feet is important for maintaining hip and knee position, for preventing deformities in the ankles, and for distributing pressure. If the feet are left to hang or are positioned too low, pressure increases under the anterior thigh area and can cut off blood flow. Positioning the feet too high places excess pressure on the ischial tuberosities and the sacrum and can cause formation of a pressure ulcer. It is recommended that the feet be positioned flat and with 90 degrees of ankle flexion (Taylor and Trefler, 1984). Support surfaces for the feet can be one or two platforms and in different sizes, depending on the person's needs. Increasing the thickness of the foot support under the shorter leg serves to accommodate unequal lower leg length. Foot platforms can be angled to accommodate fixed plantar flexion contractures of the ankle. Straps across the top of the foot, behind the heel, and across the ankle can aid in positioning. If more support is needed, there are components that completely support the foot and ankle.

**Trunk.** Once the desired position in the pelvis and lower extremities has been obtained, the trunk is considered. An upright position with the trunk aligned in midline is desirable. This position may not be attainable if the individual has fixed deformities. Possible spinal deformities are

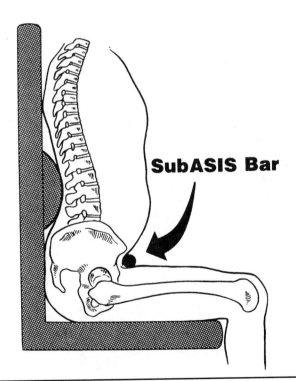

Figure 6-12   SubASIS bar. (From Margolis SA, Jones RM, Brown BE: The subASIS bar: an effective approach to pelvis stabilization in seated positioning, *Proc RESNA 8th Annual Conf,* pp 45-47, June 1985.)

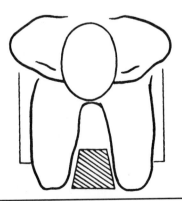

Figure 6-13   Abductor. (From Bergen AF, Presperin J, Tallman T: *Positioning for function: wheelchairs and other assistive technologies,* Valhalla, NY, 1990, Valhalla Rehabilitation Publications.)

(1) scoliosis, (2) lordosis, (3) kyphosis, or (4) a combination of these. **Scoliosis** of the spine occurs when there is lateral bending of the trunk. Scoliotic curves are further defined according to the anatomical site in the vertebral column that is involved, that is, cervical, thoracic, or lumbar. Compensatory (or secondary) curves develop as a result of the head's attempting to maintain its upright position (Figure 6-14, *A*) (Cailliet, 1975). Figure 6-14, *B*, shows an uncompensated curve with the spine unbalanced and the head lateral to the center of gravity. Rotation of the vertebrae is also frequently found in scoliosis and can cause greater respiratory difficulty than lateral curving (Cailliet, 1975).

The amount of trunk support required depends on the control the individual has of her trunk. As in the pelvis, trunk support can be provided from behind, at the side, or in front. The amount of support provided from behind is related to back height and contouring. The height of the back can be varied, depending on the amount of upper body support needed. Someone who requires minimal support

can use a lower backrest height, whereas a higher backrest is necessary for the individual with a need for greater support. Contouring allows us to accommodate the individual's body shape and provide optimal support. If the person has a kyphosis, the back needs to be recessed so that he is not pushed forward in the seat. For a lordosis, lumbar support can be added to bring the seat back in contact with the person. In cases where the shoulders are retracted, wedged blocks can be added to the back to position the shoulders forward.

When a person has difficulty maintaining a midline position (side to side) of the trunk, lateral support is provided (Figure 6-15). The positioning of the lateral supports depends on how much control the person has. Lateral supports placed high on the trunk and close to the body provide greater control than those placed lower on the trunk (Bergen, Presperin, and Tallman, 1990). Because the forces placed on the body by the lateral supports can be great, care should be taken in placement of these components and selection of materials (well padded) to prevent tissue damage. If there is scoliosis, the application of force at three positions on the body can prevent further deformity. This three-point system uses the principles of equilibrium of forces (described in the section on biomechanical principles) to stabilize and align the trunk. As shown in Figure 6-15, one pad is applied under the apex of the curve on the convex side *(F₃)*, with two other pads opposing it to provide resistance ($F_1$ and $F_2$). One of these pads is placed up high under the armpit and the other point is on the pelvis (Trefler, Hobson, and Taylor, 1993). For individuals with

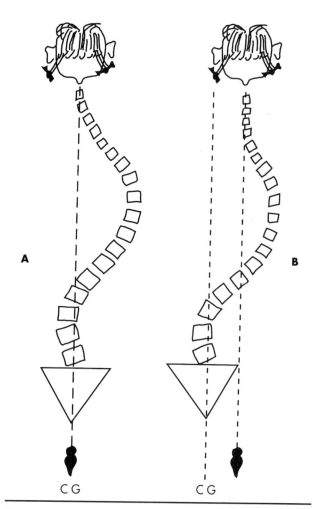

Figure 6-14    **A**, Development of compensatory curve in scoliosis. **B**, Uncompensated scoliotic curve. *CG*, center of gravity. (From Cailliet R: *Scoliosis: diagnosis and management*, Philadelphia, 1975, FA Davis Co.)

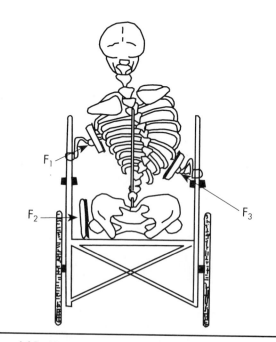

Figure 6-15    Three-point system of control for reducing the effects of scoliosis. (From Nwaobi OM: Biomechanics of seating. In Trefler E, editor: *Seating for children with cerebral palsy: a resource manual*, Memphis, 1984, University of Tennessee.)

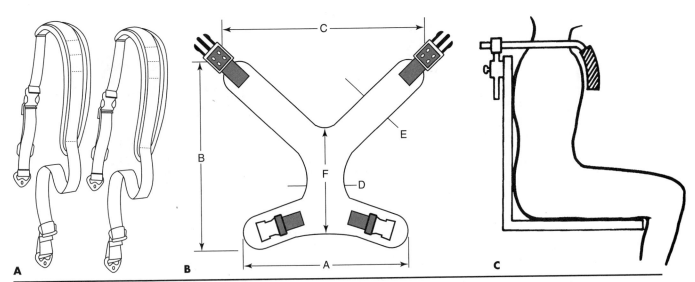

**Figure 6-16**    **A,** An example of a chest strap that attaches to the seat back below shoulder level, comes up over the shoulders, and attaches to the seating system near the hips. (Courtesy Bodypoint Designs, Inc., www.bodypoint.com.) **B,** Solid chest panel in an X design. (Courtesy Daher Manufacturing, Inc., www.daherproducts.com.) **C,** Rigid shoulder supports. (From Bergen AF, Presperin J, Tallman T: *Positioning for function: wheelchairs and other assistive technologies,* Valhalla, NY, 1990, Valhalla Rehabilitation Publications.)

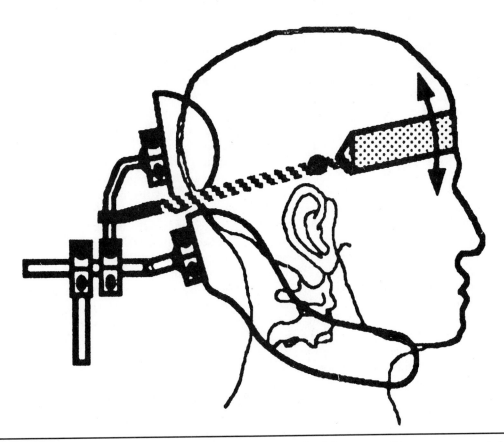

**Figure 6-17**    Head positioning components include headrest, lateral supports, and headband. One or more of these components are included in head supports. (Courtesy Whitmyer Biomechanix, Inc.)

spinal deformities, low tone, decreased strength in the trunk, or poor head control, tilting the seating system back slightly can eliminate some of the effects of gravity and also help the individual maintain a more symmetrical posture. Components such as lateral supports are more effective and more comfortable when the individual is tilted back slightly, since the force of gravity is reduced. The force required to keep the body at midline is reduced. There are wheeled bases that allow the person's orientation in space to be varied (see Chapter 10). These are useful if a person requires different positions for different activities. This feature is also useful in assisting with initial positioning and repositioning. When a person is tilted back, it is important to evaluate the affect of the tilt on vision, eating, and other functional tasks.

When control is required to prevent forward trunk flexion, anterior supports can be used. This type of support is necessary for individuals who need to be in an upright position for a functional or therapeutic activity but do not have the ability to maintain this position independently. The most common approaches used are straps, chest panels, and rigid shoulder supports. One simple approach is to use straps that are attached to the seat back below shoulder level, come up over the shoulders, and attach to the seating system near the hips (Figure 6-16, *A*). The chest strap should not be attached to the pelvic positioning belt (Bergen, Presperin, and Tallman, 1990). Another approach is a solid chest panel in a butterfly, X, or I shape with straps that attach to the seating system as above (Figure 6-16, *B*). The final approach is to use rigid shoulder components (Figure 6-16, *C*) that come over the clavicle and hold the shoulder girdle back against the seating system. These components should be adjustable and well padded to ensure stabilization without excessive pressure.

**Head and neck.** With the pelvis, lower extremities, and trunk positioned, the head and neck position are considered next. The position of the head is important in inhibiting abnormal reflexes and maximizing the visual skills of the individual. In some cases a headrest is necessary only part of the time, for example, when the individual becomes fatigued or during transportation. The most common problems leading to the need for positioning of the head include hyperextension of the neck, weak neck musculature, lateral neck flexion, and neck rotation. In addition, support may be required when the person has been reclined to right the head. As in the positioning of other body segments, posterior, anterior, or lateral components are used for support. Figure 6-17 shows examples of components for each of these types of support. Posterior support can range from a high backrest (for those requiring minimal support) to headrests of different types. With any posterior head support, it is important to avoid triggering extension or pushing the head forward into flexion. Anterior support is typically provided by headbands, which are used in conjunction with posterior head supports. Elastic materials or pulleys provide

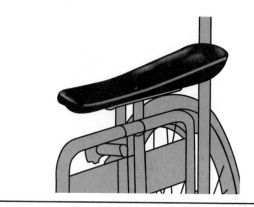

**Figure 6-18**    Arm trough. (Courtesy Otto Bock, www.ottobockus. com/products/r_wheel.htm.)

a dynamic type of support. This allows movement of the head within a limited range. Lateral supports can be incorporated into a headrest or provided as separate components. They can be applied at the temporal area, at the neck, or at the side of the face just in front of the ear.

**Upper extremities.**    Support of the upper extremities is an essential component of the seating system. A lack of support for the arms can adversely affect the head and neck position. Additionally, arms that are left to hang can sustain injury if caught on something or can acquire subluxation of the glenohumeral joint of the shoulder. Using an upper extremity support surface such as a lap tray helps with positioning of the head and neck, reduces the likelihood of damage to the arms and shoulder joints, and places the hands in a midline position that facilitates bilateral manual activities. The height of the lap tray depends on the needs of the consumer. Commonly the tray is mounted so that it allows the forearms to rest on it with the elbows bent at a 90-degree angle. For individuals with spasticity, a tray mounted up higher will help to reduce upper extremity tone (Trefler, Hobson, and Taylor, 1993). Individuals with athetosis or who are self-abusive may benefit from having their arms held in place under a tray. Some individuals do not want a lap tray but still require positioning of the upper extremities. For these situations, there are individual arm troughs (Figure 6-18) available that are mounted to the armrests of the wheelchair and provide channeling and support of the arms.

## ■ TECHNOLOGIES FOR POSTURAL CONTROL AND DEFORMITY MANAGEMENT

There are several technological approaches that can be used to implement the positioning principles described in the previous section. These approaches vary in the degree of support they provide. An approach is selected for each individual based on the amount of support required. A direct relationship exists between the amount of contact that the body has with the support surface and the degree of support it provides (Bergen, Presperin, and Tallman, 1990). We categorize the technological approaches according to a hierarchy of support that they provide: planar, standard contoured modules, and custom contoured. There are multiple technologies available within each of these categories. Some are fabricated completely on-site, whereas others utilize a central fabrication facility. Sources such as www.rehabcentral.com, www.abledata.com, and www.wheelchair.net can provide an up-to-date listing of suppliers of seating equipment. Besides the type of support surface to be used, comfort, appearance, and ease of use are also important factors to consider when selecting a particular technology.

## Planar

**Planar** technologies are flat surfaces that support the body only where it easily comes in contact with the body, such as at bony prominences. In general, they are appropriate for individuals who require minimal support. To this basic structure other positioning components can be added if additional support is required.

**Prefabricated.** Prefabricated planar components are made in standard sizes to fit a wide range of individuals. The back and seat surfaces are generally plywood or molded plastic pieces to which foam has been attached. Lateral supports and an abductor for pelvic and hip support can be attached with hardware to the basic seat, and lateral supports for trunk stability can be attached to the back section (Figure 6-19). The seat and back are attached to the wheelchair frame with interfacing hardware once the upholstery has been removed. Much of the hardware that interfaces the various components can be adjusted for angle, width, and depth. Some systems, such as the Mulholland Growth Guidance System,* consist of an integrated planar seating surface and a wheeled base that has many adjustable components. The advantage of having adjustable components is that they allow the system to be modified for growth or postural changes.

**Custom fabricated.** Custom-fabricated planar systems are made of similar materials and design as prefabricated systems, but the dimensions of the seating surface and components are customized to fit the individual. These systems can be fabricated on-site directly with the consumer, or specifications of the consumer's measurements can be sent to a manufacturer for fabrication. The density of

*Mulholland Positioning Systems, Inc., Chico, Calif (www.mulhollandinc.com).

---

CASE STUDY 6-1

POSTURAL CONTROL

Jillian is a happy 5-year-old girl with cerebral palsy, resulting in severe motor impairment. Jillian is nonverbal and uses a smile or an eye blink to indicate yes. She is very alert and aware of her environment. She will be attending kindergarten in the fall. She does not have a wheelchair and has never been evaluated for a seating system. Her parents carry her from place to place or use an umbrella stroller for her as needed. She receives therapy with a neurodevelopmental treatment approach 3 times a week. When they made the initial phone referral, Jillian's parents stated to you that they have put off getting a seating system for Jillian because they did not want her to "look handicapped." With Jillian soon to be attending school, they have decided it is time to get her a wheelchair and seating system.

Jillian has mixed tone. Her lower extremities, particularly her ankles, have increased tone. The tone in her upper extremities is increased as well. Her trunk and neck are hypotonic. She exhibits a startle reflex and the symmetric tonic neck reflex. She does not have any apparent orthopedic deformities. She is unable to keep her head up for any length of time unless she is reclined back slightly. Jillian can use a switch with her right hand when her head is held upright. She can also use the touch screen on the computer, but she needs help with sitting. Jillian is dependent for mobility and all other functional activities.

**QUESTIONS:**

1. From the information you have so far, what might be the goals of seating for Jillian?
2. Write a list of interview questions you would ask of her parents and therapists.
3. How would you proceed with a seating evaluation for Jillian?
4. Based on the information you know about Jillian at this time, what technological approaches would you consider for her and why? What type of positioning accessories would you consider and why?
5. List potential funding sources for Jillian's seating system. How would you justify her system to the funding source (refer to Chapter 5)?

---

the foam pieces can also be selected to accommodate the needs of the individual. Lateral supports, headrests, abductors, and other components are added to the basic foam and plywood (or plastic) structure. This approach can be highly labor intensive and is being replaced at many facilities as a result of the advent of a large array of off-the-shelf technologies.

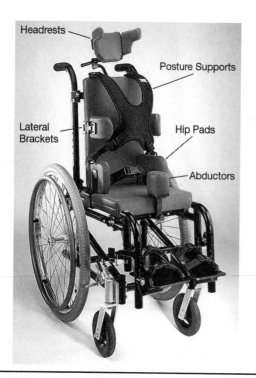

**Figure 6-19** Planar seating system with positioning components. (Courtesy Adaptive Engineering Lab, Inc., www.aelseating.com.)

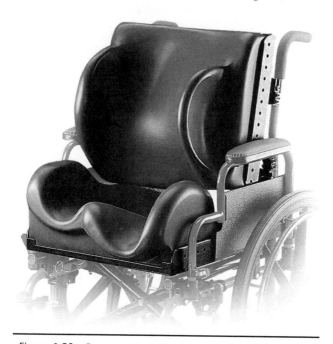

**Figure 6-20** Custom-contoured seating system. (Courtesy Invacare.)

## Standard Contoured Modules

Planar systems provide adequate support for many individuals who have relatively good motor control, fair trunk support, and spinal curvatures or fixed deformities; however, for individuals with less control, the planar surface does not provide enough support. Contoured technologies use curved

surfaces that, depending on the specific approach, more closely match the shape of the human body. By contouring the seating surface to the person's body, we increase the amount of contact that the body has with the seating surface. This provides increased support and control.

For a significant number of individuals, there is a need for contouring, but it is not necessary to contour the cushion to the exact shape of the body. Several manufacturers produce seat and back modules with standard contours in an array of sizes to fit children and adults. Generally, closed-cell foams (see the section later in this chapter on properties of cushion materials) are used with a vacuum forming manufacturing process. The foam is covered with either vinyl or cloth, which is also vacuum formed, so it closely adheres to the foam. The cushions are generally supported by some type of metal or plywood base, which is then attached with mounting hardware to the wheelchair frame. This type of cushion is useful for the individual with mild to moderate physical impairment, including a symmetrical posture and few (if any) deformities (Hobson, 1990).

## Custom Contoured

The cushion that provides the greatest amount of body contact and therefore support is one that has been shaped, or custom contoured, to the individual's body. A number of technologies have been developed to achieve a custom-contoured system. One example is shown in Figure 6-20. These types of systems differ primarily in terms of the fabrication techniques used and whether the fabrication is completed on-site or in a central location. The disadvantages of custom-contoured support surfaces include the following: Transfers to and from the system are more difficult; the system is static and has no dynamic properties, thus limiting the individual to one fixed position; and there is limited ability within the system to allow for growth of the individual.

Hobson (1990) identifies five distinct custom-contouring approaches, each of which uses a different fabrication technique. These approaches include hand-shaped foam, foaming, vacuum consolidation, modified orthotic, and shapeable matrices.

**Hand-shaped foam.** With the *hand-shaped foam* approach, seating components are shaped on-site by layering various types of foam and carving out body contours as needed. Typically a block of rigid Ethafoam is used as the base layer for stability. Less dense foams are added to this to imitate the body contours. With this type of system, the consumer often uses a temporary cover, such as sheepskin, and takes the seating component home for a trial period. Once the desired shape is achieved, the foam is covered with vinyl or cloth. This was the first approach used for obtaining a custom-contoured system. This approach is labor intensive and requires quite a bit of technical skill (Hobson, 1990). It is also possible to provide specifications to a central manufacturer who then fabricates a seating system that is contoured to fit the consumer. Taking accurate measurements of the consumer is essential when using this approach.

**Foaming.** The *foaming* approach uses a foam mixture that has two parts, both of which are liquid at room temperature. When mixed, these two elements combine to form a solid foam base or expand to envelop a shape. Polyurethane foams are manufactured in two components, which expand when mixed. The expansion is due to the production of $CO_2$, which causes the foam to rise. The rising foam can then be used to fill a mold, which is contoured to the body shape of the person. Two approaches are used: (1) the foam is shaped directly to the person's body; or (2) a mold (usually plaster bandage) is taken of the person, and the foam is used to fill the mold and make the seating system.

The first method is often called *foam-in-place* because the person is present as the foam components are added and allowed to rise.* This approach can be used on-site, and a seating system can be completed in 1 day or less. For this method the person is placed in a frame that has a flexible covering over one side. This covering is matched to the shape of the person, and she is positioned in the most desirable seated posture. The foam materials are then added to the frame and allowed to expand to contour to the person's shape. The person is removed from the frame, and the foam is allowed to harden for several hours. Once the foam hardens, the flexible covering is removed and the foam is encased in a cloth or vinyl cover. The foam can then be attached to a solid backing (usually plywood or plastic) and mounted to the wheeled base.

The second approach to foaming is called *foam-in-box* or *indirect* (Hobson, 1990). In this case a plaster mold is made of the individual and the mold is used to shape the expanding foam. This process may be done on-site, but more often the plaster cast is shipped to a central facility where the cushion is fabricated. When done centrally, the finished foam cushion can be covered with a vacuum-formable vinyl or cloth covering, which contours closely to the cushion shape and adheres strongly. This process can take several weeks.

**Vacuum consolidation.** The vacuum consolidation method of contouring uses a bag filled with small particles (similar to a beanbag chair), such as the one shown in Figure 6-21, to make the basic shape for the contoured cushion. The person to be fitted is seated in the bag and placed in the optimal position. A vacuum pump is used to draw air out of

*For example, foam-in-place from Dynamic Systems, Inc. (www.sunmatecushions.com/).

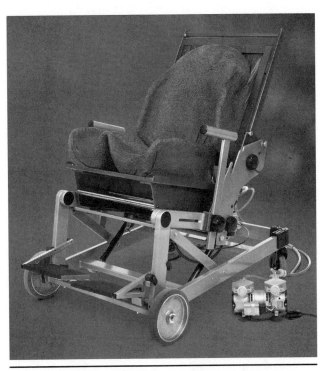

Figure 6-21    Molding frame for vacuum consolidation. (Courtesy Invacare.)

the bag, which forces the particles in the bag to compress and closely match the person's shape. As the amount of vacuum in the bag is increased, the pliability of the bag decreases. There is a point at which the bag can be manipulated and will retain its shape just like clay. This allows the ATP to contour the shape to the person's body. Once the proper position is obtained and the contour is as desired, all the air is withdrawn from the bag by the vacuum pump and the bag containing the particles becomes rigid. At this point in the process there are several alternatives to convert the form that is defined by the bag into a cushion.

The first approach is similar to the foaming process and is called *direct vacuum consolidation* (Hobson, 1990). In this process the particles in the bag are foam pellets and a glue is added to the bag before attaching the vacuum pump. The glue hardens slowly enough that the pellets can be shaped to the person's body. After the glue has hardened, a softer foam is placed over the contoured seat and back cushions and a cover is added to keep the foam clean and dry. The entire cushion is attached to plywood, plastic, or aluminum backing pieces and then attached to a wheeled base. This approach can be used on-site, and a cushion can be completed in about 12 hours.

The second approach to vacuum consolidation is called *indirect.* In both cases, latex is used for the bag and polyethylene beads are used for filling. The process of molding the bag to the person's contour is the same as for the direct method. The major difference is that no glue is placed inside the bag. Once the final shape is obtained, there are two primary techniques used for fabricating the cushion from the molded bag. The first of these involves making a plaster cast of the bag, which captures the contours. This mold is then generally sent to a central facility where the cushion is fabricated from the mold.* The major advantages of this approach include the relatively low cost of materials, the accuracy of the physical plaster cast, and the uniformity in central production. The necessity of shipping the plaster mold to a central facility and the delays encountered in central fabrication are the major disadvantages.

An alternative indirect vacuum consolidation process is to digitize the shape of the finished molded bag using a computer and digital probe.† This digitized image can be sent via a computer to a central facility, and there is no need to ship a plaster cast. This process is based on computer-aided design (CAD). CAD uses mechanical or electronic sensors that measure the contours of the body shape acquired with the simulator. This information is transferred to a computer program, which designs the appropriate seating system. The shape of the seating system can be viewed on the computer screen and certain points can be chosen and modified if needed. Once the desired cushion shape is obtained, the data are downloaded to a central facility. Using a computer-aided manufacturing (CAM) process, these data are then used to operate cutting tools, which carve the desired shape from blocks of foam. The finished seat and back cushions are covered and then returned to the on-site facility for fitting to the consumer. The major advantages are that no plaster cast needs to be made, the information regarding contours can be sent electronically instead of shipping a bulky plaster mold, and the contours of individuals can be saved in computer data files, which takes up less space than storage of physical molds. With the data stored in the computer, it is a simple process to make modifications to the cushion if it does not fit correctly or a new cushion is needed.

**Modified orthotic.** Orthotic devices are often fabricated by making a plaster cast of the body segment that is to be supported and then using that cast to mold a plastic support. This approach has been adapted to seating and positioning systems (Hobson, 1990). A negative mold of the body segment (e.g., the trunk) is obtained. Filling the negative impression with plaster then creates a positive mold. This shape closely approximates the individual's contours, and it can be used as the mold for a plastic appliance. Often

*For example, Invacare Contour U System (www.invacare.com/ product_catalog/).
†For example, the custom contoured seating system from Signature 2000, Inc. (www.signature2000.net/home.html).

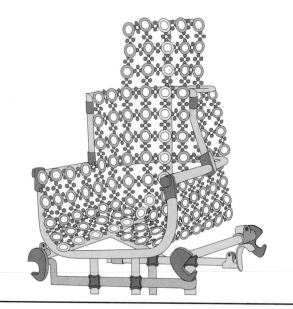

**Figure 6-22** Shapeable matrices.

plastics that are flexible at higher temperatures are used to make the appliances. These plastics are heated and then shaped over the plaster mold, and a vacuum pump is often used to obtain as close a shape as possible. As Hobson points out, although this approach provides the most intimate fit to actual body contours of all the contoured approaches, it should only be attempted by trained orthotists. Other limitations include lack of growth potential and difficulty in independently adjusting seat and back components if a single body mold is used.

**Shapeable matrices.** Seating systems that use shapeable matrices consist of an array of small components, which can be linked, shaped, and then locked to retain the desired contour (Cooper, Foort, and Hannah, 1983). The interlocking components are usually purchased in sheets.* Each element in the array can be moved over a 360-degree range, and this allows virtually any shape to be created. The matrix is shaped to the individual's contour, and then each element is tightened (Figure 6-22). A 7-inch × 3-inch sheet of this material contains six individual matrix elements, and an average seating system could have 100 or more elements, each of which needs to be adjusted. Positioning and adjustment of these systems can take several days of tedious effort. The obvious advantage of this approach is the ability to shape the system to fit any contour. The disadvantage is that this system is time intensive and may require frequent adjustments. The shapeable matrix approach can be useful for making custom components, which need to be contoured. Custom components include headrests, lateral sup-

*Matrix System, Indianapolis, 800-253-6217.

ports, and foot supports. This method has also been shown to be useful for very young children and infants, for whom molds cannot be created using other techniques.

## Hybrid

As Hobson (1990) discusses, many of these approaches can be combined into a system for a given individual. For example, a custom-contoured seat (needed for adequate pelvic control) could be combined with a foam and plywood planar back for one individual. In any case, the choice of technological approach must be driven by a thorough clinical assessment, and it must be consistent with the consumer's needs and goals.

## Interfacing Components

Seating systems are typically attached to a wheeled base. This attachment is referred to as *interfacing*. The use of appropriate interfacing hardware is important for the proper functioning of the whole system. Many methods are used, and the choice of one is based on the technological approach used for the seating system itself, the type and style of wheelchair, and personal preferences of the ATP providing the system. All manufacturers of seating systems provide interfacing components, and several other companies provide these and other accessories.

It is critical that all interfacing hardware and positioning accessories be securely attached to both the wheelchair and the seating system. In the process of attaching the hardware, it is important that the structural integrity of the wheelchair be maintained.

## ■ PRINCIPLES OF SEATING FOR PRESSURE MANAGEMENT

Another major area of need in seating is pressure management. The emphasis in this area is to manage sitting pressure and maintain the skin in healthy condition so that pressure ulcers are prevented. A **pressure ulcer** is a lesion that develops as a result of unrelieved pressure to the area and results in damage to underlying tissue (Panel for the Prediction and Prevention of Pressure Ulcers in Adults, 1992). Pressure ulcers usually occur over bony prominences, with the sacrum, coccyx, ischial tuberosities, trochanters, external malleoli, and heels being the areas most commonly affected. These lesions have also been referred to as decubitus ulcers, bedsores, pressure sores, and dermal ulcers. Because pressure is the major factor influencing the development of these lesions, it is recommended that the term *pressure ulcer* be used to describe these lesions (NPUAP, 1992).

Pressure ulcers are classified in stages according to clini-

cal manifestations. A widely accepted criterion used to classify pressure ulcers is the National Pressure Ulcer Advisory Panel (NPUAP) Staging System (NPUAP, 1989 and 1998), which defines four stages of pressure ulcers:

- Stage I: An observable pressure-related alteration of intact skin whose indicators as compared with the adjacent or opposite area on the body may include changes in one or more of the following: skin temperature (warmth or coolness), tissue consistency (firm or boggy feel), and sensation (pain, itching). The ulcer appears as a defined area of persistent redness in lightly pigmented skin, whereas in darker skin tones the ulcer may appear with persistent red, blue, or purple hues.
- Stage II: Partial-thickness skin loss involving epidermis, dermis, or both. The ulcer is superficial and presents clinically as an abrasion, blister, or shallow crater.
- Stage III: Full-thickness skin loss involving damage to or necrosis of subcutaneous tissue that may extend down to but not through underlying fascia. The ulcer presents clinically as a deep crater with or without undermining of adjacent tissue.
- Stage IV: Full-thickness skin loss with extensive destruction, tissue necrosis, or damage to muscle, bone, or supporting structures (e.g., tendon, joint capsule). Undermining and sinus tracts may also be associated with Stage IV pressure ulcers.

Although the clinical manifestations present themselves in the order described above, studies have shown that this is not actually the sequence in which degeneration of the tissue occurs. A study of dogs found that degeneration took place simultaneously in all levels of tissue from the bone to the skin (Kosiak, 1959). A study involving swine found that degeneration occurred initially in muscle and, as the amount of pressure or time increased, progressed toward the skin (Daniel, Priest, and Wheatley, 1981).

The staging criteria are used to define the maximal depth of tissue involvement after necrotic tissue has been removed. Healing of a pressure ulcer does not occur by replacing the same structural levels of body tissues (e.g., muscle, subcutaneous fat, and dermis) that were destroyed. Instead the pressure ulcer is filled with granulation tissue. Therefore it is not appropriate to use these staging criteria for reverse staging to describe improvement in a pressure ulcer (NPUAP, 2000). The NPUAP recommends that the healing process of an ulcer should be documented by noting improvement in wound characteristics such as size, depth, and amount of necrotic tissue.

There has been much research done attempting to determine the various factors that contribute to the development of pressure ulcers and to identify tools and strategies for preventing their occurrence. However, it is difficult to isolate all the variables that affect individuals as they go through their daily lives and to make substantive conclusions for a population as a whole based on this research. Each person must be considered individually, and a comprehensive program of risk assessment and prevention must be developed to address his or her needs. The ATP needs to be aware of the role of seating, as well as all the other variables, in order to prevent pressure ulcers.

## Incidence and Costs of Pressure Ulcers

Individuals who are bedridden or in a wheelchair and have limited ability to reposition themselves are at risk of developing pressure ulcers. In particular, individuals with spinal cord injury are at a high risk because they lack sensation and have limited movement below the level of the lesion. It is estimated that more than 50% of individuals with spinal cord injury will encounter some type of tissue breakdown during their lifetime (Salzberg et al, 1996; Rodriguez and Garber, 1994) and that 36% to 50% will have repeat pressure ulcers within the first year after initial healing (Niazi et al, 1997; Salzberg et al, 1996). Other populations with a high incidence of pressure ulcers include individuals with hemiplegia caused by stroke; multiple sclerosis; cancer; the elderly; and individuals who have had a femoral fracture.

It is difficult to ascertain the overall incidence and prevalence of pressure ulcers because of the number of different variables. Studies are typically limited to one particular setting. In *acute care settings* the reported incidence (new cases appearing within a specified period) of pressure ulcers varies from 2.7% (Gerson, 1975) to 29.5% (Clarke and Kadhom, 1988). In an extensive study of acute care facilities, Meehan (1990) surveyed 148 hospitals and found a prevalence (the cross-sectional count of the number of cases at a specified point in time) of pressure ulcers of 9.2%. A number of subpopulations appear to be at higher risk than the general hospital population, such as the reported 60% prevalence in hospitalized patients with quadriplegia (Richardson and Meyer, 1981) and an incidence of 66% for orthopedic patients hospitalized for femoral fractures (Versluysen, 1986). Another high-risk hospital subpopulation is critical care patients, with a reported 33% incidence (Bergstrom, Demuth, Braden, 1987) and 41% prevalence (Robnett, 1986). Through the use of the Minimum Data Set (MDS), the Health Care Financing Administration regularly collects data on a state by state basis of the percentage of residents in skilled nursing facilities who have been assessed with a Stage 1 to 4 pressure ulcer. In the most recent data the average prevalence of pressure ulcers in U.S. skilled nursing facilities was 9.8%, with states ranging from 5.6% to 14.9% (MDS National Quality Indicator System, 2000).

Pressure ulcers can be life threatening. The comparative mortality of those with pressure ulcers has been noted to be five times higher than those without ulcers (Young and Dobrzanski, 1992). In one study of patients who had been admitted to geriatric wards, pressure ulcers were listed as the primary cause of death in as many as 6% and as a major contributing factor in a further 6% (Young and Dobrzanski, 1992). The problem may be gravely underestimated because pressure ulcers are not often listed as a cause of death on death certificates.

Pressure ulcers are costly in terms of the amount of money spent on healing or surgical repair, as well as the time lost from work and other activities. Estimates for medical costs alone for treatment of pressure ulcers vary depending on the number and the severity. Miller and Delozier (1994) estimated that in 1992 the total cost of pressure ulcer treatment in the United States exceeded $1.335 billion. In their investigation it was estimated that for patients with a primary diagnosis of pressure ulcers the mean hospital charge was $21,675 and physician charges were $2900 per case. They also compared hospital charges for patients with hip fractures with and without pressure ulcers. On average, an additional $10,986 in hospital charges was ascribed to the pressure ulcers. Miller and Delozier also estimated that cost of pressure ulcer care in skilled nursing facilities and home care settings was $335 million and $60 million, respectively.

In addition to the costs for medical care, there are social costs, which have a greater effect (Krouskop et al, 1983). Krouskop et al (1983) identify these costs as including (1) time lost from work, which affects the person and his or her family; (2) time lost from school; (3) time away from family, which can affect the person's social development; and (4) loss of personal independence and productivity, which results in decreased self-esteem and self-worth.

## Origins of Pressure Ulcers

There are many factors that contribute to the development of pressure ulcers; these are shown in Figure 6-23. External forces applied to a localized area are considered to be the primary cause. With application of external pressure, the normal flow of blood and oxygen to tissue in that area is reduced. If this situation is sustained, changes occur in the tissue cells, and these changes eventually lead to death of the cells. Individuals who have limited movement and lie in bed or sit in a wheelchair for prolonged periods generate compression forces that reduce the blood supply to the tissues and make the individuals prone to pressure ulcers.

As we have mentioned, the areas that most commonly develop pressure ulcers are the tissues over weight-bearing bony prominences. The reason for the high incidence of pressure ulcers over bony prominences relates back to the principle discussed earlier that states that any force applied over a small area generates more pressure than the same force applied over a larger area.

The amount of external pressure sufficient to restrict the

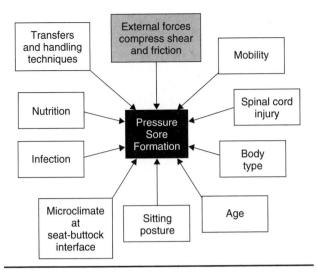

Figure 6-23    Factors that contribute to pressure ulcer development.

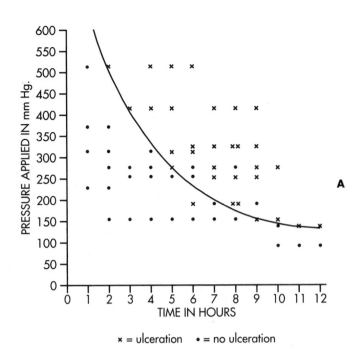

× = ulceration    • = no ulceration

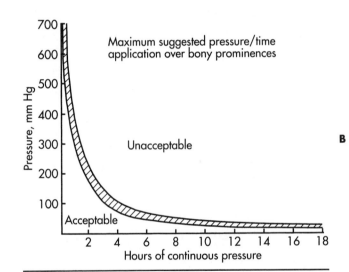

Figure 6-24    **A,** Relationship between applied pressure and time. Most points above the curve result in ulceration. (From Kosiak M: Etiology of decubitus ulcers, *Arch Phys Med Rehab* 42:19-29, 1961.) **B,** Allowable pressures versus time of application for tissue under bony prominences. (From Reswick JB, Rogers JE: Experience at Rancho Los Amigos Hospital with devices and techniques to prevent pressure sores. In Kenedi RM, Cowden JM, Scales JT, editors: *Bedsore biomechanics,* Baltimore, 1976, University Park Press.)

blood flow enough to cause tissue damage has been a point of discussion over the years. The average blood pressure in capillaries ranges from 12 mm Hg in the venous limb to 32 mm Hg in the arteriolar limb (Landis, 1930). External pressure on the weight-bearing surface that exceeds these pressures produces obstruction of the capillaries. When sitting pressures of subjects on various types of surfaces were measured, it was found that the pressure generated by each surface under the ischial tuberosities greatly exceeded capillary blood pressure (Kosiak et al, 1958). A contoured, alternating pressure chair was the only surface that provided intermittent reduction (in the down position) of pressure to levels in the range of capillary blood pressure. Because most of the seating surfaces in this study generated pressures that exceeded capillary pressure, investigators were led to question whether that is the primary cause of pressure ulcer formation or if other factors are involved.

The duration of pressure is a significant variable in the development of pressure ulcers. Kosiak (1959) determined that there is an inverse relationship between the amount of pressure sustained and the time over which it is applied. In a study involving dogs, Kosiak found that a pressure of 600 mm Hg produced ulceration in approximately 1 hour and a pressure of 150 mm Hg produced ulceration in 12 hours. The results of this study are shown in Figure 6-24, *A.* Microscopic tissue changes were found after application of as little as 60 mm Hg of pressure over 1 hour. This finding is consistent with the theory that exceeding the capillary pressure deprives the cells of enough important nutrients to cause damage at some level.

Time as a variable in pressure ulcer development is taken into consideration with the broad guidelines developed by Reswick and Rogers (1976). These guidelines, based on years of clinical experience with individuals who have spinal cord injury, establish allowable amounts of pressure that

tissue surrounding bony prominences can endure over certain periods. They recommend that pressures on the ischial tuberosities remain in the range of 30 to 60 mm Hg, as shown in Figure 6-24, *B.* Tissues that are not susceptible to the internal pressure exerted by bony prominences can tolerate higher skin surface pressures or lower pressures for longer periods.

Up to this point we have been discussing the effects of

sustained perpendicular (compression) pressure forces on tissue. Parallel (or shear) forces play a significant role in the formation of pressure ulcers as well. Shear forces are generated when two surfaces move across each other in opposite directions, for example, when an individual slides his hips forward in a wheelchair and assumes a sacral sitting posture. In this position the skin remains in contact with the seat surface and the superficial fascia is interlocked with the skin. The deeper portion of the superficial fascia, however, is mobile and slides forward. The blood vessels in this area are stretched and angulated, which causes occlusion. Resulting tissue damage is at a deeper level and typified by a large area of undermining around the base of the ulcer (Reichel, 1958). Bennett et al (1979) believe it is the combination of pressure and shear that is so effective in occluding blood flow. They found that when sufficient shear was present, only half as much pressure was needed to cause occlusion. Unfortunately, because of the difficulty in measuring shear, there is still uncertainty regarding the extent to which shear contributes to the development of pressure ulcers.

Friction, the force between two surfaces at rest or in motion, is another component of shear and the development of pressure ulcers. Friction leads to injury and ulceration of the surface of the skin. A typical friction injury to the skin occurs when it moves across a rough surface such as bedding. Dinsdale (1974) found that the skin's susceptibility to pressure ulcer development is increased with friction. When pressure alone was applied, 290 mm Hg was required to produce ulceration. With the application of pressure *and* friction, ulcerations were produced with pressure levels as low as 45 mm Hg. Moisture, heat, or properties of materials such as clothing can increase frictional forces.

## Other Factors That Contribute to Pressure Ulcer Development

Some individuals can be exposed to the mechanical forces of pressure and shear without developing pressure ulcers, whereas others have very little tolerance to these mechanisms. Although compression and shear forces are typically considered to be the chief causes of pressure ulcers, there are several other factors that contribute to skin breakdown and cause some individuals to be more susceptible than others.

**Mobility.** Moving to relieve pressure over an area is how the body typically responds to prevent tissue damage. If you were to pay attention to your movements while sitting, you would probably be surprised at how many times you adjusted and readjusted your seated position. Nondisabled subjects make side-to-side weight oscillations several times per minute while sitting (Tredwell and Roxborough, 1991). Normally, when there is a lack of oxygen and chemical irritation, pain signals from the nerve endings trigger postural changes and there is little tissue damage. Individuals

who lack normal sensation, such as those who have sustained a spinal cord injury, are unable to recognize and respond to these pain signals and are particularly susceptible to developing pressure ulcers (Grogan, Morton, and Murphy, 1986).

Exton-Smith and Sherwin (1961) recorded body movements of patients over the age of 65 who were admitted to a hospital during a 7-hour overnight period. They found that among the 10 individuals who moved the least during the night (from 4 to 20 times), 9 developed pressure ulcers. Out of 12 individuals who moved between 23 to 50 times during the night, 1 developed pressure ulcers. Those individuals who moved more than 54 times during the night did not develop any pressure ulcers. They also found that movement was less frequent in the patients who were very ill and too weak to move or those who had motor paralysis or were heavily sedated.

Individuals whose ability to reposition themselves or whose activity is limited to bed or any chair should be assessed for their risk of developing a pressure ulcer. There are scales available that determine the magnitude of risk by measuring the degree to which mobility and activity levels are limited. Two commonly used scales that assess these factors are the Norton Scale (Norton, McLaren, and Exton-Smith, 1975) and the Braden Scale (Bergstrom et al, 1987). In addition to mobility, these scales also assess other factors that place a person at risk for developing pressure ulcers, such as incontinence, impaired nutritional status, and altered level of consciousness. Individuals should be assessed using a validated systematic risk assessment tool upon admission to acute care and rehabilitation hospitals, nursing homes, home care programs, and other health care facilities, as well as at other periodic intervals. Identified risk factors can be reduced through intervention, and the development of pressure ulcers might be prevented.

**Spinal cord injury.** As discussed above, loss of sensation and limitations in mobility put individuals with spinal cord injury at great risk for development of pressure ulcers. In addition, some researchers speculate that other changes in the body as a result of the denervation caused by the spinal cord injury increase a person's susceptibility to pressure ulcers. In a study of normal and paraplegic rats, no differences were found in their susceptibility to pressure (Kosiak, 1961). Constantian (1980) concludes that there is not adequate objective evidence that individuals with denervated tissue are predisposed to the development of pressure ulcers nor that denervated tissue heals more slowly or differently than skin with normal enervation. On the other hand, there is evidence that after spinal cord injury there may be tissue alterations (e.g., loss of collagen, abnormal vascularity, tone changes) and changes in hormonal response to stress that place a person more at risk for developing pressure ulcers and impair the normal healing process (Whimster, 1976; Pfeffer, 1991; Patterson et al, 1992).

Differences in circulatory tissue perfusion between persons who have a spinal cord injury and those who do not have been documented (Patterson et al, 1992). With externally applied pressures of 32 mm Hg, it was found that the partial pressure of oxygen (an indicator of the perfusion of the tissue) was significantly lower in spinal cord–injured subjects than it was for nondisabled subjects. In order to evaluate the *response* of the peripheral circulation to externally applied pressure, Patterson et al (1992) cycled the pressure loads on and off. Although oxygen perfusion was lower during both on and off periods for the spinal cord–injured persons, it was only during the on period that these differences were statistically significant. At higher external pressures (75 mm Hg), the differences in oxygen perfusion for the two groups were not statistically significant. The difference between the two groups at the lower pressure was attributed to a lack of vascular autoregulation in the spinal cord–injured subjects (Patterson et al, 1992). Autoregulation requires a minimal pressure difference between internal pressure and external. At 75 mm Hg autoregulation cannot occur because the external pressure is near the arterial pressure. Measurements of blood volume showed significant differences between two groups at both external pressures. This study indicates that there are tissue perfusion changes in spinal cord injury that significantly impair the response to external pressure loads.

Measurement of these factors, although improving, makes it difficult to specify their particular effects on pressure ulcer development. However, it is likely that there are intrinsic changes in the body as a result of spinal cord injury that cannot be ignored. These changes may result in tissue with different properties and a reduced tolerance to external pressure.

**Body type.** The body type of the individual has some effect on pressure distribution. A thin person has less subcutaneous fat to act as padding and therefore forces per unit area of the skin are increased. An overweight individual has more padding over which to distribute pressure. However, it may be more difficult for the overweight individual to perform pressure relief exercises. Caregivers may also have more difficulty moving an overweight individual, and this may make shearing and friction forces a greater possibility.

**Nutrition.** Inadequate nutrition is often associated with weight loss and muscular atrophy, both of which reduce the amount of tissue between the seat surface and the bony prominences. Inadequate dietary intake, which results in anemia; decreased protein levels; and vitamin C deficiency are also known to interfere with the normal integrity of the tissue (Berecek, 1981; Breslow, 1991) and have been linked not only to pressure ulcer development but also to delayed healing. An increased intake of protein and calories has been shown to improve the healing rate of pressure ulcers (Breslow, 1991).

**Infection.** Torrance (1983) identifies three reasons why infection may contribute to pressure ulcer development. First, fever caused by infection increases the metabolic rate, which increases the demand for oxygen, which in turn endangers areas that are ischemic. Second, severe infection can also affect the nutritional balance of the body. Finally, localized bacteria increase the demand on metabolism in a localized area.

**Age.** As we age, our skin loses some of its elasticity and muscles atrophy, which increases our vulnerability to friction or shearing. Vascular and neurological diseases associated with aging (e.g., diabetes, renal disease) affect the circulation and may also increase an individual's susceptibility to skin breakdowns.

**Sitting posture.** Posture and deformity can affect the pressure distribution of the seat/buttock interface and can potentially contribute to skin breakdown. Two specific postures that pose a risk for pressure ulcer formation are pelvic obliquity and sacral sitting. Pelvic obliquity, which was discussed in detail in a previous section, results in increased pressure and shear under the affected lower ischial tuberosity and the posterior aspect of the lower greater trochanter (Zacharkow, 1984, 1988; Hobson, 1989). The loss of lumbar lordosis when sitting is another risk factor. This occurs as a result of limited hip mobility for flexion or decreased spinal mobility for extension (Zacharkow, 1984). Consequently, a sacral sitting posture is typically assumed, and this position results in significant amounts of pressure being placed on the sacrococcygeal region.

**Microclimate at the seat/buttock interface.** The microclimate between the body and the seating surface is a critical factor that is often overlooked. The temperature of the skin and the presence of moisture both affect the formation of pressure ulcers. An increase in skin temperature of 1° C is accompanied by a 10% increase in the metabolic demands of tissue (Fisher et al, 1978; Stewart, Palmieri, and Cochran, 1980). In tissue that already has limited oxygenation as a result of pressure, the potential for breakdown is exacerbated. Moisture, from perspiration or incontinence, also increases the risk of skin breakdown for a number of reasons. Wet skin is weaker than dry skin and therefore more likely to incur damage as a result of compression and friction (Stewart, Palmieri, and Cochran, 1980). Additionally, moisture increases the potential for bacterial growth and infection. Keeping the skin clean and dry is important for these reasons.

The material of the seat cushion, as well as its cover, can alter the temperature and the amount of moisture at the seat/buttock interface. Foam cushions have been found to cause an increase in skin temperature, whereas water-filled cushions reduced skin temperature (Stewart, Palmieri, and Cochran, 1980; Fisher et al, 1978). Excessive moisture can also be a problem and varies with the cushion, its cover, and the user. Gel and water cushions have been found to increase the amount of humidity at the seat/buttock interface by 23% and 20%, respectively (Stewart, Palmieri, and Cochran, 1980). Selecting cushion materials and coverings that reduce temperature and moisture accumulation is discussed later in this chapter.

**Transfers and handling techniques.** Abrasions or ulcerations can be caused by hitting objects or sliding across a surface during transfers. Whether the individual transfers independently or has someone providing assistance, care should be taken to prevent abrasions. The same holds true for mobility in bed. Pulling an individual across the bed sheets can cause abrasions or ulcerations from the friction. Caregivers should be reminded to lift an individual to move her in bed instead of sliding her across the bedding.

The development of pressure ulcers is a complex process, and there is still much to be learned about the exact mechanisms involved. Identifying factors that predispose an individual to pressure ulcers will help in developing a comprehensive pressure ulcer prevention program. A program for preventing pressure ulcers should include (1) a wheelchair and seating prescription for pressure distribution, postural alignment, and stability; (2) a pressure relief program; (3) dietary instruction and adequate nutrition; (4) instruction in proper transferring and lifting techniques; and (5) maintenance of good personal hygiene and skin care. The development and implementation of the prevention program should be considered an ongoing team effort involving the consumer, his or her therapists, and any medical personnel.

## Pressure Measurement

Because pressure is a primary factor in the development of pressure ulcers, we need to be able to measure it. When selecting a seat cushion for a given individual, we can determine the ability of potential cushions to distribute pressure by utilizing a pressure measurement system. This can be done by quantitatively measuring the individual's sitting pressures on various cushions. In measuring sitting pressure we can also determine if the individual has any evidence of asymmetry in sitting and what influence changing the seat-to-back angle or orientation in space may have. What we are measuring is the pressure at the interface between the cushion and the person's buttock. We actually would prefer to measure the pressure deep in the tissue, but this is not practical. This type of interface

pressure measurement is difficult and subject to error (Ferguson-Pell, 1989). The ideal sensor should be thin and small in diameter in order to disturb the measurement as little as possible.

There are four basic types of pressure measurements that can be made: (1) discrete sensor, single measurement; (2) multiple sensor, single measurement; (3) discrete sensor, continuous measurement; and (4) multiple sensor, continuous measurement (Ferguson-Pell, 1990). Discrete transducers measure pressure in only one spot, and measurements are taken as the transducer is moved to those areas of greatest pressure. When a discrete transducer is moved from point to point, the conditions may change from the first measurement to the last. This difference can cause misleading results, especially if a profile of pressures across the entire seating surface is desired. Multiple-sensor systems allow measurements simultaneously over the entire seating surface. This type of system has the advantage that the measurements at all points are taken at the same time and under the same sitting conditions.

Single-measurement systems provide a snapshot at one instant of the pressure at one point (discrete) or an array of points (multiple). Continuous-measurement systems provide information regarding the pressure changes that occur over a period of time, as well as the absolute pressures at specific points. As we have discussed, sitting is dynamic, and as a result, many changes in pressure distribution occur during movement of the wheelchair or during functional tasks. Another use for continuous pressure measurements is with seating surfaces that have an "accommodation period." For example, some foams take several minutes to conform to the person. By using a continuous-measurement system, we can measure pressure distribution as it changes and eventually stabilizes (Ferguson-Pell, 1989). For this reason, continuous-pressure measurement systems, although expensive, are desirable. Pfaff (1993) reviews the clinical application of continuous, or dynamic, pressure mapping systems.

The most common technology for measuring pressures at the sitting surface is the use of a bladder that is inflated (Zhou, 1991). These sensors have good repeatability, they conform to the shape of human soft tissue and the supporting medium, and they are inherently insensitive to shear forces and temperature changes. Because the bladder is inflated (causing tissue and cushion deformation) in order to make the measurement, the actual pressure at the interface is affected by the measurement process. Bladder transducers consist of a chamber (bladder) that is inflated and a switch that is activated when the bladder is empty. There is also a bulb (which is similar to those used with blood pressure measurement systems) to inflate the bladder, a pressure gauge, and an indicator to show when the bladder switch is opened. This latter signal indicates that the bladder is inflated enough to break the electrical contact. The pressure required to achieve this level of inflation is taken to be the external pressure exerted on the bladder. In multiple-sensor systems, the bladders are arranged in an array (e.g., 12 × 12) and each bladder has an electrical switch that can be monitored to determine applied pressures (Zhou, 1991). The bladders are connected in a pad, which is typically approximately 18 × 18 inches with individual bladders about 1¼ inches on a side. Zhou (1991) describes the procedures for pressure measurement using bladder-type devices.

Although bladder sensors have been most widely used, there are many other types of pressure and force transducers that can be employed (Olson, 1991). Some of these transducers measure force rather than pressure, and the area over which the measurement is made must be carefully determined to ensure an accurate pressure measurement. Recall that pressure is force divided by the area of application. Some types of pressure transducers are easily fabricated into thin polymer sheets, which do not occupy much space at the seat/buttock interface and lead to more accurate measurements. Ferguson-Pell (1989), Zhou (1991), and Olson (1991) describe the use of thin, pressure-sensitive mats that can be placed between the person and the sitting surface and that conform to the contours of both surfaces. Pressure changes can be detected by determining the electrical properties of materials. Properties most commonly used are electrical resistance (a measure of how well a material conducts electricity) or capacitance (a measure of how well a material can store electrical energy). For some materials, these parameters change when an external pressure is applied. For example, there are rubber materials whose electrical resistance changes when it is deformed (such as by the application of pressure). We can measure this change in resistance and relate it the amount of pressure applied. Semiconductor materials (like transistors) also conduct electrical current. For some semiconductors, the amount of electrical current that is conducted through the material changes when an external pressure or force is applied. This current can also be measured. Finally, strain gauges can be used. These gauges are small wire arrays. When they are deformed, the amount of electrical current through them is changed, and we can measure this change using an electronic device. Olson (1991) discusses the advantages and disadvantages of each of these pressure sensors.

Ferguson-Pell and Cardi (1992) carried out an evaluation of three computer-based pressure mapping systems. The first of these was the Force Sensing Array,* which utilizes a 15 × 15 array of force-sensing resistors. The Talley Pressure Monitor (TPM)† uses an array of bladder-type sensors. Two models were tested by Ferguson-Pell and Cardi: a 12-sensor

(TPM2) and a 96-sensor (TPM3) array. It takes about 1 second for each sensor to take a measurement, making this the slowest of the systems tested. The TPM3 can also be configured as a 48-cell array to place over a seat cushion. The final device tested was the Tekscan Seat,* which uses an array of 2056 force sensors that utilize conductive ink to measure pressure in a 48-inch × 43-inch area.

Using these systems, Ferguson-Pell and Cardi (1992) carried out "bench tests" to determine the properties of the sensors under controlled loads. They found that all the Tekscan and FSA sensors exhibited a change in pressure with constant load. This effect is called creep, and it can lead to different readings depending on the length of time the person has been sitting on the pressure transducer. Ferguson-Pell and Cardi also indicated that these two sensors are more sensitive to temperature-related variations in output than the TPM systems. Four cushions were used to evaluate the performance of each of the pressure mapping systems: (1) foam, (2) gel, (3) hybrid (Jay†), and (4) air filled (ROHO‡). A known load was applied to the sensor, and its output was measured. Then the sensor was placed on top of one of the four cushions and its pressure was measured again for the same load. For the foam and gel cushions, the FSA produced pressures 6 to 10 mm Hg higher with the cushion than without the cushion for the same known load. For the Jay and ROHO cushions, the readings were more than 10 mm Hg higher with the cushions. The Talley systems were generally less than 5 mm Hg different for all cushions; the Tekscan had less than 5 mm Hg of pressure using the foam and Jay cushions, 6 to 10 mm Hg for the gel, and more than 10 mm Hg for the ROHO. These results indicate that comparisons of pressure readings among different cushions for the same person may be subject to errors of as much as 10 mm Hg.

Finally, each system and cushion type was used with five evaluators who had spinal cord injuries. The pressure measurements for the same individuals sitting on the same cushion varied widely among the three mapping systems. In some cases there was agreement between sensors for the same evaluator and in others the same two sensors gave widely different results (more than 100 mm Hg) for the same evaluator. Despite these results, Ferguson-Pell and Cardi point out that multiple-sensor mapping systems, such as those tested, can play an important clinical role by providing relative information. For example, for a specific cushion the pressure distribution over different tissues and structures can be shown. It is also possible to display a pressure profile for a consumer and that can show how

---

*VistaMed, Winnipeg, Ont, Canada (www.vistamedical.org/).
†Talley, Inc., Romsey, England (www.talleymedical.co.uk).

---

*Tekscan, South Boston, Mass (www.tekscan.com/technology.html).
†Sunrise Medical, Carlsbad, Calif (www.sunrisemedicalonline.com/).
‡Crown Therapeutics, Belleville, Ill (www.crownthera.com/).

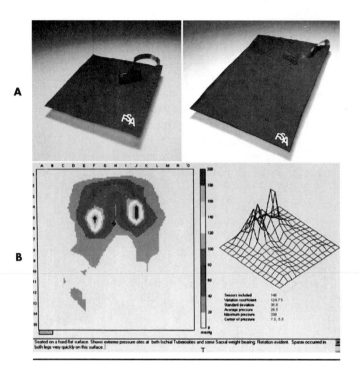

**Figure 6-25** Pressure measurement system. **A,** Map with an array of sensors. **B,** Sample display of an individual's pressure distribution profile. (Courtesy www.pressuremapping.com.)

push-ups relieve pressure if done correctly. However, absolute pressure values obtained with these systems are probably not reliable, and they must be applied with care.

Two commercial pressure-measuring systems are most commonly used clinically: The Vista Force Sensing Array* and the Crown Xsensor system.† These systems include both pressure sensing hardware and software. The hardware is a mat with an array of sensors (Figure 6-25, *A*), an electronic controller that sequentially accesses the sensor array to obtain a pressure measurement, and packaging that protects the sensor array from urine and other moisture. The software controls the measurement process, guides the clinician through the calibration and measurement, and displays a profile of the pressure distribution (Figure 6-25, *B*). Typically the profile is presented with colors depicting specific pressure. This makes it easy to identify specific areas of high pressure. The consumer being evaluated is asked to engage in movements (e.g., lean to one side, lean forward) and the pressure profile is repeated. This gives the ATP or ATS an indication of how much pressure relief will be provided under a variety of conditions. There are pros and cons to each of these systems, and often the choice comes down to the familiarity of the clinician with one type or the other and to the degree of product support provided by each supplier. Issues of durability, accuracy, and repeatability of

the measurement are most often applied to evaluation of the hardware component. Ease of use, the quality of the display, and storage of patient data (e.g., for comparison between visits) are important features of the software.

## ■ TECHNOLOGIES FOR PRESSURE MANAGEMENT

Because it is not possible to totally eliminate pressure when sitting on a support surface, it needs to be managed the best way possible so that the development of pressure ulcers is minimal. In response to the need to reduce the occurrence of pressure ulcers related to sitting in a wheelchair, an industry that designs and produces seat cushions for pressure relief and studies the effects of various types of cushions on pressure distribution has evolved. These seat cushions are typically placed on top of the sling upholstery seat of the person's wheelchair, so they can easily be removed and the wheelchair folded for transportation. Numerous studies have measured characteristics and properties of a variety of pressure-reducing devices. The majority of investigations have utilized tissue interface pressure as the basis for comparing these products. Some studies have also compared changes in transcutaneous oxygen tension and capillary blood flow. Although it has been shown that seating technologies play a significant role in pressure ulcer prevention by reducing the mechanical load on the tissue, there is no evidence that one type of pressure-reducing device works better than all others under all circumstances (Brienza et al, 2001; Conine et al, 1994; Garber, Krouskop, and Carter, 1978; DeLateur et al, 1976; Ferguson-Pell et al, 1986).

Seating technologies for pressure management can be categorized in two ways: according to the material properties of the cushion and according to the design of the cushion. Hobson (1990) categorizes the seating technologies for pressure management according to the materials used. He describes three approaches, fluid flotation, foams, and alternating pressure devices, and a fourth category, hybrid, which takes into consideration approaches that use two or more of these three types of materials. Seat cushions for pressure relief can also be categorized according to the type of design. There are two basic designs for pressure relief seat cushions: planar (flat) systems and contoured systems (Cooper, 1998).

The selection of a cushion is highly individualized and the choice of a cushion depends on the preferences and clinical needs of the consumer. The therapeutic benefit of a product should be the primary consideration when selecting a seating surface for a consumer. Other factors that should be considered when selecting a cushion include the characteristics of the context in which the cushion will be used and the characteristics of the cushion itself, such as performance,

*Vista Medical, Winnipeg, Ont, Canada (www.vistamedical.org/).
†Crown Therapeutics, Belleville, Ill (www.crownthera.com/).

Twenty years ago, at the age of 22, Alex was in a single-car accident and sustained a spinal cord injury. The lesion was at T1-T2, leaving him completely paralyzed below that level. After his initial hospitalization and adjustment to his disability, he returned to college and completed a Master's degree in vocational counseling. He has a successful private practice as a vocational counselor, which has kept him very busy. So busy in fact that he did not pay attention to his skin and ended up with a small pressure sore on his left ischial tuberosity. After weeks of medical treatment and hours spent in bed allowing the ulcer to heal, he is ready to get back to working full time again. His doctor has referred him to you for evaluation for a seating system that will manage his pressure. The physician's report states that Alex is also beginning to develop scoliosis.

Alex currently has a lightweight manual wheelchair with a sling back and a 2-inch foam cushion with a knit cover placed on top of the sling seat. He is independent with mobility, using his upper extremities. He transfers in and out of the wheelchair to all surfaces independently, including to and from his car. He is independent in all self-care activities. He is married, and his wife is responsible for all home management activities. He does admit that he has gotten into the habit of hooking his left arm behind the wheelchair push handle for stability during certain activities. He did not realize that this could be the cause of some of his problems.

QUESTIONS:

1. From the information you have so far, what might be the goals of seating for Alex?
2. Write a list of questions you would ask of Alex during your initial interview.
3. How would you proceed with a seating evaluation for Alex?
4. Based on the information you know about Alex at this time, what technological approaches would you consider for him and why? What types of positioning accessories would you consider and why?
5. List potential funding sources for Alex's seating system. How would you justify his system to the funding source (refer to Chapter 5)?

ease of use, requirements for maintenance, and cost. It is also important that the cushion does not interfere with aspects of the individual's mobility and personal autonomy (Panel for the Prediction and Prevention of Pressure Ulcers in Adults, 1992).

## Properties of Cushion Materials

An understanding of the properties of the materials used in pressure management technologies will assist in the selection of appropriate cushions. Sprigle (1992) identifies and describes five properties of cushion materials: (1) density, (2) stiffness, (3) resilience, (4) dampening, and (5) envelopment.

**Density** of a material is the ratio of its weight to its volume. A greater density generally means a more durable material but not always. Low-density materials will fatigue faster than high-density ones under the same loading conditions. **Stiffness** of a material describes how much it gives under load. In a cushion this is the distance that the person sinks into the cushion. Soft materials may bottom out, but failure to compress can also lead to an increase in seating pressures and tissue breakdown. **Resilience** is the ability of a material to recover its shape after a load is removed or to adjust to a load as it is applied. Short-term resilience is the immediate recovery when a load is altered, such as when someone shifts weight on a seat cushion. Long-term resilience is the overnight recovery of a cushion that has been loaded and then unloaded. **Dampening** is the ability of the cushion to soften on impact and is best observed by dropping a relatively heavy object on the material. If the object sinks into the material, then dampening is occurring. If it bounces off, or if the material does not react to the object, then the material is poorly dampened. This is the "shock absorber" feature of cushion materials. **Envelopment** is the degree to which the person sinks into the cushion and the degree to which the cushion surrounds the buttocks. Good envelopment promotes stability and helps reduce peak pressures.

## Flotation Cushions

Air, water, viscous fluid, and elastomer gels are the media that have been used in flotation cushions (Figure 6-26) (Hobson, 1990). The purpose for using these fluids in the cushion design is to allow for adjustment in the individual's body movement and to allow for changing pressures. By creating this flexible seating surface, the stability provided by the surface generally is reduced.

**Air filled.** Air-filled cushions consist of a sealed receptacle that holds air. The cushion may be configured to allow the air to circulate within the whole receptacle, or it may be divided into compartments to better control the airflow. Air-filled cushions distribute pressure from high-pressure areas, such as the ischial tuberosities, to areas where there is less pressure. These cushions have good long-term and short-term resilience. The pressure-relieving properties of this type of cushion are typically good; however, the ability of this cushion to envelop the user and thus its effectiveness are dependent on the amount of inflation. An air-filled cushion that is overinflated will not envelop the buttocks

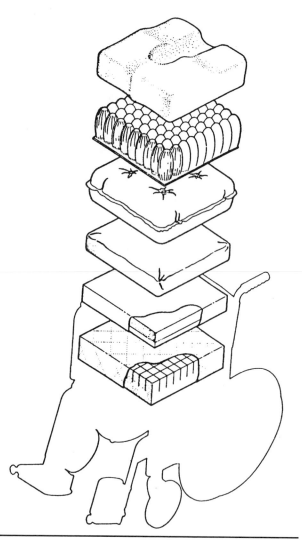

**Figure 6-26**    Types of cushions used for pressure management. *Top to bottom:* Standard contoured, air filled, water filled, elastomeric gel, planar viscoelastic foam (multidensity), planar polyfoam (serrated). (From Hobson DA: Seating and mobility for the severely disabled. In Smith RV, Leslie JH, editors: *Rehabilitation engineering*, Boca Raton, Fla, 1990, CRC Press.)

and will result in increased pressure at bony prominences and reduced sitting stability. Underinflation of the cushion can result in the air being pushed away from the high-pressure areas, allowing them to "bottom out" against the hard sitting surface of the seat. Persons who lack sensation may not be able to feel whether the cushion is underinflated.

Commonly used air-filled cushions are the ROHO* and Bye Bye Decubiti.† The original ROHO cushion consists of a number of 4-inch-high rubber-balloon cells that are interconnected at the base to allow for airflow among cells

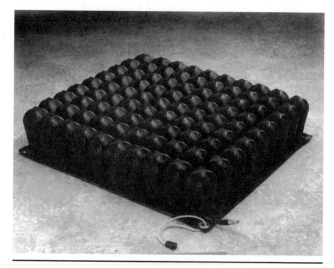

**Figure 6-27**    The ROHO High Profile air-filled cushion. (Courtesy Crown Therapeutics.)

(Figure 6-27). This type of cushion is also available in a low-profile model with shorter cells or with the option of restricting the airflow within individual compartments. The multiple compartments allow the air to be regulated in each compartment separate of the other compartments. Air-filled cushions are generally lightweight, and the materials they are made of do not deteriorate over time. The disadvantages of air-filled cushions are that they may be punctured or torn and that changes in air pressure may occur, reducing the cushion's effectiveness and requiring frequent monitoring.

**Elastomeric gels.**    Gel cushions consist of an elastomeric gel contained in a membrane. This membrane may affect the properties of the overall cushion. The gel functions much like air to equalize the pressure over the seating surface (Cooper, 1998). When discussing fluid-filled cushions, the concept of viscosity is important. Basically, viscosity in a fluid is analogous to friction on a surface. Viscosity represents the degree to which fluid molecules move across each other. A highly viscous fluid will not flow easily because the molecules don't easily slide across each other. A low-viscosity fluid or nonviscous fluid (such as water) will flow easily. Elastomeric gels are actually very high viscosity fluids, which have practically no flow (Hobson, 1990). High viscosity means that envelopment is poor and short-term and long-term resilience is poor. Gel cushions can also be affected by changes in external temperature. In cold weather some gels will freeze. However, these items have good dampening and thermal properties (they conduct heat away from the body) and provide a more stable base than an air cushion. An example of this type of cushion is the Royale Luxury Cushion.*

**Water filled.** Another type of flotation cushion is filled with water. Because of the low viscosity of these types of cushion, they have good envelopment and good short-term resilience. Dampening depends on the container and how much it is filled. These cushions have the advantage of cooling the body by conducting heat away. The structure of the water-filled container is usually rather flexible and, if placed on top of a sling seat by itself, does little to overcome the hammocking effects. In general, these cushions are heavy (averaging 15 pounds) and subject to puncture. Consequently, they are not commonly used. The AquaEase* is an example of a water-filled cushion.

**Viscous fluid filled.** Between the very high viscosity elastomeric gel and the very low viscosity, water-filled cushion are cushions filled with moderate-viscosity fluids. These moderate-viscosity cushions are sometimes called lightweight gels and have the properties of whipped cream (Cooper, 1998). This lighter weight gel has greater shock-absorbing properties than elastomeric gels. These fluids have some flow, and they provide good dampening. Resilience is poor, again because of the limited flow of the material. Envelopment can be good, depending on the membrane that encompasses the fluid. As with elastomeric gels and water, there is good conduction of heat away from the body. Often these cushions are placed in oversized, flexible membranes, which allow redistribution of the fluid during sitting (Hobson, 1990). If placed on a precontoured support surface, viscous fluid-filled cushions can also provide good support (see the section on hybrid cushions). These cushions have largely replaced water-filled types (Sprigle, 1992).

## Honeycomb

Honeycomb cushion material is made from an array of thermoplastic elastomers (TPEs) that combine the properties of rubber and plastics. The honeycomb is bonded using a fusion-bonding process instead of adhesives. The material consists of layers of interconnected open cells that flex when pressure is applied. The open cells allow air to flow through, which keeps the cushion cooler and prevents moisture. Reducing heat and moisture is important in preventing pressure ulcers. The combination of the upholstery and the honeycomb design also reduces sliding forward in the seat. The material used in this cushion is antifungal and antibacterial. A unique feature of this cushion material is that it can be cleaned in a washing machine. The manufacturer of this material produces a line of different cushions using this fusion-bonding technology.† The cushions are available in

either a planar design or a standard contour. At approximately 3 pounds, the cushions are fairly lightweight.

## Foam Cushions

Over the years, foams have been the material most commonly used in the fabrication of cushions. Polyurethane or latex foams come in a variety of thicknesses and densities, and are often characterized by their cell structures. There are two commonly used cell structures for foams: open cell and closed cell. Each type has certain advantages, and they are often combined in the same cushion to accomplish different functions. Open-cell foams have interconnected, perforated membranes that permit airflow between the cells and result in better ventilation (Tang, 1991). This type of foam is often less dense because of the air captured in the open cells. However, the size of the cells can be controlled, and this affects the density of the foam as well. Open-cell foams absorb fluids, which makes them difficult to clean. Closed-cell foams are composed of individual structures encased in a membrane. These foams are generally less compliant than open-cell foams, and airflow is restricted. Some foams have a combination of open-cell and closed-cell structures, and they are identified by the percentage of open-cell configuration (Tang, 1991).

Foam cushions are typically lightweight and inexpensive. Foams compress with the application of weight, which results in good envelopment. The amount of compression depends on the stiffness of the foam. Although soft foam will compress and allow the person to sink in more, a foam that is too soft might bottom out. Because foams have a tendency to trap heat near the body, their thermal features are considered to be poor. In general, the short-term and long-term resilience of foam is good, but again this varies depending on the structure and density of the foam. The two main disadvantages of using foam are that it (1) is prone to deterioration from light and moisture and (2) has a tendency to loose its resilience over time. Replacement of the foam depends on the type of foam and how much time the user spends sitting on the cushion. The life expectancy of a foam cushion is between 6 and 12 months (Hobson, 1990). It is recommended that foam cushions be checked periodically and replaced when warranted.

In addition to the polyurethane and latex foams, there are viscoelastic foams, which were originally developed by NASA for space travel. These foams,* because of their high viscosities, tend to resist deformation if pressed quickly, but they will accommodate slowly to a constant load. They also have memory, which delays their return to the original shape. This time-dependent property is the most distinguishing feature of this type of foam. Viscoelastic foam also

---

*Lumex, Bayshore, NY, 800-645-5272.
†The Stimulite Classic, Slimline, Contoured, and Pediatric Cushions from Supracor, Inc., (www.supracor.com).

---

*For example, Sunmate Foam and Pudgee from Dynamic Systems, Inc. (www.sunmatecushions.com/).

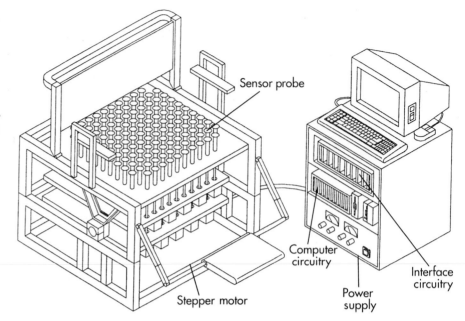

**Figure 6-28** Components of a CAD/CAM system that measures pressure and generates a contoured cushion to match. (From Kwiatkowski R, Inigo R: The design of a computer aided seating system, *Proc RESNA Int 92*, pp 216-217, 1992.)

has good thermal properties and good envelopment. The resilience and dampening properties are variable depending on the density and other properties (Sprigle, 1992).

One reason foam has achieved such popularity is because a cushion made from foam can be custom fabricated or instantly modified in the clinical setting to fit the user. Foam cushions can also be ordered ready to use from a manufacturer. Foams are used in the fabrication of three basic types of cushion designs, depending on the needs of the person.

**Planar.** Planar foam cushions, as shown in Figure 6-26, are designed from flat blocks of foam, which can be highly adaptable. These blocks can be fabricated using one layer of a selected thickness (up to 4 inches) and selected density of foam, or they can be fabricated using multiple densities and varying thicknesses of foam (Hobson, 1990). In the latter case, for example, a piece of a stiff foam that is 1 to 2 inches thick might be used on the bottom to provide a stable base and a 3/4- to 1-inch-thick piece of soft foam could be placed on top for pressure relief. Planar foams can also be adapted by cutting out (e.g., under the ischial tuberosities) or building up areas as necessary for pressure distribution or postural management. Zacharkow (1984, 1988) and Ferguson-Pell (1990) describe the fabrication of these cushions.

**Standard contoured.** The intention of standard-contoured cushions (see Figure 6-26) is to provide a generic contoured cushion that will distribute pressure across the seating surface and will fit people within a certain size range. The cushions are manufactured using standard molds that are injected with a polyurethane foam (Hobson, 1990). This type of cushion works well for individuals who are at low risk for pressure ulcer development. This approach is also generally less costly than a custom-contoured cushion. The Combi Cushion* is one example of a standard contoured cushion.

**Custom contoured.** In some instances it is necessary to custom contour the seat cushion to the shape of the individual. Custom-contoured cushions can be achieved using vacuum forming or seating contour measurement systems.

One approach, known as foam-in-place, uses a container with three solid sides and a thick rubber membrane on the fourth side. The foam-in-place process was discussed in an earlier section. The main advantages of this approach are that the foam is of uniform density and there are fewer shear stresses within the material than there are in planar types (Hobson, 1990).

CAD and CAM are technologies that are used in the fabrication of custom-contoured cushions. One product, the Silhouette,† uses a surface that mechanically senses the contour of the person in the seated position. This contour is then recorded on a form that is sent to a central fabrication facility for manufacturing using a CAM technique. There is also software available that allows the ATP to view and modify the three-dimensional shape of the cushion on the computer. Other approaches, most of which are experimental, use an array of pressure transducers, which determine the contour to be manufactured by the CAD system (Sposato et al, 1990). A typical system, shown in Figure 6-28, consists of an array of 128 pressure probes; stepper

*Sunrise Medical, Carlsbad, Calif (www.sunrisemedicalonline.com/).
†Invacare Corp., Elyria, Ohio (www.invacare.com).

motors, which provide loading of the probes; interface circuitry; and a computer (Kwiatkowski and Inigo, 1992). When a person sits on the sensor array, the probes are displaced vertically according to the local pressure generated. By adjusting the resistive force of each sensor through the stepper motors, it is possible to simulate the resistive force of a "desired" cushion, and the final displacement profile of the sensor array is used to fabricate the contour of the seat cushion. This CAD/CAM approach offers the potential of closely matching the cushion contour to reduce areas of high pressure.

## Alternating Pressure Cushions

Research (Kosiak, 1959; Reswick and Rogers, 1976) has documented a relationship between amount of pressure applied and its duration and the development of pressure ulcers. In a study described earlier, it was found that the alternating pressure cushion was the only seating surface to intermittently bring pressures within the range of capillary blood pressure (Kosiak et al, 1958). All the cushions described thus far are static cushions, which have been designed on the premise that (1) they redistribute pressure over the sitting surface, and (2) the individuals using them also need to follow through with pressure relief activities. Alternating pressure devices are designed on the basis that weight-bearing surfaces can tolerate high pressures for a time if alternated with increments of no pressure.

The principle of intermittent pressure relief is implemented in commercially available cushions by using an oscillating pump to alternately inflate bellows arranged in rows (Hobson, 1990). Each individual elastomeric bellow (typical cushions have arrays of 48 arranged in 8 rows of 6) can be inflated individually or in groups. Generally rows are inflated together. One approach* couples every third row of the array of bellows. During operation, two of the couples rows are inflated and one is deflated, which relieves pressure over one third of the seating surface; then the next third of the array is deflated, and so on. An alternative approach automatically cycles only the back four rows (out of 8 total) under the ischial tuberosities. Each row is sequentially inflated and deflated to provide intermittent pressure relief to local tissue. These cushion systems use a recycling air pump powered by a battery to inflate the bellows. If the pressure pump should fail to operate in these systems (e.g., the battery becomes discharged), the cushion can still be used as an air-filled cushion. Because of the added weight, the need for recharging of the battery, and the cost, these seating devices have not been as widely distributed as other cushion types.

## Hybrid Cushions

Hybrid cushions consist of a combination of the materials described above. The most typical combination is a closed-cell foam base with a membrane that contains gel, viscous fluid, or air that is placed on top or inserted in a cutout. This method provides a combination of good envelopment, good thermal properties, and pressure relief (because of the flotation materials), as well as good support and dynamic properties, which are provided by the foam base (Sprigle, 1992). The series of Jay cushions* are commonly used hybrid cushions that consist of a combination of a standard-contoured, high-density foam base with a gel-filled pad that sits atop the foam base. The pad can be purchased in different configurations, such as an overfilled pad or pads with the gel sectioned off into quadrants, which prevents the pooling of gel into certain areas. The Varilite Solo Cushion† is an example of a hybrid cushion that has a foam and air-holding membrane that sits on top of a standard-contoured foam base. The overall properties of these types of cushions depend on the type of container, as well as the properties of the foam base.

## Cushion Covers

The application of a cover over a cushion needs to be carefully considered. All the pressure distribution, moisture, and heat properties of the cushion could be altered with the cover. A cover that is not the right size or shape for the cushion can cause problems. For example, a cushion covering that is pulled tightly across the surface of the cushion will not allow the individual to sink down into the cushion and can thereby reduce the enveloping properties of the cushion material. A cover that is too large will wrinkle on the surface and can result in increased shear. A stretchy cover that contours to the surface of the cushion is recommended.

The cushion cover should also permit air exchange, limit moisture accumulation, and be easy to clean. Cushion coverings with nonporous covers, such as vinyl or plastic, do not absorb moisture and allow moisture to build up at the seating surface. Recommended fabrics include Lycra, cotton, and certain polyknits (Sprigle, 1992).

## Seating for Pressure Distribution and Postural Support

Individuals who are at risk for development of pressure ulcers can benefit from proper positioning in the wheelchair as well. In fact, it is recommended that positioning be addressed first, since postural alignment often results in changes in pressure distribution (Minkel, 1990). Through

---

*For example, the Pegasus Altern8 Therapeutic Seating System, model 3600 (www.pegasus-airwave.com/us/index.html) or the Microsolo 900T (www.biologics900t.com/biologic.htm).

---

*Sunrise Medical, Carlsbad, Calif (www.sunrisemedicalonline.com/).
†Varilite, Seattle, Wash (www.varilite.com/).

postural alignment, pressure can be distributed more evenly; postural deformities, such as pelvic obliquity, scoliosis, and kyphosis, can be prevented; back pain can be alleviated; and stability can be increased. In turn, this will influence the individual's mobility, energy expenditure, and function.

Many of the principles we have described regarding sitting posture and postural control apply to this population as well. Some of the technologies used with the cerebral palsy population for postural control have transferred to the population with spinal cord injuries, and new technologies that specifically address the needs of this population have been developed as well. We describe some basic strategies for positioning for postural management for this population.

A cushion that is by itself and is placed in the seat will not totally eliminate the hammocking effect, and eventually the sling seat stretches further and the cushion conforms more to the sling. Simply installing a solid seat can minimize the hammocking affect of the sling upholstery. Solid seats can be made from a ³/₈-inch sheet of plywood or plastic seats can be purchased from many cushion manufacturers. Any of the cushions described earlier can then be placed on the solid seat. Inclining the seat 10 degrees prevents the buttocks from sliding forward, reduces shear, maintains the pelvic position, distributes pressure more evenly, and prevents a kyphotic posture of the spine (Zacharkow, 1984). The seat incline can be achieved with a tapered foam wedge seat cushion, by raising the front casters, adjusting the rear axles (available on certain wheelchairs), or using a power tilt mechanism (Latter and Dehoux, 1991). A lap belt is also recommended for maintaining the neutral pelvic position.

The hammock back of the wheelchair does not provide lumbar support and promotes a sacral sitting position with kyphosis of the spine. The hammock back can be replaced with a solid, contoured back that is commercially available (e.g., Varilite Evolution Back* or J2 Back†) or custom made of foam (see Zacharkow, 1988, for description). The seat back should be assessed for appropriate height and seat-to-back angle. It is recommended that the back be reclined approximately 15 degrees to help stabilize the trunk and prevent forward loss of balance. The back height is determined by the amount of support needed by the individual. An appropriate back height for individuals with function at C6 level or better is typically half an inch to 1 inch below the scapulae (Zacharkow, 1984). Many paraplegics have adequate trunk strength and wish to preserve mobility (particularly for sports), so they prefer lower backs on their wheelchairs and prefer not to use trunk-positioning components. Quadriplegics (C4 and C5) with less trunk control can benefit from a higher seat back that supports all or part of the scapulae, and those with C1 to C3 spared will require headrests (Zacharkow, 1984). For quadriplegics, contoured

*Varilite, Seattle, Wash (www.varilite.com).
†Sunrise Medical, Carlsbad, Calif (www.sunrisemedicalonline.com).

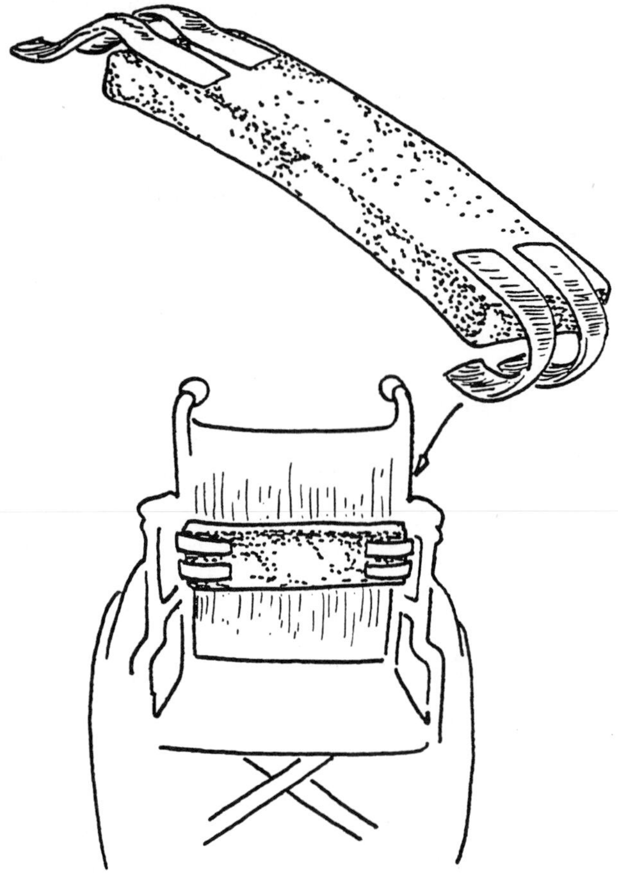

Figure 6-29  A lumbar pad made of firm polyurethane foam attached to a wheelchair. Typical dimensions are 4 to 6 inches high, 2 to 3 inches wide, and 1¹/₂ to 2¹/₂ inches thick. (From Zacharkow D: *Wheelchair posture and pressure sores,* Springfield, Ill, 1984, Charles C Thomas.)

back support and reclining of the back to 20 degrees is recommended. If a side-to-side trunk position is difficult for the individual to maintain or if scoliosis is present, the application of lateral trunk supports, as discussed in an earlier section, is necessary to prevent further deformity.

A lumbar pad on the back is also recommended. Shields and Cook (1988) found a decrease in six areas of high pressure, including the ischial tuberosities, with the use of a lumbar support. If the person has lumbar mobility, a lumbar pad (as illustrated in Figure 6-29) can be placed on the seat back. It is recommended that the lumbar pad be placed slightly below the posterior iliac crests. Placing the lumbar pad lower than this will push the pelvis forward; placing it higher than this will mean that the lower lumbar spine is supported. Placing a solid backing on the lumbar pad or using it with a solid seat back will make it more effective. Otherwise the lumbar pad will tend to sag with the sling back and diminish its effectiveness. With a combination of the recommended seat and back angles and the lumbar pad, it is possible to closely duplicate the lordotic upright sitting posture that was described in an earlier section (Zacharkow, 1984).

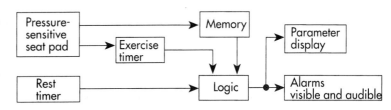

Figure 6-30    Block diagram of major components used in pressure relief monitors. (From Bellahsene BE, Cook AM: Aids for the tactilely impaired. In Webster JG et al, editors: *Electronic devices for rehabilitation*, New York, 1985, John Wiley & Sons.)

A cushion added to a wheelchair seat is going to increase the seat height, and often armrests are inadvertently left in the same position without accounting for this increased height. Adjustable armrests on the wheelchair allow the height to be changed, so the individual can use them for weight bearing. Weight bearing on the armrest can remove some of the pressure from the seating surface. Gilsdorf, Patterson, and Fisher (1991) found that paraplegic subjects applied an average of 8% to 9% of their body weight to the armrests and quadriplegic subjects applied approximately 5%. Armrests that are too low either are not used for weight bearing or, if they are, the individual has to lean to reach one side, which then promotes an asymmetrical posture. Armrests that are too high place the scapulae in elevation and may cause shoulder and neck problems. Appropriately placed armrests also aid the individual during pressure relief activities.

The height of the footrest affects postural stability and the amount of pressure exerted on the seat surface. Footrests adjusted so that the thighs are horizontal are in the optimal position (Ferguson-Pell, 1990). Footrests that are too low increase pressures under the thigh and encourage sacral sitting. Footrests that are too high cause an undue amount of pressure to be placed on the ischial tuberosities.

## Pressure Relief Activities

Even with an appropriate cushion and positioning to distribute pressure, it is still required that the individual carry out pressure relief activities. For individuals who lack the ability to perform automatic posture adjustments, activities to relieve pressure on weight-bearing surfaces should be a part of their prevention program. For individuals who are bedridden, it is recommended that care staff follow a regular schedule of turning the person every 2 hours and repositioning them in bed (Norton, McLaren, and Exton-Smith, 1981; Torrance, 1983). Individuals who sit in a wheelchair for any length of time also need to perform pressure relief activities at regular intervals throughout the day. It is recommended that pressure relief be performed every 10 to 20 minutes for a duration of at least 3 seconds (Torrance, 1983; Merbitz et al, 1985).

There are a number of ways in which pressure relief can be accomplished. A person who has adequate strength in the upper body can place both arms on the armrests and push the whole body up off the seating surface; lean forward in the wheelchair with forearms resting on the thighs; or alternately rock to one side (using the armrest for support) to relieve the weight on the opposing buttock. It is advocated that the forward leaning method be used because this is less conspicuous than the other methods, less fatiguing, more stable, and reported to be more effective in relieving pressure (Zacharkow, 1988).

For individuals who lack the strength and trunk stability to perform pressure relief, a reclining or a tilt-in-space wheelchair is used. In a reclining wheelchair the back goes down, placing the person in a supine or nearly supine position. This relieves the pressure from under the buttocks and redistributes it to the trunk area. However, the action of reclining the back and then returning it to an upright position can produce detrimental shearing forces on the buttocks. Zero-shear reclining wheelchairs, which reduce this shearing mechanism, have been designed. With a tilt-in-space wheelchair, the total seating surface is tilted backward while maintaining the back-to-seat angle. Again this acts to redistribute the pressure away from the buttocks to the trunk. These wheelchairs and their special features can be either manually or power controlled. These features are described in greater detail in Chapter 10.

Several methods for monitoring the frequency and the duration of pressure relief activities have been developed. Akbarzadeh (1991) cites four purposes for taking these measurements: (1) determining the relationship between pressure relief behavior and pressure ulcers, (2) training individuals to develop pressure relief habits, (3) assessing the effectiveness of training programs, and (4) identifying those individuals who are at risk for developing pressure ulcers. He also describes several studies related to these purposes and the different techniques used for monitoring pressure relief behavior.

Pressure relief monitoring devices are used during rehabilitation to train individuals with newly acquired spinal cord injury to develop the habit of carrying out pressure relief activities. These devices are also used with individuals who need assistance to remember to perform pressure relief. Based on Bellahsene and Cook (1985), a general approach used in pressure monitoring devices is shown in Figure 6-30. A sensor used to detect pressure is placed on the seating surface or on the armrests of the wheelchair. The sensor is triggered when the person is in the chair, and this trigger starts a timer. When the person performs an adequate pressure relief, the timer is reset. If the pressure relief is not completed for the designated frequency or duration, a visual, tactile, or auditory alarm is activated.

The use of alarms can have adverse effects on the person's behavior. Visual displays and buzzers can cause embarrassment and are noticeable when placed on the wheelchair. Klein and Fowler (1981) observed problems with carryover in pressure relief behavior when the person went home and stopped using the alarm. They also found that in many cases the alarm was viewed as punishment and was disabled when nursing staff was not around. Some of the suggestions made by Akbarzadeh (1991) are that the ideal monitoring device should be inconspicuous, it should not be used as punishment, it should not disrupt daily life activities, it should be cost effective and easily adjustable for use with different persons, it should be convenient to connect and disconnect, it should be durable, and it should not require frequent maintenance.

## ■ PRINCIPLES AND TECHNOLOGIES OF SEATING FOR COMFORT

In this section we consider the need for comfort in seating and technologies that address that need. There are three distinct populations that can benefit from seating technologies for comfort: (1) wheelchair users who have sitting discomfort and pain (e.g., individuals with postpolio syndrome [PPS], amyotrophic lateral sclerosis [ALS], and multiple sclerosis [MS]); (2) the elderly; and (3) individuals suffering from low-back pain, which can keep them from effectively performing their jobs. For individuals in any one of these populations, discomfort in seating can lead to a decreased ability to participate in activities of daily living. In cases of severe discomfort, the individual may find it necessary to be restricted to bed for some or all of the day. This further reduces the individual's ability to function and can lead to medical problems as well. There are unique technologies for each of these populations, but the commonality is that they enhance comfort in the seated position.

In comparison to the other two categories of need we have discussed, the technologies available to meet the comfort seating needs of individuals falls far short. There are a number of reasons for this. One is that equipment that is deemed necessary for comfort typically is not paid for by third-party funding sources because it is not considered a medical necessity. Another reason is that there is very little agreement among researchers on how to define and assess comfort and discomfort (Hobson and Crane, 2001). Although much research has been done to assess comfort, it is a difficult variable to objectively measure because it can be highly subjective and involve multiple factors. A cushion that is described as comfortable by one individual may feel uncomfortable to another. Researchers have also been unsuccessful in tying discomfort to quantitative measures such as posture, muscle fatigue as indicated by electromyogram

(EMG) measurements, or seat interface pressure (Hobson and Crane, 2001). The lack of outcomes relating to the effectiveness of seating products said to promote comfort make it necessary for clinicians to use a trial-and-error approach to recommending equipment for the consumer. This can be costly and is often not funded by third-party sources. In turn, without funding at the clinical level for such products, there is no financial incentive for manufacturers to address this unmet need. It is necessary that those involved in this industry determine the best way to assess the many factors of discomfort and comfort. Only then can the efficacy of the current technologies for this population be carefully evaluated and new technologies be developed.

## Technologies to Enhance Sitting Comfort for Wheelchair Users

In a study that assessed the satisfaction of wheelchair users, comfort was rated as the most important variable for a wheelchair seating aid (Weiss-Lambrou et al, 1999). At the same time, comfort was rated as the least satisfying variable among these wheelchair users. The reasons stated for dissatisfaction related to comfort included seat cushions that caused pain and discomfort; fatigue; uncomfortable headrests and thoracic supports; sliding in wheelchair seat caused by discomfort; and poor posture as a result of unsuitable installation. Comfort is also related to the contact surface between the seating system and the person. For example, materials that provide good air exchange and maintain an even temperature and control moisture are more likely to provide a comfortable sitting climate.

The needs of this population are currently not being met. Wheelchair users who experience discomfort and chronic pain need seating systems that allow persons to relieve the discomfort and participate fully in activities of daily living. Technologies such as tilt or recline systems were developed to manage pressure or control posture, not to relieve discomfort (Hobson and Crane, 2001). Utilizing systems such as these to relieve discomfort often limits the individual's function (Hobson and Crane, 2001).

The Rehabilitation Engineering Research Center (RERC) on Wheeled Mobility at the University of Pittsburgh is addressing the issue of seating discomfort through *Research Task-2: Investigation of Dynamic Seating for Comfort*. The focus of this research task is dynamic sitting to relieve discomfort in wheelchair users who are unable to independently attain normal relief from chronic sitting discomfort or pain (RERC on Wheeled Mobility, 2001). The results of this task will identify the characteristics of a dynamic seating device that best meet the needs of this population. The ultimate goal is the development of a prototype for a dynamic seating device. This device would be used by individuals to self-adjust the characteristics of the seating support surface (e.g., shape and resiliency) in order to attain acceptable levels of relief from discomfort and increase the amount of time the user can participate in daily activities.

## Technologies That Increase Ease of Sitting for the Elderly

People are living longer, which means that the number of well elderly, and those in need of supervised care, is growing considerably. As an individual ages, mobility may be reduced as a result of acute illnesses or trauma, such as stroke, hip fracture, or progressive conditions such as arthritis. Consequently, it is likely that the amount of time the individual spends sitting increases. The goal of seating in this category depends on the individual's needs and skills, as it does for the other categories. Just as there is a range of needs for the elderly population, there is also a range of seating technologies. Seating technologies for the aging population can be matched to the level of functional mobility the individual has: (1) ambulatory (2) mobile, nonambulatory, and (3) dependent mobile (Fernie and Letts, 1991). Chairs are needed that promote comfort, safety, ease of ingress and egress, and propulsion if necessary. Table 6-1 shows each of these types of users, the related technologies, and the desired outcomes to be achieved.

**Static lounge chairs.** The typical user of a static lounge chair ambulates independently or with the use of a cane or crutches. The major concern for seating for those who are mobile is getting in and out of different chairs safely and easily. A second concern is that the seat provides a safe, comfortable surface on which to sit (Fernie and Letts, 1991). Figure 6-31 shows three examples of static lounge chairs. The height, depth, and angle of the seat, the type of armrests, and the backrest on the chair can make a big difference. A seat height that is too low to the ground will make egress from the chair difficult. Similarly, on many chairs the depth of the seat is too long, which makes it hard

**TABLE 6-1**    **Types of Chairs and Users**

| Type of User | Type of Chair | Features To Be Achieved |
|---|---|---|
| Ambulatory | Static lounge chair | Ease of ingress/egress, comfort, healthy posture |
| Mobile, nonambulatory | Self-propelled chair | Ease of propulsion, comfort, and safe transfer |
| Dependent mobile | Mobile reclining lounge chair | Comfort and support, ease of transfer |

Fernie G, Letts RM: Seating the elderly. In Letts RM, editor: *Principles of seating the disabled,* Boca Raton, Fla, 1991, CRC Press.

for the individual to come to a standing position. An incline on the front of the seat helps to prevent sliding forward, but it should not be so much that the person has difficulty standing up. There are lifting seats (Figure 6-31, *C*) that can be purchased and integrated into a regular chair or used as a component that is placed on top of an existing chair. These lifting seats can assist the individual in standing up from the seating surface and are either mechanically or electronically operated.

It is preferable to have a high back on chairs for this population, typically one that comes to the height of the shoulders. A contoured back with a slight amount of lateral support is helpful. Lumbar support, which is typically a need for the younger population, should be decreased or eliminated. With the aging population, the spine is not as mobile and excessive padding in the lumbar area may only be uncomfortable and force the person forward in the chair. Armrests assist the individual in coming forward in the seat in preparation for standing and for actually standing. These armrests should be at a height that provides the user with the best mechanical advantage for these tasks, not too high and not too low.

**Self-propelled wheelchairs.** This category represents those individuals who are primarily nonambulatory but are able to independently propel a wheelchair. Desirable features for a wheelchair for this population include ease in propelling and folding, comfort, and ability to transfer safely to and from the sitting surface. It is estimated that there are 600,000 wheelchair users older than 65 residing in skilled nursing facilities in the United States (Shaw and Taylor, 1991). In one city alone, it was found that more than 80% of elderly residents in skilled nursing facilities experienced at least one problem with sitting in their wheelchairs related to discomfort, hampered mobility, or poor posture (Shaw and Taylor, 1991). Furthermore, it was found that in most cases these problems could be resolved using existing technologies tailored to each individual's needs. It was concluded that appropriate service delivery mechanisms are needed for educating care providers, matching the technology, and locating funding.

Typically, conventional wheelchairs with sling upholstery are provided for this population, and all the common problems we discussed as resulting from this lack of proper seating occur (see Figure 6-7). Pressure distribution, postural control, and deformity management are all important considerations in seating for elderly persons who use a wheelchair. The principles and technologies described in this chapter can be applied to this population as well. Providing the individual with a firm, planar padded seat or a moderately contoured cushion will improve the person's sitting posture, distribute pressure, and be much more comfortable. Existing technologies have been demonstrated to be appropriate for this population, but a coordinated effort of service

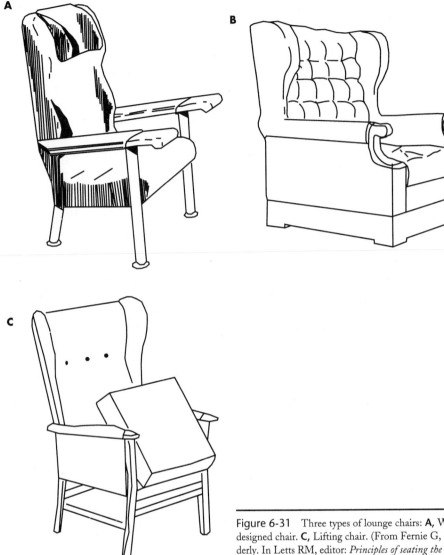

Figure 6-31    Three types of lounge chairs: **A,** Well-designed chair. **B,** Poorly designed chair. **C,** Lifting chair. (From Fernie G, Letts RM: Seating the elderly. In Letts RM, editor: *Principles of seating the disabled,* Boca Raton, Fla, 1991, CRC Press.)

delivery is required (Shaw and Taylor, 1991). Education seems to be a primary factor, and it is important that care providers understand the need for better support and posture with this population. Care provider training should also include instruction in checking the shape of cushions on a regular basis to determine if the cushion has bottomed out (Ham, Aldersea, and Porter, 1998).

**Attendant-propelled wheelchairs.** The third category applies to users who are unable to or have no need to independently propel a wheelchair. These chairs are frequently used in skilled nursing facilities when the goal is to be able to have the individual safely sitting in an upright position in something other than the bed. These chairs are commonly referred to as *Geri* or *stroke chairs* (see Chapter 10, Figure 10-13). These chairs look like conventional easy chairs but have small caster wheels so an attendant can move

them. Unfortunately, because they are designed to fit a wide range of people, for some individuals they fit poorly and are uncomfortable. Newer designs allow for smaller individuals and for postural accommodation (Hobson, 1990).

## Seating Individuals in the Workplace

It is estimated that approximately 45% of American workers work in offices, and sitting is the work position most commonly assumed (Reinecke, 1990). Many individuals experience adverse effects, primarily low-back pain, as a result of the seated position. Those who sit in a static posture most of the day are more prone to back problems than those whose jobs allow changes in position. The area of ergonomic seating has emerged as an area of specialization and has grown rapidly. When selecting a seating surface for an individual in the workplace, the worker's gender, age,

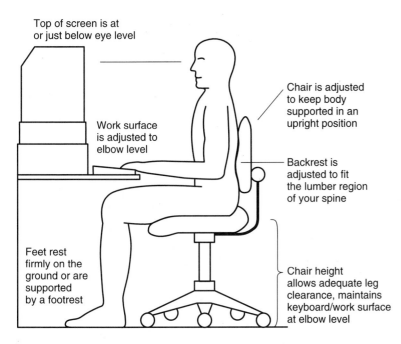

Top of screen is at or just below eye level

Work surface is adjusted to elbow level

Chair is adjusted to keep body supported in an upright position

Backrest is adjusted to fit the lumber region of your spine

Feet rest firmly on the ground or are supported by a footrest

Chair height allows adequate leg clearance, maintains keyboard/work surface at elbow level

**Figure 6-32**   Ergonomic sitting posture. (Courtesy Hewlett-Packard Co., 1994.)

physical attributes, and type of activities to be performed need to be taken into consideration. There are many technologies available, and selecting an appropriate chair should be taken seriously. The consumer should spend more than a few minutes trying out various chairs. A tool such as the Ergonomics Seating Evaluation Form (found at http://ergo.human.cornell.edu/ahSEATING.html) can be helpful in systematically gathering information and assessing the effectiveness and quality of different chairs for a specific consumer.

Many of the principles discussed in the biomechanics section relate to this seated posture and can be applied when selecting and adjusting an office chair. Figure 6-32 shows principles of good ergonomic positioning while sitting at a computer. Regardless of the type of work being performed, the chair should be comfortable, provide good seat and back support, and allow the user to change positions throughout the day. Figure 6-33 shows an office chair in which the controls are within the user's reach and allow easy adjustment of the angle of the seat and back and the height of the chair and armrests.

When addressing seating for the office worker, the "ABCs" (Armrests, Backrest, Chair Height, and Seat) of sitting in a chair, as shown in Box 6-4, will help with achievement of the appropriate seated position. When applying these principles, remember that all the parts of the body work together and modifying one area may affect another. For example, decreasing the seat height so that the worker may rest his feet on the floor may result in the worker's straining his neck to view the monitor unless the height of the monitor is adjusted as well. No matter how ergonomically sound the design and position of the office seat is, the individual still needs to take breaks periodically,

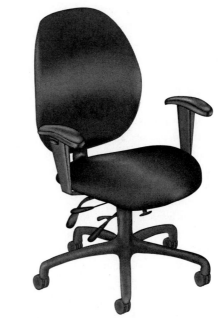

**Figure 6-33**   Office chair with controls to adjust the armrests, seat and back angle, and chair height. Seat pan with a rounded, "waterfall" edge.ergonomic_22.htm.)

change position often, get up and move around, and carry out some simple exercises.

## ■ SUMMARY

This chapter has shown the potential outcomes that can be achieved through seating in three primary areas of need: postural control and deformity management, pressure

---

**BOX 6-4**   **The ABCs of Seating for Office Workers**

**ARMRESTS**
- The chair should have armrests that allow for adjustment.
- The armrests should support both forearms while the worker performs tasks and should not hinder movement.
- The armrests should be adjusted correctly for height so that the user's shoulders are relaxed when resting on the armrests and not hunched or elevated.

**BACKREST**
- The height of the backrest should be sufficient to provide support to the worker's torso.
- The chair back should be at an angle between 100 to 110 degrees so that the individual's torso is supported.
- The backrest of the chair should have good lumbar support in the appropriate area for the worker's shape and size of back. If there is an adjustable support, use this to get the best position. If not, use a rolled towel or a cushion to improve lower back support (Hedge, 2001).

**CHAIR HEIGHT**
- The height of the chair should be adjusted correctly so that the individual's knees are slightly higher than the seat of the chair and the feet are flat on the ground or on a solid surface such as a footrest. This prevents pressure under the thighs and behind the knees and allows adequate circulation to the legs and feet.
- The chair height should also allow adequate clearance under the desk so that the legs and feet fit comfortably under the desk.

**SEAT**
- The seat pan needs to be the right size for the particular individual, not too small and not too large.
- The front of the seat pan should have a rounded "waterfall" edge to it so that it doesn't press behind the user's knees.
- A seat pan with angle adjustment is also desirable. This allows the worker to adjust the tilt of the seat as needed to maintain proper support in different positions.

---

management, and comfort. Procedures for evaluation and matching of device characteristics to the individual's needs were presented. Basic principles of biomechanics frequently used in seating and positioning were discussed. Principles and technologies related to each area of need were also presented.

## Study Questions

1. What are potential outcomes of seating and positioning?
2. Based on the needs of consumers, what are the three areas of seating that can be addressed by assistive technologies?
3. What are the three types of force, and why are they relevant to seating and positioning?
4. What is the difference between force and pressure?
5. Distinguish among tension, compression, and shear.
6. What is meant by the *center of gravity,* and how does it relate to seating and positioning systems?
7. Describe the typical population served by seating for postural control and the basic premises underlying the provision of these technologies.
8. What are possible asymmetrical postures acquired in the pelvis?
9. Describe the major approaches used to obtain alignment and control of the pelvis.
10. Describe the three spinal deformities that may occur.
11. List three methods used to support the trunk in postural control seating systems, and describe when each method is indicated.
12. What does *three-point positioning* mean and how is it applied to spinal deformities?
13. Describe how the head can be positioned posteriorly, anteriorly, and laterally. What factors lead to the use of each of these?
14. What are the major technical approaches used for seating for postural control?
15. Describe the primary methods of fabricating a custom-contoured seating system.
16. What is the major cause of pressure ulcer development? What are other factors that contribute to the development of pressure ulcers?
17. What are the major technical approaches used for seating for pressure relief? List one advantage and one disadvantage for each approach.
18. What is a honeycomb cushion? What advantages does it have over other approaches?
19. How do gel and foam cushions differ? List an advantage and disadvantage of each.
20. What are the four techniques used to measure sitting pressures? What are the limitations of pressure measurement?
21. What are the two primary systems used for interface pressure measurement in seating systems? Which of the four techniques do they use?
22. In addition to supplying a cushion to distribute pressure, what else should be involved in a pressure management program?
23. What are the primary populations for whom comfort is the major goal in developing a seating system?
24. Identify the reasons why there are limited technolo-

gies available for populations for whom comfort is the major goal.

25. Identify seating needs particular for the aging population and the three types of technology that address these needs.

26. What are the major factors involved in selecting a chair for maximal comfort and support in the workplace?

## References

Adrian MJ, Cooper JM: *Biomechanics of human movement,* Indianapolis, 1989, Benchmark Press.

Akbarzadeh MR: Behavior for relieving pressure. In Webster JG, editor: *Prevention of pressure sores,* Bristol, England, 1991, IOP Publishing.

Bellahsene BE, Cook AM: Aids for the tactilely impaired. In Webster JG et al, editors: *Electronic devices for rehabilitation,* New York, 1985, John Wiley & Sons.

Bennett L et al: Shear vs pressure as causative factors in skin blood flow occlusion, *Arch Phys Med Rehabil* 60:309-314, 1979.

Berecek KH: Etiology of decubitus ulcers. In Horsley JA, editor: *Preventing decubitus ulcers,* New York, 1981, Grune & Stratton.

Bergen AF, Presperin J, Tallman T: *Positioning for function: wheelchairs and other assistive technologies,* Valhalla, NY, 1990, Valhalla Rehabilitation Publications.

Bergen AF, Presperin J, Tallman T: Evaluation criteria, *Team Rehabil Rep* 2(4):34-35, 1991.

Bergen AF, Presperin J, Tallman T: Planning intervention, *Team Rehabil Rep* 3(2):38-41, 1992.

Bergstrom N, Demuth PJ, Braden BJ: A clinical trial of the Braden Scale for Predicting Pressure Sore Risk, *Nurs Clin North Am* 22(2):417-428, 1987.

Bergstrom N et al: The Braden Scale for Predicting Pressure Sore Risk, *Nurs Res* 36(4):205-210, 1987.

Breslow R: Nutritional status and dietary intake of patients with pressure ulcers: review of the research literature 1943 to 1989, *Decubitus* 4:16-21, 1991.

Brienza D et al: A preliminary report regarding the clinical evaluation of pressure-reducing seat cushions for elderly patients: www.rst.pitt.edu/Res/SSBL/ResearchProjects/pressred(prelim).html, June 20, 2001.

Brown BE: *The influence of postural adjustment of physically handicapped children on teachers' perceptions,* thesis, Madison, 1981, University of Wisconsin.

Cailliet R: *Scoliosis: diagnosis and management,* Philadelphia, 1975, FA Davis.

Clarke M, Kadhom HM: The nursing prevention of pressure sores in hospital and community patients, *J Adv Nurs* 13(3):365-373, May 1988.

Conine T et al: Pressure ulcer prophylaxis in elderly patients using polyurethane foam or Jay wheelchair cushions, *Int J Rehabil Res* 17:123-137, 1994.

Constantian MB: Etiology: gross effects of pressure. In Constantian MB, editor: *Pressure ulcers: principles and techniques of management,* Boston, 1980, Little, Brown.

Cooper DG, Foort J, Hannah RE: Structural matrices for use in rehabilitation, *Prosthet Orthot Int* 7:25-28, 1983.

Cooper RA: *Wheelchair selection and configuration,* New York, 1998, Demos.

Daniel RK, Priest DL, Wheatley DC: Etiologic factors in pressure sores: an experimental model, *Arch Phys Med Rehabil* 62:492-498, 1981.

DeLateur BJ et al: Wheelchair cushions designed to prevent pressure sores: an evaluation, *Arch Phys Med Rehabil* 57(3):129-135, 1976.

Dinsdale SM: Decubitus ulcers: role of pressure and friction in causation, *Arch Phys Med Rehabil* 55:147-152, 1974.

Exton-Smith AN, Sherwin RW: Prevention of pressure sores: significance of spontaneous bodily movements, *Lancet* 2:1124-1126, 1961.

Ferguson-Pell MW: Body-support pressures and sitting, *Proc Fifth Int Seating Symp,* pp. 204-209, February 1989.

Ferguson-Pell MW: Seat cushion selection, *J Rehabil Res Dev Clin Suppl* 2:49-72, 1990.

Ferguson-Pell M, Cardi M: Pressure mapping systems, *Team Rehabil Rep* 3(7):28-32, 1992.

Ferguson-Pell MW et al: A knowledge-based program for pressure sore prevention, *Ann N Y Acad Sci,* 1986.

Fernie G, Letts RM: Seating the elderly. In Letts RM, editor: *Principles of seating the disabled,* Boca Raton, Fla, 1991, CRC Press.

Fisher SV et al: Wheelchair cushion effect on skin temperature, *Arch Phys Med Rehabil* 59:68-72, 1978.

Garber SL, Krouskop TA, Carter RE: A system for clinically evaluating wheelchair pressure-relief cushions, *Am J Occup Ther* 32(9):565-570, 1978.

Gerson LW: The incidence of pressure sores in active treatment hospitals, *Int J Nurs Stud* 12(4):201-204, 1975.

Gilsdorf P, Patterson R, Fisher S: Thirty-minute continuous sitting force measurements with different support surfaces in the spinal cord injured and able-bodied, *J Rehabil Res Dev* 28(4):33-38, 1991.

Grogan S, Morton K, Murphy M: Skin breakdown. In Woll NM, editor: *Nursing spinal cord injuries,* Totowa, NJ, 1986, Rowman & Allanheld.

Ham R, Aldersea P, Porter D: *Wheelchair users and postural seating: a clinical approach*, New York, 1998, Churchill Livingstone.

Hedge A: Back care for sitting work: www.spineuniverse.com/, June 5, 2001.

Hobson DA: Contributions of posture and deformity to the body-seat interface variables of a person with spinal cord injury, *Proc Fifth Int Seating Symp*, pp. 153-171, February 1989.

Hobson DA: Seating and mobility for the severely disabled. In Smith RV, Leslie JH, editors: *Rehabilitation engineering*, Boca Raton, Fla, 1990, CRC Press.

Hobson DA, Crane B: State of the science white paper on wheelchair seating comfort, February 2001: www.rerc.pitt.edu/RERC_PDF/Comfort.pdf, May 15, 2001.

Hobson DA, Nwaobi OM: Specialized seating and positioning. In *Wheelchair mobility: a summary of activities at University of Virginia Rehabilitation Engineering Center 1983-1987*, Charlottesville, 1987, University of Virginia Press.

Hulme JB et al: Effects of adaptive seating devices on the eating and drinking of children with multiple handicaps, *Am J Occup Ther* 41(2):81-89, 1987.

Kangas KM: Seating, positioning, and physical access, *Developmental Disabilities Special Interest Section Newsletter, Special Issue on Assistive Technology* 14(2):2-3, 1991.

Klein RM, Fowler RS: Pressure relief training device: the microcalculator, *Arch Phys Med Rehabil* 62:500-501, 1981.

Kosiak M et al: Evaluation of pressure as a factor in the production of ischial ulcers, *Arch Phys Med Rehabil* 39:623-629, 1958.

Kosiak M: Etiology and pathology of ischemic ulcers, *Arch Phys Med Rehabil* 40:6262-6269, 1959.

Kosiak M: Etiology of decubitus ulcers, *Arch Phys Med Rehabil* 42:19-29, 1961.

Krouskop TA et al: The effectiveness of preventive management in reducing the occurrence of pressure sores, *J Rehabil Res Dev* 20(1):74-83, 1983.

Kwiatkowski R, Inigo R: The design of a computer aided seating system, *Proc RESNA Int 92 Conf*, pp 216-217, 1992.

Landis EM: Micro-injection studies of capillary blood pressure in human skin, *Heart* 15:209-228, 1930.

Latter JE, Dehoux E: Seating and the spinal cord injured. In Letts RM, editor: *Principles of seating the disabled*, Boca Raton, Fla, 1991, CRC Press.

Letts RM, editor: *Principles of seating the disabled*, Boca Raton, Fla, 1991, CRC Press.

MDS National Quality Indicator System: MDS quality indicator report for skin care, Health Care Financing Administration, January/March 2000: www.hcfa.gov/projects/mdsreports/qi/qi3.asp?group=11&qtr=1, June 18, 2001.

Meehan M: Multisite pressure ulcer prevalence survey, *Decubitus* 3(4):14-17, 1990.

Merbitz CT et al: Wheelchair push-ups: measuring pressure relief frequency, *Arch Phys Med Rehabil* 66:10-34, 1985.

Miller H, Delozier J: Cost implications of the pressure ulcer treatment guideline. Columbia (MD): Center for Health Policy Studies; 1994. Contract No. 282-91-0070. 17 p. Sponsored by the Agency for Health Care Policy and Research.

Minkel JL: Seating SCI clients, *Proc Sixth Northeast RESNA Regional Conf*, 1990.

National Pressure Ulcer Advisory Panel (NPUAP): Pressure ulcers: incidence, economics, risk assessment. Consensus development conference statement, *Decubitus* 2(2):24-28, 1989.

National Pressure Ulcer Advisory Panel (NPUAP): Stage I assessment in darkly pigmented skin, 1998: www.npuap.org/positn4.htm, June 15, 2001.

National Pressure Ulcer Advisory Panel (NPUAP): Statement on pressure ulcer prevention, 1992: www.npuap.org/positn1.htm, June 15, 2001.

National Pressure Ulcer Advisory Panel (NPUAP): The facts about reverse staging in 2000: the NPUAP position statement, 2000: www.npuap.org/positn5.htm, June 15, 2001.

Niazi ZBM et al: Recurrence of initial pressure ulcers in persons with spinal cord injuries, *Adv Wound Care* 10(30):38-42, 1997.

Norton D, McLaren R, Exton-Smith AN: *An investigation of geriatric nursing problems in hospital*, London, 1975, Churchill Livingstone. Original work published in 1962.

Norton D, McLaren R, Exton-Smith AN: Pressure sores. Part I: a study of factors concerned in the production of pressure sores and their prevention. In Horsley JA, editor: *Preventing decubitus ulcers*, New York, 1981, Grune & Stratton.

Nwaobi OM: Biomechanics of seating. In Trefler E, editor: *Seating for children with cerebral palsy: a resource manual*, Memphis, 1984, University of Tennessee.

Nwaobi OM: Effect of different seating orientations on upper extremity function in children with spastic and athetoid cerebral palsy, *Proc 10th Annu Conf Rehab Technol*, pp 264-265, 1987.

Nwaobi OM, Hobson D, Trefler E: Hip angle and upper extremity movement time in children with cerebral palsy, *Proc 8th Annu Conf Rehabil Technol*, pp 39-41, 1985.

Nwaobi OM, Smith PD: Effect of adaptive seating on pulmonary function of children with cerebral palsy, *Dev Med Child Neurol* 28:351-354, 1986.

Olson J: Conventional pressure transducers. In Webster JG, editor: *Prevention of pressure sores*, Bristol, England, 1991, IOP Publishing.

Panel for the Prediction and Prevention of Pressure Ulcers in Adults: *Pressure ulcers in adults: prediction and prevention* (Clinical Practice Guideline No 3, AHCPR Pub No 92-0047), Rockville, Md, 1992, Agency for Health Care Policy and Research, Public Health Service, U.S. Department of Health and Human Services.

Patterson R et al: The physiological response to repeated surface pressure loads in the able bodied and spinal cord injured, *Proc RESNA Int 92 Conf,* pp. 205-206, June 1992.

Pfaff K: Seating science, *Team Rehabil Rep* 4(5):31-33, 1993.

Pfeffer J: The cause of pressure sores. In Webster JG, editor: *Prevention of pressure sores,* Bristol, England, 1991, IOP Publishing.

Presperin JJ: Seating and mobility evaluation during rehabilitation, *Rehabil Manage,* pp 53-57, April/May 1989.

Rehabilitation Engineering Research Center (RERC) on Wheeled Mobility: R-2: investigation of dynamic seating for comfort, January 29, 2001: http://www.rerc.pitt.edu/RERC_Res/research.html, June 17, 2001.

Reichel SM: Shearing force as a factor in decubitus ulcers in paraplegics, *JAMA* 762-763, February 15, 1958.

Reinecke S: Seating, *Proc Sixth Northeast RESNA Regional Conf,* 1990.

Reswick JB, Rogers JE: Experience at Rancho Los Amigos Hospital with devices and techniques to prevent pressure sores. In Kenedi RM, Cowden JM, Scales JT, editors: *Bedsore biomechanics,* Baltimore, 1976, University Park Press.

Richardson RR, Meyer PR Jr: Prevalence and incidence of pressure sores in acute spinal cord injuries, *Paraplegia* 19(4):235-247, 1981.

Robnett MK: The incidence of skin breakdown in a surgical intensive care unit, *J Nurs Qual Assur* 1(1):77-81, 1986.

Rodriguez GP, Garber SL: Prospective study of pressure ulcer risk in spinal cord injury patients, *Paraplegia* 32(3):235-247, 1994.

Salzberg CA et al: New pressure ulcer risk assessment scale for individuals with spinal cord injury, *Am J Phys Med Rehabil* 75(2):96-104, 1996.

Shaw G, Taylor SJ: A survey of wheelchair seating problems of the institutionalized elderly, *Assist Technol* 3:5-10, 1991.

Shields RK, Cook TM: Effect of seat angle and lumbar support on seated buttock pressure, *Phys Ther* 68(11):1682-1686, 1988.

Sposato BA et al: Prescribing customized contoured seat cushions by computer-aided shape sensing, *Proc 13th Ann RESNA Conf,* pp 103-104, 1990.

Sprigle S: The match game, *Team Rehabil Rep* 3(3):20-21, 1992.

Stewart SFC, Palmieri BS, Cochran GVB: Wheelchair cushion effect on skin temperature, heat flux, and relative humidity, *Arch Phys Med Rehabil* 61:229-233, 1980.

Tang S: Seat cushions. In Webster JG, editor: *Prevention of pressure sores,* Bristol, England, 1991, IOP Publishing.

Taylor SJ: Evaluating the client with physical disabilities for wheelchair seating, *Am J Occup Ther* 41(11):711-716, 1987.

Taylor SJ, Trefler E: Decision making guidelines for seating and positioning children with cerebral palsy. In Trefler E, editor: *Seating for children with cerebral palsy: a resource manual,* Memphis, 1984, University of Tennessee Press.

Torrance C: *Pressure sores: aetiology, treatment and prevention,* London, 1983, Croom Helm.

Tredwell S, Roxborough L: Cerebral palsy seating. In Letts RM, editor: *Principles of seating the disabled,* Boca Raton, Fla, 1991, CRC Press.

Trefler E, Hobson DA, Taylor SJ: *Seating and mobility for persons with physical disabilities,* Tucson, Ariz, 1993, Therapy Skill Builders.

Versluysen M: How elderly patients with femoral fracture develop pressure sores in hospital, *Br Med J (Clin Res Ed)* 17, 292(6531):1311-1313, 1986.

Weiss-Lambrou R et al: Wheelchair seating aids: how satisfied are consumers? *Assist Technol* 11(1):43-52, 1999.

Whimster IW: The trophic effects of nerves on skin. In Kenedi RM, Cowden JM, Scales JT, editors: *Bedsore biomechanics,* Baltimore, 1976, University Park Press.

Young JB, Dobrzanski S: Pressure sores: epidemiological and current management concepts, *Drugs & Aging* 2:42-57, 1992.

Zacharkow D: *Posture, sitting, standing, chair design & exercise,* Springfield, Ill, 1988, Charles C Thomas.

Zacharkow D: *Wheelchair posture and pressure sores,* Springfield, Ill, 1984, Charles C Thomas.

Zhou R: Bladder pressure sensors. In Webster JG, editor: *Prevention of pressure sores,* Bristol, England, 1991, IOP Publishing.

# CHAPTER 7

# Control Interfaces for Assistive Technology

## Chapter Outline

## Learning Objectives

Upon completing this chapter you will be able to:

1. Describe the elements of the human/technology interface and its role within the assistive technology component of the HAAT model
2. Describe the characteristics of control interfaces
3. Identify and define the basic selection methods
4. Describe the means by which the user's physical control can be enhanced
5. Discuss a framework for control interface decision making
6. Identify technologies for direct selection
7. Identify technologies for indirect selection
8. Discuss the outcomes that can be achieved through implementation of a motor training program and how technology can be used to improve motor response

## Key Terms

Acceptance Time
Activation Characteristics
Automatic Scanning
Circular Scanning
Coded Access
Command Domain
Continuous Input
Control Enhancers
Control Interface
Direct Selection

Directed Scanning
Discrete Inputs
Distributed Controls
Group-Item Scanning
Indirect Selection
Input Domain
Integrated Control
Inverse Scanning
Linear Scan

On-Screen Keyboard
Rotary Scanning
Row-Column Scanning
Scanning
Selection Methods
Selection Set
Sensory Characteristics
Spatial Characteristics
Step Scanning

The human/technology interface is a major part of the assistive technology component of the Human Activity Assistive Technology (HAAT) model. Bailey (1989, p. 170) defines an interface as "the boundary shared by interacting components in a system" in which "the essence of this interaction is communication, the exchange of information back and forth across the boundary." The human/technology interface, therefore, is the boundary between the human and the assistive technology across which information is exchanged. This exchange of information is bidirectional and includes both the interface from the person to the device used to control the assistive device and the interface that provides feedback regarding the device's operation from the device to the person.

The exchange of information in the form of input to operate the device takes place by way of a control interface between the user and the device. This may vary from someone who needs an enlarged light switch to turn a light off and on, to someone who needs to access a portable communication system with a single switch, to someone who needs to control a powered wheelchair with a joystick.

The exchange of information from the device to the person takes place through a visual or auditory display. These displays have an important role in providing feedback to the user and are also considered a component of the human/technology interface. The role of displays in specific assistive technology applications is discussed in subsequent chapters.

In this chapter we discuss the various control interfaces, their characteristics, and the control methods that provide the link between the person with a disability and the device being controlled. A framework for matching these control interfaces, control methods, and enhancement techniques to the user's needs and skills is also presented.

### ■ ELEMENTS OF THE HUMAN/ TECHNOLOGY INTERFACE

The human/technology interface is more than just a piece of hardware that inputs into the device. There are actually *three* elements of the human/technology interface that contribute to the operation of a device: the control interface, the selection set, and the selection method. These three elements are interrelated, and careful attention must be given to each element to have an effective human/technology interface.

## Control Interface

The **control interface** (e.g., keyboard, joystick) is the hardware by which the human in our assistive technology system operates or controls a device. It is sometimes also referred to as an *input device*. The control interface generates from one to an infinite number of independent inputs, or signals, defined as the **input domain** (Morasso et al, 1979). The input domain may be either discrete or continuous.

A control interface with **discrete inputs** is one in which each location has a fixed value representing a distinct result with no intermediate steps. For discrete interfaces, the size of the input domain is equal to the total number of targets available to the user. For example, a computer keyboard may have more than 100 keys, each representing a different letter or symbol, which is the signal that is sent to the processor. Whereas a single switch has only one signal in its input domain, a dual switch has two signals. With a **continuous input** interface the inputs are ongoing, with an infinite number of values. Interfaces that are continuous either vary in quantity along a range, as with a volume control, or maintain an even quantity while providing a continuous input, such as driving straight ahead using a steering wheel to make small adjustments. A proportional joystick and a computer mouse both have a continuous input domain in which there can be an infinite number of possible input signals.

## Selection Set

The **selection set** is the items available from which choices are made (Lee and Thomas, 1990). Selection sets can be represented by traditional orthography (e.g., written letters, words, and sentences), symbols used to represent ideas, computer icons, line drawings or pictures, or synthetic speech. The modalities in which the selection set is presented can be visual (e.g., letters on the keyboard), tactile (e.g., braille), or auditory (e.g., spoken choices in auditory scanning).

The size, modality, and type of selection set chosen are based on the user's needs and the desired *activity output*. An electronic aids to daily living (EADL) or a powered wheelchair typically has fewer items in the selection set than an augmentative communication device. The size may also vary according to the user's skills. For example, an individual who spells and has good physical control has the skills to use the selection set of a standard keyboard, which consists of all the letters and function keys. Another individual who is working on developing language and communication skills may

have a selection set consisting of only two picture symbol choices displayed on a lap tray. Selection sets are discussed further in Chapter 9.

## Selection Methods

There are two basic methods in which the user makes selections using the control interface. We refer to these as **selection methods.** They are direct selection and indirect selection. Currently used indirect selection methods include scanning, directed scanning, and coded access.

**Direct selection.** With **direct selection** the individual is able to use the control interface to randomly choose any of the items in the selection set. The consumer indicates his choice by using voice, finger, hand, eye, or other body movement. In this method of selection the user identifies a target and goes directly to it (Smith, 1991). At any one time, all the elements of the selection set are equally available for selecting; that is, they are not time dependent. Typing on a keyboard or even picking a flower from the garden are considered direct selection. Physically, direct selection requires refined, controlled movements and is the most difficult. Cognitively, there is an immediate, direct result from the selection made; therefore direct selection is more intuitive and easier to use. Figure 7-1 shows the input that is made using direct selection to obtain the letter *S.* The various types of control interfaces that allow the individual to use direct selection are described in the section on selecting a control interface for a user.

**Indirect selection.** As the term suggests, with **indirect selection** there are intermediary steps involved in making a selection. Probably the most common indirect selection method is scanning. With **scanning,** the selection set is presented on a display and is sequentially scanned by a cursor or light on the device. When the particular element that the individual wishes to select is presented, a signal is generated by the user. With an assistive device, the control interface used for scanning is a single switch or an array of two switches. Depending on the needs of the user, scanning can vary in the format used for the selection set and in the manner in which the control interface is used to make the selection. These various techniques are discussed later in this chapter.

Scanning requires several more steps than direct selection. Good visual tracking skills, a high degree of attention, and the ability to sequence are requirements for scanning. The advantage of scanning is that it requires very little motor control to make a selection. With training it is possible for an individual to acquire the skills necessary for scanning.

**Directed scanning** is a hybrid approach in which the user activates the control interface to select the direction of the scan, vertically or horizontally. Then the selection set is

## Direct Selection

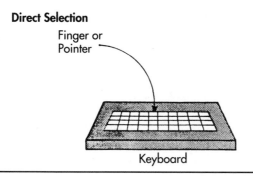

| Input | Output |
|-------|--------|
| Press S | S |

**Figure 7-1**    This figure shows the input required to obtain the letter *S* using direct selection. (From Smith RO: Technological approaches to performance enhancement. In Christiansen C, Baum C, editors: *Occupa-* *tional therapy: overcoming human performance deficits,* Thorofare, NJ, 1991, Slack.)

## Directed Scanning

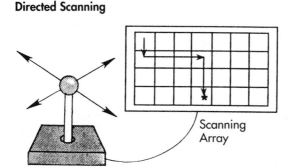

| Input | Output |
|-------|--------|
| Move Joystick:<br>Down<br>Right<br>Right<br>Right<br>Down | S |

**Figure 7-2**    Directed scanning showing the input required to select the letter *S*. The user selects the direction of the scan and the items in the selection set are scanned sequentially by the device. When the desired item is reached, the user makes the selection. (From Smith RO: Technologi- cal approaches to performance enhancement. In Christiansen C, Baum C, editors: *Occupational therapy: overcoming human performance deficits,* Thorofare, NJ, 1991, Slack.)

scanned sequentially by the device. When the desired choice is reached, the user sends a signal to the *processor* to make the selection. This signal is generated either by pausing at the choice, an **acceptance time,** or by activating another control interface to indicate the choice. In directed scanning, both the type of movement made and the point when the movement is made contribute to the selection (Vanderheiden, 1984). A joystick or an array of switches (two to eight switches) are the control interfaces used with directed scanning. Figure 7-2 gives an example of the input required to select the letter *S* using directed scanning with a four-position joystick.

Directed scanning requires more steps than direct selection but fewer steps than single-switch scanning. The user needs to be able to activate and hold the control interface and to release it at the appropriate time. If the individual can produce the movements required to use this method, the outcome is faster entry of the desired selections into the device.

Another form of indirect selection is **coded access.** In coded access the individual uses a distinct sequence of movements to input a code for each item in the selection set. Like the other two methods of indirect selection, intermediate steps are required for making a selection. The control interface used is a single switch or an array of switches configured to match the code. Morse code is one example of coded access, wherein the selection set is the alphabet but an intermediate step is necessary in order to obtain a letter. Morse code was developed to be very efficient. This was achieved by assigning the most frequently used letters the shortest codes. This efficiency can be useful in written or conversational communication. In addition, Morse code does not require that a selection set be displayed. The codes are usually memorized, although visual displays, diagrams, or charts can be used to aid in recalling the codes. Morse code and other coded access methods are described in greater detail later in this chapter.

Like scanning, coded access requires less physical skill than direct selection. The advantage of coded access over scanning, however, is that the timing of the input is under the control of the user and is not dependent on the device. The disadvantage is that it takes more cognitive skill, especially memory and sequencing, than direct selection.

Fortunately, most current devices can be accessed by more than one type of control interface and selection method. The selection set on most devices also can be varied to match the user's needs. From a manufacturing perspective, versatility of a device allows it to be applicable to a wider population. From a consumer's perspective, this helps to contain the cost of the device and makes it possible to adapt to changing user needs and skills.

## The Processor: Connecting the Human/ Technology Interface to the Activity Output

When the control interface is activated by the user, information is sent via a signal to the *processor*. The processor interprets the information and generates two signals that are converted to (1) feedback to any display that is being used and (2) an activity output, depending on the functions of the assistive technology system. The set of device functions is referred to as the **command domain** (Morasso et al, 1979). For example, the command domain of a joystick on a powered wheelchair is typically configured so that the signal for the UP input is transformed into forward movement of the wheelchair, DOWN into reverse movement, LEFT into movement to the left, and RIGHT into movement to the right. That same joystick can be used to control a television set in which the same input domain of UP, DOWN, LEFT, RIGHT becomes a command domain of television volume up, volume down, channel up, channel down. In an electric feeder the command domain includes lifting up the spoon, rotating the plate, and putting the spoon back down. In a communication device the command domain is the meaning assigned to each input selection, including functions such as print and speak.

For every element in the command domain there must be a corresponding element in the *selection set*. The selection set is presented to the user via the selection method. For example, with direct selection each item in the selection set is labeled on the target itself. In direct selection the size of the input domain (number of independent signals) is equal to the size of the command domain. With indirect selection, the input domain has fewer signals than the number of elements in the command domain. With scanning, each item in the selection set is presented sequentially by the device. Thus we can see how the selection method connects the human/technology interface to the command domain of the processor.

To use many of the alternative control interfaces to access a computer, such as an expanded keyboard or a single switch, there must be a bridge between the control interface and the computer. Sometimes this bridge is built into the control interface and other times it is separate. Because the control interface itself is only a switch (or set of switches in a keyboard) pressing a switch or key does not generate any meaningful information for the computer or other assistive device. To make the information meaningful, a *decoder* must be used (Anson, 1997). This decoder may be built into the control interface (particularly keyboards), it may be accomplished through software in the computer, or it may require an additional component. When an external component is required, it is often referred to as a *general input device-emulating interface* or *GIDEI*. The GIDEI is a special-purpose processor that translates (i.e., decodes) the signals from the control interface so they match the command domain requirements of the computer. For example, if the computer application requires the use of ESC or DEL keys, then the GIDEI must provide a way for the control interface to generate these key commands. This may require sending special signals from the GIDEI to the computer. How GIDEIs work and how to choose them for a specific application is discussed in Chapter 8.

## ■ CHARACTERISTICS OF CONTROL INTERFACES

Before we can discuss the specific types of control interfaces and the selection of a control interface for the user, we need to have an understanding of their characteristics. Controls differ according to their spatial, sensory, and activation characteristics (Barker and Cook, 1981). When selecting a control interface for an individual, these characteristics should be taken into consideration. We need to consider the placement and size of the control interface (spatial characteristics), how it is activated (activation characteristics), and what feedback is obtained as a result of its activation (sensory characteristics).

### Spatial Characteristics

The **spatial characteristics** of a control interface are (1) its overall physical size (dimensions), shape, and weight; (2) the number of available targets contained within the control interface; (3) the size of each target; and (4) the spacing between targets. Control interfaces can be grouped into broad categories based on their spatial characteristics. For example, a single switch has one target, and the target size is the dimension (height and width) of the switch. Typically a single switch can accommodate an individual who has limitations in range and only gross resolution for activation. Switch arrays (including joysticks) have two to five switches, each representing a different target. The user's range required to access a switch array needs to be larger than for a single switch but still relatively small, depending on the spacing between the switches. The user's resolution needs to be more refined than that required for a single switch and less refined than that for a keyboard. A contracted keyboard has keys (targets) of small size in close proximity to each other. Its overall size is also small. The keys on these keyboards range in size from 0.5 to 1.5 cm, and they require relatively fine resolution from the user. The requirement for the user's range is moderate (less than 15 cm in both horizontal and vertical directions). Standard or commonly used keyboards require moderate range and

**TABLE 7-1    Method of Activation**

| Signal Sent, User Action (What the Body Does) | Signal Detected | Examples |
|---|---|---|
| 1. Movement (eye, head, tongue, arms, legs) | 1a. Mechanical control interface: activation by the application of a force | 1a. Joystick, keyboard, tread switch |
| | 1b. Electromagnetic control interface: activation by the receipt of electromagnetic energy such as light or radio waves | 1b. Light pointer, light detector, remote radio transmitter |
| | 1c. Electrical control interface: activation by detection of electrical signals from the surface of the body | 1c. EMG, EOG, capacitive, or contact switch |
| | 1d. Proximity control interface: activation by a movement close to the detector but without contact | 1d. Heat-sensitive switches |
| 2. Respiration (inhalation-expiration) | 2. Pneumatic control interface: activation by detection of respiratory airflow or pressure | 2. Puff and sip |
| 3. Phonation | 3. Sound or voice control interface: activation by the detection of articulated sounds or speech | 3. Sound switch, whistle switch, speech recognition |

*EMG*, Electromyographic; *EOG*, electroculographic.

relatively fine resolution of the user. Finally, expanded keyboards have large overall size and enlarged target size, requiring relatively large range and fine resolution. Switch arrays and keyboards can have from 2 to more than 100 targets.

## Activation and Deactivation Characteristics

There are many characteristics related to the activation of the control interface. The **activation characteristics** of a control interface consist of the method of activation, effort, displacement, flexibility, and durability and maintainability. Deactivation, or the release, of a control interface is another characteristic that needs to be considered.

**Method of activation.** The *method of activation* is the way in which a signal sent by the user is detected by the control interface and activates the processor. Table 7-1 shows the methods of activation. The first column identifies the three ways the user can send a signal to the control interface: movement, respiration, and phonation; the middle column shows how each of these signals is detected by the control interface; and the column on the far right provides examples of each type of control interface.

Movements by the user can be detected by the control interface in three basic ways. The movement may generate a force, external to the body, that is detected by the control interface. These are *mechanical control interfaces*, and they represent the largest category of control interfaces. Most switches, keyboard keys, joysticks, and other controls that require movement or force for activation (e.g., mouse,

trackball) fall into this category. Force is always required to activate a mechanical control interface; however, mechanical displacement may or may not occur. For example, force-controlled joysticks and membrane keyboards have very little displacement when activated. *Electromagnetic control interfaces* do not require contact from the user's body for activation. They detect movement at a distance through either light or radio frequency (RF) energy. Examples include head-mounted light sources or detectors and transmitters used with EADLs for remote control (similar to garage door openers). Another example of an electromagnetic control interface is the use of a light beam in a manner similar to the system in many retail stores in which a customer interrupts a light beam when entering or leaving the store. *Electrical control interfaces* are sensitive to electric currents generated by the body. One type, called a capacitive switch, detects static electricity on the surface of the body. This is similar to the game children play when they attempt to shock someone with static electricity. A common example of this type of interface is seen in some elevator buttons. The switches require no force, and they are therefore useful to individuals who have muscle weakness. Other electrical control interfaces use electrodes attached to the skin to detect underlying muscle electrical activity. The electromyographic (EMG) signal associated with muscle contraction is the most commonly used signal. Electrodes placed near the eyes can measure eye movements and generate an electroculographic (EOG) signal based on them. *Proximity control interfaces*, the last type of interface that detects movement, are also active at a distance, but they detect heat or other signals without coming into contact with the body. Although infrequently used, body heat sensors have been successful as control interfaces when force cannot be generated. In summary, mechanical and electrical switches both require contact with the body, and mechanical types also require the generation of force. Electromagnetic and proximity switches do not require contact with the body.

The second type of body-generated signal shown in Table 7-1 is *respiration*. The signal detected is either airflow or air pressure. The use of this type of control interface, generally called a puff-and-sip switch, requires that the user be able to place and maintain her lips around a tube and produce good control of airflow. When sound or speech is produced by the airflow, we call it *phonation* (see Chapter 3). This is a method of activation that has developed rapidly over the last few years with speech recognition interfaces. Individuals who have physical involvement that makes other means of activating a control interface difficult may be able to produce sounds, letters, or words consistently enough to activate a control interface.

**Effort.** The *effort* required by the user to generate the signal from the control interface is the next activation characteristic to consider. Activation effort varies from zero upward to a relatively large amount. For a mechanical interface, this is the force required to cause switch activation. For an electromagnetic interface, the effort is the minimal distance of movement sufficient to cause activation of the sensors. For example, an individual using a light pointer to choose from an array of different items must have sufficient head movement (the effort) to move the light beam from one element (represented by a sensor) to another element (which has a different sensor) and enough stability to hold the light beam on that element. Electrical interfaces require a range of effort from zero (for a capacitive switch) to relatively high for muscle force activation of an EMG. The EMG is measured by electrodes placed on the surface of the skin. The magnitude of the electrical signal is proportional to the amount of force generated by the muscle (the effort). Depending on the muscle and the sensitivity of the measurement system, this can vary from a small force to a large force. The level of effort for proximity switches is the distance of movement required for activation. An example is waving a hand close to a heat-sensitive switch. The activation effort of pneumatic control interfaces is the amount of exhalation or inhalation required for activation. This can be either how hard (pressure) or how fast (flow) air is exhaled or inhaled. For example, some powered wheelchair processors utilize a system in which a hard puff (large effort and high pressure generated) is forward, a soft puff (small effort and low pressure generated) is a right turn, a hard sip is reverse, and a soft sip is a left turn. The difference in these control signals is based primarily on effort generated. Phonation signals also have a level of effort related (at the simplest control interface level) to volume or loudness.

Noise-activated or sound-activated switches are similar to those found on some toys. For speech recognition control interfaces, the effort also includes proper pronunciation, since the detection is based on identification of a particular word (see the section on speech recognition later in this chapter).

**Displacement.** Another characteristic that needs to be considered apart from effort is *displacement*. Displacement is how far a control interface travels from its original position to its activated position and is unique to mechanical control interfaces. Some mechanical interfaces, such as a force-activated joystick, respond to force and require no displacement (Spaeth and Cooper, 1999). In this case the amount of force that the user exerts determines the output of the joystick. If more force is exerted, the output is greater. Because force is detected, rather than amount of travel or displacement of the joystick, the demands placed on the user change. For individuals who can exert a force over a small distance, this type of joystick is ideal. It also provides more tactile feedback to the user. Many mechanical control interfaces require movement and force for activation. The displacement of these control interfaces provides kinesthetic (movement) feedback, as well as tactile and proprioceptive feedback (see Chapter 3). This increased amount of sensory feedback is often a benefit to the user. For example, membrane keyboards have very small displacement, and the forces to activate them are often larger than for switches, which have greater displacement. Without the sensory feedback provided by the displacement, however, users frequently press harder than necessary, thinking that more force is needed to activate the keys.

**Deactivation.** Although we have focused on the activation of control interfaces, we need to keep in mind that there is also a force required to release, or *deactivate*, some control interfaces. Muscle contraction is necessary to remove, or release, the body part from the interface. Weiss (1990) measured both activation and deactivation forces for several mechanical interfaces and found that force was required to release the control interface in all cases, but the deactivation force was approximately one third to one half that required for activation.

**Flexibility.** The *flexibility* of the control interface, or the number of ways in which it can be operated by a control site, also needs to be considered. There are many types of keyboards, joysticks, and switches and just as many ways in which they can be activated by the user. Among individuals with physical disabilities, wide differences in motor performance exist. Depending on the nature of the disability, an individual may or may not have deficits in strength, range of motion, muscle tone, sensation, or coordination. For example, the quality of movement may be smooth or uncoordinated, reflex patterns may dominate movement or be absent, sensory deficits may or may not be present, muscle tone may be normal or increased or decreased, or there may be limitations in range of motion at any joint. Thus one person may push a key with a finger, another may use a thumb, a third a head pointer. Control interfaces that allow for various ways of activation are considered to be flexible. In general, control interfaces that are activated by movement can typically be activated by several body sites and are considered to be flexible in comparison to control interfaces that are limited to activation by respiration and phonation. Within the category of movement-activated controls, the flexibility varies, for example, from a lever* switch, which is most commonly activated by head movement, to a tread† switch, which is routinely used for activation by the foot, knee, hand, head, or chin. Some control interfaces, such as the touch switch,‡ have an adjustment for the amount of effort required to activate them. This type of control can be useful for evaluation purposes or for an individual who has fluctuating endurance or a degenerative condition.

The ways in which the control interface can be mounted or positioned for use also contribute to its flexibility. Being able to mount a control interface at the optimal position in the individual's workspace facilitates activation. Some control interfaces, such as a computer mouse, are not intended for mounting and need to be used on a table or other flat surface, whereas other control interfaces, such as a joystick, can usually be mounted in a variety of locations and can therefore be activated by the chin, hand, or foot. Mounting systems are discussed later in this chapter.

**Durability and maintainability.** The *durability* of the control interface is a characteristic that needs consideration as well. Gathering information during the assessment regarding how often the interface is to be used and the amount of force that is to be generated on the interface by the user assists the assistive technology practitioner (ATP) in making recommendations that correspond with the durability of the control interface. If the control interface is to be used by someone who exerts a great deal of pressure on it because of uncontrolled movements, it must be constructed so it can withstand this type of use. Switches and keyboards made out of plastic, for example, may not hold up well under these circumstances. In the long run it may be cost effective to buy a more expensive interface that is made out of metal and will last longer.

A final consideration is the maintainability of the control interface. It is important to consider whether the interface can be easily cleaned and how it should be cleaned so as not to damage any components. Other considerations are whether any of its components need to be replaced periodically and, if so, how difficult a procedure it is. For example,

certain switches require a battery in order to operate, and when the battery dies, it must be replaced. It also helps to know who will be able to repair the control interface if it breaks down and, if it is in need of repair, whether there is a loaner available for the consumer to use in the interim.

## Sensory Characteristics

The auditory, somatosensory, and visual feedback produced during the activation of the control interface comprise its **sensory characteristics.** Some control interfaces provide auditory feedback in the form of a click when activated. For example, keyboards that use mechanical switches for each key usually click when pressed, thus providing auditory feedback. Other keyboards have a smooth membrane surface that does not provide any auditory feedback. Somatosensory feedback is the tactile, kinesthetic, or proprioceptive response sensed on activation of the control interface. For example, the texture or "feel" of the activation surface provides tactile data. The position in space of the control site when the user activates the switch provides proprioceptive data. The data generated as a result of movement provide kinesthetic feedback to the user. When the interface is within the consumer's visual field, visual data are obtained through observation of the placement and the movement of the control interface. For some individuals the type of visual data will mean the difference between successful and unsuccessful use of a control interface. For example, someone who has difficulty attending to objects in the environment may be more attentive to a switch that is large and bright red or yellow.

There is usually a direct relationship between the sensory data provided by the control interface and the amount of effort required to activate it. A contact switch that is activated by an electric charge from the body (i.e., requiring only touch) does not provide the user with any somatosensory feedback. There is no force required and therefore little proprioceptive or visual feedback is provided. The contact switch is also silent, so auditory feedback is absent as well. In some instances we can alter the feedback generated by a control interface. For example, adding a beep to a contact switch provides auditory data or placing a distinguishing texture over the surface of a membrane keyboard provides feedback through the tactile system. Other switches, such as the tread, wobble,* and rocker†, provide abundant feedback in terms of having a certain feel to them (tactile), an observable movement of the mechanism (visual), and an audible click (auditory).

Generally interfaces that provide rich sensory feedback facilitate performance. On occasion, sensory feedback may be detrimental to the user's performance. For example, a

---

*Zygo Industries, Portland, Ore. (www.zygo-usa.com).
†Zygo Industries, Portland, Ore.
‡Zygo Industries, Portland, Ore.

*Prentke Romich Co., Wooster, Ohio (www.prentrom.com/index.html).
†Prentke Romich Co., Wooster, Ohio.

control interface with an audible click may trigger a startle reflex in the user that interferes with motor movement. The user may eventually adjust to the sound and ignore it, but the ATP may want to consider an alternate control interface.

It is clear that the interrelationship of spatial, sensory, and activation characteristics of control interfaces plays an important role in the design of an assistive technology system. Each of these characteristics must be carefully considered to make effective selections that meet the needs of the consumer.

## ■ SELECTING CONTROL INTERFACES FOR THE USER

Selecting a control interface for an individual can be a complex process. Understanding the characteristics of control interfaces as described above and following a systematic process to determine the user's skills and evaluate the effectiveness of control interfaces can make this process easier. Figure 7-3 outlines a framework to guide the ATP through the decision-making process, ultimately leading to the selection of a human/technology interface that matches the user's needs and skills. Based on information acquired from the needs identification and physical-sensory components of the evaluation process described in Chapter 4, the ATP makes a decision to pursue further evaluation on one of two paths: (1) interfaces for direct selection or (2) interfaces for indirect selection. In general, control interfaces for direct selection typically have greater numbers of targets and require more refined resolution skills. Control interfaces for indirect selection have eight or fewer targets and are more suitable for individuals with gross motor control. To make an informed decision regarding the most appropriate control interface for a user, the ATP needs to understand the alternatives that are available and evaluate and compare the consumer's ability to operate them. In the following sections we describe specific control interfaces for both direct and indirect selection and factors that influence the selection of one particular interface over another.

### Applying the Outcomes of Needs Identification and Physical-Sensory Evaluations to Control Interface Selection

In Figure 7-3 we list specific information related to human/technology interface selection that is an outcome of the needs identification process. The information gathered reveals particular factors that should be considered during the interface selection process. For example, identifying the activity the consumer wants to perform provides us with information on how large an input domain is required and possible control interfaces to consider. If the consumer is in

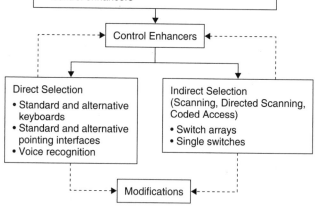

Figure 7-3    Framework for control interface decision making.

need of a powered wheelchair and is not interested in using a computer, for example, it is not necessary to determine whether he can use a keyboard. Alternatively, the consumer may need to perform several functional activities (e.g., communication, mobility, and environmental control). This also affects the way in which we pursue selection of an interface. In situations such as this, we need to consider whether a different control interface for each function or a single integrated control for all the functions is to be used.

The information gathered during the physical-sensory skills evaluation gives us a profile of the user's skills in these areas, specifically those shown in Figure 7-3. This information can be used to determine the acceptable parameters for potential control interfaces. The *range measurement* determines the consumer's minimal and maximal comfortable reach and defines the geometric requirements for the individual's workspace. This parameter provides an indication of the possible locations for placement of a control interface (or interfaces) and the maximal distance between the extreme outer edges of the interface (e.g., the overall size of a keyboard or switch array). The *resolution measurement* provides data on the consumer's ability to control her movement to select targets.

Given this information on the consumer's skills, we can select potential candidate control interfaces that have similar characteristics in terms of the number and spacing of the targets and the size of individual switches or keys. Once candidate interfaces have been selected, comparative testing is conducted. The purpose of comparative testing using the control interfaces is to provide the ATP with information on how fast the consumer can input using the control interface, as well as the accuracy of that input. Methods for carrying out comparative testing are described in Chapter 4. During comparative testing, it is also critical that the ATP gather subjective information from the consumer on each interface that is evaluated. This information includes the ease or difficulty of use.

## Control Enhancers: Interface Positioning, Arm Supports, Mouthsticks, Head Pointers, and Hand Pointers

**Control enhancers** include aids and strategies that enhance or extend the physical control (range and resolution) a person has available to use a control interface. In some cases a person's control may be enhanced to the extent that his range and resolution make it possible for him to select directly. In other cases, control enhancers make it physically easier and minimize fatigue for an individual. These control enhancers include strategies, such as varying the position or the characteristics of the control interface, and devices such as mouthsticks, head and hand pointers, and arm supports.

The person and the control interface should both be positioned to maximize function. In Chapter 6 we talked about the importance of proper positioning to maximize an individual's function. A person's position should be observed before and during the control interface evaluation. If inadequate positioning appears to be affecting the person's ability to control an interface, it should be addressed before continuing with the evaluation. The position of the control interface can also affect the person's ability to activate it. Changing the height or the angle of the control interface even slightly may enhance the person's ability to control it.

As control interfaces become more sophisticated through the utilization of electronics, control-enhancing features are becoming part of the interface. For example, certain joysticks have a feature, called tremor dampening, that allows adjustment of the joystick for people who have tremors. Tremor-dampening joysticks are able to distinguish between tremors, which are faster and smaller, and intentional movements, which are slower and larger. The joystick is adjusted so that the tremors are disregarded and only intentional movements are detected. This enhances the ability of an individual, who might otherwise be unable to operate a joystick, to control a powered wheelchair. A

---

### CASE STUDY 7-1

#### COMPARATIVE EVALUATION

Max is an 18-year-old male who has cerebral palsy. He lives in a residential facility and attends a work program through United Cerebral Palsy. Max has been referred to ABC Assistive Technology Center for a communication device. He currently communicates with others using a manual communication board and eye blinks for yes and no.

Through evaluation of Max's range and resolution, it has been determined that his best control sites are his right hand and his head. However, he does not have fine enough control at either site to use direct selection. You decide to perform comparative interface testing using a tread switch with his hand and a lever switch at the side of his head. Data collected during the comparative testing phase of the evaluation show that Max is more accurate and faster activating the switch with his head (versus his hand). However, Max has indicated a preference for using his hand instead of his head.

**QUESTIONS:**

1. Given Max's limited verbal communication, how would you gather information from him regarding his opinion on the hand and the head switches?
2. What type of subjective information would you want to gather from Max regarding his use of and preference for each of these two switches?
3. Your data indicates that Max is faster and more accurate using the head switch. However, Max has indicated to you that he prefers the hand switch. What would your recommendation be and why?

---

similar feature, called *filter keys,* is employed in Windows. When the filter keys feature is activated in Windows, brief keystrokes are ignored and the rate at which keys repeat when being pressed is delayed.

Individuals who have weakness in the arm may not have enough strength to access the full range of a keyboard adequately. A mobile arm support (Figure 7-4, *A*), which props the arm and assists in arm movements by eliminating some of the effects of gravity, may then allow the individual to access a keyboard. For the individual who has the gross motor ability to move her arm and hand around a keyboard but has difficulty extending and isolating a finger to depress a key, a pointing aid may help. There are commercially available aids that can be strapped on to the hand to assist in pointing, such as the typing aid shown in Figure 7-4, *B*. In some cases it is necessary to custom fabricate a pointing aid in order for it to fit the consumer's hand appropriately.

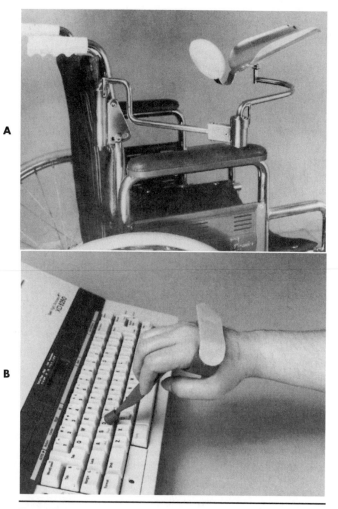

Figure 7-4   Control enhancers. **A,** Mobile arm support used to enhance the control in the upper extremity for accessing a control interface. **B,** Typing aid used to enhance a person's ability to point and access a keyboard. (Courtesy Sammons Preston Co., Bolingbrook, Ill.)

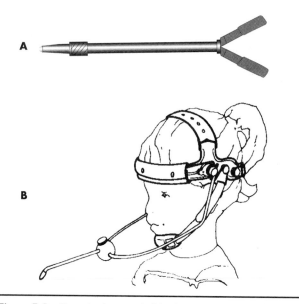

Figure 7-5   Control enhancers. **A,** Mouthstick. **B,** Head pointer.

These custom-fabricated aids can range from complex hand splints to simple tools such as a dowel with a rubber tip on the end.

For individuals who lack functional movement in their arms and hands, a mouthstick or head pointer (Figure 7-5) can be used with head and neck movement to access a keyboard or perform other types of manipulation tasks (e.g., dialing a telephone number or turning pages in a book) (Chapter 11). For a head pointer, a rod with a rubber tip is attached to a band that is worn around the top of the head. The individual can then use the end of this rod to depress keys. Besides being able to move the head vertically and horizontally, the individual must have the ability to produce a third dimension of movement to depress keys using a head pointer: forward and backward. There are also light pointers that can be worn on the head or held in the hand to control devices. One advantage of head-controlled light pointers is that it is not necessary for the user to move the head forward or backward. Light pointers are described in greater detail in the section on pointing interfaces.

Mouthsticks are often used by individuals who are quadriplegic as a result of a spinal cord injury. A mouthstick consists of a pointer attached to a mouthpiece. The user grips the mouthpiece between his teeth and moves his head to manipulate control interfaces or other objects. The shaft of the mouthstick can be made from a wooden dowel, a piece of plastic, or aluminum. In some cases, interchangeable tips for different functions (e.g., painting, writing, typing) can be inserted into the distal end of the shaft. The mouthpiece can be a standard U shape that is gripped between the teeth or a custom-made insert. Puckett et al (1988) identify a number of criteria for design of a mouthstick. Mouthsticks are also available from several suppliers.* Use of a mouthstick requires good oral-motor control; later in this chapter we discuss training to develop these skills.

The consumer's range and resolution with the control enhancer can be determined using the same methods discussed in Chapter 4. In some cases, particularly if there is a need to extend the consumer's range (e.g., when the head is the likely control site), it is apparent at the beginning of the evaluation that the consumer will benefit from using a control enhancer. When the user has adequate range but resolution is in question, it may not be obvious during the physical-sensory evaluation whether a control enhancer will be beneficial. In these cases it is recommended that comparative testing of candidate interfaces with and without the use of control enhancers be completed. This provides the ATP with objective data regarding the effectiveness of the control enhancer. Certain control interfaces, however, cannot be activated using a control enhancer. These include

---

*For example, Sammons Preston, Bolingbrook, Ill. (www.sammonspreston.com) and Extensions for Independence, Imperial Beach, Calif.

displays specially designed to be used with light pointers, eye-controlled systems, or capacitive switches requiring skin contact for activation (Lee and Thomas, 1990).

## ■ CONTROL INTERFACES FOR DIRECT SELECTION

The most rapid selection method is direct selection; this method is therefore preferred over the use of indirect selection methods. Control interfaces for direct selection include various types of keyboards, pointing interfaces, speech recognition, and eye-controlled systems. The critical questions presented in Box 7-1 can assist the ATP in determining the consumer's ability to use any keyboard. As each question is considered, a yes answer means that the evaluation is proceeding on the correct pathway and the ATP should continue with the next question. Affirmative responses to all seven questions indicate that the control interface by itself is likely to meet the consumer's needs.

The answer to the first question is determined by asking the consumer to reach the keys at each corner of the keyboard. To obtain an answer to the second question, have the consumer press several keys located in different areas of the keyboard. The consumer's rate of input can be timed for entering characters. Accuracy can be measured by monitoring errors made during these tasks. In some situations, speed is of primary importance (e.g., in a work setting). In general, speed and accuracy are in opposition; that is, as speed increases, accuracy decreases. In some cases, to be accurate the consumer may make selections so slowly and deliberately that the use of the control interface under investigation becomes impractical. For example, if it takes several seconds to select a key, this may be equivalent to the use of scanning to make a selection. Because scanning takes much less physical effort, it should then be considered as an alternative to direct selection. Computer-assisted methods to measure speed and accuracy data are described in Chapter 4. The criterion for accuracy is somewhat subjective and

subject to clinical judgment. We recommend that at least three out of four selections (75%) be correct.

If the answer to any of the questions in Box 7-1 is determined to be no, then the use of a control enhancer, the use of modifications, or a less limiting keyboard should be considered. For example, if a standard keyboard cannot be used because of a targeting problem, we may consider the following: (1) an enlarged keyboard with larger targets (less limiting), (2) a keyguard (modification), or (3) a typing aid (a control enhancer). Modifications apply to all types of keyboards and are addressed after we discuss the different types of keyboards.

### Keyboards

For written communication, a keyboard is typically considered the most efficient means of inputting information. The standard keyboard is the first choice for computer access. However, many individuals with disabilities are unable to use a standard keyboard. Fortunately there are a number of alternatives. Table 7-2 provides examples of some commercially available alternatives to the standard keyboard.

**Standard keyboards.** Some individuals may have difficulty writing because of fatigue or minimally impaired motor control. A standard keyboard on a computer may be all that is needed to allow them to complete writing tasks effectively. Because it is readily available, the standard 101 key keyboard is the most desirable interface for direct selection for text entry. For general purpose computer use, the standard keyboard typically has a full alphanumeric array consisting of letters, numbers, punctuation symbols, and special characters such as \@#$%. Most general-purpose computer keyboards also have special keys. Some of these always have the same effect, such as END, which moves the cursor to the end of a line, or DEL, which erases a previous entry. Other special keys (e.g., a print command in a word processing program) can be assigned to special functions dictated by a software application. These are called function keys. In addition, most computer keyboards contain modifier keys such as SHIFT, CONTROL, and ALT. When one of these keys is held down and another key is pressed, the meaning of the second key is modified. Familiar examples are the use of SHIFT to obtain capital letters or to obtain # as a shifted 3. Key size, spacing, and amount of distance the keys travel vary depending on the type and manufacturer of the keyboard. To keep the overall size down, laptop computers in particular have smaller keyboards. For this reason, it is wise to have the consumer try the particular type of keyboard she will be using.

**Ergonomic keyboards.** The term *repetitive strain injury* (RSI) encompasses several musculoskeletal disorders that develop as a result of sustained, repetitive movements (Bear-Lehman, 1995). Carpal tunnel syndrome is the most

---

| BOX 7-1 | Critical Questions for Evaluating Keyboard Use |
|---|---|

1. Can the consumer reach all the keys on the keyboard?
2. Are the size, spacing, and sensory feedback of the keys appropriate?
3. Is the consumer's speed of input adequate for the task?
4. Does the consumer target keys with approximately 75% accuracy?
5. Is the consumer able to simultaneously hold down the modifier key and select another key?
6. Is the consumer able to control the duration for which a key must be pressed before it repeats itself?
7. Does the consumer effectively use the standard keyboard layout?

**TABLE 7-2**  Alternative Keyboards for Direct Selection

| Category | Description | Device Name/Manufacturer |
|---|---|---|
| Expanded keyboards | Generally membrane keyboards that have enlarged target areas, often programmable so that key size can be customized; useful for individuals with good range and poor resolution; also useful for individuals with limited cognitive/language skills or visual impairment. | IntelliKeys (IntelliTools); WinKing Keyboard (TASH, Inc.); Expanded Keyboard (EKEG Electronics Company, LTD); Key Largo (Don Johnston Developmental Equipment); Concept Keyboard (Penny & Giles Computer Products) |
| Contracted keyboards | Miniature, full-function keyboards, typically with membrane overlay; useful for individuals with limited range of motion and good resolution. | WinMini Keyboard (TASH, Inc.); Mini Keyboard (EKEG Electronics Co. Ltd.); The Magic Wand Keyboard (In Touch Systems) |
| Touch screens/touch tablets | Activated by either breaking a very thin light beam or by a capacitive array that detects the electrical charge on the finger; the electrode array used to detect where the finger or pointer is touching is transparent; touch screen can be placed over the face of a monitor. | Touch Window (Edmark Corp.); MagicTouch (Laureate Learning Systems, Inc.) |
| TongueTouch Keypad | Battery-operated, radio frequency-transmitting device with nine pressure-sensitive keys activated by tongue; universal controller processes information sent from keypad to receiver. | UCS 2000 with TongueTouch Keypad (newAbilities, Inc.) |
| Special-purpose keyboards | Keyboards on special-purpose devices, such as augmentative communication and environmental control devices; available keys may be much more limited in number or may be specific in function compared with standard keyboard. | See Chapter 9, Table 9-6 |

Data from Don Johnston Developmental Equipment, Wauconda, IL (www.donjohnston.com); Edmark Corp, Redmond, WA (www.edmark.com); EKEG Electronics, Vancouver, Canada; Laureate Learning Systems, Inc. Winooski, VT (www.laureatelearning.com); newabilities, Inc., Palo Alto, CA (www.newabilities.com); Intelli-Tools, Petaluma, CA (www.intellitools.com); In Touch Systems, Spring Valley, NY (www.magicwandkeyboard.com); Penny & Giles Computer Products (www.penny-gilescp.co.uk); TASH, Ajax, Ontario, Canada, or Richmond, VA (www.tashinc.com).

common RSI. It is thought that the use of a standard keyboard with horizontal rows on a flat platform may contribute to RSI in some individuals. Standard keyboards place the hands in an unnatural position with the forearms pronated and the wrists extended and ulnarly deviated. This position causes strain on the tendons and nerves. Numerous alternatives to the standard keyboard have been developed in attempts to reduce this strain on the wrist and hands. These alternatives range from minor rearranging of the keys to major redesign of the keyboard shape and configuration. Here we discuss ergonomic keyboards, those keyboards that have been designed with the intent of minimizing the risk of RSIs. These ergonomic keyboards all use the QWERTY keyboard layout (see Figure 7-12, A) with the keys repositioned in some way. Later in this section we talk about modifications to the standard QWERTY keyboard layout.

Ergonomic keyboards attempt to reduce the strain placed on the hands and wrists during the repetitive motion of keying by putting the forearms, wrists, and hands in a neutral position, which is more natural and more comfortable for the typist. There are three basic ways in which the standard keyboard has been redesigned. The first and most

common type of ergonomic keyboard is the fixed-split keyboard. In this type of keyboard the layout of the keys is split into two different sections. The center of the keyboard may also be slightly raised with a small slope toward each side. The difference between these keyboards and standard keyboards is that the keys are spaced farther apart and the keyboard is curved, so that the hands are placed in a more neutral position. Many of these keyboards have a built-in wrist rest to support the wrists while typing. The Tru-Form Keyboard* shown in Figure 7-6, A, is one example of this type of keyboard.

The second basic type of ergonomic keyboard is the adjustable-split keyboard. This type also splits the keyboard layout into two parts. A mechanism on the keyboard allows one or both sides of the keyboard to be adjusted horizontally and vertically to the position where it is most comfortable. Each section of the split keyboard typically adjusts from 0 to 30 degrees. A user who is a 10-finger typist and does not need to look at the keyboard may be able to take advantage of this range of adjustment. However, for those individuals who need to have the keyboard in their visual field, adjust-

*Adesso Inc., Culver City, Calif (www.adessoinc.com).

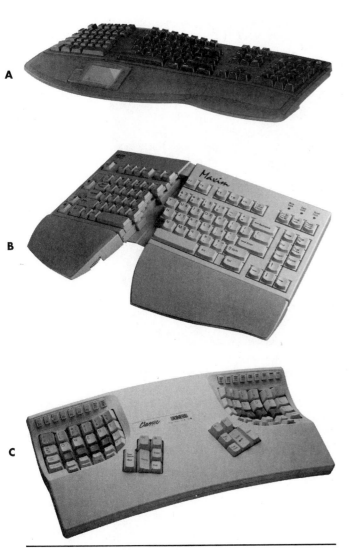

**Figure 7-6**   Ergonomic keyboards. **A,** The Tru-Form Keyboard. **B,** The Maxim Adjustable Keyboard. **C,** The Contoured Keyboard. (**A,** Courtesy Adesso Inc., www.adessoinc.com; **B** and **C,** courtesy Kinesis Corporation, www.kinesis-ergo.com.)

ing the angle too far may make it difficult to see the keys. An example of this type of keyboard is the Maxim Adjustable Keyboard* shown in Figure 7-6, *B.*

The third type of ergonomic keyboard uses a concave keywell design. The keyboard layout again is split into two sections, but in this design the keys are arranged in a well such as that shown on the Contoured Keyboard† in Figure 7-6, *C.* The principle behind this design is that finger excursion is reduced by having the keys arranged at the same distance from each of the finger joints (Anson, 1997). Other products for all three types of ergonomic keyboards can be found at www.tifaq.org/keyboards.html.

Manufacturers of ergonomic keyboards claim that their keyboards reduce the strain placed on the wrist and hands.

However, the use of ergonomic keyboards in reducing symptoms of RSI has not been demonstrated in controlled studies. For this reason, it is advised that ergonomic keyboards *not* be recommended for the purpose of preventing RSI (Anson, 1997; Tessler, 1993). Situations in which an ergonomic keyboard may be recommended for a consumer include (1) meeting the needs of consumer with physical limitations (e.g., limits in range of motion) and (2) when the consumer finds the ergonomic keyboard more comfortable to use than a standard keyboard. The most critical factor to consider when selecting a keyboard is the user's level of comfort with the different keyboards (Anson, 1997).

**Expanded keyboards.**   Individuals who do not have sufficient resolution to target the keys on a standard keyboard but still have adequate resolution to select directly may be able to use an expanded keyboard. Expanded keyboards are generally membrane-type keyboards that have enlarged target areas from which the individual can select directly (Figure 7-7, *A*). The minimal size of the target areas on an expanded keyboard is 1 inch square. If the person still has difficulty targeting this size of key, the expanded keyboard can be customized by grouping keys together to form larger keys. In this way the keyboard can be redesigned to match the skills of the user.

Expanded keyboards vary in overall size and can be chosen depending on the size of the selection set needed by the individual and the key size the individual is able to target accurately. IntelliKeys* has a large surface area that can be configured for a variety of key sizes and shapes. It comes with several standard keyboard overlays, such as the one shown in Figure 7-7, *B.* This overlay is an example of an layout that has been configured with different sizes and different shapes of keys on the same keyboard. The IntelliKeys can also be customized to match specific applications by using the companion Overlay Maker software.† The keys can be labeled with letters, words, symbols, or pictures. Because they can be customized, expanded keyboards are also useful with individuals who have a cognitive or visual impairment. Examples of expanded keyboards are shown in Table 7-2.

**Contracted keyboards.**   Some individuals may have sufficient resolution but lack the range of movement to reach all the keys on a standard keyboard. In this situation a contracted, or mini, keyboard may be the solution. These keyboards use either raised keys or a membrane surface. For computer use, contracted keyboards must meet the requirement that all keys of the standard keyboard be represented. This is accomplished by using additional modifier keys. Figure 7-8 shows a consumer being evaluated using a mouthstick with the WinMini keyboard.‡ This keyboard is

*Kinesis Corporation, Seattle, Wash (www.kinesis-ergo.com).
†Kinesis Corporation (www.kinesis-ergo.com).

*IntelliTools, Petaluna, Calif. (www.intellitools.com).
†IntelliTools, Petaluna, Calif.
‡Tash Inc., Richmond, Va (www.tashinc.com).

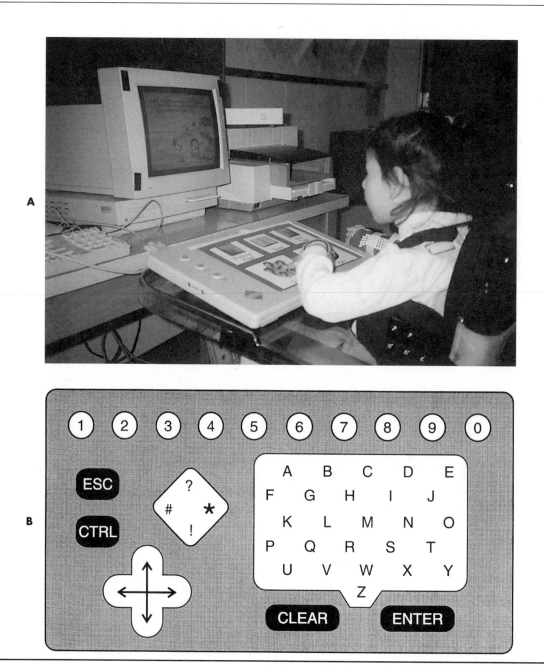

Figure 7-7  **A,** Consumer using an expanded keyboard with thumb. **B,** Expanded keyboard showing configuration with different sizes and shapes of keys on the same keyboard.

approximately 7 ¹/₂ × 4 ³/₄ inches in overall size, with the size of each key approximately one half inch square. Several of the keys have multiple functions, depending on which modifier key is pressed first. The functions corresponding to various modifiers can be colored to match the modifier key. The selection set (the alphabet) in Figure 7-8 is not placed in the QWERTY format typical of standard keyboards. The letter placement is based on a "frequency of use" system in which the letters most commonly used in the English language are placed toward the center, with the less commonly used letters placed in the outer edges of the keyboard. This particularly makes sense to use on a con-

tracted keyboard where the individual's range of motion is restricted. Because of the small key size and closeness of the keys, the user of a contracted keyboard must have good fine motor control. Persons using contracted keyboards type with either a single digit, a handheld typing stick, or a mouthstick.

**Special-purpose keyboards.** Keyboards are also used on special-purpose devices, such as augmentative communication and environmental control devices. In these cases the available keys may be much more limited in number or they may be very specific in function compared with the standard

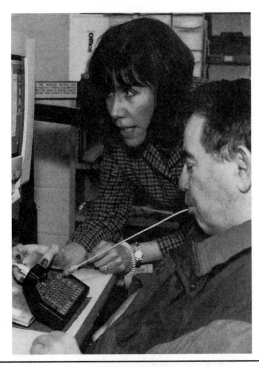

**Figure 7-8**  Consumer being evaluated using the WinMini Keyboard and a mouthstick.

keyboard. For example, in portable augmentative communication devices such as the AlphaTalker,* the keyboards have membrane keys and are restricted to a total of 32 keys (see Chapter 9). These keys are not assigned any specific character or function when manufactured but can be programmed to represent just about anything the user would like. Other devices come with certain keys that have been designated to be specific functions. For example, a key may be designated "SPEAK," and pressing it will cause whatever was entered to be spoken. In all these cases, however, the keyboard provides the same function: direct selection input from the user to the processor.

Dedicated communication devices can also be used as input devices for a general-purpose computer. The communication device is connected to the computer through a special interface (see Chapter 8). This connection allows the communication device to send characters to the computer as if they were typed from the computer keyboard. Because the user of the communication device is familiar with the keyboard on the communication device, it is easy for him to use it for computer entry and he does not have to learn another keyboard arrangement. Another advantage is that any words or phrases that are stored in the communication device can be sent to the computer as words or phrases as well. A standard has been developed to allow all keyboard characters to be sent to the computer, even if the communication device

does not have that character. For example, computer keys such as DEL may not be on the communication device, but the user can send a sequence of characters that the computer interprets as the DEL key. Character codes for a number of keys are shown in Chapter 8. Selection of a special-purpose keyboard for a consumer also requires careful consideration of the items presented in Box 7-1.

## Touch Screens and Touch Tablets

There are touch screens available on augmentative communication devices and for Apple, Macintosh, and MS-DOS computers that the user activates by pointing directly to the selection set on the screen. Using a touch screen makes selection cognitively easier for many users, particularly young children, because it is more direct and intuitive. These interfaces are activated by either breaking a very thin light beam or by a capacitive array that detects the electrical charge on the finger. The electrode array used to detect where the finger, or pointer, is touching is transparent, and the touch screen can be placed over the face of a monitor. In either detection method an array of horizontal and vertical sensors is arranged so that an object the size of a finger will be detected. The position in the array determines what the interpretation of the pointing action will be, just like the specific key on a keyboard determines what the input will be. Touch screens can either be attached to the computer monitor or used on a tabletop or other flat surface. The selection set varies with the application program being used.

## TongueTouch Keypad*

One of the most recent developments in control interfaces is the TongueTouch Keypad, shown in Figure 7-9 with the components necessary for its operation. This keypad consists of nine separate small switches incorporated into a dental mouthpiece that fits in the roof of the mouth. It is a battery-operated, radio frequency-transmitting interface that activates a processor that sends infrared signals to the computer. Each of the nine switches corresponds to one choice on a menu presented on a computer screen. The first menu provides choices of environmental control (e.g., television, lights), computer access (keyboard emulation), and wheelchair control. Once one of these categories is chosen, nine more choices pertaining to that category are presented, such as volume and channel control for the television; letters, keyboard array, and mouse movement directions for computer entry; or numeric choices for telephone dialing. This approach is useful for individuals who do not have motor control in their limbs but have good head, neck, and oral-motor control. In particular, the user must have good

*Prentke Romich Co., Wooster, Ohio (www.prenrom.com).

*New Abilities Systems, Inc., Mountain View, Calif. (http://members.aol.com/UCS1000/index.html).

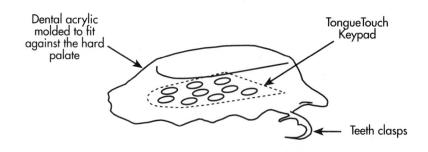

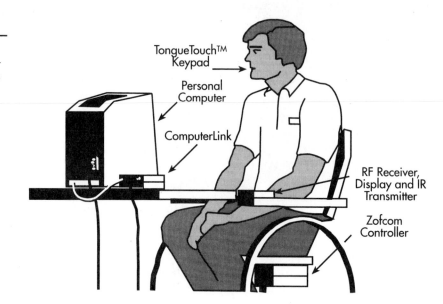

Figure 7-9    Components of the TongueTouch Keypad. *IR, Infrared.* (From Lau C, O'Leary S: Comparison of computer interface devices for persons with severe disabilities, *Am J Occup Ther* 47(11):1022-1029, 1993.)

elevation of the tip of the tongue to activate the individual keys efficiently (Lau and O'Leary, 1993).

## Standard and Alternative Electronic Pointing Interfaces

The other commonly used control interface for direct selection in general-purpose computers is a *mouse.* There are also alternative pointing interfaces that can replace the mouse, such as a trackball, a head sensor, a continuous joystick, and the use of the arrow keys on the keypad (called

*mouse keys).* Box 7-2 identifies the critical questions to consider when assessing an individual for using any type of pointing interface.

It is necessary to determine whether the consumer can use the pointing interface to reach the items in the selection set (targets) and stay fixed on the target while executing the action needed to make a selection. These all imply that the selection targeted is accurate. The person may be able to get to a target area on the screen, but the size of the target may affect her ability to maintain that position while selecting it. Any location on the screen can be a target, and these can be of different sizes. Depending on the software program, the size of the target may be fixed or it may be possible to modify the size to meet the user's needs. The user can employ one of two techniques to make a selection. Utilizing an *acceptance time selection technique,* the user pauses at the selection for a predetermined period (which is adjustable) and that pause signals the selection. With the *manual selection technique,* the user activates another switch to let the device know that the selection has been made. The second approach provides more control for the user, but it also requires additional user motor control.

Pointing interfaces vary in terms of the tactile and proprioceptive feedback they provide, and this may affect the user's performance. Using a pointing interface also requires a significant amount of coordination between the body site executing the movement of the cursor and the eyes following the cursor on the screen and locating the targets. Finally, it should be determined whether the layout of the items in the selection set is beneficial or detrimental to the user's performance. The selection set and its layout will vary depending on the pointing interface and the software being used. It is important to know whether the layout of the selection set can be modified for a particular pointing interface and what type of modifications will benefit the user.

**Mouse.** The standard computer mouse is a solid box that rides on top of a ball. As the mouse is gripped by the user and moved across a flat surface, the ball rotates, causing the cursor on the screen to move. As the mouse moves, the computer screen shows a pointer that follows the mouse movement. The *graphic user interface* (GUI) is used as the selection set. In this type of selection set, the screen contains a list of options, either written words or icons. If the mouse is moved to the option and a button is pressed (usually called *clicking*), then that item is chosen. Two rapid clicks are used to run, or execute, the program related to the icon. If the mouse button is held down while the mouse is pointing to a menu item and then the mouse is moved down the list (called *dragging* the mouse), a new list of choices appears. The GUI reduces the number of keystrokes and provides a prompting display for the user. The GUI does not require a mouse (e.g., the arrow keys can be used), but the mouse does require a GUI. The GUI has other characteristics and capabilities that are also important, and they are discussed in Chapter 8. Sometimes the GUI is oriented to a specific task such as drawing, and in other cases it is more general.

The mouse is ideally suited for functions such as drawing, moving around in a document, or moving a block of text. The mouse can be a useful tool for individuals with disabilities who cannot otherwise draw using a pen or pencil. However, mouse use requires a high degree of eye-hand coordination and motor coordination and a certain amount of range of motion. Standard computer mice are available in many different shapes and sizes. If a consumer is having difficulty using the mouse that came with the computer, the solution may be as simple as finding a mouse that fits his hand better. The standard mouse requires a great deal of motor control, however, and many individuals with disabilities find that the use of a standard computer mouse is difficult or impossible. Another option is to try a different control site for mouse use. If the consumer has better control of his feet than his hands, his foot can be used with a foot-controlled mouse such as the No Hands Mouse.* There are also alternatives to mouse

*Hunter Digital, Los Angeles, Calif. (www.earthlink.net/
~footmouse).

## CASE STUDY 7-2
### EVALUATION AND SELECTION OF A POINTING INTERFACE

David is a 21-year-old male who has muscular dystrophy. He would like to be able to access the family computer for educational and recreational purposes. David would like to play computer-based games and use drawing programs that typically require a mouse. He lacks movement in his four extremities, with the exception of wrist and finger movement. He is able to reach with each hand from within 3 inches of his body to 8 inches out from his body. With his right hand he can reach approximately 5.5 inches to the right of midline and with his left hand he can reach 3 inches to the left of midline. He cannot cross midline with either hand.

A contracted keyboard was tried by David, and he was able to point to keys in a restricted range near the middle of the keyboard. He was unable to access other areas of the keyboard without assistance for repositioning of his arms. He was able to move a continuous joystick in all four directions and use it with the on-screen keyboard software, but this was difficult for him. A trackball was also used with the on-screen keyboard software to determine whether David could use it. He could easily use the trackball as a pointing device to point to the keys shown on the screen. Using a drawing program and the trackball, he was able to direct the cursor to various parts of the screen with enough precision to draw lines and shapes. However, he was unable to hold the trackball in place with the cursor on the desired selection and simultaneously press the button on the trackball with the same hand to make his selection. The acceptance time selection technique was shown to him, and he was able to easily use this technique.

### QUESTIONS:

1. From the data given, would you recommend a contracted keyboard for David?
2. From the information given, what would be the optimal control interface for David? Is there other information you would like to find out regarding David's needs and skills that might influence your recommendation?
3. What other software will David need to operate the recommended control interface?

use that are easier for many persons with disabilities. Any control interface that can imitate the two-dimensional movement (up/down, left/right) of the mouse can be made to look to the computer like a mouse. Table 7-3 lists the major alternatives to mouse input, as well as sample technologies. Examples of several of these approaches are shown in Figure 7-10.

**Keypad mouse.** For those individuals who are able to use a standard keyboard but have difficulty using a standard mouse, the first alternative to evaluate is the keypad mouse. A numeric keypad is embedded in most standard computer keyboards. When used with Windows 95 and later versions, when the NUM LOCK key is engaged, each key on the numeric keypad functions as the number to which it is assigned (1 to 9). When the NUM LOCK key is disengaged and "mousekeys" (see Chapter 8) is running, these keys can perform the same functions as a mouse. The 5 key serves as a mouse click, and the surrounding number keys move the mouse in vertical, horizontal, or diagonal directions.

There are also keypad mice that are external to the standard keyboard, such as the Micro Pad.* The advantage of external keypads is that they can be placed in any position in the workspace. The disadvantage is that they take up more space on the work surface. External keypad mice are also available with enlarged keys, such as the Expanded Keypad† and the Big Blue Mouse,‡ both of which have

---

*Micro Innovations, Avenel, NJ.
†EKEG Electronics Co Ltd, Vancouver, BC, Canada.
‡EKEG Electronics Co Ltd, Vancouver, BC, Canada.

---

| TABLE 7-3 | Alternative Electronic Pointing Interfaces | |
|---|---|---|
| Category | Description | Device Name/Manufacturer |
| Keypad mouse | Mouse movement is replaced by keys that move the mouse cursor in horizontal, vertical, and diagonal directions. One or more keys perform the functions of the mouse button (click, double-click, drag). | Big Blue Mouse and MacRat (EKEG Electronics Co. Ltd.); R.A.T. (Adaptivation, Inc.); see Chapter 8 for software solutions |
| Trackball | Looks like an inverted mouse; a ball is mounted on a stationary base. Included on the base are one or more buttons that provide the functions of the standard mouse buttons. The base and hand remain stationary and the fingers move the ball. Requires minimal range of motion and less eye-hand coordination. | Thumbelina Mini Trackball (Appoint); Trackman Marble Plus (Logitech); EasyBall (Microsoft); Roller Trackball (Penny & Giles Computer Products) |
| Continuous input joysticks | Joysticks (continuous input and switched) are used as direct selection interfaces for powered mobility. For computer use, movements are similar to wheelchair control; easy to relate cursor movement (direction, speed, and distance) to joystick movement. | Jouse (Prentke Romich Co); Roller Joystick (Penny & Giles Computer Products); all manufacturers of powered wheelchairs have their own joystick, which is supplied with wheelchair |
| Head-controlled mouse | An interface controlled through head movement; the user wears a sensor on the head, which is detected by a unit on the computer. Movement of the head is translated into cursor movement on the screen. | Head Master Plus (Prentke Romich Co.); Head Mouse (Origin Instruments Co.); Tracker (Madentec Ltd. Communications) |
| Light pointers and light sensors | These devices either emit a light beam that can be used to point to objects or as a control interface, or they receive light and provide an output when the light is reflected from an object or the light beam is interrupted. | Light-operated Ability Switch (Ability Research, Inc.); Viewpoint Optical Indicator (Prentke Romich); Infrared/sound/touch switch (Words+ Inc.) |

Data from Ability Research, Inc., Minnetoka, MN (www.skypoint.com/~ability/contacts/html); Adaptivation, Sioux Falls, SD (www.adaptivation.com); Appoint, Pleasanton, CA; Logitech, Fremont, CA (www.logitech.com); Madentec Limited, Edmonton, Alberta, Canada (www.madentec.com); Microsoft, Redmond, WA (www.microsoft.com); Origin Instruments, Grand Prairie, TX (www.orin.com); Prentke Romich Co., Wooster, OH (www.prenrom.com); Words+ Inc. (www.words-plus.com).

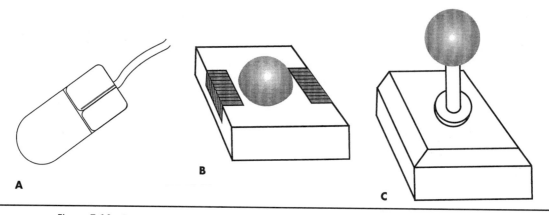

Figure 7-10    Pointing interfaces. **A,** Standard computer mouse. **B,** Trackball. **C,** Proportional joystick.

1.5-inch square membrane keys. Input using mouse keys is discussed in greater detail in Chapter 8.

**Trackball.** Use of a trackball is one approach that was developed for the able-bodied population but has often been found to be helpful for persons who cannot use the mouse. This device looks like an inverted mouse; a ball is mounted on a stationary base. Included on the base are one or more buttons that provide the functions of the standard mouse buttons. The ball is rotated by moving the hand or finger across it, causing the cursor to move on the screen. Because the base and hand remain stationary and the fingers move the ball, this approach requires less range of motion than the standard mouse and is easier for some disabled users. It is also possible to use the trackball easily with other body sites such as a chin or foot. On most trackballs the user can latch the mouse button. This allows single-finger or mouthstick users to perform "click and drag" functions without having to hold down a button while simultaneously moving the mouse. Trackballs are available in a variety of sizes, shapes, and configurations. There are trackballs (such as the Trackman Marble Plus*) in which the ball is positioned on the side where it can be controlled by the thumb. There are also very small trackballs such as the Thumbelina Mini Trackball† that fit in the palm of the hand. Having the consumer try the different types of trackballs is important, even if this means taking a trip to a local computer store that has different models available for demonstration.

**Continuous input joysticks.** A joystick provides four directions of control and is thus ideally suited for use as another alternative to the mouse. There are two types of joysticks: proportional (continuous) and switched (discrete). A proportional joystick has continuous signals, so that any movement of the control handle results in an immediate response by the command domain in that direction. Using a proportional joystick, the individual can control not only direction of movement, but also the rate of that movement. Proportional joysticks are most commonly used with powered wheelchairs. The farther the wheelchair joystick moves away from the starting point, the faster the wheelchair goes. The proportional joystick is also more likely to be used as a mouse substitute, since the direction and rate of cursor movement can be controlled by the user. The Jouse‡ is a joystick-operated mouse that is controlled with the chin or mouth. Mouse button activations can be made using a puff-and-sip switch that is built into the joystick. Just like the proportional joystick used for wheelchair control, the joystick used for a mouse substitute will cause the mouse

pointer to move faster the farther away it gets from the center position. A major difference between mouse and trackball use and the use of a joystick is that the joystick is always referenced to a center point, whereas the mouse cursor movement is relative to the current position. This can cause difficulties for the consumer when first using the joystick. The user must spend some time learning how to use this control interface in order for it to be an effective alternative to the mouse (Anson, 1997).

**Head-controlled mouse.** For individuals who lack the hand or foot movement to operate a mouse or joystick, there are alternative pointing interfaces that are controlled using head movement (Figure 7-11, *A*). The user wears a sensor that is attached either to the forehead directly with adhesive, to a pair of glasses, or to a band or headset worn on the head. Through the sensor, a tracking unit on the computer detects head movement and translates it into a signal that the computer interprets as if it were sent by a mouse. By moving the head (with the sensor on it), the person moves the cursor on the screen. For mouse-related tasks (e.g., selecting an icon, opening a window), the head-controlled interface is a direct replacement. Clicking and double-clicking are done by using either an acceptance (or dwell) time (which can be adjusted to meet the user's needs) or a switch. When a switch is used, it is often a puff-and-sip switch that is attached directly to the headset. The person generates a single puff to click and two puffs to double-click. To perform the drag function the user must produce sustained pressure on the puff switch. Some individuals may not have the breath control to perform the drag function. In this case there are software programs that can be used; we discuss these in Chapter 8. For typing, the head-controlled interface must be used with an on-screen keyboard program (also see the section regarding on-screen keyboards in Chapter 8).

In general, head-controlled mouse systems operate by using a tracking unit that senses and measures head position relative to a fixed reference point. This reference point is the center of the screen for the cursor. As the head moves away from this point in any direction, the cursor is moved on the screen. The technology that is used to sense the head movement differs from one system to another and may be ultrasound, infrared, or image recognition. Each of these relies on transmission of a signal to the sensor on the user's head and detection of a reflected signal that is sent back. Different commercial systems implement this reflective measurement in a variety of ways. In early versions of head-controlled interfaces, the headset worn by the user was connected with a wire to the computer. This made it difficult for the user to come and go from the computer independently. Most of the systems currently available have a wireless connection, which allows the user to move around more freely. Several devices require only a reflective dot to be placed on the user's face (usually the

---

*Logitech, Fremont, Calif. (www.logitech.com).
†Appoint, Pleasanton, Calif.
‡Prentke Romich Co., Wooster, Ohio (www.prenrom.com).

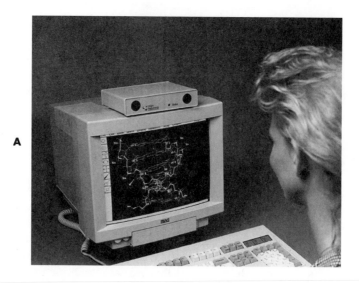

**A**

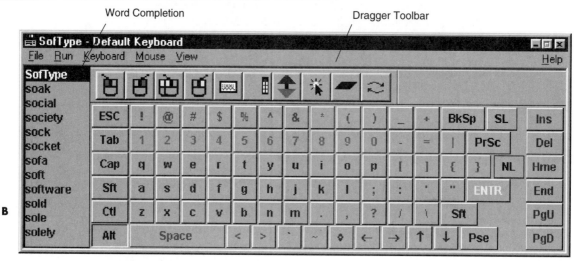

Word Completion                    Dragger Toolbar

**B**

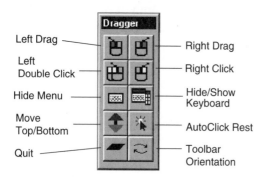

Left Drag

Left
Double Click

Hide Menu

Move
Top/Bottom

Quit

Right Drag

Right Click

Hide/Show
Keyboard

AutoClick Rest

Toolbar
Orientation

Figure 7-11    **A,** Head-controlled mouse. **B,** An example of an on-screen keyboard screen for Microsoft Windows. (Courtesy Origin Instruments Corporation, www.orin.com.)

forehead). This eliminates the bulky head pointer used in earlier devices.

These systems are intended for individuals who lack upper extremity movement and who can accurately control head movement. For example, persons with high-level spinal cord injuries who cannot use any limb often find these head pointers to be rapid and easy to use. On the other

hand, individuals who have random head movement or who do not have trunk alignment with the vertical axis of the video screen often have significantly more trouble using this type of input device.

**On-screen keyboards.** Much work has been done to make the many useful features of keyboards available to individuals who are unable to use any of the keyboards described earlier. We use the term **on-screen keyboard** to refer to keyboard emulation methods (discussed in Chapter 8) that employ the use of an image of the keyboard on the video screen, together with a cursor. The keyboard image, shown in Figure 7-11, *B,* is divided into "keys," each of which is labeled with an alphanumeric character, special character, or function. All the possible keys on the computer keyboard being emulated are included within the on-screen keyboard display. In order to enter a character or select a function, the user of the on-screen keyboard positions the cursor inside the desired "key" on the screen. Movement of the cursor can be by mouse, trackball, joystick, switch array, or head-controlled mouse. Once the cursor is located inside the targeted key, the user makes the selection either by activating another switch or by holding the cursor on the choice until it is accepted by the device.

In general, on-screen keyboards are designed for text entry only, and they do not provide access to graphics-based software. Not all on-screen keyboards are the same, and there are choices of format, image size (some take the whole screen, others only a small part), choice of input devices, amount of memory used, and price. The ATP should thoroughly evaluate all possible options based on consumer needs and skills.

**Light pointers and light sensors.** A visible light beam may be used as a pointing interface for direct selection. In a simple form the light can be pointed at objects in a room or at letters on a piece of paper. The effectiveness of the light pointer is directly related to how bright it is, and this in turn affects size and weight. Light pointers are most commonly attached to a band worn on the head, but they can also be held in the hand.

To use a light beam with an electronic device, we need to have a light sensor that can detect that the light has been shined on it. Any number of light sensors can be used, but typically we use an array of light sensors, one for each element in the selection set. Then the light pointer is used to point to any element.

It is also possible to reverse the role of the light detector and the light pointer. This has some advantages because the detectors are smaller and weigh less than the lights. In this approach an array of lights is rapidly turned on and off in sequence from the upper left corner of the array to the lower right corner, one light at a time. As a result of sensory memory and persistence of the image on the retina (see Chapter 3), the user has the perception that all the lights are dimly lit. The light sensor, usually worn on the head, is aimed at one of the lights, and when that light is turned on, it is detected by the sensor. The device knows which light is on at any time, and it can relate the sensor output to a specific light. When a light is chosen, it is turned on for a longer period and it becomes brighter to the user. This

approach has the major disadvantage that the sensor worn on the head does not emit light, and the user cannot see where she is pointing, except by the feedback from the selected light. This approach is used with the Vantage* and the Vanguard.†

## Speech Recognition

Speech recognition is an alternative method for keyboard input developed for the able-bodied population that is becoming widely used by individuals who have disabilities. With speech recognition systems, the individual uses sounds, letters, or words as a selection method. Speech recognition systems detect the pressure waveforms produced by speech and generate a signal that is transformed into output (Baker, 1981).

Two basic types of speech recognition systems exist. With a *speaker-dependent system,* the user trains the system to recognize his voice by producing several samples of the same element. The method in which the training is handled varies among systems. Some systems average the words spoken during training and compile them into a single template, whereas other systems keep each voice sample separate (Baker, 1981). The system analyzes these samples so that it can recognize variations in the user's speech and generate a signal. The disadvantage, of course, is that even after the system has been trained using several speech samples, there likely will be times when the system does not recognize the user's speech and does not produce a response. Recognition accuracy is steadily increasing as advances are made in the computer algorithms used for analysis. Rates can be greater than 75% for general input and nearly 100% for isolated word applications (e.g., command and control, database, spreadsheet). Speaker-dependent systems can be further divided into continuous and discrete categories. Comerford, Makhoul, and Schwartz (1997) describe the development of automatic speech recognition (ASR) systems and describe the technical aspects of these systems. They predict growth in use of ASR systems for application with the Internet, dictation, and general telephone use; most computer activities will be possible via ASR by the year 2005. These advances will create a sufficient demand for these systems to ensure low cost and high functionality. Persons with disabilities will be the beneficiaries.

*Speaker-independent systems* recognize speech patterns of different individuals without training (Gallant, 1989). These systems are developed using samples of speech from hundreds of people and information provided by phonologists on the various pronunciations of words (Baker, 1981). The tradeoff with this type of total-recognition system is that the vocabulary set is small. In assistive technology

---

*Prentke Romich Co., Wooster, Ohio.
†Prentke Romich Co., Wooster, Ohio.

## CASE STUDY 7-3

### EVALUATION AND SELECTION OF SPEECH RECOGNITION

Marilyn Abraham is a 44-year-old woman who has been diagnosed as having reflex sympathetic dystrophy (RSD) of both wrists. Apparently caused by vasospasm and vasodilation, RSD is a reaction to pain after an injury (Kasch, Poole, and Hedl, 1998). It results in edema; shiny, blotchy skin; and pain. Ms. Abraham is a secretary in a large state office, which she shares with other co-workers. She uses the computer for much of the day. The RSD ensued in her right wrist as a result of the repetitive motion she uses in performing her job. After this injury she received retraining to transfer her hand dominance to her left hand and the Dvorak one-handed keyboard layout was recommended (see Figure 7-12). Subsequently she broke her left wrist in a motor vehicle accident, which also resulted in RSD. She is able to type or use the mouse for only 10 minutes before her hands and forearms swell. Ms. Abraham has tried different positions and adaptations when typing. For example, she used a pointer held by a cuff in her palm to type so that her forearm remained in a neutral position. This still resulted in swelling and pain. She also experiences neck pain when using the keyboard.

Ms. Abraham first tried using a trackball with her hand and the on-screen keyboard. After using the trackball for a short time, Ms. Abraham found that it also caused pain. Ms. Abraham next tried using her right foot with an expanded keyboard and then a trackball. There were concerns about the utility of both these approaches because of potential neck strain from looking down and that possibility that the repeated movement of her ankle to input characters using the trackball might lead to repetitive motion problems with her foot.

Next Ms. Abraham tried a head-controlled interface that was worn on a band and attached to her head. She used this interface with an on-screen keyboard and acceptance time to make a selection. She was able to control this interface without difficulty but thought that after a period of use her neck would become tired.

### QUESTIONS:

1. What other control interfaces could you try with Ms. Abraham?
2. If you evaluate automatic speech recognition for Ms. Abraham, what issues will you need to take into consideration?

applications, speaker-independent systems are primarily used for environmental and robotic control (Chapter 11) and powered mobility (Chapter 10).

The earliest types of speech recognition systems were discrete types. These systems require the user to pause between each word in order for recognition to occur. This is a very unnatural type of speech, and there have been reports of voice problems associated with the use of discrete speech recognition systems (Kambeyanda, Singer, and Cronk, 1997). These are due to the abrupt starting and stopping of speech required for these systems, coupled with the monotone quality required for good recognition, both of which are unnatural speech patterns. In an attempt to make the systems easier to use and to avoid some of the vocal stress problems, continuous automatic speech recognition systems were developed. These systems allow the user to speak in a more normal manner, without major pauses. The rates of input are getting faster, but they still are barely within the range of normal rates of human speech (150 to 250 words per minute). This means that it is still necessary for the speaker to adjust her speech pattern to maximize recognition. Although the possibility of damage to the vocal folds is reduced with these systems, it is not totally eliminated. Because the discrete systems are more accurate for single-word recognition, they are sometimes used for commands and control in applications like spreadsheets and databases. Some manufacturers (e.g., Dragon Systems*) provide both continuous (e.g., Naturally Speaking) and discrete (e.g., Dragon Dictate) automatic speech recognition, sometimes bundled into the same package. Currently used speech recognition systems are listed in Table 7-4. The majority of these use continuous recognition.

Speech recognition can be used for computer access, wheelchair control, and EADLs. The systems shown in Table 7-4 allow the consumer to use his speech to enter text directly into a computer application program. Recognition of control words, such as "save file," used in a word processor are also trained. System vocabulary is also growing rapidly. Early systems had recognition vocabularies (the list of words the system can recognize when spoken) in the 1000 to 5000 range. Current systems have vocabularies of 50,000 words or more. The faster speech rate, larger vocabularies, and continuous recognition all place significant demands on the speed and memory of the host computer. Continuous speech recognition systems require large amounts of memory and high-speed computers. As the cost of this added computer functionality continues

---

*Newton, Mass. (www.dragonsys.com).

**TABLE 7-4** Speech Recognition Interfaces

| Category | Description | Device Name/Manufacturer |
|---|---|---|
| Speaker-dependent systems | Recognition depends on the system's learning the user's speech patterns and building a user vocabulary. | Naturally Speaking and Dragon Dictate (Dragon Systems); Via Voice (IBM); Voice Xpress (Lernout and Hauspie); Free Speech98 (Phillips Electronics N.V.); Voice Commander Pro (Applied Voice Recognition, Inc); Voice Pilot Global (Voice Pilot Technologies) |
| Speaker-independent systems | The operation is similar to continuous speech recognition systems, but there is no training required. Generally limited to small, application-specific vocabularies. | Used in special-purpose assistive devices for environmental control or robotic control (see Chapter 11) and wheelchair control (see Chapter 10). |

to decline, these additional requirements will be less important. However, ASR systems do require more computer resources than other alternative input methods (Anson, 1999).

There are other hardware issues that are important in ASR as well. Foremost of these is the microphone. Anson (1997) discusses considerations in the choice of a microphone for ASR. Although the microphones supplied with ASR systems are satisfactory for use by nondisabled users, they are not adequate when the user has limited breath support, special positioning requirements, or low-volume speech. Most ASR systems use a standard headset microphone. Individuals who have disabilities may not be able to don and doff such microphones independently, and desk-mounted types are often used. Current ASR systems do not require separate hardware to be installed in the computer, and they utilize commonly available sound cards (Anson, 1999).

EADLs may also utilize speech recognition to access their functions (see Chapter 11). In such devices the individual can instruct the system to turn lights off and on or perform other functions using her voice. She can train the system to execute these commands with just about any sound, letter, or word.

The questions listed in Box 7-3 can be used to determine the usefulness of speech recognition for a given consumer. The key for success in using speech-activated systems is that the user be able to produce a *consistent* vocalization or verbalization. Differences in speech production are found not only among individual speakers, but also within the same speaker. Variability in the user's speech can cause problems with recognition. For this reason, this type of control interface may not be effective for individuals who have dysarthria. Individuals who have had a spinal cord injury and have no functional use of the upper extremities yet have good speech control are potential candidates for a speech recognition system. It is important when considering a speech recognition system to determine whether the user's voice pitch, articulation, and loudness change or fatigue over time. Other noises or voices in the area where the speech-

**BOX 7-3** Critical Questions for Evaluating Use of Speech Recognition Interface

1. Can the consumer consistently utter all the sounds necessary to access the speech recognition system?
2. Is the recognition vocabulary adequate?
3. Is the consumer's voice articulation, pitch, and loudness consistent enough for accurate selection?
4. Is there likely to be background noise in the consumer's context that will interfere with the speech recognition system?
5. Would an alternative template or vocabulary be beneficial?

activated system is being used can also confuse the system. This results in either an incorrect selection or the system having difficulty registering any selection, causing the user to repeat the vocalization several times.

## Eye-Controlled Systems

A final type of control interface for direct selection is a system that detects the user's eye movements. Manual eye-controlled communication systems have been in use for a long time. In manual systems the user communicates yes or no though eye blinks or uses the eyes to point to letters on an alphabet board to spell utterances. This manual form of using eye movement as a means of input has recently been translated to electronic eye-controlled systems.

There are currently two basic types of eye-controlled systems. One type employs an infrared video camera mounted below a computer monitor. An infrared beam from the camera is shined on the person's eye and then reflected by the retina. The camera picks up this reflection of the individual's eye as he looks at the on-screen keyboard appearing on the computer monitor. Special processing software in the computer analyzes the images coming into the camera from the eyes and determines where and for how long the person is looking on the screen. The user makes a selection by looking at it for a specified period, which can be

| TABLE 7-5 | Modifications to Keyboards and Pointing Interfaces | |
|---|---|---|
| **Need Addressed** | | **Approach** |
| User's speed not adequate for task prediction software* | | Modify keyboard layout, macros, rate enhancement software, word |
| User has problems making accurate selections | | Keyguard, template, shield, delayed acceptance* |
| User has difficulty holding down the modifier key while pressing another key | | Mechanical latch, software latch* |
| User cannot release key before it starts to repeat | | Keyguard, careful selection of keyboard characteristics; software to disable key repeat function* |

*Software modifications are discussed in Chapter 8.

adjusted according to the user's needs. The EyeGaze System* and Quick Glance† are examples of two eye-controlled systems of this type. The other type of eye-controlled system utilizes a head-mounted viewer that tracks the movements of one eye. This viewer is attached to one side of the frame of a standard pair of glasses so that it is in front of one eye. The movements from the eye are viewed and converted into keyboard input by a separate control unit. One example of this type of system is VisionKey.‡ Both types of eye-controlled systems provide the user with computer access for written or verbal communication, Internet access, environmental control, and telephone operation. To operate either type of eye-controlled system the user must have good vision and control of at least one eye; good head control, including the ability to keep the head fairly stationary; and the cognitive ability to follow instructions.

An eye-controlled system is beneficial for individuals who have little or no movement in their limbs and may also have limited speech, for example, someone who has had a brainstem stroke, has amyotrophic lateral sclerosis (ALS), or has high-level quadriplegia. Some disadvantages of eye-controlled systems are that sunlight, bright incandescent lighting, and contact lenses may interfere with system tracking, and the cost of such systems is still rather high in comparison with other input methods. For some individuals, however, this may be the only reliable means of control.

## Modifications to Keyboards and Pointing Interfaces

There are several problems that may be experienced by individuals with a physical disability in using any of the control interfaces just described. As mentioned earlier, if a consumer is having difficulty using a particular control interface, there are three paths to pursue. A control enhancer may resolve the difficulty (e.g., when the user has limited range for accessing the interface). Modification of

the interface being evaluated is another alternative, and trying a less limiting interface is the third approach. Before introducing a less limiting control interface, modification of the method being evaluated should be considered. Table 7-5 lists the areas of need for which modification of a control interface may be beneficial and approaches that can be used. Each of these difficulties in using a keyboard can be addressed by either hardware or software modifications. Here we discuss hardware approaches, and in Chapter 8 we discuss software solutions to these problems.

**Keyboard layouts.** The QWERTY keyboard layout (Figure 7-12, *A*), the one most familiar to people, was originally designed more than 100 years ago to slow down 10-finger typists using a manual typewriter so the keys would not jam. The QWERTY layout requires much excursion of the fingers and assumes that two hands with 10 fingers will be used. With an increasing number of individuals using computers, there has been a substantial increase in repetitive strain injuries to the hand. Redefining the layout of the characters on the keyboard can reduce the amount of finger movements required by the user to access the keys and may reduce fatigue and the likelihood of an individual's incurring a repetitive strain injury. Furthermore, there are alternative keyboard layout designs that have been developed to accelerate typing speed, such as when the individual is using only one hand or a mouthstick. With computer keyboards, the definition of the keyboard layout is determined by software in the computer and the keys are labeled with the corresponding characters. The keyboard hardware (other than labeling of the keys) is not modified with any of the alternative keyboard layouts.

Developed in the 1930s by University of Washington Professor August Dvorak, the Dvorak keyboard layout was designed to reduce fatigue and increase speed by placing letters that are most frequently used on the home row of the keyboard. On the left side of the home row are all the vowels, and five of the most used consonants are on the right side of the home row. There are three Dvorak keyboard layouts: one for two-handed typists (Figure 7-12, *B*), one for right hand-only typists (Figure 7-12, *C*), and one

*LC Technologies, Inc., Fairfax, Va. (www.lctinc.com/).
†EyeTech Digital Systems, Mesa, Ariz. (www.eyetechds.com/).
‡H.K. EyeCan Ltd., Ottawa, Canada (www.cyberbus.ca/~eyecan).

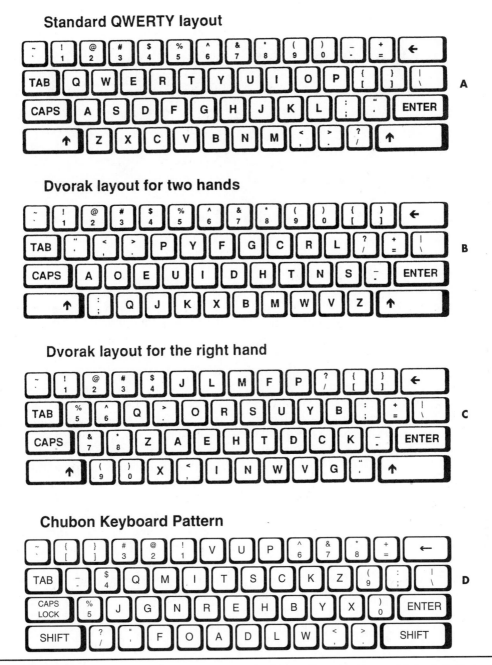

**Figure 7-12    A,** Standard QWERTY layout. Dvorak keyboard layouts: **B,** two-hand layout; **C,** one-hand layout, right hand; **D,** Chubon keyboard layout for a typist who uses a single digit or a typing stick.

for left hand-only typists (similar to that shown for right hand-only typists but flipped). Information on how to redefine the computer keyboard as a Dvorak layout can be found at this Web site: web.mit.edu/jcb/www/Dvorak/index.html.

The Chubon keyboard is a layout pattern that was designed to be used by the single-digit or typing-stick typist (Chubon and Hester, 1988). In this layout (Figure 7-12, *D*) the letters in the English language that are used most frequently are arranged near each other in the center. This

layout also places letters that are most frequently used together (e.g., *r* and *e*) in close proximity. This reduces the amount of movement required by the user for entering text and helps to increase the rate of input. For individuals who use a mouthstick or typing stick, an alternative keyboard layout that reduces the amount of travel to keys can significantly increase efficiency.

Another alternative keyboard layout is an alphabetical array. Often individuals who are nonverbal and have been using a manual communication board to spell have learned

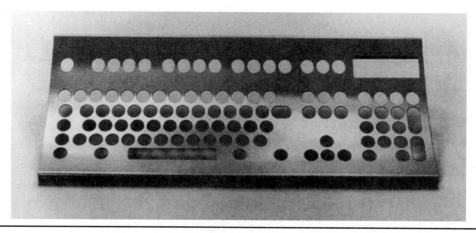

Figure 7-13   Keyguard. (Courtesy TASH, Ajax, Ontario, Canada.)

to use an array in which the letters are placed in alphabetical order. They are very familiar with this arrangement and may be very efficient in selecting characters. For these individuals, it often does not make sense to have them learn a completely new letter arrangement. In this case the keyboard can be redefined, using software, to have an alphabetical arrangement.

When selecting a keyboard pattern, several factors need to be considered. The first factor to consider is whether the user is already familiar with one particular keyboard layout. If this is the case, it is important to keep in mind that the time needed for retraining to use a new keyboard pattern is estimated at 90 to 100 hours (Anson, 1997). Another factor to consider is whether the keyboard is shared with other individuals. It is possible to have the computer keyboard defined to use two keyboard patterns (e.g., QWERTY and Dvorak) and to label the keys so that the standard keys are not obscured (e.g., via a clear overlay with the new key labels on them, so when placed over the standard keys the original labels are still visible). However, this can be confusing to all typists. Finally, there are little data to support the claims that alternative keyboard patterns increase speed or reduce injury. Selecting an alternative keyboard, like other technologies, depends on the needs and skills of the user and which layout she feels most comfortable and efficient using.

**Keyguards, shields, and templates.** Some persons may be able to select individual keys directly, but they may occasionally miss the desired key and enter the wrong key. For individuals who have difficulty in accurately targeting and activating keys, a keyguard (Figure 7-13) placed over the keyboard helps by isolating each key and guiding the person's movement. A keyguard is also useful for individuals who produce a lot of extraneous movement each time they bring their hand off the keyboard in their attempt to target a new key. Instead of moving away from the keyboard to make the next selection, the person can rest his hand on top of the keyguard without activating any keys and make

relatively isolated, controlled (and thus faster) selections. Although keyguards have been shown to increase the user's accuracy, speed is typically compromised (McCormack, 1990). In nearly all situations a clear keyguard is preferred, so that there is minimal obstruction of the labels on the keys. Still, the position of the keyboard with a keyguard needs to be assessed to ensure that the key labels are not being obstructed from the user's view. Keyguards are commercially available for the common computer keyboards. There are cases, though, where an individual uses a special terminal in a work setting and would benefit from a keyguard. In these instances a keyguard can easily be custom fabricated out of clear plastic to fit the desired terminal.

Similar to the use of a keyguard is the use of a shield on the keyboard to block out certain keys. This is typically done with children who are just beginning to use computers and are using software programs that only require the use of a few select keys. To guide the child to the correct keys and increase her chances of success with the program, a shield is placed over the keys that are not being used.

A template used on a joystick to guide the individual's movement is akin to the use of a keyguard for a keyboard. The template has four channels that guide the movement of the joystick. The shape of the channel may vary depending on the template, and this can be a factor in the individual's ability to control the joystick. For example, an individual using the cross-shaped template in Figure 7-14, *A*, may need more precise movement to enter the desired channel but once in one of these channels will be able to stay easily. If the template is like the one in Figure 7-14, *B*, it will be easy for the individual to enter one of the channels but difficult to stay. A compromise solution is to use a template similar to the one shown in Figure 7-14, *C*. In this case, because the entrance to each arm of the cross has been widened, it is easier to move in each direction. Because the end of the slot in each direction retains the cross shape, it is easier to keep the joystick in one direction. We can also improve the performance of the star template (Figure

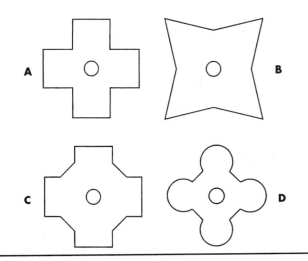

Figure 7-14    **A-D**, Four different shapes of joystick templates to maximize user's skills.

7-14, *B*) by restricting the travel at the end of the channel once the movement has been made in a direction. This change is shown in Figure 7-14, *D*. For some individuals, the use and type of joystick template means the difference between success or failure in the operation of a powered wheelchair.

**Technologies for reducing accidental entries.** Many keyboards produce multiple entries of characters by prolonged pressing of the key. This is called *key repeat*. Although this is useful to nondisabled users (e.g., to obtain multiple spaces or underlines), it can present a problem for persons with disabilities who may not be able to release the key fast enough to prevent double entry. There are a number of ways this can be avoided. Certain types and sensitivities of keyboards may increase or decrease double entries, and auditory feedback (e.g., a beep) when a key is activated may also cue the user to release the key in a timely manner. Both of these are sensory characteristics of control interfaces, described earlier in this chapter, that need to be considered as part of the overall assessment. Sometimes the presence of a keyguard helps to diminish the double entries. If the double entries remain a problem, there are software applications that disable the repeat key feature; these are discussed in Chapter 8.

### ■ CONTROL INTERFACES FOR INDIRECT SELECTION

When an individual's physical control does not permit him to select directly, indirect selection methods are considered. Indirect methods of selection use a single switch or an array of switches and require that the consumer be able to carry out a certain set of skills. Box 7-4 shows the critical questions to pose during the evaluation to determine whether the consumer has the basic set of skills for switch use.

During the evaluation, it is first necessary to determine whether the user can *activate* the switch. This determines whether there is a match between the sensory, spatial, and activation (e.g., force) requirements of the switch and the physical-sensory skills of the user. If activation is possible, it is necessary to look at other skills related to the way the switch is to be used for indirect selection. The first of these is whether the consumer can *wait* for the desired selection to be presented. This requires that the consumer have sensory skills for awareness of the selections being presented. Depending on the consumer's sensory abilities, selections can be presented visually or auditorily. An inability to wait can result from problems with central processing or motor control. If the consumer is having difficulty waiting, determining the underlying cause (i.e., sensory, central processing, or motor) may make it possible to modify the task. However, this is not always easy to determine. The consumer must also be able to *reliably activate the switch at the right time* (i.e., when the desired selection is presented).

Another critical condition is that the consumer be able to *hold* a switch in its closed position for the time it takes the signal from the control interface to register. This time is a variable of the control interface and may differ from switch to switch. In addition, applications such as Morse code input, inverse scanning, and wheelchair mobility require the user to hold the switch closed. Within each of these applications, the length of this hold time varies. For example, for the person using one-switch Morse code, the hold time varies from shorter to longer depending on the input signal (dot or dash). Inverse scanning (see next section) and wheelchair mobility are other applications that require the user to hold down the switch for varying lengths of time. With inverse scanning, the switch is held until the right choice appears; for wheelchair mobility, the switch is held down until the user wants the chair to stop. If the user cannot carry out precise holding of the switch, it can result in frustration, embarrassment, and possibly serious injury in the case of mobility. If the consumer is having difficulty activating or holding the switch, the switch may require too much force or displacement for activation or the sensory

Mrs. Antonelli is a 30-year-old woman who has spastic quadriplegia as a result of meningitis at age 10. She lives with her husband and 2-year-old daughter. Mrs. Antonelli was referred for an evaluation for an augmentative communication system for conversation and writing. She has limited functional speech and communicates primarily by finger spelling with her left hand. Her husband interprets the finger spelling, but many others with whom Mrs. Antonelli would like to communicate do not understand her finger spelling. She independently uses a powered wheelchair that she controls by a joystick with her left hand.

Mrs. Antonelli showed limited range using either hand, and her resolution seemed fair; therefore her ability to use keyboards was assessed using a contracted keyboard with each hand. She copied words with a great deal of effort and was less than 50% accurate.

Because Mrs. Antonelli uses a switched joystick to control her powered wheelchair, a switched joystick was tried with an electronic communication device in a directed scanning mode. Mrs. Antonelli used her left hand with the joystick in approximately the same position as her wheelchair joystick. She was able to move this joystick in all four directions. However, when asked to hold and release the joystick on a specific target, Mrs. Antonelli had difficulty. She was able to do this, but it required significant effort and several attempts to successfully select the desired target.

The pad switch,* a pneumatic switch, and a rocker switch† were then tried to evaluate the potential for Mrs. Antonelli to use coded access. The switches were positioned one at a time on the right wheelchair armrest and used with her right hand. Both a single-switch approach, in which a short switch hit produces a dot and a long switch hit produces a dash, and a dual-switch approach (one side produces dots and the other dashes) were tried. Mrs. Antonelli had difficulty with the one-switch mode because she was unable to consistently hold the switch for the appropriate length of time. In the two-switch mode, Mrs. Antonelli was able to move easily between the two parts of the rocker switch to generate dots and dashes. Mrs. Antonelli pressed one side of this switch with her index finger and one side with her middle finger. Mrs. Antonelli felt that the single switches were more difficult to operate than the rocker switch. Mrs. Antonelli also indicated a preference for the dual switch over the joystick for communication. She wanted to continue using her left hand to operate the joystick on her powered wheelchair and use her right hand for Morse code input into her communication device. Mrs. Antonelli acquired the communication system and, with a period of training, quickly memorized the Morse code; her rate of input became rapid.

*TASH, Ajax, Ontario, Canada.
†Prentke Romich Co., Wooster, Ohio.

feedback it provides may be inadequate. If this is the case, having the consumer experiment with less limiting switches is recommended. *Releasing* the switch in a timely manner is the next criterion. Inability to release the switch causes inadvertent selections. It is easier for some individuals to activate and hold the switch than to release it. Finally, it should be determined whether the consumer is able to carry out these sets of skills repeatedly.

The ATP can begin evaluating the consumer's skills by using simple technology such as a tape recorder or battery-operated toy as an output when the switch is activated. Once it is determined that the consumer can use the switch on command to control this output, switch activation, holding, and release can be evaluated using software programs designed for that purpose (see Chapter 4). Frequently the use of more than one body control site and candidate interface is considered for a given consumer. Using the critical questions to evaluate each pairing (control site and interface) will help the ATP to make a comparison among them and develop a recommendation. If the consumer has difficulty

with any of these skills, there are certain techniques that can make selection easier.

## Selection Techniques for Scanning

The action required by the user to activate the switch to make a selection during scanning and directed scanning usually can be varied to accommodate the user's skills. Table 7-6 lists the three scanning techniques and the level of skill required by the technique for each of the motor acts described earlier. This is helpful in matching the scanning technique to the user's skills. With **automatic scanning,** the items are presented continuously by the device at a rate that can be set and adjusted according to how fast the user can respond. When the desired selection is presented, the user selects the choice by activating the switch and stopping the scan. Automatic scanning requires a high degree of motor skill by the user to wait for the desired selection and to activate the switch in the given time frame. It also requires a high degree of sensory and cognitive vigilance for

**TABLE 7-6**  Selection Techniques for Scanning and Directed Scanning

|  | Automatic Scanning | Step Scanning | Inverse Scanning |
| --- | --- | --- | --- |
| Wait | High | Low | Medium |
| Activate | High | Medium | Low |
| Hold | Low | Low | High |
| Release | Low | Medium | High |
| Motor Fatigue | Low | High | Low |
| Sensory/Cognitive Vigilance | High | Low | High |

Modified from Beukelman D, Mirenda P: *Augmentative and alternative communication*, Baltimore, 1992, Paul H. Brookes, p 129.

**BOX 7-5**  Scanning Formats

**SELECTION SET FORMATS**
Linear
Circular
Matrix

**ADAPTATIONS TO FORMATS FOR INCREASING RATE OF SELECTION**
Group-item
Row-column
Halving
Quartering
Frequency of use placement

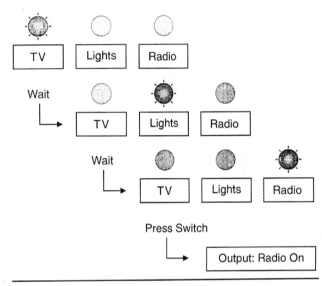

Figure 7-15   In linear scanning, choices are presented vertically or horizontally one at a time.

attending to and tracking the cursor on the display. With **step scanning,** the user activates the switch once for each item to move through the choices in the selection set. When the user comes to the desired choice, there are two possibilities for selecting it. Either an additional switch is used to give a signal to select that choice or an acceptance time is used. Step scanning allows the user to control the speed at which the items are presented. The ability to wait is not required for the scan but it may be for the acceptance of the selection. The ability to activate the switch repeatedly, however, is highly important for step scanning. Motor fatigue can be high because of repeated switch activation.

The last technique is **inverse scanning.** In this type of scanning the scan is initiated by the individual's activating and holding the switch closed. As long as the switch is held down, the items are scanned. When the desired choice appears, the individual releases the switch to make the selection. For accuracy, inverse scanning requires a high level of skill to hold the switch and release it at the proper time. For individuals who require lots of time to initiate and follow through with movement, inverse scanning may be easier than automatic scanning, which requires activation of the switch within a specified time frame. Like automatic scanning, motor fatigue is reduced over step scanning because of fewer switch activations; however, sensory and cognitive fatigue is higher because of the vigilance required to attend to the display.

Many devices are capable of providing each of these

scanning techniques as options for the user. Angelo (1992) performed a study with six subjects that compared these three scanning techniques. This study found that subjects with spastic cerebral palsy performed poorly using the automatic scanning technique. Step scanning was found to be the most difficult for subjects with athetoid cerebral palsy. In determining which technique is most suitable, it is helpful for the consumer to try each of these selection techniques to experience the subtle differences among them.

## Selection Formats for Scanning

In scanning, there are a number of formats in which the items in the selection set can be presented to the user for selection (Box 7-5). In a **linear** format, as shown in Figure 7-15, the items in the selection set are presented in a vertical or horizontal line and scanned one at a time until the desired selection is highlighted and selected by the user. With **circular,** or **rotary, scanning** (Figure 7-16), the items are presented in a circle and scanned one at a time. Because of the slowness inherent in both these types of scanning, Vanderheiden and Lloyd (1986) recommend that the array be limited to 15 choices.

To increase the rate of selection during scanning, **group-item scanning** can replace the singular-item scan. In this case there are several items in a group and the groups are sequentially scanned. The individual first selects the group that has the desired element. Once the group has been selected, the individual items in that group are scanned

until the desired item is reached. When there are a large number of items, a *matrix* scan can be used. In this type of scanning the *group* is a row of items and the *items* are located in columns; thus it is called **row-column scanning.** In row-column scanning there may be several rows of items and each complete row lights up sequentially. The row with the desired item is selected; then each column in that row lights up until the desired item is selected. Figure 7-17 shows the input required using a single switch with row-column scanning to produce the letter *S*.

There are other ways that scanning formats can be adapted to increase the user's rate of selection. *Halving* is a group-item approach in which the total array is divided in halves. Each half is scanned until the user selects the desired half. The scanning then proceeds in a row-column format as described above until the desired item is reached. This same concept can be used in a *quartering format,* in which the array is divided into fourths. Another method used to increase rate of selection is to place the selection set elements in the scanning array according to their frequency of use. For example, if letters are being used as the selection set, placement of *E, T, A, O, N, I* (the most frequently used letters) in the upper left positions of the scanning array results in a significant increase in rate of selection (Vanderheiden and Lloyd, 1986). The application of these principles to augmentative communication is discussed in Chapter 9.

## Coded Access

Coded access is another indirect selection input method that requires an intermediate step. As we discussed earlier, one of the most common and most efficient methods of coded access is Morse code. Figure 7-18 shows the symbols for international Morse code. The required sequence of movements for obtaining the letter *C* is dash, dot, dash, dot. In two-switch Morse code, one switch is configured to represent a dot and the other switch a dash. Figure 7-19

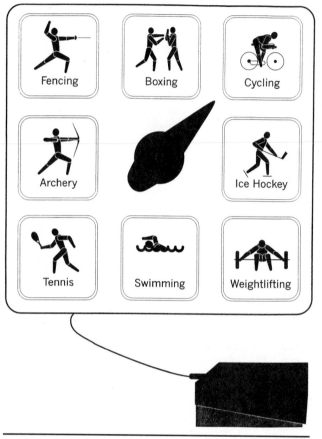

**Figure 7-16**   In rotary scanning, choices are presented one at a time in a circle.

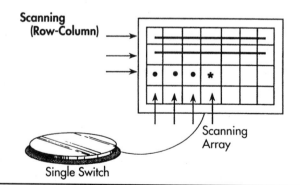

**Figure 7-17**   Row-column scanning showing the input required for selecting the letter *S*. The rows are first scanned and the user selects the row with the desired item. Then each item in that row is scanned until the desired item is selected. (From Smith RO: Technological approaches to performance enhancement. In Christiansen C, Baum C, editors: *Occupational therapy: overcoming human performance deficits,* Thorofare, NJ, 1991, Slack.)

shows the steps required for obtaining the letter *C* using two-switch Morse code. In single-switch Morse code the system is configured so that a quick activation and release of the switch results in a dot and holding the switch closed for a longer period before releasing it results in a dash. Letter boundaries are distinguished by a slightly longer pause than between dots and dashes within one letter.

Another example of coded access is Darci code. This selection method, used with the DARCI TOO* to control a computer (see Chapter 8), uses an eight-way switch code. An eight-way switch is similar to a four-position switched joystick, with the diagonal positions utilized as additional switch positions (Figure 7-20, *A*). Using this code, the letter *C* is generated by moving the switch to position 2, then to

*The Darci Institute of Rehabilitation Engineering, Farmington, Utah (www.darci.org/).

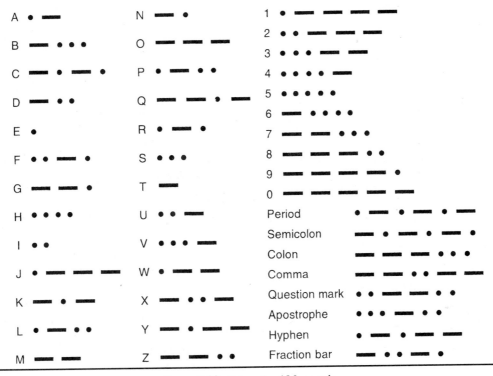

Figure 7-18    International Morse code.

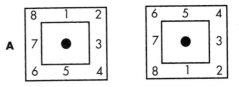

| Input | Morse Code | Output |
|---|---|---|
| Press Switch 1 | ▬ | |
| Press Switch 2 | ● | |
| Press Switch 1 | ▬ | |
| Press Switch 2 | ● | C |

Figure 7-19    The input required for selecting the letter *C* using Morse code.

| | Input | Output |
|---|---|---|
| **B** | Move joystick to position 2 | |
| | Move joystick to position 1 | |
| | Move joystick back to center | C |

Figure 7-20    **A,** Two alternatives for designating the light switch locations. **B,** The input required for selecting the letter *C* using Darci code.

**TABLE 7-7     Examples of Single-Switch Interfaces**

| Category | Description | Switch Name/Manufacturer |
|---|---|---|
| Mechanical switches | Activated by the application of a force; generic names of switches include paddle, plate, button, lever, membrane | Pal Pads (Adaptivation Corp.); Big Buddy Button, Microlight Switch, Grasp Switch (TASH); Big Red and Jelly Bean Switches (AbleNet Inc.); Leaf and Tread Switches (Zygo Industries); Wobble Switch (Prentke Romich Co.) |
| Electromagnetic switches | Activated by the receipt of electromagnetic energy such as light or radio waves | Infrared/sound/touch switch (Words +) |
| Electrical control switches | Activated by detection of electrical signals from the surface of the body | Taction Pad (Adaptivation Corp.) |
| Proximity switches | Activated by a movement close to the detector, but without actual contact | Airtouch Switch (Adaptivation Corp.); ASL 204 and 208, Proximity Switch (Adaptive Switch Laboratories, Inc.); Untouchable Buddy (Tash Inc.) |
| Pneumatic switches | Activated by detection of respiratory airflow or air pressure | LifeBreath Switch and Sip and Puff Switch (Toys for Special Children); ASL 308 Pneumatic Switch (Adaptive Switch Laboratories); PRC Pneumatic Switch Model PS-2 (Prentke Romich Co.); Pneumatic Switch Model CM-3 (Zygo Industries); Wireless Integrated Sip/Puff Switch (Madentec) |
| Phonation switches | Activated by sound or speech | Voice Activated Switch (Enabling Devices—Toys for Special Children); Infrared/Sound/Touch Switch (Words +) |

Data from Ablenet Inc., Minneapolis, MN (www.ablenetinc.com); Adaptive Switch Laboratories, Inc., Spicewood, TX, www.asl-inc.com; Adaptivation Co Sioux Falls, SD (www.adaptivation.com); Madentec Limited, Edmonton, Alberta, Canada (www.madentec.com); Prentke Romich, Wooster, OH (www.prenrom.com); TASH, Ajax, Ontario, Canada or Richmond, VA (www.tashinc.com); Enabling Devices—Toys for Special Children, Hastings-on-Hudson, NY (www.enablingdevices.com); Words + Inc., words-plus.com; Zygo, Portland OR (www.zygo-usa.com).

position 1, then to the center (Figure 7-20, *B*). It is this sequence of movements that tells the processor that the desired entry is the letter *C*. Using this access method, it is also possible to emulate mouse movements and to access whole words. Other eight-switch (sometimes called *eight-way*) codes have been used in augmentative communication devices (Chapter 9).

## Types of Single Switches

There are numerous single switches that are commercially available. It is also possible to custom fabricate switches, but this is not advised for a number of reasons. Although it may seem less inexpensive to purchase the materials to make a switch, when you factor in the time it takes to make the switch the cost involved increases significantly. In addition, custom-made switches are not as durable as commercially available switches and will not hold up over time.

When selecting a switch for an individual, it is important to consider the spatial, activation-deactivation, and sensory characteristics discussed earlier. Single switches come in many different sizes and shapes and have diverse force and sensory requirements. It is critical that the consumer have the opportunity to try out any switches being considered for a control interface.

We can categorize the types of switches by using the activation-deactivation characteristics of control interfaces described earlier. Single-switch interfaces can be activated by body movement, respiration, or phonation. Table 7-7 summarizes the types of single-switch interfaces and gives a sampling of switches that are available.

The switches that are activated by body movement detect the movement in one of four ways: mechanical, electromagnetic, electrical, or proximity. Switches that are mechanical in nature are activated by force applied by any part of the body. Mechanical switches are the most commonly used type of single switch, and they can be of various shapes and sizes. Paddle switches (Figure 7-21, *A*) have movement in one direction. On some types of paddle switches the sensitivity can be adjusted according to the user's needs. Wobble (Figure 7-21, *B*) and leaf switches (Figure 7-21, *C*) have a 2- to 4-inch shaft that can be activated by the user in two directions. The wobble switch makes an audible click when activated and the leaf switch does not, making the wobble switch more desirable when the switch is out of the user's visual range, such as during head activation. Lever switches (Figure 7-21, *D*) are similar to wobble switches with the exception that they can only be activated in one direction. This type of switch usually has a round, padded area at the end of a shaft and produces an audible click, which also makes it desirable for activation by the head. There are also various types of button switches that come in different sizes,

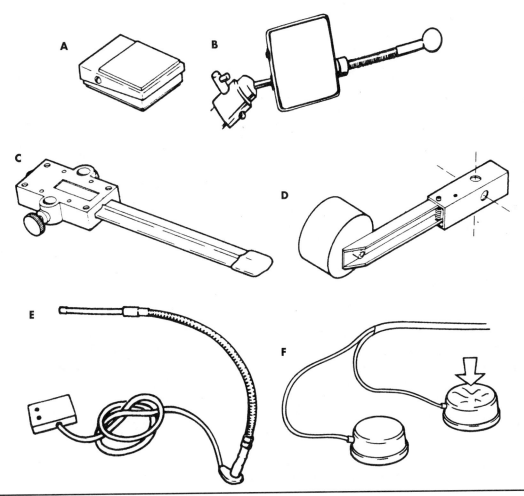

Figure 7-21    Examples of single switches. **A,** Paddle switch. **B,** Wobble switch. **C,** Leaf switch. **D,** Lever switch. **E,** Puff-and-sip switch. **F,** Pillow switch. (**A, C,** and **D,** Courtesy Zygo Industries, Portland. **B, E,** and **F** from Bergen AF, Presperin J, Tallman T: *Positioning for function: wheelchairs and other assistive technologies,* Valhalla, NY, 1990, Valhalla Rehabilitation Publications.)

from a large, round switch such as the Big Red switch,* to a small button switch that can be held between the thumb and the index finger, such as the Cap switch.† Membrane switches consist of a very thin pad, which also requires some degree of force to activate. These pads are available in various sizes, from as small as 2 inches × 3 inches to as large as 3 inches × 5 inches. The advantage of these membrane pads are that they are flexible, can be paired with an object (by being directly attached to it), and can be used to teach the user to make a direct connection between the object and the switch. The main disadvantage of membrane switches is that they provide poor tactile feedback. This can lead to extra activations or failure to apply enough force to activate the switch. All these switches are activated by body movement that produces a force upon the switch. They are considered *passive switches* because they do not require any outside power source.

There are also switches that are activated with body movement but do not require force or even contact with the switch. These are referred to as *proximity switches.* The switch is activated when it detects an object within its range. The activation range of these types of switches varies from nearly touching the switch to 3 feet away and usually is adjustable. Near Switches* are a series of switches that do not require contact for activation. The switches in this series utilize different technology to detect the movement, from photoelectric to fiber optic. These switches are *active,* meaning they require an outside power source, such as a battery, to operate.

*Pneumatic switches* are activated by detection of respira-

*AbleNet, Minneapolis, Minn. (www.ablenetinc.com).
†TASH, Richmond, Va. (www.tashint.com).

*Adaptive Switch Laboratories, Inc., Spicewood, Tex. (www.asl-inc.com).

tory airflow or pressure and include puff-and-sip and pillow switches. Puff-and-sip switches (Figure 7-21, *E*) are activated by the individual's blowing air into the switch or sucking air out of it. The individual can send varying degrees of air pressure to the switch, which provides different commands to the processor. Pillow switches (Figure 7-21, *F*) respond to air pressure when squeezed (such as with a hand bulb) or when pressure is applied to a cushion.

## Switch Arrays, Discrete Joysticks, and Chord Keyboards

Switches are commercially available in preconfigured arrays (two to eight), and any of the single switches we have discussed can be used to design a custom array to meet the needs of the consumer. These offer the advantages of multiple signals while retaining the requirement of low resolution typical of single switches.

Paddle switches are often used in switch arrays when two to five input signals are desirable. A type of paddle switch that provides dual input from one control is called a *rocker switch* (Figure 7-22, *A*). A rocker switch is like a seesaw and does exactly what it says, it rocks from side to side around a fulcrum. This allows the user to maintain contact with the switch and perform a rotating movement with the control site to activate each side. This type of dual-switch array is often used for Morse code input, with one side signaling dots and the other side dashes. The Slot Switch* (Figure 7-22, *B*) is one example of a commercially available paddle switch array that is already configured. The switches in this array are mounted on a base piece that has dividers between the switches. The purpose of the dividers is to help the user isolate the appropriate switch. This array is typically used with the hands or feet by someone who has gross motor skills and a fairly large range. The isolation of each switch helps when the user may not be able to locate the switch visually. There are other switch arrays that are mounted and activated using the head. Switch arrays are often used for powered wheelchair control; we discuss them in greater detail in Chapter 10.

At the other extreme, in terms of size, is the Penta switch array.† This array consists of five switches, each approximately a quarter inch in diameter. Its overall size is 2 inches in diameter, and it is small enough so that it can be held in the palm of the hand and be activated by the thumb.

A discrete joystick is also considered an array of switches. It consists of four or five switch input signals (UP, DOWN, LEFT, RIGHT, and ENTER) that are either open or closed (off or on), with nothing in between. To close the switch, the control handle is moved in the direction of one

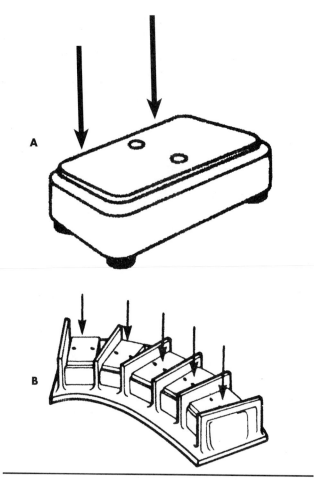

**Figure 7-22**    Examples of switch arrays. **A,** Dual rocker switch. (Webster JG et al, editors: *Electronic devices for rehabilitation,* New York, 1985, John Wiley and Sons.) **B,** Slot switch. (Courtesy Zygo Industries, Portland.)

of the other switches. Switched joysticks require limited range but moderate resolution by the user. They are available with a variety of displacements, forces, and handles to accommodate different grasping abilities of the user. If there is a maximum of five items (e.g., directions of a powered wheelchair) in the selection set, the joystick functions as an interface for direct selection. When the selection set is more than five, indirect selection is required using directed scanning. Using the joystick with this method, the individual selects the direction and the device determines the speed of cursor movement.

A chord keyboard is also an array of switches or keys (typically five), each of which is intended to be pushed by one finger. Two-handed versions have 10 or more switches or keys (some have multiple keys for thumb use), and one-handed versions have five or more. The name of these keyboards is derived from the manner in which they are used for text entry. To make an entry, one or more (usually at least two) of the switches are pushed simultaneously. This

---

*Zygo, Portland, Ore. (www.zygo-usa.com).
†Tash Inc., Richmond, Va.

is analogous to the playing of several notes together on a piano to make a musical chord. The most commonly used chord keyboard is the one used by court stenographers. Using this keyboard, a stenographer can transcribe speech as it is spoken. This amounts to more than 150 words per minute. For this reason, chord keyboards have often been proposed for rapid text entry by persons with disabilities. However, unless the person has good fine motor control and good coordination of the fingers, this approach is not viable. The degree of finger travel when using a chord keyboard is greatly reduced, since generally only the thumb moves from key to key (usually to press a different key to change meaning of the other four keys). It would follow, therefore, that chord keyboards would reduce the incidence of repetitive strain injuries. However, the fingers still need to move to activate the keys. Like the modified keyboard layouts described earlier, there are no studies that demonstrate that chord keyboards reduce the incidence of RSIs.

The chord keyboard is used in a coded access method. Each letter, number, and special symbol is entered by pressing a combination of keys (switches). This combination is interpreted as that character by the processor. For example, to enter the letter *C*, keys 1 and 3 may be pressed together. The codes for each selection must be learned because it is not possible to label the keys with the necessary codes. Therefore the individual using a chord keyboard needs to have good memory skills in addition to good motor skills.

## ◼ OTHER CONSIDERATIONS IN CONTROL INTERFACE SELECTION

### Multiple versus Integrated Control Interfaces

A long-standing goal of rehabilitation engineers and others is the integration of systems for augmentative and alternative communication (AAC), powered mobility, environmental control, and computer access (Barker, 1991; Caves et al, 1991). One of the major reasons for this emphasis is to allow the use of the same control interface for several applications, called **integrated control**. This can free the individual from multiple controls, and it can reduce the jumble of electronic devices surrounding the person.

With recent advances in technology, it is now possible to operate several devices through one processor. The processor is capable of operating only one device at a time, and a method is set up in which the user designates the mode in which she would like to function. For example, there are several powered wheelchairs* with processors that allow the consumer to use one interface, such as a joystick, to control

*Invacare, Elyria, Ohio; Permobil, Woburn, Mass.; Everest & Jennings, St. Louis, Mo.

many functions. By selecting the drive mode, the person uses the joystick to propel the wheelchair in all directions. The person can exit the wheelchair drive mode, select the mode designated for environmental control, and turn the lights on and off in the house.

There is an inherent value in the simplification that can result from this type of integration; however, there are also many situations in which separate control interfaces (called **distributed controls**) and devices for each of the functions are warranted. Before deciding whether to use an integrated control or distributed controls, the implications of each method for the consumer should be carefully deliberated. As a guideline, Guerette and Sumi (1994) recommend that integrated controls be used when (1) the person has one single reliable control site; (2) the optimal control interface for each assistive device is the same; (3) speed, accuracy, ease of use, or endurance increases with the use of a single interface; and (4) the person or his family prefers integrated controls for aesthetic, performance, or other subjective reasons.

In some cases the consumer may have only one body site that she can control, and she may also have limited range and resolution of this control site. Trying to position more than one control interface for use by this site could be problematic. Using the same control interface for multiple functions would simplify this situation. Next, consider what is the optimal way for the consumer to operate each assistive device. Let's say, for example, that you are evaluating a consumer for control of both a powered wheelchair and an AAC device. If the consumer can easily control a joystick, that would be the optimal control interface for the powered wheelchair. If this is also the easiest control interface for the consumer to use for controlling an AAC device, it would stand to reason that an integrated control (the joystick) to operate both devices would be beneficial. However, if this person is able to use direct selection with an expanded keyboard for controlling an AAC device, the keyboard would be the optimal control interface for AAC. Integrating the control interfaces by using the joystick for both functions would not make sense in this situation.

Another reason to implement an integrated control interface is the user's preference. The consumer ultimately has the final input into the selection of a control method. The consumer's preference may be based on a sense of having better performance with one method over the other, aesthetic reasons, or the importance of independence in going from one function to another. Because integrated controls combine interfaces into one unit, they typically require less hardware and tend to look better than multiple control interfaces. Integrated controls also provide increased independence for the consumer in accessing multiple assistive devices (Guerette, Caves, and Gross, 1992). The consumer does not have to depend on others to set up a different control interface or device. Some consumers place higher value on these issues than other consumers, and what is of importance to the individual consumer must be identified.

Although there are apparent advantages to using integrated controls, there may be circumstances in which distributed controls are preferred. Guerette and Nakai (1996) identify situations where integrated control may not be appropriate: "(1) when performance on one or more assistive devices is severely compromised by integrating control, (2) when an individual wishes to operate an assistive device from a position other than from a powered wheelchair, (3) when physical, cognitive, or visual/perceptual limitations preclude integrating, (4) when it is the individual's preference to use separate controls, and (5) when external factors such as cost or technical limitations preclude the use of integrated controls" (p. 64). In the example of Mrs. Antonelli (see Case Study 7-4), it was easy for her to control her powered wheelchair using the joystick with her left hand. However, this was not the easiest method for her to use to operate the communication device. She had the option, however, of using another body site, and it turned out that the "best" way for her to access the communication device was by using a dual rocker switch with her right hand. If the controls had been integrated and she was to use the joystick for both powered mobility and AAC, her activity output for communication would have been significantly compromised. The decision was made to use distributed controls, and her performance in communication was much improved.

In a study that measured consumer satisfaction with integrated controls, Angelo and Trefler (1998) reported that the majority of respondents indicated they were either very satisfied or satisfied with their integrated control device. An increase in independence and the ability to control other equipment such as televisions and computers were reasons the respondents gave for being satisfied with their integrated control devices.

## Mounting the Control Interface for Use

In all situations it is necessary to address the position and placement of the control interface so that it is optimally accessed by the user. Most keyboards are connected with a cable to the computer, which allows some latitude in positioning them so they are accessible. Keyboards can be placed on stands that raise them (e.g., for mouthstick use) or easels that tilt them (e.g., for easier hand access or foot access). Some keyboards (e.g., contracted keyboards) can be mounted to wheelchairs.

It is also necessary to mount single switches, joysticks, and switch arrays in a convenient location. The most common mounting locations are attachments to a table or desk, to a wheelchair, and to the person's body. There are

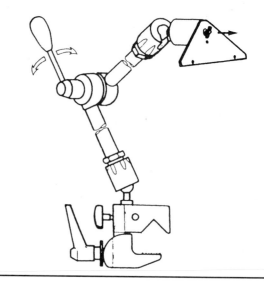

**Figure 7-23**   Flexible mounting system. (Courtesy Zygo Industries, Portland, Ore.)

commercially available mounting systems* for table and wheelchair mounting. Some mounting requirements are more challenging than others. For example, it is generally more difficult to position a joystick for foot or chin use than it is to place it for hand use.

There are flexible and fixed mounting systems. Flexible mounting systems (Figure 7-23) can be adjusted and placed in various positions. This is advantageous in settings where more than one person needs a switch mounting. Costs can be controlled by using the same mounting system at different times for several people. This type of mounting system is also advantageous for individuals who require changes in the position of their control interface because of fluctuating skill or need. The disadvantage of flexible mounting systems is that the position for the control interface must be determined each time it is put in place. Sometimes even a slight fluctuation in the position of the switch can make a significant difference in the individual's ability to access it. Other mounting systems are fixed and are designed for use of a specific control site and switch. The advantage of this approach is that the mounting system is not as likely to get out of position and require adjustment.

Switches are also attached to the individual by straps. Attachment to the body has the major advantage of not being as affected by the person's change in body position. If a switch is mounted to the wheelchair and the person shifts his position even slightly, the switch may no longer be reachable or the new position may make it difficult to generate enough force to activate the switch.

The majority of control interfaces have a cable that connects them to the device being used. However, there are wireless keyboards, pointing interfaces, and switches. There

*AbleNet, Minneapolis, Minn.; Zygo, Portland, Ore.

are also separate wireless links that can be used with most switches. These links consist of a transmitter that is plugged into the switch and a receiver that plugs into the device. When the switch is pressed, the signal is transmitted to the receiver and the device. Thus the switch is not physically connected to the device. Wireless control interfaces communicate with the processor via infrared signals such as those used with television remote controls. Obvious advantages of a remote control interface are that there is one less wire for the user to become tangled in and that it looks better. It can also be advantageous to have a wireless control interface when the interface is mounted on the person's wheelchair. This allows the person to move to or away from the device being used without having to connect or disconnect the interface. In many situations the person with a disability needs a personal attendant to assist with connecting the cable of the interface to the computer. The use of a remote control interface allows the person to come and go independently, so an attendant is not needed for this task.

## ■ DEVELOPMENT OF MOTOR SKILLS FOR USE OF CONTROL INTERFACES

In some situations it is necessary to establish a program that develops the individual's motor skills. Three outcomes can be achieved by such a program: (1) the individual can broaden his repertoire of motor capabilities and the number and type of inputs that can be accessed; (2) the individual can refine the motor skills she has in using an interface to increase speed, endurance, or accuracy; and (3) the individual who lacks the motor capabilities to use any interface functionally can develop these skills. The amount of training needed will vary in each of these circumstances, depending on the person and the desired outcome. In some cases, such as when the individual has never had the opportunity to control objects physically, this training can be carried out over a period of years. In comparison, a person who needs to develop tolerance for using a mouthstick may require a minimal amount of training. In general, training programs should be interesting, be graded according to the user's skill level, and be age appropriate.

What is initially chosen as the best control site and method for an individual may not necessarily remain constant over time. Kangas (1989) advises that the initial control site and method be considered just that, a starting place for the individual, and that the practitioner remain open to the individual's trying alternative sites and methods for control. Horn and Jones (1996) present a detailed case study in which both direct selection and scanning were used with a child. Although the initial assessment indicated a preference for single-switch scanning based on physical assessment, the child was later able to effectively utilize direct selection. This unexpected result is discussed by Horn

and Jones in terms of the physical and cognitive skills required for these two selection methods. Their results point out the importance of ongoing assessment (see Chapter 4) and the role of training in matching the skills of the user to the control interface.

Kangas (1988) recommends that practitioners encourage users to develop a repertoire of control methods, so that they broaden the potential number of devices they can access. For example, if a child who previously used a single switch becomes proficient in the use of a joystick, both these control options can be maintained through different activities. The joystick can be used to play computer games or activate a communication device, and the single switch can still be used to turn on some music. Similar to the concepts presented by Kangas is the *parallel interventions model* (Angelo and Smith, 1989; Smith, 1991). This model proposes that the individual use an initial control interface for accessing a device while simultaneously participating in a motor training program to maximize his ability to operate control interfaces. Broadening the person's repertoire allows access to a greater number of devices and may allow the user to lessen her reliance on assistive technology. For example, after a period of training, the user may be able to progress from using a single switch to a switch array or from an expanded keyboard to a standard keyboard.

An individual may have the prerequisite motor skills to use a control interface with a device but require training to refine those skills. Refining these motor skills may result in an increased rate of input, fewer errors, or increased endurance for using the control. For example, a person may be able to select directly but need training to learn to use a specific keyboard layout to reduce fatigue or increase speed. There are software programs available, such as the Five Finger Typist program,* that help a person acquire one-handed keyboard skills. Additionally, there are a number of Web sites that provide information on training with different types of keyboard layouts, such as http://home1.gte.net/bharrell/index.htm or www.dgp.toronto.edu/people/ematias/papers/ic93. Refinement of motor skills for mouse use is another example. Again there are many software programs available that have been developed to gradually improve a person's ability to use a mouse or an alternative to a mouse. These programs include activities for developing targeting skills and mastering point-and-click and click-and-drag skills.

Use of mechanical and electronic pointers worn on the head typically require substantial training to gradually build the consumer's tolerance and effectiveness in using the control enhancer. Similarly, strengthening of the person's existing neck, facial, and oral musculature and a gradual development of tolerance for the mouthstick should take place before having him perform tasks such as writing or

---

*Tash Inc., Richmond, Va.

---

**TABLE 7-8**  **Sequential Steps in Motor Training for Switch Use**

| Goal | Tools Used to Accomplish Goal |
|---|---|
| 1. Time-independent switch use to develop cause and effect | Appliances (fan, blender)<br>Battery-operated toys/radio<br>Software that produces a result whenever the switch is pressed |
| 2. Time-dependent switch use to develop switch use at the right time | Software that requires a response at a specific time to obtain a graphic or sound result |
| 3. Switch within specified window to develop multichoice scanning | Software requiring a response in a "time window" |
| 4. Symbolic choice making | Simple scanning communication devices<br>Software allowing time-dependent choice making that has a symbolic label and communicative output |

---

typing. Playing simple board games, painting, or batting a balloon are examples of activities that can be used to develop skills for mouthstick or head pointer use. Many games can also be adapted so that a person using a light pointer can play them and get practice with that interface.

Assistive technology provides many individuals with physical disabilities with their first opportunity to perform a motor act to access communication, mobility, and environmental control. Before this technology became available, those individuals with severe physical disabilities had few or no opportunities to utilize their existing motor movement. For this reason, there are many instances in which an individual may have a control site and the ability to activate a single switch, but the ability to activate this control interface is not consistent enough to justify the purchase of an assistive device such as a wheelchair, computer, or augmentative communication system. The intervention then becomes one of improving the individual's motor control.

In these cases a graded approach using technology as one of the modalities for improving the individual's motor skills can and should be implemented. Table 7-8 illustrates some general steps and tools involved in such an approach. The technology then becomes a tool to meet short-term objectives aimed at reaching the long-term goal of using assistive technology. It is important that this be kept in mind so that the ATP reevaluates the individual at periodic intervals and allows her to move beyond the use of this technology as a tool and into functional device use.

In situations such as those just described, frequently the individual is not able to communicate verbally and the question of whether he has the cognitive-language skills to access assistive technology also becomes an issue. Therefore this approach (see Table 7-8) starts with evaluating *cause and effect* and providing training at that level as needed. This is the ability of the individual to understand that he can control things in his environment and can make something happen. It encompasses the prerequisite skills of attention

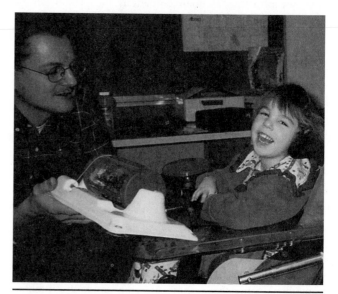

**Figure 7-24**  Child using a single switch with a battery-operated toy as a reinforcer.

and object permanence. The individual must be able to attend to and be aware of his environment and the permanence of objects in that environment. Information can be gathered on the individual's ability to understand cause and effect through the use of a single switch.

At the first stage, the goal related to assistive technology use is for the individual to be able to activate the switch at any given time and associate the switch activation with a result. The individual is asked to use a control site to activate a single switch that is connected to some type of reinforcer. Caregivers can provide initial information on what the individual enjoys and finds reinforcing. Objects that can be adapted for switch input and that may be of interest include battery-operated toys, a radio, a blender, or a fan. The child shown in Figure 7-24 is using a switch with a battery-operated toy for the reinforcer. Levin and Scherfenberg (1987) make suggestions of activities for all age groups.

Typically the individual who is aware that she has generated an effect will show some type of response, such as smiling, crying, or looking toward the reinforcer.

If there is success with these activities, computer software programs can be used as an alternative type of reinforcement. These programs provide interesting graphics, animation, and auditory feedback each time the switch is activated. Individuals of all age groups find the programs enjoyable. For each switch activation, data can be collected, including (1) time from prompt to activation, (2) whether the individual activates the switch independently or whether verbal or physical prompting was needed, and (3) the consumer's attention to the result. There are a number of companies* that sell software programs to be used at the different stages described in this section.

At the second stage, the goal is for the individual to activate his switch consistently at a specific time. This can also be considered one-choice scanning, in which the switch is either hit or not—choice making at its most fundamental level (Cook, 1991). For example, with some computer games the individual needs to activate the switch for an object to move or to carry out an action such as shooting a basket, hitting a target, and so on. With some programs, as long as the individual successfully activates the switch, the movement of objects on the screen speeds up. Any data provided by the program (e.g., speed, number of correct hits, errors) and data regarding the individual's success in activating the switch at the correct time and whether prompts have been needed are recorded. Burkhart (1987) makes suggestions for computer-based and non-computer-based activities that can be used for motor training. One suggestion for a non-computer-based activity is to use a battery-operated toy fireman that climbs a ladder as long as the switch is activated. To make this a time-dependent activity, a picture of a reinforcer is attached somewhere along the ladder and the individual is asked to release the switch to stop the fireman at the picture and receive the reinforcement.

During the third phase of this training program, the time window becomes more defined as the individual is asked to use the switch to choose from two or more options. Toys, appliances, and computer software programs are also used at this stage. The goal is to increase the number of elements in an array that can be reliably selected by the individual. This is important if scanning is to be used for communication or environmental control. One approach is to highlight loca-

tions on the screen in sequence. When the switch is hit on a highlighted item, the program provides an interesting result. In some programs the highlighted areas can be limited so that only one is correct. This helps the consumer develop scanning selection skills in the absence of language-based tasks. In addition to the data that have been collected in the previous stages, data on the minimal scan rate the individual can successfully use are recorded.

If the need is for powered mobility, then the next step is to use software specifically designed for developing skills in using a joystick. Alternatively, scanning training software aimed at single-switch or dual-switch wheelchair use can be used for training at this stage.

In the final training phase for communication, symbolic representation is added to the choice making. Development of the individual's language skills may have been taking place in conjunction with the motor skills training, and this linguistic step may follow naturally. Selection of symbol systems is discussed in Chapter 9. Through this phase the individual makes the transition from object manipulation (environmental control) to concept manipulation (communication) (Cook, 1991). The individual now has greater resources to use to convey needs, wants, and other information. Simple scanning communication devices can be used at this stage or the type of program with multiple choices described earlier can be used for further skill development as a precursor to a scanning communication device.

Given repetition of any motor act, we assume that people will improve. It is possible that the quality and speed of their movement may improve, and even the number of movement patterns (e.g., head movement and hand movement) available to them increase. Hussey and Cook (1992) documented the progress of two young women following the implementation of a motor training program similar to the one described in Table 7-8. Initially, both Janice and Marge lacked the head control to activate even a single switch. The initial control site for both of them was flexion at the elbow, in one case to activate a mercury switch and in the other case, a leaf switch. After extensive training using the approach just described, Janice and Marge are now able to select directly from a limited array using a light pointer worn on the head with a portable augmentative communication device. These two cases are representative of the skills that individuals can gain from a systematic motor training program so that use of assistive technology for a functional activity can be achieved.

■ **SUMMARY**

In this chapter we have defined the elements of the human/technology interface and its relationship to the other components of the assistive technology. The elements of the

---

*Academic Software, Inc., Lexington, Ky. (www.acsw.com); R.J. Cooper, Dana Point, Calif. (www.rjcooper.com); Don Johnston, Volo, Ill. (www.donjohnston.com/); Edmark, Redmond, Wash. (www.edmark.com/); Judy Lynn Software, Inc., East Brunswick, NJ (www.intac.com/~judylynn/); IntelliTools, Novato, Calif.; Laureate Learning Systems, Inc., Winooski, Vt. (www.laureatelearning.com); SoftTouch, Bakersfield, Calif.

human/technology interface include the control interface, the selection method, and the selection set. The selection set encompasses the items in the array from which the user can choose. There are two basic methods by which the user makes selections: direct selection or indirect selection. Indirect selection encompasses a subset of selection methods known as scanning, directed scanning, and coded access. Each selection method applies to a different set of consumer skills.

With advances in technology, there is a wide range of control interfaces available for use by persons with disabilities. Control interfaces can be characterized by their sensory, spatial, and activation-deactivation features. Understanding these characteristics can help the ATP sort through the maze of control interfaces. This chapter also described a framework that provides the ATP with a systematic process for matching the interface to the needs and skills of consumers. Critical questions were identified that relate to the user's skills needed to control particular types of interfaces. Addressing these questions during the evaluation can facilitate the selection of an appropriate control interface for the consumer.

## Study Questions

1. What is the function of the control interface? Describe the difference between a discrete and a continuous input with examples for each.
2. Define the elements of the human/technology interface and how they are related to the processor and the output.
3. What is a selection set?
4. What are the two basic selection methods used with control interfaces?
5. What are the scanning formats that can be used to accelerate scanning?
6. Why is coded access an indirect selection method? What is the selection set for Morse code?
7. What are the somatosensory characteristics of control interfaces that need to be considered when selecting an interface for a consumer?
8. Describe three control interface activation characteristics.
9. How are sensory and activation characteristics of control interfaces related?
10. What two measurements obtained from the consumer during the initial assessment provide us with information that will assist us in identifying spatial characteristics of the control interface?
11. What is a control enhancer? List several examples.
12. Describe tremor dampening.
13. Compare the user profile for a standard, an ergonomic, an expanded, and a contracted keyboard. What user skills would lead you, as the ATP, to select one of these over the others?
14. What are the major design goals of ergonomic keyboards?
15. What are the primary considerations that would lead to the choice of speech recognition as an alternative direct selection method?
16. Describe the difference between continuous and discrete speech recognition systems.
17. What is the difference between speaker independent and speaker dependent automatic speech recognition systems?
18. What are the most common alternatives to a computer mouse? List at least one advantage and one disadvantage of each.
19. What is an on-screen keyboard?
20. List three types of modifications to keyboards and pointing devices, and give an example of the problems that each solves.
21. Describe the three different selection techniques used with scanning and directed scanning. Which one provides the user with more control and why?
22. Review the description of control interface flexibility in the section on characteristics of control interfaces. Pick three switches from those described in the section on selecting control interfaces, one that is very flexible, one that is moderately flexible, and one that is not flexible. Justify your choices.
23. Describe distributed and integrated control. What are the advantages and disadvantages of each?
24. What outcomes can be achieved through the implementation of training programs for development of motor skills?
25. Describe the steps taken in a training program to develop motor control.

## References

Angelo J: Comparison of three computer scanning modes as an interface method for persons with cerebral palsy, *Am J Occup Ther* 46(3):217-222, 1992.

Angelo J, Smith RO: The critical role of occupational therapy in augmentative communication services. In American Occupational Therapy Association, editors: *Technology review '89: perspectives on occupational therapy practice*, Rockville, Md, pp 49-53, 1989.

Angelo J, Trefler, E: A survey of persons who use integrated control devices, *Assist Technol* 10:77-83, 1998.

Anson D: Speech recognition technology, *OT Practice*, pp 59-62, January/February 1999.

Anson DK: *Alternative computer access: a guide to selection*, Philadelphia, 1997, FA Davis.

Bailey, RW: *Human performance engineering*, ed 2, Englewood Cliffs, NJ, 1989, Prentice Hall.

Baker JM: How to achieve recognition: a tutorial/status report on automatic speech recognition, *Speech Technol*, pp 30-31, 36-43, Fall 1981.

Barker MR: *Integrating assistive technology: communication, computers, control and seating and mobility systems*. Presented at Demystifying Technology Workshop, CSUS Assistive Device Center, 1991, Sacramento, CA.

Barker MR, Cook AM: A systematic approach to evaluating physical ability for control of assistive devices, *Proc 4th Ann Conf Rehabil Eng*, 287-289, June 1981.

Bear-Lehman J: Orthopedic conditions. In Trombly CA, editor: *Occupational therapy for physical dysfunction*, ed 4, Baltimore, Md, 1995, Williams & Wilkins.

Beukelman D, Mirenda P: *Augmentative and alternative communication*, Baltimore, Md, 1992, Paul H Brookes.

Burkhart LJ: *Using computers and speech synthesis to facilitate communicative interaction with young and/or severely handicapped children*, College Park, Md, 1987, Linda J. Burkhart.

Caves K et al: The use of integrated controls for mobility, communication and computer access, *Proc 14th RESNA Conf*, pp 166-167, June 1991.

Chubon RA, Hester MR: An enhanced standard computer keyboard system for single-finger and typing-stick typing, *J Rehabil Res Dev* 25(4):17-24, 1988.

Comerford R, Makhoul J, Schwartz R: The voice of the computer is heard in the land (and it listens too), *IEEE Spectrum* 34(12):39-47, 1997.

Cook AM: Development of motor skills for switch use by persons with severe disabilities, *Developmental Disabilities Special Interest Newsletter* 14(2): 1991.

Gallant JA: Speech-recognition products, *EDN*, pp 112-122, January 19, 1989.

Guerette P, Caves K, Gross K: One switch does it all, *Team Rehabil Rep* pp 26-29, March/April 1992.

Guerette PJ, Nakai RJ: Access to assistive technology: a comparison of integrated and distributed control, *Technol Dis* 5:63-73, 1996.

Guerette P, Sumi, E: Integrating control of multiple assistive devices: a retrospective review. *Assist Technol* 6:67-76, 1994.

Horn EM, Jones HA: Comparison of two selection techniques used in augmentative and alternative communication, *Augment Altern Commun* 12:23-31, 1996.

Hussey SM, Cook AM, Whinnery SE, Buckpitt L: A conceptual model for developing augmentative communication skills in individuals with severe disabilities, *Proc RESNA Int 92 Conf*, 287-289, June 1992.

Kangas K: Assessment and training of methods of access and optimal control sites, *Assist Device News* 5(1), 1988.

Kangas K: The optimal position, *Assist Device News* 5(4), 1989.

Kambeyanda D, Singer L, Cronk S: Potential problems associated with the use of speech recognition products, *Assist Technol* 9:95-101, 1997.

Kasch M, Poole SE, Hedl M: Acute hand injuries. In Early MB editor: *Physical dysfunction practice skills for the occupational therapy assistant*, St. Louis, 1998, Mosby.

Lau C, O'Leary S: Comparison of computer interface devices for persons with severe disabilities, *Am J Occup Ther* 47(11):1022-1029, 1993.

Lee KS, Thomas DJ: *Control of computer-based technology for people with physical disabilities: an assessment manual*, Toronto, 1990, University of Toronto Press.

Levin J, Scherfenberg L: *Selection and use of simple technology in home, school, work, and community settings*, Minneapolis, 1987, Ablenet.

McCormack DJ: The effects of keyguard use and pelvic positioning on typing speed and accuracy in a boy with cerebral palsy, *Am J Occup Ther* 44(4):312-315, 1990.

Morasso P, Penso M, Suetta GP, Tagliasco V: Towards standardization of communication and control systems for motor impaired people, *Med Biol Eng Comput* 17:481-488, 1979.

Puckett AD et al: Development of an improved mouthpiece for a mouthstick, *Proc Int Conf Assn Adv Rehabil Tech*, pp 100-101, June 1988.

Smith RO: Technological approaches to performance enhancement. In Christiansen C, Baum C, editors: *Occupational therapy overcoming human performance deficits*, Thorofare, NJ, 1991, Slack.

Spaeth DM, Cooper RA: Designing a variable compliance joystick for control interface research, *Proc RESNA 99 Conf*, pp 131-133, June 1999.

Tessler FN: The Apple adjustable keyboard, *MACWORLD*, November 1993.

Vanderheiden GC: *A unified quantitative modeling approach for selection-based augmentative communication systems,* doctoral dissertation, Madison, 1984, University of Wisconsin.

Vanderheiden GC, Lloyd LL: Communication systems and their components. In Blackstone S, Bruskin D, editors: *Augmentative communication: an introduction,* Rockville, Md, 1986, American Speech Language and Hearing Association.

Webster JG et al, editors: *Electronic devices for rehabilitation,* New York, 1985, John Wiley and Sons.

Weiss PL: Mechanical characteristics of microswitches adapted for the physically disabled, *J Biomed Eng* 12:398-402, 1990.

## CHAPTER 8

# Computers As Extrinsic Enablers for Assistive Technologies

## Objectives

Upon completing this chapter you will be able to:

1. Describe the computer user interface
2. List the major components of a computer system and give the function of each
3. Define what is meant by *operating systems* and describe how they relate to adaptations of computers for use by persons with disabilities
4. Describe the major approaches to keyboard and mouse emulation
5. Describe how computer outputs are adapted for individuals with visual or auditory limitations
6. Describe the major approaches to Internet access for persons with disabilities.

---

## Key Terms

Accessibility Options
Central Processing Unit (CPU)
Compact Disk-Read-Only Memory
 (CD-ROM)
Concept Keyboards
Easy Access
Emulation

General Input Device-Emulating
 Interface (GIDEI)
Graphical User Interface (GUI)
Internet
On-Screen Keyboard
Parallel Port
Multitasking

Serial Port
Screen Readers
Transparent Access
Random Access Memory (RAM)
Read-Only Memory (ROM)
Universal Access
User Agent
Windows

---

Computers are used in two rather distinct ways with assistive technologies. *Computer workstations* are general-purpose desktop or portable computers that are adapted to make them applicable to the needs of persons who have disabilities. These computers are used for many of the same tasks for which nondisabled persons use computers. However, we often make modifications in the computer to facilitate use by persons with disabilities. The second way in which computers are used in assistive technologies is by incorporation into other devices that are specifically designed to perform one type of function. For example, powered wheelchair controllers, augmentative communication devices, and electronic aids to daily living (EADLs) are generally based on special-purpose computers. A set of basic principles applies to both these uses of computers in terms of what the computer can offer. Functionally, the most useful characteristics of computer-based systems are (1) flexibility (multiple options with the same hardware), (2) adaptability (e.g., as users' skills change over time), (3) customization to a specific user and need (e.g., settings of scanning rate in augmentative communication, acceleration rate on powered wheelchair), and (4) specific applications or upgrades based on software rather than hardware (e.g., augmentative communication application software and upgrades, specific user profile of speed and acceleration parameters in a powered wheelchair controller). In this chapter we describe these basic principles, as well as how general-purpose or stand-alone computers can be adapted to the needs of persons with disabilities. Special-purpose computer applications are discussed in later chapters.

### BASIC COMPONENTS OF A COMPUTER-BASED SYSTEM

Because all assistive technology applications of computers involve a human operator, it is important to understand the computer/user interface. There are several characteristics that distinguish this interface from other human/device applications. One of the most important of these is that human/computer interaction is two way; that is, information is transferred both from the user to the computer and from the computer to the user (Bailey, 1989). Although this type of bi-directional transfer of information is typical of many electronic assistive technologies, computer use requires greater attention to both *input* to the computer from the user and *output* from the computer to the user. The two-way transfer of information requires that all the intrinsic enablers that describe the human operator (see Figure 3-1) be considered when evaluating the use of computers by persons with disabilities. Sensory and perceptual abilities are required for the processing of computer outputs. Motor control and effector capabilities are essential for generating input to the computer. Cognitive skills, including problem solving and decision making, memory, language, motivation, and developmental level are also important to successful use of a computer. The potential user's skills in all these areas must be carefully determined when a computer configuration that is to be used as part of an assistive technology system is designed.

It is not necessary for the assistive technology practitioner (ATP) to be a computer scientist or engineer, but it is important to have a general understanding of the major components of a computer and how they relate to functional performance. This understanding will allow the ATP to specify the major parts of a computer system (Figure 8-1) for a particular person who has a unique need. It is expected that you are familiar with this information, or that you know where to obtain it. There are many reference books that describe the basic structure of computer systems.

To apply computer systems effectively to meeting the needs of persons with disabilities, it is necessary to have an understanding of the major *functional* components. Many of these components are part of any computer, whether designed for a special purpose or for general use. Others are present only in general-purpose computers. We will make

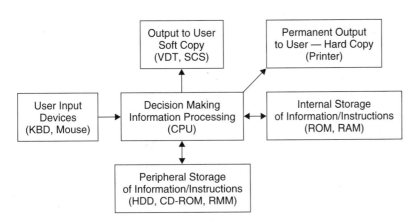

Figure 8-1   The basic components of a computer system are shown. Not all these components are included in every computer system. *CD-ROM*, Compact disk-read-only memory (optical storage of programs and data; some current CD-ROMs are read-and-write); *CPU*, central processing unit; *HDD*, hard disk drive (permanent magnetic storage); *KBD*, keyboard; *RAM*, random access memory (temporary electronic storage); *RMM*, removable magnetic media (removable permanent magnetic storage, e.g., floppy disk drive, Zip disk drive); *ROM*, read-only memory (permanent electronic storage); *SCS*, sound card and speakers (sound and speech output); *VDT*, video display terminal.

this distinction in the following discussion. In this chapter we discuss two basic types of general-purpose computers. The Apple Macintosh computer is widely used in kindergarten through twelfth grade education. For business applications and postsecondary education, computers based on IBM's original design are used. We refer to these systems as **Windows** computers because of their basic operating system. These computers are also often used in high schools.

## Functional Structure of Computer Systems

Figure 8-1 shows the major functional components of a standard (nonadapted) computer system. Each of these components contributes to the characteristics of the total computer, and any one computer may have different individual components.

**Control and processing.** At the heart of any computer system is the **central processing unit (CPU).** This portion of the computer is capable of executing a set of instructions assembled in the form of a program, accepting input and sending output, and transferring information among the components. The heart of the CPU is an electronic integrated circuit known as a *microprocessor*, frequently referred to as the "computer chip."

**Computer storage.** Computers are able to store information, data, and instructions in electronic circuits, on magnetic media, or on optical disks. Broadly speaking, there are two types of electronic circuits used for storage. Temporary storage is in circuits called **random access memory (RAM).** When the power to the computer is turned off, the information in RAM is lost. This is the type of memory that is used to specify the size of a computer's internal storage and is one important consideration when specifying a computer for use by a consumer. The other type of electronic memory is called **read-only memory (ROM).** This type of memory differs from RAM in that it cannot be erased and reprogrammed. It is used for permanent commands and instructions that are required for the computer

to function (e.g., boot the disk). In addition, there are hybrid types of memory that can be altered but that also hold information when the power is turned off. One type, used in augmentative communication systems and other assistive technology applications, is called *electrically erasable programmable read-only memory (EEPROM).* This type of memory is programmed by electrically enabling it, and it can be altered (erased) by applying a different electrical signal. In contrast to RAM, stored information remains after the power is turned off. Unlike ROM, it can be altered.

All general-purpose and some special-purpose computers also have some type of removable storage that utilizes magnetic media. Most commonly, the magnetic media are in the form of disks. However, some systems use tapes for either primary storage or backup. Disks are referred to as either *floppy* disks or *hard* disks. Floppy disks are 3 1/2 inches in size and hold approximately 1.5 megabytes (MB) of data. Zip disks are larger and hold 100 MB or more of data. Disks are read and written to using disk drives. One disk can be removed from the drive and replaced with another to change applications, to load or save files or data, or to transfer data from one computer to another. Hard disks are generally built into the computer, and they constitute the largest and most often used permanent storage area.

Hard disks offer fast, reliable storage of large amounts of data. There are also miniature hard disk drives that are incorporated into special-purpose computers such as for augmentative communication. The hard drive and floppy disk storage determines the number or programs and amount of data that can be stored on the computer. The amount of floppy and hard disk storage is an important characteristic that must be specified when designing an assistive technology system.

Another form of storage is optical, rather than magnetic. **Compact disk-read-only memory (CD-ROM)** uses lasers to read and write data to optical disks. These disks are similar to the CDs used for audio recording, and they can store music and pictures, in addition to large amounts of data. The large data capacity is equivalent to a 10-million word or 20-volume encyclopedia (Church and Glennen,

1992). Church and Glennen (1992) cite several advantages of CD-ROMs, in addition to the large storage capacity. First, optical disks are protected from spills and scratches by a plastic coating, and they are not susceptible to erasing by magnetic fields. Second, CD-ROMs are easily and inexpensively mass produced. This process, also used in the music industry, results in considerable savings over magnetically distributed materials (e.g., mass-produced floppy disks). Many materials are available on CD-ROM, including multimedia educational materials, books, and encyclopedias. Most application programs (e.g., word processing, databases) are also delivered on CD-ROM.

In recent years, several writeable formats for CDs have been developed. The earliest of these was the write-once read-many (WORM) disk (Buddine and Young, 1987). Once data are written to these disks, they become read only. These are intended for archiving data or creating large custom databases. Erasable CD-ROMs that can be used repeatedly are commercially available. These disks can be used in interactive learning situations that require data to be collected and stored while allowing large amounts of data to be available as well (e.g., student's responses to guided instruction and statistics on learning). Erasable CD-ROM disks can also be used in interactive databases in which large amounts of data are stored but the data change. In assistive technology an example of this type of use is in consumer files utilized in service delivery and in product databases (Attigupam et al, 1993). Currently, erasable CD-ROMs are slower than hard disk drives; continued development will likely lead to widespread use of this technology in PCs. In summary, there are three types of CDs currently available: (1) those that can only be *read* by a computer (CD-ROM), (2) those that can be *written to once* and read many times (WORM), and (3) those that can be *read from and written to* many times (erasable CD-ROM).

**Input devices.** The most common user input to general-purpose computers is provided via either a keyboard or a mouse. There are many alternatives to both the keyboard and the mouse that use different control interfaces and different selection methods (see Chapter 7). The type of adaptation is usually related to the severity of the physical limitations the user has. Keyboards are found on special-function computers such as those used for environmental control, augmentative communication, or adjustment of parameters on powered mobility, as well as on general-purpose computers.

**Output devices.** There are several different types of output devices used in computer systems. User output from the computer is generally provided by a visual display. This type of display is also referred to as *soft copy*. For both general-purpose computers and special-purpose computers built into assistive devices with displays, video display

terminals (VDTs) and liquid crystal displays (LCDs) are generally used as output devices. The other type of output from a computer is in a permanent form, or *hard copy*, using a printer. Finally, computers also provide auditory outputs in sound, music, or synthetic speech. These outputs are important to individuals who have visual impairments.

## Communication with Peripheral Devices

Computers may use one or more ports for data input and output. The two most common that are used for devices such as printers and voice synthesizers are **parallel** and **serial ports.** Serial data transfer is most commonly used in assistive technologies (e.g., augmentative communication devices or powered wheelchair controllers and environmental control systems) because the serial port is bi-directional (data can be fed *into* the device as well as *out of* the device) and because the serial port requires only a two- or three-conductor cable as opposed to a bulky 10- to 12-conductor cable for parallel ports. Other ports used for assistive technology applications include keyboard ports on both Windows-based and Macintosh computers, the Apple data bus (ADB) on Macintosh computers, and the universal serial bus (USB) ports on all computers.

## Graphical User Interface

In order for a human to interact with a computer, there must be an effective communication channel. The most commonly used channel today, the **graphical user interface (GUI),** is established for nondisabled users through the keyboard or mouse for input and the VDT or speakers for output. What makes these peripheral elements into a user interface is the way in which they interact with the internal computer programs. Input of data, storage and processing, and output are all handled by the computer operating system. Some types of user interfaces are more suitable for adaptation of the computer to provide physical or visual access to the computer. The ATP must understand the various types of user interfaces and how they affect access.

The GUI has three distinguishing features: (1) a mouse pointer, which is moved around the screen; (2) a graphical menu bar, which appears on the screen; and (3) one or more windows, which provide a menu of choices (Hayes, 1990). Movement of the mouse or a mouse equivalent (e.g., keystrokes, trackball, head pointer, or joystick) causes the pointer to move around the screen. There are two primary characteristics of GUIs that are particularly important in assistive technology applications: (1) the use of graphical menus and icons to which the user can point and click for input instead of using the keyboard, and (2) multitasking capabilities, which allow more than one program to be loaded and run simultaneously. The creation of a graphical environment can save typing, reduce effort, and increase accuracy, and the use of icons generally helps with recall and ease of use. The GUI allows the use of windows, which partition the screen into smaller screens, each showing a particular application. When an application or function is opened or run by clicking (or sometimes double-clicking), a feature (e.g., a calculator) or application (e.g., a word processor) is displayed in a window. Several windows may be open at the same time. Figure 8-2 shows multiple windows open and examples of menus and dialog boxes used for manipulating data and information. Specific implementations of GUIs have slightly different modes of operation, but the basic principles are similar to those described here.

The GUI has both positive and negative implications for persons with disabilities. The positive features are those that apply to nondisabled users. The major limitation of GUI use in assistive technology is that the user may not have the necessary physical (eye-hand coordination) and visual skills. In addition, adaptation for alternative input or output devices is often difficult and adaptations must be redone when changes are made to the basic operating system. The GUI is the standard user interface because of its ease of operation for novices and its consistency of operation for experts. The latter ensures that every application behaves in basically the same way (e.g., screen icons for the same task look the same, operations such as opening and closing files are always the same). We discuss adaptations of the GUI for persons with disabilities in following sections.

## Application Software

The computer only becomes useful when we look beyond its internal operation to the programs it can run. There are many types of application programs that are useful to everyone. However, for persons who cannot use pencil and paper to write, many of these programs are essential. These include business software such as word processing; academic programs for mathematics or language skill development; scientific and engineering software such as computer-aided design, data plotting, and statistical analysis; games for leisure time; and Internet access. The operating system and user interface manage the interaction between application programs and the internal operation of the computer.

Most application programs are loaded and run directly. However, some programs (generally utilities) are loaded into memory, remain there, and are run only when a specific set of conditions exist. This configuration is often used in computer adaptations for persons who have disabilities, and it is important for the ATP to understand the basic operation. In contrast to a standard application, many of these utility programs will not run until a specific key sequence is entered, such as hitting the SHIFT key five times to turn on StickyKeys (Table 8-1). At this time, the accessibility program stops execution of the application program (e.g., a word processor) and runs itself; for example, StickyKeys will allow SHIFT, ALT, or CONTROL to be pressed in sequence with the affected key, rather than pressing them together. The computer appears to be running two programs, but in reality only the accessibility program is running and the word processor has been temporarily halted. When the user is finished with the accessibility program, she presses another key sequence. This concept is fundamental to many of the computer adaptations for meeting the needs of persons with disabilities.

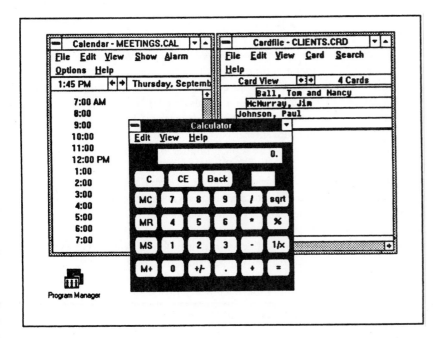

Figure 8-2    An example of a graphical user interface with several windows open for different applications. (From *Microsoft Windows manual*, Microsoft Corp., Seattle, Wash.)

| TABLE 8-1 | Minimal Adaptations to the Standard Keyboard and Mouse* |
| --- | --- |
| **Need Addressed** | **Software Approach** |
| Modifier key cannot be used at same time as another key | StickyKeys† |
| User cannot release key before it starts to repeat | RepeatKeys† |
| User accidentally hits wrong keys | SlowKeys,† BounceKeys,† FilterKeys† |
| User cannot manipulate mouse | MouseKeys† |
| User wants to use augmentative communication device as input | SerialKeys† |
| Hardware approaches are discussed in Chapter 7 | |

*Easy Access (part of Universal Access) in Macintosh operating system, Apple Computer, Cupertino, Calif.; Accessibility Options in Windows, Microsoft Corp., Seattle, Wash.

†Software modifications developed at the Trace Center, University of Wisconsin, Madison. These are included as before-market modifications to the Macintosh operating system or Windows in some personal computers and are available as after-market versions in others. The function of each program is as follows:

*StickyKeys:* user can press modifier key, then press second key without holding both down simultaneously.

*RepeatKeys:* user can adjust how long key must be held before it begins to repeat.

*SlowKeys:* a delay can be added before the character selected by hitting a key is entered into the computer; this means that the user can release an incorrect key before it is entered.

*BounceKeys:* prevents double characters from being entered if the user bounces on the key when pressing and releasing.

*FilterKeys:* the combination of SlowKeys, BounceKeys, and RepeatKeys in Microsoft Windows.

*MouseKeys:* substitutes arrow keys for mouse movements.

*SerialKeys:* allows any serial input to replace mouse and keyboard.

## BASIC PRINCIPLES OF ADAPTED COMPUTER INPUTS

In this section we describe the major ways in which computers can be adapted to allow individuals who have difficulty in using the keyboard or mouse to utilize the full range of its capabilities. Many of these adaptations are mandated by the legislation described in Chapter 1 (e.g., those listed in Table 8-1). Our approach is to begin with the simplest modifications designed for the most minimal of physical limitations on the part of the user. We then progress to more complex adaptations designed to accommodate even the most severely limited potential user.

We use the term **transparent access** to describe two fundamental concepts that apply to all levels of computer adaptation: (1) 100% of the functions of the computer must be adapted if the user who has a disability is to have full access; and (2) all application software that runs on the unmodified computer must also run on the adapted computer. For example, all the keyboard keys, including modifier and special function keys, must be available. Likewise, all the mouse functions, such as point, click, and drag, must

be available on the adapted input system. If a word processing program works with the standard computer, then it should work with the adaptations. The adaptations also have to be consistent with the operating system (e.g., Windows) of the computer. The Trace Center developed the term **general input device-emulating interface (GIDEI)** to describe emulation of the mouse or the keyboard or both. We use the term in this chapter to describe the use of alternatives for keyboard or mouse input.

## Adaptations to the Standard Keyboard

There are several problems that persons with disabilities have in using a standard keyboard. Software adaptations for these problems are shown in Table 8-1, together with typical solutions. Hardware adaptations are discussed in Chapter 7. These software adaptations are built into Windows* and Apple Macintosh† operating systems. Collectively these are called **Accessibility Options** in Windows and **Universal Access** for the Macintosh. They are accessed and adjusted for an individual user through the control panel. Universal Access for the Macintosh includes **Easy Access** and CloseView. Easy Access features are those shown in Table 8-1. CloseView is described later in this chapter. When StickyKeys is used, the modifier keys are converted to sequential rather than simultaneous use. Recall that other effectors (e.g., for the head and foot) can also be used to access standard keyboards. In many cases there is also a need for StickyKeys (Windows and Macintosh) and FilterKeys (Windows) or SlowKeys (Macintosh) adaptations. FilterKeys includes the functions of BounceKeys, SlowKeys, and RepeatKeys.

Microsoft has added some additional accessibility features to Windows 2000. Two new utilities are Narrator and an on-screen keyboard. Narrator is a text-to-speech utility for people who are blind or have low vision. This program reads text that is displayed on the screen in an active window or menu options or text that has been typed into a window. The on-screen keyboard operates in a manner similar to those described later in this chapter. Two modes of entry are available when an on-screen key is highlighted by mouse cursor movement: clicking and dwelling. In the latter the user keeps the mouse pointer on an on-screen key for an adjustable, preset time and the key is entered. The on-screen feature also allows entry by scanning using a hot key or switch-input device. Several keyboard configurations are included, and an auditory click may be activated to indicate entry of a character. Windows 2000 combines these two new options, the Magnifier program from earlier Windows versions (discussed later in this chapter), and a Utility

---

*Microsoft Corp., Seattle, Wash. (microsoft.com).

†Apple Computer, Cupertino, Calif., Education and Disability Resources (www.apple.com/education/k12/disability/).

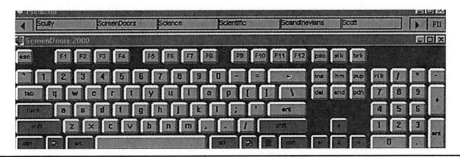

**Figure 8-3**   Typical on-screen keyboard display. All keyboard characters are included. (Courtesy Madentec, Edmonton, Alberta, Canada.)

Manager in its Accessibility menu, which is accessed through the Start menu in Windows 2000.

## Alternatives to the Standard Keyboard

We often use expanded or contracted keyboards when an individual with physical disabilities cannot use a standard keyboard (see Chapter 7). Current approaches to these adapted keyboards include both the hardware necessary for input to the computer and software allowing the keyboard alternative to replace the standard keyboard. The electrical connection to the computer is provided via a cable that connects the computer to the Apple desktop bus (ADB) or USB port (Macintosh) or serial port, keyboard port, parallel port, or USB port (Windows computer).

## Alternatives to the Standard Mouse

It is possible to use the arrow keys on the keyboard to simulate mouse movement. This software interprets the arrow keys as mouse input when the mouse-emulating software is active and interprets them as arrow keys when it is not active. One version of this is called *MouseKeys* and is included in the Accessibility Options for Windows and in the Macintosh operating systems. MouseKeys allows adjustment of the mouse speed (distance the cursor moves with each arrow key press) and acceleration (the rate at which the cursor moves).

When a trackball, joystick, or other hardware alternative is substituted for the mouse, a software program called a *driver* is also required. The mouse emulator is a software driver program that provides an input to the computer that causes the mouse cursor to move as though a real mouse has been used. If the mouse emulator allows switched joystick control, then any array of four switches can be used (see Chapter 7). Both trackball and joystick approaches must also accommodate the mouse buttons, including clicking (rapid press and release), double-clicking, and dragging (holding the button while moving the mouse). To accomplish all these functions, both hardware connections to the computer and software programs that interact directly with the computer's operating system are required. There are software programs that replace these mouse button func-

tions with dwelling on the selection and by selecting which mouse button function is required.

## On-screen Keyboard Software

The term **on-screen keyboard** is used to refer to those keyboard **emulation** methods that employ a video image of the keyboard on the video screen, together with a cursor.* A typical on-screen keyboard display is shown in Figure 8-3. On-screen keyboards use mouse (point-and-click) approaches to make selections. Any of the mouse alternatives described in Chapter 7 can be used. All approaches require both a hardware interface and a software program. The software places the keyboard image on the screen, detects the mouse cursor position, relates the position to the key label of the on-screen keyboard image, and inserts that character into the keyboard routine of the computer, so it is treated as a typed character.

Various types of on-screen keyboards allow changes in the keyboard arrangement, size of the on-screen keys, location of the keyboard on the screen, and methods by which this customization can be accomplished. Many of the on-screen keyboard systems also include other characteristics. One of the most common is a word prediction feature that displays frequently used words as the first few characters are typed. Each word may be in a key location or on a list presented in a window. This type of input acceleration is discussed in more detail in Chapter 9. Other features that can be used to optimize performance include horizontal and vertical cursor movement speed, keyboard layouts, and location of the keyboard image on the screen (e.g., top or

*Discover: Screen, Don Johnston Developmental Systems, Wauconda, Ill. (www.donjohnston.com); EZ Keys, Words Plus, Lancaster, Calif. (www.words-plus.com); HandiKey and HandiKey Deluxe, Cyber Patrol, The Learning Company Framingham, Mass. (www.cyberpatrol.com); Liason, Apt Technologies, Shreve, Ohio (www.apt-technology.com); On Screen, RJ Cooper, Dana-Point, Calif. (www.rjcooper.com); ScreenDoors, Madentec Communications, Inc., Edmonton, Alberta, Canada (www.madentec.com); Reach Interface Author, San Antonio, Tex. (www.aht-net.com/reach); SofType, Origin Instruments Corp., Grand Prairie, Tex. (www.orin.com); WiVik, WiVik2, and WiVik2 Scan, all available from Prentke Romich Co., Wooster, Ohio (www.prentrom.com).

bottom, depending on the type of application program that is running). Anson (1997) describes several commercial approaches to both hardware and software for on-screen keyboards.

## Automatic Speech Recognition As an Alternative Keyboard

Automatic speech recognition technology can be applied to computer access by allowing the user to speak the names of keys or key words and have these spoken utterances interpreted by the computer as if they had been typed. This approach is appealing because human speech is so rapid and voice control is so natural. Automatic speech recognition systems that are extremely reliable, flexible, and easy to use are available for use as full-function GIDEIs. These systems also allow the user to speak. For example, if a word processing program is being run, then control functions such as Delete, Move, and Print, as well as the most common vocabulary the person normally uses, a greeting and ending for a business letter, and other similar vocabulary items can be used. If the user changes to a spreadsheet program, he can use vocabulary that contains items specific to that application.

## Cognitive Access via Concept Keyboards

**Concept keyboards** replace the letters and numbers of the keyboard with pictures, symbols, or words that represent the concepts being used or taught. When the user presses on the picture, the correct character is sent to the computer to create the desired effect. As an example, a child who is having difficulty with basic arithmetic and monetary concepts may be more successful using a concept keyboard in which each key displayed is a coin of a particular denomination, rather than the value (number) or name of the coin (letters). The child can push on the coin and have that number of cents entered into the program. A simple program that asks the child to make change could be used to encourage the child to develop subtraction skills while also learning the value of specific coins. This approach is more motivating for some children and it is easier to press on a key labeled with a quarter than to enter "2" and "5."

Very simple programs may require only two keys. For example, the SPACE key can move a cursor to different matching choices and the RETURN key can select the desired one. This concept can be used to match shapes or numbers or to control any two-choice task. It functions as a keyboard, even though only two keys are used.

Another approach to concept keyboards is the use of specially designed software together with special-input keyboards. These systems do not require the use of a special input interface because they plug directly into a serial, parallel, USB, or ADB port. The software also comes with overlays for the keyboard. For example, a program to teach

language concepts can be implemented by placing pictures of the concepts on specific keys and having the child generate words by pressing the correct key, causing the concept to be spoken and the picture to be repeated on the screen. When the child plays with the objects described, she learns to label her actions, as well as the objects. Concept keyboards provide a direct relationship between the task and the child's action. For example, by using a picture of the body as the "keyboard" and each body part as a "key," a child can touch the body part when the program instructs him to do so. When he does, the program can repeat the body part name and cause it to be moved on the screen. The Intellikeys keyboard* is often used as a concept keyboard.

An even more direct concept keyboard is the Touch Window.† With this device the user merely touches the screen at the proper place and the touch screen enters the information as though it has been typed. Monitors with built-in touch screens are also available for Macintosh and Windows computers. Moving the finger on the screen can also be used to draw. This device can be placed horizontally on a table or lap tray and used as a concept keyboard with an appropriate overlay.

## Switch-Controlled Keyboard and Mouse Emulation: Scanning and Morse Code

When the use of a keyboard of any type (including on-screen keyboards and automatic speech recognition) is not practical, we use scanning or coded access, as discussed in Chapter 7. When considering using scanning for computer access, it is important to keep in mind that a scanning display of some sort must be used to present the choices to the user. Typically the scanning array resembles an on-screen keyboard, and it may occupy up to half of the screen. This results in the user's having two windows open, one for the scanning array and one for the application program.

On-screen keyboards can also be used with scanning. In this case, additional hardware is required to accept from one to five switches as input. The scanning hardware plugs into the computer through a parallel, serial, or USB port (Windows) or the ADB or USB port (Macintosh). The scanning operation of the on-screen keyboard is similar to that of other scanning applications such as augmentative communication devices (see Chapter 9). One or more of the scanning approaches described in Chapter 7 may be used. Once a scanning choice is made, the on-screen keyboard software performs the same tasks as in the direct selection (mouse-pointing) case described earlier.

Software adaptations that allow scanning control of mouse functions are also available. In one approach, a line moves slowly down the screen when the user presses the

---

*Intellitools, Richmond, Calif. (www.intellitools.com).
†Edmark, Redmond, Wash. (www.edmark.com).

**TABLE 8-2  Nonstandardized Morse Codes Used for Computer Access**

| Character | Ke:nx* | Darci Too† | HandiCode‡ |
|---|---|---|---|
| ESC | ---. | ..-.. | ---- |
| ENTER | .-.- | .-.- | .-.- |
| DELETE | ..-.. | -..-. | -- |
| TAB | -.-.- | -.--... | ...... |
| . | .-.-. | .-.-. | .-.-. |
| ! | .-..- | .-.-.. | ---..- |
| $ | .-.-. | -....-. | -..-- |
| SPACE | ..-- | ..-- | .-.- |
| , | --..-- | --..-- | --..-- |
| ". | -.-- | -..-- | --.-- |
| ( | ..-.-. | .--..-.. | ---.- |
| ) | ..-.- | ...---. | ..---. |
| UP ARROW | --.-- | -.-.-.- | .-..- |
| DOWN ARROW | --..- | -.--.-. | .-... |
| LEFT ARROW | ---- | -.-.-.. | .-.-.. |
| RIGHT ARROW | ..-..- | -.-.-. | .-.-. |
| SHIFT | ....-. | ..-.- | ....-. |

NOTE: Standard alphanumeric Morse code characters are shown in Chapter 7.
* Ke:nx for Macintosh computers, Don Johnston Developmental Systems, Wauconda, Ill.
†Darci Too for Windows-based computers, WesTest Engineering, Bountiful, Utah.
‡HandiCode for Windows-based computers, Microsystems Software, Inc., Framingham, Mass.

scanning switch.* As it scrolls down the screen, the line intersects various on-screen icons. If the switch is pressed a second time, a pointer moves across the screen. When the pointer is located over the desired screen icon, a third switch press selects that icon as though the mouse button had been pressed. These programs also allow the user to select what mouse button function (click to select, double-click to open and run the application, or drag to move) is activated with the third switch press.

The other major option for single- or dual-switch users is coded access (see Chapter 7), including Morse code and Darci code.† Because codes are typically memory based, they do not require a selection display (a set of characters on the screen) as is needed for an on-screen keyboard or scanning array. This allows the entire screen to be used for the application software being run. Recall that one of our basic principles for computer adaptation to be successful is that 100% of the keys on the keyboard must be available to the user. When Samuel Morse invented his code in the late 1880s there were no computers, and therefore basic Morse code (see Chapter 7) does not include ESC or RETURN keys on the computer or characters such as punctuation or \@#$%. Even more important, Morse saw no need for a SPACE character. He just told his key operators to wait a

*Cross Scanner, RJ Cooper, DanaPoint, Calif. (rjcooper.com).
†Darci Too, WesTest Engineering Corp., Bountiful, Utah (www.darci.org).

**CASE STUDY 8-1**

**AAC AS COMPUTER INPUT**

You are working with a teenager who has an augmentative and alternative communication (AAC) device that she uses very well (see Chapter 9). She has come to you for development of computer access for writing in school. Which of the Accessibility Options would you use to interface with her AAC device? What questions would you ask about her AAC device, and what capabilities would it need to have to be functional in this application? What character strings would need to be available in the AAC device for her to be able to input the RETURN, ALT, and SHIFT characters in her word processing program?

little longer between dots and dashes (a dot [.] is a short sound and a dash [-] is a longer sound). Unfortunately for us, the computer requires that a specific ASCII character be sent for SPACE. The absence of standardized codes for anything other than alphanumeric characters presents a problem with using Morse code for computer access. Examples of codes developed for computer use by several different manufacturers are listed in Table 8-2. Note that in some cases the codes for the same characters are different for the three systems and in other cases they are the same. This makes it difficult for the consumer to change from one communication device or adapted input device to another. Once the set of codes is learned and the motor patterns developed, it is very difficult to change to a new set of codes. Computer access using either scanning or Morse code can be accomplished by software programs, hardware adaptations, or combinations of both.

## Communication Devices As Alternative Inputs

Many augmentative communication devices (see Chapter 9) can also function as alternative keyboards for computer access. This approach has the advantage that the operator of the communication device can use the same control interface and selection technique for computer access as she uses for communication. This reduces training and skill development time (e.g., no need to learn two keyboard layouts) and allows the user to concentrate on learning how to operate the computer. Another advantage is that any vocabulary (e.g., words or phrases or complete computer commands) stored in the communication device can be sent from the communication device to the computer as a whole using a serial port. In many currently available communication devices, computer control is a built-in feature. In others it must be added as an option. Accessibility Options (Windows) and Universal Access (Macintosh) provide for input from the communication device via serial keys (see Table 8-1).

| TABLE 8-3 | Trace Standard for Computer Input Via Augmentative Communication Systems and Other GIDEIs | |
| --- | --- | --- |
| Key Designation | ESC Sequence | Computer* |
| DEL | [ESC]del. | A |
| DELETE | [ESC]delete. | I, M |
| CONTROL | [ESC]control. | All |
| DOWN ARROW | [ESC]down. | All |
| LEFT ARROW | [ESC]left. | All |
| ENTER | [ESC]enter. | M, I |
| RETURN | [ESC]ret. | A, M |
| TAB | [ESC]tab. | All |
| BACKSPACE | [ESC]backspace. | I, M |
| SHIFT | [ESC]shift. | A, I, M† |
| ALTERNATE | [ESC]alt. | I† |
| CONTROL | [ESC]ctrl. | A, I,† M† |
| ESCAPE | [ESC]esc. | All |
| RESET | [ESC]reset. | A |
| FUNCTION + # | [ESC]f# | I‡ |
| INSERT | [ESC]insert. | I |
| HOME | [ESC]home. | I |
| END | [ESC]end. | I |
| PAGE UP | [ESC]pageup. | I, M |
| PAGE DOWN | [ESC]pagedown. | I, M |
| KEYPAD | [ESC]keypad. | I, M§ |
| SCROLL | [ESC]scroll. | I, M |
| PRINT SCREEN | [ESC]print. | I |
| OPTION | [ESC]option. | A, M |

*A, Apple II series; M, Apple Macintosh; I, Windows PC.
†Some computers have both left and right shift, control, or alternate keys; use left or right key. For example, LEFT SHIFT = [ESC]lshift., RIGHT ALT = [ESC]ralt., LEFT CONTROL = [ESC]rctrl.
‡This sequence is used for each function key, with the key number substituted for the # sign; for example, function key #1 = [ESC]f1.
§On Macintosh and Windows PCs, the keypad keys are all preceded by kp; for example, 7 on keypad = [ESC]kp7.

There are, however, some disadvantages to this approach. One of these is that in many cases the communication device needs to be physically connected to the computer; that is, a cable must be physically plugged in to the computer. An alternative approach is to use wireless links to replace the cable. Most wireless systems use infrared (IR) links, which are similar to the IR environmental control links described in Chapter 11.

The second potential problem is that most communication devices are not able to generate all the possible ASCII codes needed for general-purpose computer access. For this reason, a special standard* has been developed for establishing interaction between the computer and the communication device. Table 8-3 lists examples of the character strings used in this standard. All these codes begin with the ESC (escape) code and end with a period (.), and they are intended to be transmitted over a cable to the computer

*Available from the Trace Center, University of Wisconsin, Madison, Wisc. (www.trace.wisc.edu).

serial port. Unfortunately, not all currently available communication devices support this standard, and it may be necessary for the ATP to program the communication device manually to allow use of the computer. For example, one square on a communication device may have the sequence of characters "[ESC]ret." stored; when this square is selected, the computer responds as though the RETURN key has been pressed. These characters must be programmed into the communication device, together with the other sequences in Table 8-3.

Referring to Table 8-3, to cause a TAB key to be entered, a GIDEI that adheres to the Trace standard looks for the five-character string [ESC]TAB., and when it is received, the program running on the computer reacts as if the TAB key has been pressed by itself from the keyboard. For example, in a word processing program, pressing the TAB key moves the cursor five spaces to the right. Another example from Table 8-3 is the entry of a function key. The Trace standard uses the four characters [ESC]F1. as the character string for function key number 1. When this string is sent from the communication device, the computer acts as if the key F1 has been pressed from the keyboard. In many programs, entering this key results in a help menu, and the character string has the same effect as pressing the F1 key.

## ■ KEYBOARD- AND MOUSE-EMULATING INTERFACES

In this section we describe the characteristics of typical GIDEIs. Like all other computer hardware and software, commercial GIDEIs change rapidly, and we emphasize the general characteristics of these devices in this section. Commercial products may be implemented with features that include some or all of the general characteristics discussed here.

In general, the less flexible the host computer is, the more the GIDEI must do. Thus early GIDEIs developed for computers such as the Apple II series required maximal hardware and software to implement the needed functions. Systems designed for Windows computers or the Macintosh rely much more on the flexibility of the host computer and primarily require a software approach for implementation.

### Characteristics of General Input Device-Emulating Interfaces

It is important to think of the GIDEI as having a set of features that allows the computer to be altered for a given application and a specific person with a disability. This set of features is called a *setup*, a concept that originated with the Adaptive Firmware Card (AFC) for the Apple II series of computers (Schwejda and Vanderheiden, 1982). As

| BOX 8-1 | Major Features of Commonly Used General Input Device-Emulating Interfaces |

**A setup consists of the following three parts:**
1. Input method
   Keyboard:
   • Assisted
   • Contracted
   • Expanded
   • Virtual
   • Normal
   Morse code:
   • One switch
   • Two switch
   ASCII*:
   • Parallel
   • Serial
   Scanning:
   • Linear or row-column
   • Auto, inverse, or step
   • Single, dual, four, or five switch
   • Switched joystick
   Proportional:
   • Mouse
   • Trackball
   • Joystick
2. Overlay: all three of the following may be the same or they may be different

User: the selection set arrangement from which the user chooses
Computer: the character or string of characters sent to the application program when the user chooses
Speech: synthetic speech used as a prompt to the user or as feedback when a selection is made
3. Options
   Abbreviations: text-based codes
   Autocaps: CAP and 2 spaces after ., !, or ?
   Key repeat rate
   Levels: like a shift, can be many levels on one setup; equivalent in scanning is branching
   Macros: codes can include control characters and functions
   Mouse emulation: move, drag, click, and tab
   Multitasking: can interrupt one mode for another
   Predictive entry: previous characters determine user overlay
   Rate: how fast or slow the user can input to the GIDEI
   Screen selection display location: where on the screen the user overlay appears
   Slowdown of programs
**Application program or disk:**
The business, education, or recreational program being used

*Sometimes used with AAC, environmental control units, or powered wheelchair controllers (see text).

shown in Box 8-1, a setup consists of three basic elements: (1) an input method (see Chapter 7), (2) overlays, and (3) a set of options. The features of the setup may be implemented in hardware (electronic circuits) or software (a program) or both. Storage of a setup may be in memory within the GIDEI hardware or resident in the computer RAM. Setups are also usually stored on the computer hard disk drive or in the peripheral device (e.g., an adapted keyboard). This allows them to be loaded into the computer or the GIDEI as needed. As shown in Box 8-1, the setup is used with an *application program.*

Several examples of setups that may be used with numerous application programs are shown in Figure 8-4. The setup shown in Figure 8-4, *A,* is intended to be used for text entry in a business environment. The application software can be a word processor, a spreadsheet, or a database. The major function is the entry of text characters, and the setup includes several options to make this process more efficient. Auto capitalization automatically enters two spaces and latches the shift function following sentence-ending punctuation (i.e., .?!). Abbreviations allow a few characters to be used as a code for a longer word or phrase. The user of the GIDEI stores both the sequence of characters and their corresponding abbreviation. When the abbreviation (code) is entered, the GIDEI automatically expands it into the whole stored word or phrase. For example, typing the two letters *MN* (for "my name") followed by an abbreviation

key would result in the user's name and address being entered. Several methods of abbreviation expansion and other types of rate enhancement are discussed in Chapter 9. The setup also includes *macros,* which are codes similar to abbreviations. The macros differ, however, in that they are often used to control application program functions. For example, assume that the word processor requires that the following keys be pressed to set a margin (such as for typing an address on an envelope): SHIFT F8 (shifted function key number 8) 174 ENTER, a total of 6 keystrokes (if SHIFT and F8 are pressed in sequence). A macro for this key sequence could be defined as [ALT]E. This would save four keystrokes (if ALT and E were pressed in sequence), and it would also be easier to remember these two keys than the entire key sequence. It is also possible to store mouse functions and "replay" them with one command. Another way to save keystrokes is for the computer to anticipate the words based on previous characters entered. For example, if a *T* is typed, then an *H* is very likely to follow. Likewise, it is possible to predict whole words rather than just letters. This method of input acceleration is called *word prediction* or *word completion.* In some cases the GIDEI software program keeps track of the words that the user inputs most frequently, and the choices presented is in the order of frequency of use for the specific person utilizing the GIDEI. We discuss word prediction further in Chapter 9. Many of these options are available for both the

|   | Method | Overlay | Options | Application |
|---|--------|---------|---------|-------------|
| **A** | Virtual keyboard | User:       QWERTY Layout<br>Computer: Same<br>Speech:    No | Speed of mouse<br>•<br>• | Business, productivity software (word processing, spreadsheet, etc.) |
| **B** | Single-switch scanning | User:       ETA Array<br>Computer: Same<br>Speech:    No | Rate<br>•<br>• | |
| **C** | Expanded keyboard | User:  ⇨ 🛑<br>Computer: Arrow, Return<br>Speech:    "This one,"<br>             "Next one" | Speech Slowdown<br>•<br>• | Early education matching task with arrow and return |
| **D** | Single-switch scanning | User:  ---> OK<br>Computer: Arrow, Return<br>Speech:    "This one,"<br>             "Next one" | Rate<br>Speech<br>Slowdown | |

Figure 8-4   A GIDEI setup consists of three parts: input method, overlay, and options. **A-D,** Four examples of GIDEI setups for different consumers and different applications are shown.

Windows (see http://microsoft.com/enable/) and Macintosh (see www.apple.com/education/k12/disability/) operating systems. Additional information is available from the manufacturers' Web sites listed here.

This set of options can be used with any of the input methods shown in Box 8-1. The particular input method determines the overlays. For example, if the individual is using an on-screen keyboard, the display of the keyboard layout on the screen can contain key locations for use as macros and it can be arranged to make selections as fast as possible (see Figure 8-4, *A*). For a single-switch user, the overlay on the screen may be a scanning array with special characters included, as shown in Figure 8-4, *B*.

A second setup, shown in Figure 8-4, *C* and *D,* is for a young child who is using any of a wide range of software programs that require selection of an answer by matching a cursor (pointer) location with the correct item (Figure 8-5). The task may be to match numbers, letters, shapes, words, or pictures. Often the software requires that one key (e.g., RIGHT ARROW) be used to move the cursor and another key (e.g., RETURN) to select the one that the student believes is correct. Two setups are shown in Figure 8-4 for this application. In this case the user and computer overlays are different, and we also have included a speech overlay. Because the user is not likely to have learned to read yet, we use the speech overlay to help identify the choices to be made. We also use speech as a reinforcer when the choice is made. This is shown as a second speech overlay in Figure 8-4, *C.* This setup is for use with an expanded keyboard. In

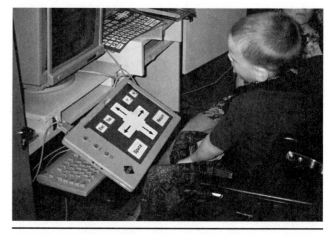

Figure 8-5   A GIDEI overlay for cursor-controlling movement using arrows. This is being used with an expanded keyboard and an educational software program.

this case a visual overlay that utilizes symbols can be used. An example is shown in Figure 8-6. Another overlay, Figure 8-4, *D,* uses scanning on the screen, and we are restricted to text characters. We can generate an arrow with two dashes and the greater than (>) sign. We chose to use "OK" as the label for "this is the one I want" (the student's choice). For both these setups we use the speech, scanning rate, and program slowdown options. However, for the second (scanning) we also include an option that allows us to place the scanning array on any line of the display monitor. This is

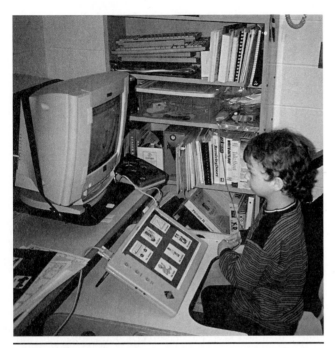

**Figure 8-6**   A symbol-based GIDEI overlay for use with an expanded keyboard and an educational software program.

---

**CASE STUDY 8-2**

**DESIGN OF A GIDEI FOR SCANNING**

Assume that you are working with a child who is using a program that requires the four arrow keys to move between on-screen locations and a "choose key" to pick the desired alternative. Design a scanning GIDEI setup for this child. Include all of the elements shown in Figure 8-4. What labels would you use for the GIDEI overlay? How would this GIDEI differ if the child were using direct selection on an enlarged keyboard?

---

important because the scan line can hide part of the program if it is in a fixed location.

Many GIDEIs allow other features, such as mouse emulation and the use of macro instructions and multitasking. Mouse emulation substitutes a set of keys, a scanning array, or Morse code characters for mouse functions (similar to MouseKeys, described earlier). Macros can be used to return the mouse cursor to a specific location based on stored information. This can save time when scanning is the mode used for mouse emulation. **Multitasking** is the ability to pause while running one software program to run another program. For example, if a person is writing using a word processor and someone interrupts him, he can convert

to his communication program, talk to the person, and then resume his word processing program without having to exit one program and start the next. All these features can be incorporated into a setup that can be loaded when it is necessary or desirable to use the mouse. Anson (1997) describes the characteristics of several GIDEIs for both Windows and Macintosh operating systems.

### Examples of Commercial GIDEIs

There are many commercially available GIDEIs. Some are designed for Windows-based computers, some for the Macintosh computer, and some for both. All GIDEIs have a software component, and some also have hardware that is used for emulation. All also have provisions for attachment of control interfaces (alternative keyboards, switches, etc.). Because many alternative input methods discussed in Chapter 7 include their own built-in decoding to make them function like the standard keyboard, they do not require an external GIDEI. There are, however, some hardware GIDEIs that perform additional functions not possible in a software-only approach. The simplest of these is the attachment of a switch for use with scanning or encoded access. The current situation in adapted computer input is one in which a great variety of approaches exist in commercial systems. These do, however, fall into several categories. First are adapted inputs that have all the necessary hardware for storage and use of setups (as described above) built into their hardware. These may also have software that is loaded into the computer and facilitates the creation of setups. A second approach is stand-alone GIDEIs that accept a range of adapted inputs and provide the necessary support for setups, as well as the decoding required for the computer to accept the input as if it came from the keyboard. These devices will also often have a software component that is loaded into the computer and is used for setup creation, implementation, or both. Finally, there are software-only systems that utilize the standard computer input ports and provide the capability for customization via setups. Devices in all these categories are available for both Windows and Macintosh operating systems.

**Adapted inputs with built-in GIDEIs.** Many of the adapted inputs described in Chapter 7 include decoding, which allows them to provide input to the computer as though it has been typed from the keyboard or generated by mouse actions. Examples of such systems are listed in Table 7-2. The operation of these adapted input devices is discussed in Chapter 7. In general, these systems also require a software program to be loaded into the host computer. This software may be used as part of the emulation process, and it also supports specialized setups for the adapted input device,

**Stand-alone GIDEIs.** The first GIDEI to be widely available was the Adaptive Firmware Card. The original version of this device was intended for use in the Apple II+ computer (Schwejda and Vanderheiden, 1982). The features incorporated in the AFC are still fundamental to most current GIDEIs. In a very real sense, virtually all the basic GIDEI capabilities have their origins in the AFC. The major advances in GIDEI design have been the result of advances in the host computer, rather than fundamental insights into the process of keyboard and mouse emulation.

Many of the stand-alone GIDEIS also allow for synthetic speech feedback through the use of "talking setups" that allow the user to receive auditory, as well as visual, prompting and feedback. This is useful for young children who may not be able to read, for visually impaired individuals, and as an added input modality for persons with learning disabilities.

The Ke:nx* was designed to provide alternative input to the Macintosh. Ke:nx incorporates scanning, alternative keyboard, and on-screen keyboard functions. The Ke:nx is installed in the system folder of the Macintosh desktop, and it can either be enabled at startup (when the power is turned on) or activated by clicking on a Ke:nx icon once the computer has booted. Some of the most useful features of this GIDEI are those that are specifically aimed at the GUI. It is possible with the Ke:nx, for example, to set tabs on the screen where the mouse is to point, and then store the tab as a code (or macro). When the code is entered (using any of the basic selection methods and control interfaces), the mouse carries out the movement stored. By saving a series of mouse movements, it is possible to move to a menu, open it, select a specific entry, and then double-click (to start execution), all with one command. This not only saves many mouse movements, but it also avoids errors during tedious and complex movements. These errors could require that the entire sequence be reentered. Ke:nx also provides row-column scanning with visually enhanced scanning arrays. Other useful features include digitized speech, on-screen keyboards, touch windows, and development and printing of keyboard overlays for use with expanded keyboards. The features of Ke:nx are also available in the Discover Switch (scanning), Discover Screen (on-screen keyboard), and Discover Board (expanded keyboard) systems.

The Darci Too† provides for alternative mouse, alternative keyboard, joystick, and switch input to Windows-based and Macintosh computers. Input to the computer is through the serial port and conforms to the Trace standard for GIDEI design. Both a hardware component for attaching the external device to the computer and software to accept that input are included. Two versions of the Darci Too are available. One uses an external hardware box that connects to a serial port on the computer. Five operating modes are available with the Darci Too: scanning, Morse

code, Darci code (see Chapter 7), matrix keyboard, and communication device. The Darci USB supports alternative input similar to the Darci Too on a portable computer.

**Software-based GIDEIs.** All the hardware approaches we have described are relatively expensive, and software-only approaches are less expensive. The process by which a computer can be adapted using a software program is described by Hortsman, Levine, and Jaros (1989). Programs in this category range from those implementing the basic features of Table 8-1 to the use of alternate control interfaces and selection methods (Gorgens, Bergler, and Gorgens, 1990). The programs described by these authors and others provide access to Windows and or Macintosh operating systems.* Anson (1997) describes these and other approaches.

Shein et al (1991) describe some of the challenges, as well as approaches that solve some of the problems in the development of GIDEIs for Windows. They indicate that any visual keyboard in a GUI should have several features. First, selecting keys (e.g., with an on-screen keyboard and head pointer) from the visual keyboard should not transfer the internal computer keyboard routines to the new selection, but should keep the computer looking for input from the visual keyboard. Typically the most recently opened window is "on top" of the others. If the keyboard image is in a window, then it must stay on top even if selections from it open another window. Second, the visual keyboard array should send keystroke input information to the application that is active at any given time. Finally, Shein and co-workers state that the visual keyboard should support a range of layouts. These authors have developed one software-based GIDEI for the Windows and OS/2 GUIs.† Several other commercially available products for Windows are available. These products include a variety of input methods (on-screen keyboard with pointing device, scanning in several modes, Morse code), output options (voice synthesis, enlarged screen characters), and optional features (e.g., word prediction, communication device pop-up windows, environmental control interfaces to telephone and appliances). Just like other computer-based products, changes occur frequently in these software-based GIDEIs.

## ■ BASIC PRINCIPLES OF ADAPTED COMPUTER OUTPUTS

As we have stated, computer interaction is bi-directional, and the ATP must also understand how computer outputs can be adapted for persons with sensory impairments. Stan-

---

*Don Johnston Developmental Systems, Wauconda, Ill. (www.donjohnston.com).
†WesTest Engineering Corp., Bountiful, Utah (www.darci.org).

*HelpWare, World Communications, Fremont, Calif; HandiWare, Microsystems Software, Framingham, Mass.; Prentke Romich Co., Wooster, Ohio (www.prentrom.com); Regenesis Development Corp., North Vancouver, B.C., Canada; Words Plus, Lancaster, Calif.
†WiVik, WiVik2, and WiVik2 Scan, all available from Prentke Romich Co., Wooster, Ohio (www.prentrom.com).

dard computer outputs (visual display devices and printers) are not suitable for use by persons who have visual impairments. We use the term *low vision* to indicate that the individual is able to use her visual system for reading, but the standard size, contrast, and/or spacing are inadequate. We use the term *blind* to refer to individuals for whom the visual system does not provide a useful input channel for computer output displays or printers. For individuals who are blind, we must use alternative sensory pathways of either audition (hearing) or touch (feeling) to provide input. Because low-vision and blindness needs are so different from each other, we discuss them separately. Persons who are deaf or hard of hearing also may experience difficulties in recognizing auditory computer outputs such as sounds or speech. Adaptations that facilitate some of these functions and that are included in Accessibility Options in Windows* are shown in Table 8-4. ToggleKeys generates a sound when CAPS LOCK, NUM LOCK, or SCROLL LOCK key is pressed. ShowSounds displays captions for speech and sounds. SoundSentry generates a visual warning when the system generates a sound.

In Chapter 12 we discuss assistive technologies for general-purpose reading and mobility for persons who are blind or have low vision. Some of the devices (e.g., reading machines or refreshable braille displays) can be used to provide both output from and input to a computer. In this section, however, we focus primarily on assistive technologies that have been designed and developed specifically to provide persons with visual impairments access to information normally presented on computer video displays.

## Alternatives to Visual Displays for Individuals with Low Vision

For individuals with low vision, the major problem with visual computer displays is that the on-screen text and graphics are not easily readable. There are three factors that affect the readability of text (see the section on sensory function in Chapter 3): (1) size (vertical height), (2) spacing (horizontal distance between letters and width of letters), and (3) contrast (the relationship of background and foreground color). These apply to all types of monitors (black and white, monochrome, and color). Thus the problem we must solve is to alter the size, spacing, or contrast of the soft copy display to make the characters readable to the individual with low vision.

Screen-magnifying software that enlarges a portion of the screen is the most common adaptation for people who have low vision. We refer to the unmagnified screen as the *physical screen*. The screen magnification program takes one section of the physical screen and enlarges it to fit the whole display screen. Thus at any one time the user has access to only the portion of the physical screen that appears in this

| TABLE 8-4 | Simple Adaptations for Sensory Impairment* | |
|---|---|---|
| Need Addressed | | Software Approach |
| User cannot see ToggleKeys lights (for showing status of CAPS LOCK, NUM LOCK, etc.) | | ToggleKeys |
| User cannot hear beeps used to signal change of operation or error during program operation | | SoundSentry |
| User cannot hear speech or sounds made by programs | | ShowSounds |

*Software modifications developed at the Trace Center, University of Wisconsin, Madison. These are included as before-market modifications to DOS, OS/2, or Windows in some personal computers and are available as after-market versions in others.

magnified viewing window. The size of the text in this window is referred to as the *magnification* and varies from 2 to 32 times or more in current magnifier programs. The viewing window must track any changes that occur on the physical screen. This means that the window must move to show the portion of the physical screen in which the changes are occurring. Commercial screen readers move the viewing window to any point on the GUI where input is required or where a change has occurred. For example, if a navigation or control box is active, then the viewing window highlights that box. If mouse movement occurs, then the viewing window tracks the mouse cursor movement. If text is being typed in, then the viewing window highlights that portion of the physical screen. Scrolling allows the user to slowly move the viewing window over the physical screen image. This may be automatic or manual.

Brown (1989) has identified the capabilities that an ideal screen magnification utility should have. These are listed in Box 8-2. As stated earlier in this chapter, the major goal of computer access for persons with disabilities is to provide the same computer capabilities to them as are available to the rest of the population. This is the intent of the legislation discussed in Chapter 1, and it is addressed by the capabilities listed in Box 8-2. Compatibility with all commercially available software is the hallmark of equal accessibility. If the adaptations provided work with only a few commercial applications, then the user with low vision becomes relegated to second-class user status. However, it is also important that the adaptations not prevent a nondisabled person from using the computer. This is important, for example, in data processing applications, where several shifts of workers may use the same computer workstations at different times of the day. If the adaptation prevents this type of use, then it is much less likely to be accepted by the employer. Thus the low-vision adaptation must also make it easy to shift to the normal screen. Finally, the standard computer user interface is a GUI, and it is important that

*Microsoft Corp., Seattle, Wash. (microsoft.com/enable).

this and other graphical representations be made available in adaptations for low vision.

Also shown in Box 8-2 are user interface capabilities that are important in low-vision adaptations of computer outputs. Because the visual skills of individuals vary widely, it is important to have a variety of sizes of text and foreground-background color combinations. These are two of the three factors that influence visibility of text for reading. The ability to adjust these parameters is also important because persons with low vision often experience fluctuations in their visual capabilities throughout the day. Because the text and graphics in an application program may appear anywhere on the physical screen, it is important that the enlarged viewing window be movable to any location on the screen and not be confined to the top left corner (for example). Once again, this location should be under the control of the user.

A final set of capabilities shown in Box 8-2 relate to the operation of the low-vision adaptation and interaction with the computer. Brown (1989) recommends that the adaptation be software based instead of consisting of a combination of software and hardware, primarily because it can be easily installed in any computer. In educational or vocational settings, where one person may use several computers, software-based adaptations can be more easily moved from one computer to another. Also, a consumer can carry the magnifier software to school or a job and install it on the educational or work computer easily. Although these factors are important, hardware adaptations are often more flexible and provide better results than software-only systems. If hardware adaptations are used, Brown recommends that they be contained completely within the computer (such as

on a plug-in circuit board). Ease of use and maintenance emphasize that the method of adaptation be simple in concept and that the interface presented to the user should not require extensive training to use it. One way to address this is to make the adapted system operation as similar to the procedures required for the standard computer (which the user must learn anyway) as possible. Brown (1989) recommends that systems to be used in educational or business settings require no more than 30 minutes of training.

Visual input depends on a stable image, and text that is jerky or erratic is not easily read. Because low-vision systems provide a continually moving window that enlarges a portion of the text, it is important that the movement of this window be smooth. Likewise, when the user moves the viewing window from one location to another, the low-vision system should be able to follow and update the window rapidly. Finally, the low-vision adaptation should be cost effective. Note that we said *cost effective*, not inexpensive. When considering cost effectiveness, we must include both the benefits received (e.g., access to a computer and perhaps an education or a job) and the cost of making the adaptations. As we have emphasized throughout this text, there are many ways to solve almost all problems, and picking the one that meets the person's needs at the lowest cost is one of the roles of the ATP.

Adaptations that allow persons with low vision to access the computer screen are available in several commercial forms. Lazzaro (1999) describes several potential methods of achieving computer access. The simplest and least costly are built-in screen enlargement software programs provided by the computer manufacturer. One system for the Macintosh, built in to the operating system, is CloseView.* This program allows for magnification from 2 to 16 times and has fast and easy text handling and graphics capabilities (Brown, 1989). Magnifier (included in Windows†) displays an enlarged portion of the screen (from 2 to 9 times magnification) in a separate window. Options include having the window follow mouse cursor movement, follow the text editing, or follow keyboard entry. In addition, both inverted (e.g., black background, white letters) and high-contrast modes are available. For individuals who need only the high contrast option, that is also available in Accessibility Options for Windows. High contrast uses color combinations for text, background, windows, and other GUI features. None of these built-in options are intended to replace full-function screen magnifiers.

Screen magnifying lenses that are placed over the monitor can also enlarge the information, but limited magnification (about 2 times) and distortion are the major problems. Increased contrast and reduced glare can be achieved with

---

| BOX 8-2 | Capabilities of an Ideal Computer Output System for Low Vision |
|---|---|

**COMPATIBILITY CHARACTERISTICS**
All commercially available software
Normal screen display
Monochrome, color, or enhanced color display
Both text and graphics

**USER INTERFACE CHARACTERISTICS**
Range of text magnifications
Adjustable, automatic scrolling of text
Movement of viewing window to any location on screen

**OPERATIONAL CHARACTERISTICS**
Software based
Easy to use and maintain
Smooth, fast display of enlarged text or graphics
Cost effective

---

Data from Brown C: *Computer access in higher education for students with disabilities,* ed 2, Monterey, Calif., 1989, US Department of Education.

---

*Human Ware, a Division of Optelec, Loomis, Calif. (www.humanware.com)
†Microsoft Corp., Seattle, Wash. (microsoft.com/enable).

filters placed over the screen. Large monitors can have the effect of increasing text and graphics size, but the magnification is fixed. Adaptations that include both hardware and software provide the greatest compatibility, but they are also the most expensive alternatives. Closed circuit television (CCTV) systems often allow access not only to print material (see Chapter 12), but also to the computer video screen. The technology is virtually the same for print or computer output. One such product is Spectrum SVGA,* which allows the screen to be split into two. One half is used for CCTV display of printed material and the other is used for enlarged computer output. This system also functions as either a computer screen magnifier only or CCTV only.

Software programs that are purchased separately rather than being built in offer wider ranges of magnification and have more features than built-in screen magnifiers. For example, the inLARGE program,† for the Macintosh, provides increased scrolling and cursor tracking features (Lazzaro, 1999). This package has a standard Macintosh-style control panel. It can be linked to the outSPOKEN program for speech output (see below).

There are also both hardware and software commercial products available for Windows-based‡ systems. The Vista PCI§ provides hardware and software enlarged display capabilities. This product enlarges text with varying magnification levels and provides a mouse-controlled moving window for enlarged text. The Vista PCI includes a card that plugs into an expansion slot in the computer and a specially designed mouse that facilitate screen navigation. Vista PCI provides graphics and multiple (up to four)

enlarged windows of different portions of the screen. The multiple windows are superimposed on the entire unmagnified screen. This gives the user a rough idea as to where he is in the text. A comparable system is the VIP Librette,* which utilizes an approach similar to the Vista PCI, using both hardware and software to achieve maximal flexibility and ease of use. The VIP Librette also includes a camera that can be used to create images of three-dimensional objects such as prescription bottles. Speech output for screen reading is also included (see next section).

There are several screen magnification utilities for Windows computers† (see also the Microsoft accessibility Web site, microsoft.com/enable, and the Screen Reader Test Page, www.magnifiers.demon.nl/testintro). Many of these programs can also run with a screen reader (speech output utility). In some cases the screen reader is bundled with the magnification software, and in other cases the screen magnifier speech output runs in conjunction with a separate screen reader. Magnification of up to 32 times or more is available. These programs also allow tracking of the mouse pointer, location of keyboard entry, and text editing. The magnification window can be coupled with one or more of these to facilitate navigation for the user. All screen images (including windows, control buttons, and other windows objects) are magnified. Automatic scrolling of the screen (left, right, up, down) is also available to make it easier to read long documents when they are magnified.

For individuals who have low vision or blindness, hard copy (printer) output is also a challenge. If the output is to be read by a person with normal vision, the text can be edited on the screen using the methods described earlier and then printed out using a standard printer font size. If, however, the user with visual impairment needs to access the hard copy output, then either enlarged or braille printout is desirable. For enlarged print, the most common approach is to use a laser printer coupled with a special software program to create larger characters.

---

*Human Ware, a Division of Optelec, Loomis, Calif. (www.humanware.com)
†ALVA Access Group, Emeryville, Calif. (www.aagi.com).
‡Microsoft Corp, Seattle, Wash. (microsoft.com/enable).
§Both Vista and Vista PCI are available from Telesensory, Sunnyvale, Calif. (www.telesensory.com).

---

### CASE STUDY 8-3

#### COMPUTER ACCESS FOR LOW VISION

Cheryl is a college student. Her visual limitations prevent her from using the standard computer display. She has asked you to help her find a way for her to use the computer. The constraints on her situation are that she must use several different computers during the day: her own home computer, a laptop that she carries to class for note taking, and the computers in the student lab. What approach would you recommend for her? Would you recommend that she buy special hardware or software to meet her needs, or can she make use of features built into Windows? How would you evaluate the success of your solution for Cheryl?

## Alternatives to Visual Input for Individuals Who Are Blind

For individuals who are blind, the problem is one of providing input via an alternative sensory pathway, auditory

---

*JBliss Imaging, Los Altos, Calif. (www.jbliss.com).
†For example, Lunar and Lunar Plus from Dolphin, Computer Access, San Mateo, Calif. (www.dolphinusa.com); Magnum and Magnum Deluxe from Artic Technologies, Troy, Mich. (www.artictech.com); Magic from Freedom Scientific, St. Petersburg, Fla. (www.freedomsci.com); VIP and ezVIP from JBliss Imaging Systems, San Jose, Calif. (www.jbliss.com); Vocal Eyes, Window Eyes, LP DOS, LP Windows, and Zoom Text from GW Microsystems, Fort Wayne, Ind. (www.gwmicro.com/gwie); Zoom Text Xtra (Level 1 and Level 2, V6 and DOS) from AI Squared, Manchester Center, Vt. (www.aisquared.com).

BOX 8-3     **Capabilities of an Ideal Computer Output System for Blind Users**

**COMPATIBILITY CHARACTERISTICS**
All commercially available software
A variety of speech synthesizers
Both text and graphics

**USER INTERFACE CHARACTERISTICS**
Utilize aviator's alphabet (e.g., a = alpha, b = bravo,
    c = charlie)
Read letters, words, or lines forward or backward
Spoken output of punctuation, spaces, text attributes (bold,
    underlined, reverse video)
Read complete sentences and screens
Optional spoken output of prompts and messages

**OPERATIONAL CHARACTERISTICS**
Easy to use and maintain
Terminal emulation
Continuous review mode
Fast and accurate cursor routing
Macro capability
User-defined windows on the screen

Data from Brown C: *Computer access in higher education for students with disabilities,* ed 2, Monterey, Calif., 1989, US Department of Education.

or tactile or both. Auditory output is provided by voice synthesizers (hardware or software based), and tactile output is generally provided by braille arrays.

Systems that provide voice synthesis output for blind users are generally referred to as **screen readers.** Brown (1989) has identified the capabilities that an ideal computer voice output system for blind individuals should have. These are listed in Box 8-3. The requirements for compatibility are the same as for the low-vision system; that is, a computer user who is blind should be able to access all the same software as a person who is sighted. As indicated in Box 8-3, this applies to graphics and text. There are a variety of commercially available speech synthesizers. Most screen reader software is compatible with all these. Some companies that make screen readers also make speech synthesizers (e.g., Artic Technologies' Artic Vision and Business Vision,* and Human Ware's Keynote Gold†). Many screen reader software packages utilize the built-in speech of Macintosh or Windows-based computers. Most screen reader systems are also compatible with the DECTalk‡ voice synthesizers (DECTalk 32 software-based, DECTalk Express standalone synthesizer, and DECTalk PC plug-in card).

The major attributes of the ideal interface for blind users

are also listed in Box 8-3. These characteristics all have to do with the manner in which the on-screen information is presented to the user. Spoken letters often sound the same (e.g., *b* and *v, p* and *b*), and the use of words that represent the letters is preferred to reduce ambiguity. The aviator's alphabet (e.g., a = alpha, b = bravo, c = charlie) is often used for this type of application in speech synthesis. Most blind users prefer to use the spoken letters rather than the aviator's alphabet. Because our goal is to emulate every aspect of the visual process for reading a screen, the adapted output system should provide similar capabilities to normal vision (Brown, 1989). The key to providing access for blind users is to allow the user to select the most desirable configuration on command, so that needed information is found quickly and easily. This includes reading either forward or backward and providing speech output for punctuation, spaces, and screen attributes (such as highlighted or underlined material and features of the graphical user interface). A sighted computer user will often scan a screen for a specific piece of information or to obtain a sense of the continuity and flow of the written material, and this includes looking for specific screen attributes. For the user who is blind, duplicating this capability requires that the adapted output system provide reading of complete sentences (which may be longer or shorter than one line on the screen) and of the entire screen. User interaction should allow pausing during reading of longer passages, and the output should take full advantage of the speech synthesizer's ability to produce highly intelligible speech. Finally, some application programs provide on-screen messages or prompts for user input during program operation. The ability to read these messages and prompts is a useful feature that should be included in an ideal adapted output system. Graphic characters should have text labels attached to them. These can be read to the consumer using speech synthesis software.

Several operational characteristics that can significantly improve the effectiveness of adapted output systems are included in Box 8-3. Screen readers and other adapted output methods for blind users are often difficult to use, and they can require a great deal of training. The basic operations necessary to read letters, words, and lines should be acquired in an hour or less, but complete familiarity and skill with the system usually requires 2 to 4 weeks of training (Brown, 1989). Several screen reader manufacturers provide training material in either audio cassette or electronic (e.g., CD-ROM) format to help the user develop skill with the software.

*Terminal emulation* refers to the use of a personal computer as if it were a terminal to a mainframe computer or the Internet. (We discuss specific issues related to Internet access in the next section.) Thus the blind user can access a larger computer via an adapted personal computer and carry out the same job functions as a sighted person using the

---

*Troy, Mich. (www.artictech.com).
†Loomis, Calif. (www.humanware.com).
‡Digital Equipment Company, Maynard, Mass.

standard terminal. For the personal computer to be utilized as a terminal, it must be configured using either hardware or software to make it function like the terminals that are normally used with the mainframe computer. Because these adaptations may also take advantage of special software, hardware, or both, care must be taken to ensure that they are compatible with the screen reader. It is also important that the software running on the host computer (e.g., an Internet browser and Web site page layouts or a company mainframe computer) have features that support accessibility.

Most screen readers have two modes: application and review. With most current screen readers, reading is normally carried out in the application mode, in which the user can utilize all the screen features, as well as the features of the application program. When screen reading is carried out in review mode, the user can utilize all the screen reading features but cannot access the features of the application program. For example, a word processor text file can be read but not edited in this mode. Current systems eliminate the use of the two modes for most applications (e.g., word processing, spreadsheets, Web browsing) and provide full review capability while in an application program. For some applications (e.g., a complex document with multiple columns or a complicated Web page), the review mode is used. *Cursor routing* is directly related to the use of the two modes in screen readers. Assume that a user is reviewing a document and she finds an error she wishes to correct in the application mode. Cursor routing allows her to mark that location so that the screen reading cursor can return to it when she exits the review mode and goes into application mode. We discussed macros earlier in this chapter. These sets of keystrokes that are stored and then recalled using one key are useful in screen reading, as well as in keyboard emulation. Because many programs, especially those employing GUIs, use a series of windows on the screen, it is important that adapted output systems include a capability for locating these areas, monitoring them for changes, and outputting information to the user if changes occur.

Screen readers are ideally suited for applications that consist of text only. The power of the screen reader is in the degree to which the other capabilities listed in Box 8-3 are successfully accomplished. For both Windows- and Macintosh-based computers, most screen readers utilize software-based speech synthesizers.

The GUI presents unique and difficult problems to the blind computer user. There are fundamental differences between the ways in which a text-only command line interface (CLI) and a GUI provide output to the video screen. These differences present access problems related both to the ways in which internal control of the computer display is accomplished and to the ways in which the GUI is employed by the computer user (Boyd, Boyd, and Vanderheiden, 1990). CLI-type interfaces use a memory buffer to store text characters for display. Because all the displayed text can be represented by an ASCII code, it is relatively easy to use a software program and to divert text from the screen to a speech synthesizer. Early screen readers operated on this principle. However, these screen readers were unable to provide access to charts, tables, or plots because they had graphical features. This type of system is also limited in the features that can be used with text. For example, all text is the same size, shape, and font. Enlarged characters or alternative graphical forms are not possible with a CLI-type of system, and this limits its usefulness to sighted users. The GUI uses a totally different approach to video display control that creates many more options for the portrayal of graphical information. Because each character or other graphical figure is created as a combination of dots, letters may be of any size, shape, or color and many different graphical symbols can be created. This is useful to sighted computer users because they can rely on "visual metaphors" (Boyd, Boyd, and Vanderheiden, 1990) to control a program. *Visual metaphors* use familiar objects to represent computer actions. For example, a trash can may be used for files that are to be deleted, and a file cabinet may represent a disk drive. The graphical labels used to portray these functions are referred to as *icons*.

Another feature of the GUI is that it provides a specific, consistent layout of controls on the screen. This aids the user (especially a novice) in accessing programs, since everything is consistent from one application program to another and within an application. Figure 8-2 illustrates a typical GUI with several windows open and an application program running. Note that the icons used are of familiar objects, and each window has a similar look and feel.

The GUI presents several problems to the blind user. First, the graphical characters are not easily portrayed in alternative modes. Text-to-speech programs and speech synthesizers are designed to convert text to speech output (see Chapter 9). However, they are not well suited to the representation of graphics, including the icons (visual metaphors) used in GUIs. Fortunately, most icons used in GUIs have text labels with them, and one approach to adaptation is to intercept the label and send it to a text-to-speech voice synthesizer system. The label is then spoken when the icon is selected.

Another major problem presented to blind users by GUIs is that screen location is important in using a GUI and this is not easily conveyed via alternative means. Visual information is spatially organized, and auditory information (including speech) is temporal (time based). It is difficult to convey the screen location of a pointer by speech alone. An exception to this is a screen location that never changes. For example, some screen readers use speech to indicate the edges of the screen (e.g., right border, top of screen). A more significant problem is that the mouse pointer location on the screen is relative, rather than referenced to an absolute standard location. This means that the only information available to the computer is how far the mouse has moved and the direction of the movement. If there is no visual information available to the user, it is difficult to know where the mouse is pointing. The Microsoft Screen Access Model is a set of technologies that facilitate the development of screen readers and other accessibility utilities for Windows. These technologies provide alternative ways to store and access information about the contents of the computer screen. The Screen Access Model also includes software driver interfaces that provide a standard mechanism for accessibility utilities to send information to speech devices or refreshable braille displays.

The commercially available screen reader outSPOKEN provides access to both Windows and the Macintosh.* This system provides spoken identification of icons, text reading, and use of sound to identify attributes of text (bold, underline, etc.). outSPOKEN is compatible with a variety of speech synthesizers, and it is fully compatible with all application software. There are two versions of outSPOKEN. One provides speech output only and the other provides either speech or braille output.

For Windows-based computers, the majority of commercial approaches include both a voice synthesizer and a software-based screen reader. These systems provide many of the features listed in Box 8-3. Most software-based screen readers are sold separately from the voice synthesizers, and they have software programs that are compatible with a variety of speech synthesizers. Many of these bundled software programs also work with computer sound boards to generate high-quality synthetic speech.

Currently available screen reader programs provide navigation assistance via keyboard commands. Examples of typical functions are movement to a particular point in the text, finding the mouse cursor position, providing a spoken description of an on-screen graphic or a special function key, and accessing help information.† Screen readers also monitor the screen and take action when a particular block of text or a menu appears (Lazzaro, 1999). This feature automatically reads pop-up windows and dialog boxes to the user. Screen readers can typically be set to speak by line, sentence, or paragraph. Other features are also available; for example, Jaws for Windows* allows the user to read the prior, current, or next sentence or paragraph in all applications by using specified keystrokes (e.g., read prior sentence = ALT + UP ARROW; read next sentence = ALT + DOWN ARROW; read current sentence = ALT + NUM PAD). The user may use the standard Windows method of switching between applications (ALT + TAB). Some screen readers also provide a "window list" in which applications that are running appear in alphabetical order. This allows the user to switch between, close, or see the state of any active application. This is a faster way to switch between applications when a user has many windows open, rather than moving the cursor to a pull-down menu or "close" box. Hal† is a screen reader designed to operate with the visible information on the screen. Hal recognizes objects by looking for distinct attributes, shapes, borders, highlights, and so on. This is in contrast to using the standard labels of Windows, and it means that Hal is independent of whether an application has obeyed the rules of Windows programming. Hal recognizes objects by their final shape on the screen, rather than their Windows attributes. The advantage of this approach is that once set up for one application, all similar-looking applications will talk correctly without any adjustment to the settings. Hal also includes a braille layout mode. Window Bridge‡ provides simultaneous synthetic speech and the braille display in a single screen reader. Both MS-DOS and Windows applications are supported, and they use identical commands for reading and navigation. Window Bridge supports a variety of braille displays, software-based speech output software, and hardware speech synthesizers. The physical layout of Windows screens can be represented on the braille display using Window Bridge. One-key commands control speech output, mouse navigation, language selection, and Internet exploration.

Screen Reader/2§ provides screen reading capability for the IBM OS/2 WARP graphical user interface. Screen Reader/2 is controlled by a dedicated 18-key keypad. This allows the keyboard to be reserved for application functions. The user can read complete screens, paragraphs, sentences, words, or individual characters. Editing allows speaking of characters, words, or lines as they are typed or as the cursor

---

*ALVA Access Group, Emeryville, Calif. (www.aagi.com).
†For example, Screen Reader2 from IBM, Special Needs Systems, Austin, Tex. (www.rs6000.ibm.com/sns); ScreenPower for Windows from Telesensory, Sunnyvale, Calif. (www.telesensory.com); WinVision from Artic Technologies, Troy, Mich. (www.artictech.co); outSPOKEN from ALVA Access Group, Emeryville, Calif. (www.aagi.com); Slimware from Human Ware, Loomis, Calif; VIP and ezVIP from Jbliss Imaging Systems, San Jose, Calif. (www.jbliss.com); Jaws for Windows from Freedom Scientific, St. Petersburg, Fla. (www.freedomsci.com); Zoom Text Xtra Level 2 from AI Squared, Manchester Center, Vt. (www.aisquared.com); Supernova and Hal from Dolphin Computer Access, San Mateo, Calif. (www. dolphinusa.com); Magnum and Magnum Deluxe from Artic Technologies, Troy, Mich.; SLIMWARE Window Bridge, Syntha-voice Computers, Inc., Stoney Creek, Ontario, Canada, (www.synthavoice.on.ca); Protalk32 for Windows, Biolink Computer, Vancouver, B.C., Canada; (www.biolink.bc.ca); Window Eyes from GW Microsystems, Fort Wayne, Ind. (www.gwmicro.com/gwie).

---

*Hunter Joyce, St. Petersburg, Fla. (www.hj.com).
†Dolphin Computer Access, San Mateo, Calif. (www.dolphinusa.com).
‡Syntha-voice Computers, Inc., Stoney Creek, Ontario, Canada (www.synthavoice.on.ca).
§IBM (Special Needs Systems), Austin, Tex. (www.rs6000.ibm.com/sns).

moves across the text. Screen Reader/2 allows creation of user-defined dictionaries for acronyms, abbreviations, and other specially pronounced words, and the program monitors the screen and alerts the user when changes occur, such as status or error messages. This program utilizes a "switch list" that allows mouse cursor movement, clicking, and dragging with the screen reader keypad. This list contains common mouse locations on the screen for a specific program. Each location can be accessed by a code entered from a special numeric keypad supplied with the program. IBM supplies switch profiles, which can be selected to match the user's work needs, for many applications. Schwerdtfeger (1991) describes the operation of this program in detail. This software also provides serial output to both refreshable braille displays and speech synthesizers, pronounces icons and application program titles, and simulates mouse movement using the keypad. These are only examples of product features; as is true for any computer application, rapid advances are common.

The other major alternative sensory output for visual information is tactile. The major approach to tactile output is braille. This requires the use of a translator program to convert text characters to braille cell dot patterns. There are three commonly used grades of braille. Grade 1 is straight letter-by-letter conversion from text to braille cells. Grades 2 and 3 utilize greater and greater amounts of contractions, and they allow substantially faster reading speeds. Computer output systems utilize either a refreshable braille display consisting of raised pins (see Chapter 12) or hard copy via braille printers. One system is the Navigator* hardware, with refreshable braille cells, a braille keyboard, controls for moving the cursor, and software that converts on-screen text to grade 2 braille or converts grade 2 braille entered from the keyboard to ASCII characters for display on the screen. The refreshable braille display consists of 20, 40, or 80 separate cells. A unique eight-dot cell format is available in which the seventh and eighth dots are used to indicate the location of the cursor and to provide single-cell presentation of higher level ASCII characters. The latter feature is necessary because the normal 6-cell braille display can only generate 64 permutations and full ASCII has 132 characters.

The ALVA† braille terminals provide 45- and 85-cell refreshable displays for desktop use and 23- and 43-cell displays for portable applications (battery operated). All four versions have eight-dot braille cells. All ALVA models also provide extra status cells that display the location of the system cursor, which line of text is displayed in braille, which attributes are active, and the relationship of those attributes to the characters on the screen. This information

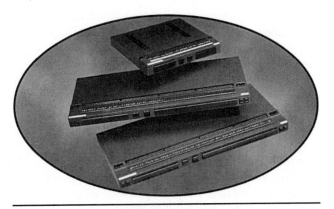

Figure 8-7   Refreshable braille cells are available with a variable number of cells. (Courtesy Freedom Scientific, St. Petersburg, Fla, www. freedomsci.com.)

can be monitored with the left hand while the right hand reads the text on the braille display. Text is provided in both grade 1 and grade 2 braille. The ALVA displays are compatible with DOS, Windows, Windows NT, UNIX, and OS/2 applications.

AccessAbility, Inc* makes the RBT 40 braille display, a small (11.7 × 4.3 × 1 inches), lightweight (less than 2 lb), and flexible unit. It was developed to provide access to multiple systems, since it can easily be moved from one workstation to another. The RBT 40 can be used with both laptop and desktop systems. The desktop keyboard or laptop rests on the RBT 40 expansion storage chassis. It works with most Windows-based software packages. The RBT 40 has six control buttons arranged vertically, three at each end of the braille display. Combinations of buttons are used to enter commands. Blaize Engineering† makes a series of refreshable braille displays shown in Figure 8-7. The PowerBraille 40 is a 40-character, 8-dot braille display for notebook or desktop computers. The PowerBraille 65 is a 65-character, 8-dot braille display for desktop computers. The PowerBraille 80 is an 81-character, 8-dot braille display for desktop computers. All these models are configured for split-window display or as programmable status cells. The latter are accessed by clicking a sensor located above one of the braille cells to instantly move the mouse pointer or cursor to a new location for editing. Grade 2 braille translation is included on all models. The PowerBraille systems are compatible with a variety of access packages for Windows, Windows NT, OS/2, and UNIX.

For computer users who are familiar with braille, this approach can be more effective than screen readers. However, a combination of approaches may be most effective with braille and speech combined. If done thoughtfully and carefully, the hardware and software

---

*Telesensory, Mountain View, Calif. (www.telesensory.com).
†ALVA Access Group, Emeryville, Calif. (www.aagi.com).

*AccessAbility, San Francisco, Calif. (www.4access.com).
†Forest Hill, Md. (www.blazie.com).

designed for braille can be used together with that developed for screen reading using speech synthesis. Supernova* provides screen magnification (2 to 32 times) and speech and braille output in one package for Windows applications. There are six different viewing modes: full-screen, split screen, window, lens, autolens, and line view (for smooth scrolling). "Hooked access" allows parts of the screen such as the current line of a word processor to be permanently displayed. Supernova also supports graphic object labeling, providing speech output and a braille layout mode.

Hard copy (printed) output also must be modified for persons who are blind. Typically, braille output is produced by *embossers*. One approach is to design and build a printer specifically for braille embossing from a computer. The VersaPoint braille embosser† prints 60 braille characters per second in either 6- or 8-dot format on 20 to 100 lb paper. Companion software allows printing of graphics for Windows and Macintosh computers. The Paragon Braille Printer‡ is an embosser that prints on tractor-feed paper from 20 to 100 pounds in weight and up to 15 inches in width. The speed of the Paragon is 40 characters per second, which enables it to print more than 120 pages per hour. Vinyl and aluminum sheets can also be embossed to signs with braille markings. The Mountbatten Brailler is a braille writer with a braille keyboard, built-in memory, auto-correction features, and extensive formatting controls. The Mountbatten can be used as an embosser for a computer or as a braille translation device. It can translate from print into braille or braille into print and is available in both electric and battery-operated models. All these embossers include internal software that accepts standard printer output from the host computer and converts it to either six- or eight-cell braille embossed on heavy paper. The Basic-S§ embosser prints at 42 characters per second on single-sided tractor-feed paper. Software for conversion of text to grade 2 braille is included. American Thermoform Corporation‖ makes a variety of braille embossers. These cover application from mass production to systems for individual users.

Braille translation programs are available from Duxbury Systems.# These programs convert ASCII text in many forms (word processor text files, spreadsheets, database files) to grade 2 braille in hard copy form. Translation of braille cells to text characters and vice versa is not typically on a one-for-one basis. Translation is especially complicated with grade 2 braille, since contractions are used. Formatting of braille pages also involves issues beyond those affecting print. Duxbury Braille Translation provides translation and for-

matting capabilities to automate the process of conversion from regular print to braille (and vice versa) and also provides word processing functions for working directly in braille, as well as print format. Braille characters can be displayed on the screen for proofreading before printing. Operation of this program has the same features (e.g., menus and screens) for Macintosh and Windows. This software is typically used both by individuals who do not know braille and those who do. The Duxbury Braille Translator allows the user to create braille for schoolbooks and teaching materials, office memos, bus schedules, personal letters, and signs compliant with the Americans with Disabilities Act (ADA). The software allows importing of files from popular word processors, including Microsoft Word and WordPerfect, and HTML sources, as well as others.

## ■ INTERNET ACCESS

As the **Internet** becomes more and more dependent on multimedia representations involving complex graphics, animation, and audible sources of information, the challenges for people who have disabilities increase. The most obvious barriers are for those who are blind; however, as the amount of auditory Web content increases, people who are deaf are also prevented from accessing information. People who have learning disabilities and dyslexia also find it increasingly difficult to access complicated Web sites that may include flashing pictures, complicated charts, and large amounts of audio and video data. It is estimated that as many as 40 million persons in the United States have physical, cognitive, or sensory disabilities (Lazzaro, 1999). Thus the importance of making the Internet accessible to all is great.

Many of the approaches to computer input and output that we have discussed in this chapter are important to the provision of access to this information for persons who have disabilities. Two useful sources of information are the World Wide Web Consortium Web Accessibility Initiative (W3C WAI; www.w3.org/WAI) and the Trace Center (www.trace.wisc.edu/world/web). Vanderheiden (1998) provides a comprehensive review of the issues related to Internet access by persons with disabilities. He gives both an overview of current approaches and prospects for future developments based on emerging technologies.

## User Agents for Access to the Internet

Access to the Internet must be independent of individual devices. This device independence means that users must be able to interact with a *user agent* (and the document it renders) using the input and output devices of their choice based on their specific needs. A **user agent** is defined as software to access Web content (www.w3.org/wai). This includes desktop graphical browsers, text and voice brows-

---

*Dolphin Computer Access, San Mateo, Calif. (www.dolphinusa.com).

†Blazie Engineering, Forest Hill, Md. (www.blazie.com).

‡ALVA Access Group, Emeryville, Calif. (www.aagi.com).

§Gammelstad, Sweden.

‖ City of Commerce, Calif. (www.atcbrleqp.com).

#Westford, Mass.

ers, mobile phones, multimedia players, and software assistive technologies (e.g., screen readers, magnifiers, GIDEIs) that are used with browsers.

Input devices that are used for Internet access include many of those described earlier in this chapter and in Chapter 7. Mouse and mouse-alternative pointing devices, head wands, keyboards and keyboard alternatives such as on-screen keyboards, braille input keyboards, switches and switch arrays, and microphones can all serve as input devices for user agents. Output devices for Internet access are also those described in this chapter. In addition to the typical computer monitor and audible output, screen readers, screen magnifiers, braille displays, and speech synthesizers are the most commonly used output devices for user agents.

The W3C WAI project is developing guidelines to inform user agent developers of design approaches required to make their products more accessible to people with disabilities. The W3C WAI project also provides practical solutions for the development of accessible user agents based on existing and emerging technologies. These resources will also increase usability for all users. The W3C initiative emphasizes the use of designs that facilitate compatibility between graphical desktop browsers and dependent assistive technologies (e.g., screen readers, screen magnifiers, braille displays, and voice input software). These developments will also benefit those who do not use the standard keyboard and mouse to access the Internet (e.g., those who are mobile and access the Web through palmtop computers, telephones, and auto terminals) (Vanderheiden, 1998).

These guidelines encourage designers of user agents to consider that users access documents in a variety of contexts. Potential users may be unable to see, hear, move, or process some types of information easily or at all. Users may also have difficulty reading or comprehending text, and they may not have or be able to use a keyboard or mouse. They define two classes of user agents. The first are commonly used graphical desktop browsers; we discuss their role in obtaining accessibility later. The second type of user agent is those that are dependent on other user agents for input or output. These include many of the technologies discussed in this chapter, such as screen magnifiers, screen readers, alternative keyboards, and alternative pointing devices. The guidelines being developed focus on interoperability between these two classes of user agents.

The W3C WAI user agent guidelines are based on several principles that are intended to improve the design of both types of user agents. The first is to ensure that the user interface is accessible. This means that the consumer using an adapted input system must have access to the functionality offered by the user agent through its user interface. Second, the user must have access to document content through the provision of control of the style (e.g., colors, fonts, speech rate, speech volume) and format of a document. Many of the approaches described earlier (e.g., easy

scrolling, and viewing windows that follow changes) help ensure access to content. A third principle is that the user agent help orient the user to where he is in the document or series of documents. In addition to providing alternative representations of location in a document (e.g., how many links the document contains or the number of the current link), a well-designed navigation system that uses numerical position information allows the user to jump to a specific link. Finally, the guidelines call for the user agent to be designed following system standards and conventions. These are changing rapidly as development tools are improved. Communication through standard interfaces is particularly important for graphical desktop user agents, which must make information available to assistive technologies. Technologies such as those produced by the W3C include built-in accessibility features that facilitate interoperability. The standards being developed by the W3C WAI provide guidance for the design of user agents that are consistent with these principles. The guidelines are available on the W3C WAI Web page (www.w3.org/wai).

## How Web Pages Are Developed

Web pages are a mixture of text, graphics, and sound. These pages are typically developed using a variety of programming languages. Hypertext markup language (HTML) has become a standard for Web design. HTML is a nonproprietary format that can be created and processed by a range of tools, from simple plain text editors in which the HTML codes are entered from scratch to sophisticated authoring tools. Many word processors convert files from the word processor format to HTML.

The W3C produces recommendations for HTML. These are specifications for developers, and they include guidelines for accessibility and multimedia (www.w3.org/MarkUp). HTML guidelines also provide access to style sheets. Cascading style sheets (CSS) allow a Web page to be viewed in any layout chosen by the user (Lazzaro, 1999). Style sheet layouts that are compatible with screen magnifiers, screen readers, and braille are available. The W3C recommends that, wherever possible, developers use a style sheet for formatting their presentation and use HTML purely for structural markup. It is important that developers include options that allow style sheets to be turned off for those people using browsers that do not support style sheets. By using HTML as a standard, problems with file incompatibilities (e.g., from different word processors) can be avoided. One example of an HTML accessibility standard is the alt="text" HTML attribute. This function associates text with each graphic object. By pressing the ALT key on the keyboard, the text associated with the object is displayed. This can also be linked to a screen reader or braille output device.

Because of its capability of allowing a programmer to

develop a single version of an application that can be used on a variety of computers and devices, the Java language (Sun Microsystems, java.sun.com) is widely used in programming for the Internet. Johnson, Korn, and Walker (1999) describe the Java platform and its accessibility features. The Java Accessibility Utilities provide linkages to help assistive technologies provide access to the GUI via toolkits that implement the Java accessibility application programming interface (API), a set of packages of software components that provide the basis for building functions such as input and output, data structures, system properties, date and time, internationalization, networking, user interface components, and applets (small application programs that can be run within other applications). Details of these accessibility functions are described by Johnson, Korn, and Walker (1999) and are available at the Java Web site.

Using the Microsoft Synchronized Accessible Media Interchange (SAMI), authors of Web pages and multimedia software can add closed captioning for users who are deaf or hard of hearing. This standard simplifies captioning for developers, educators, and multimedia producers and designers and is available to the public as an open (no licensing fees) standard. This approach is similar to the use of closed captioning for television viewers (see Chapter 12). The W3C WAI SMIL is designed to facilitate multimedia presentations in which an author can describe the behavior of a multimedia presentation, associate hyperlinks with media objects, and describe the layout of the presentation on a screen. These features allow integration of timing of multimedia presentations into HTML programs.

## Web Browsers

Web browsers for general use incorporate accessibility features to varying degrees. Because most are compatible with Windows, any other accessible products that are also compatible with Windows should work with the browser. That is, however, pure theory, because there are many features of browsers that are independent of the operating system. Thus the accessibility of browsers varies.

Lynx is a text-based browser for the Internet. As such it is useable by individuals who are blind because it is compatible with braille or screen reading software. Lynx also offers navigational functions.

One Internet browser that provides access to the Internet in an auditory or dual-mode manner is pwWebSpeak.* This browser is designed specifically to translate the information content on Web pages into speech. The user may navigate through the structure of a document based on its contents, paragraphs, and sentences, rather than having to deal with scrolling and interpreting a structured screen display.

Microsoft† Internet Explorer contains a range of features

for people with disabilities. These include keyboard navigation (among links, frames, and client-side image maps), optional display of text descriptions instead of images, multiple font sizes, and an optional disabling of style sheets so that the user's font, color, and size settings will be used. Explorer also uses the High Contrast function to increase legibility and incorporates Microsoft Active Accessibility to provide information about the document.

Many of the screen readers described earlier have features that take advantage of Internet Explorer's capabilities. Examples include Hal, JAWS for Windows, outSPOKEN, Window Bridge, Window Eyes, and WinVision. The features that provide access to the Windows operating system are also used to provide access to Web pages. Many of these screen readers are also compatible with other general-purpose browsers such as Netscape.

Netscape Navigator* allows for enlargement of fonts. The IBM Home Page Reader speaks Web-based information by combining features of the IBM's ViaVoice Outloud text-to-speech speech synthesizer and Netscape Navigator. Home Page Reader provides audible information from GUI Web pages to the user. This information includes tables, frames, forms, and alternate text for images. Home Page Reader speaks information regarding page links or ALT text for objects like images and image maps. You can navigate and read complex tables, such as television listings, using table navigation mode. In table navigation mode, you can easily read table rows, columns, and cells, including table cells that span multiple rows or columns. Marcopolo† is a plug-in for the Netscape browser that utilizes either a standard PC sound board or the DECTalk speech synthesizer to provide access to the Internet using speech and musical sounds.

The VIP InfoNet‡ talking Web browser provides screen enlargement to optimize visual displays for people with low vision. Extensive voice prompting (which can be turned off) is of use to people who are blind. Key shortcuts are described in command menus that help the user operate the system. A narrative help file is also available. VIP InfoNet includes features common to other browsers. Features are similar to the VIP screen magnification software described earlier in this chapter.

## Making Web Sites Accessible

The W3C WAI has also developed guidelines for creating accessible Web sites. Their Quick Tips are shown in Box 8-4. These guidelines particularly address the way in which Web sites are laid out and the programming that is done to create the Web site. The guidelines facilitate access to the Web page by people using alternative input or output

---

*Productivity Works, Trenton, N.J. (www.prodworks.com).
†Microsoft Corp., Seattle, Wash. (www.microsoft.com).

*Mountain View, Calif. (www.netscape.com).
†Sonicon, Boston, Mass. (www.webpresence.com).
‡JSBliss, San Jose, Calif. (www.jbliss.com).

methods and give designers guidelines for making their content accessible to individuals who have visual, auditory, or manipulation disabilities. The technical terms that appear in the guidelines (e.g., CSS, HTML, scripts, applets) are defined on the W3C WAI home page.

Vanderheiden and Chisholm (1999) describe the development of authoring guidelines for Web site development. They emphasize the concept of having pages that "transform gracefully" across users, techniques, and situations. By transforming gracefully, they mean that a Web page remains stable regardless of what user, technological, or situational constraints occur. They cite the example of a person with low vision needing to enlarge the entire screen to 36-point text. In this case the author-determined font size will be overridden. They list three guidelines to help authors create documents that transform gracefully. First, authors should ensure that all the information available on the page can be perceived entirely visually and entirely auditorially, as well as being available in text. Second, they recommend that authors separate the content of the site (what is said) and the structure of the content (how it is organized) from the way the content and structure are presented (how the content is accessed by a user). Finally, they advise Web authors to ensure that all pages are operable utilizing a variety of hardware, such as systems without mice, with small or low resolution, or with only speech or text input. They relate these recommendations to the W3C WAI authoring guidelines.

The Center for Applied Special Technology (CAST) has developed a web-based software tool called "Bobby" (www.cast.org/bobby). Bobby analyzes Web pages for their accessibility to people with disabilities. To analyze a Web site, the URL of the page to be examined is entered into the CAST Web site. Bobby displays a report that indicates any accessibility or browser compatibility errors found on the page. Once the site receives a "Bobby Approved" rating, the Bobby Approved icon can be displayed on the site. The report includes both those things that can be checked automatically and a list of questions regarding checkpoints that must be validated manually. This information must be submitted to CAST before the approval is granted.

## ■ SUMMARY

In this chapter we have looked at basic computer structure and function and at adaptations for both inputs (alternatives to keyboard and mouse) and outputs (options for video display and printer). The fundamental advantages of computer-based systems—programmability, software reconfigurability, and adaptability—are exploited in the design of specific-purpose assistive technologies. For example, powered wheelchair controllers can be programmed in the field for specific speed, acceleration, braking, and other parameters to match an individual consumer's needs. Features can be added to augmentative communication devices by changing the internal program without a need for hardware modifications. EADLs can be adapted both to the specific appliance to be controlled (e.g., a television) and to the type of control interface and method to be used. These examples and many others are discussed in succeeding chapters.

## Study Questions

1. List the major components of a computer system, briefly describe each one, and describe how the components affect the recommendation of a computer for use in an assistive technology system.
2. What is a GUI? What advantages does it provide for persons with disabilities?
3. What special problems does the GUI present for persons who are blind?
4. How are adaptations made to the GUI for persons with physical limitations? How does this differ for the Macintosh and for Windows-based PCs?
5. What are the features included in Universal Access and Windows Accessibility options?
6. What does the term *transparent access* mean, and what features are used to implement it?
7. What is an on-screen keyboard?

8. What features are important in matching a specific on-screen keyboard to an individual's needs and skills?

9. List three means of providing input to on-screen keyboards.

10. Examine Table 8-2. Which Morse codes listed in the nonstandard section are the same for all three example systems? Why do you think these particular codes happen to be the same, given that there are no standards? Why do you think that the other codes are different for different systems?

11. What is a GIDEI, and what basic functions does it perform?

12. What is included in a GIDEI setup?

13. What are the relative disadvantages and advantages of software-based and hardware-based GIDEIs?

14. List three limitations of current voice-only screen reading programs developed for visual access.

15. What are the three factors that must be considered when accommodating for low vision? How are they normally dealt with in access software?

16. Describe the relative advantages and disadvantages of software and hardware approaches to obtaining enlarged displays for persons with visual impairments.

17. What is the primary tactile method used for computer output?

18. What special adaptations are made to braille specifically for computer output use?

19. What adaptations are made to provide hard copy for users with low vision?

20. What adaptations are made to provide hard copy for users who are blind?

21. Define *scrolling* as applied to screen reader programs.

22. What does the term *navigation* mean in describing a screen magnification or screen-reading program?

23. How is *magnification* defined for a screen-enlarging program?

24. What are the primary challenges in obtaining Web access for persons who have disabilities?

25. What is the Web Accessibility Initiative?

26. What is a user agent? What are typical user agents for persons with disabilities? What guidelines are used to ensure that a user agent is accessible?

27. How are Web pages developed, and what steps are necessary to ensure that they are useable by persons with disabilities?

28. What is a Web browser? What features are necessary in a Web browser to ensure that people who have disabilities can use it?

29. List the major features of accessible Web sites. What tools are typically used to test accessibility of Web sites?

## References

Anson D: Alternative Computer Access, Philadelphia, 1997, FA Davis.

Attigupam P, Cook AM, Hussey SM, Coleman, CL: Automation of an assistive technology center, *Proc 16th Ann Conf Rehabil Eng,* pp 23-25, June 1993.

Bailey RW: *Human performance engineering,* ed 2, Englewood Cliffs, NJ, 1989, Prentice Hall.

Boyd LH, Boyd WL, Vanderheiden GC: The graphical user interface: crisis, danger, and opportunity, *J Vis Impair Blindness* 84(10):496-502, 1990.

Brown C: *Computer access in higher education for students with disabilities,* ed 2, Monterey, Calif, 1989, US Department of Education.

Buddine L, Young E: *The Brady guide to CD-ROM,* New York, 1987, Brady.

Church G, Glennen S: *The handbook of assistive technology,* San Diego, 1992, Singular Publishing Group.

Gorgens RA, Bergler PM, Gorgens DC: HandiWare: powerful, flexible software solutions for adapted access, augmentative communication and low vision in the DOS environment, *Proc 13th Ann Conf Rehabil Eng,* pp 43-44, June 1990.

Hayes F: From TTY to VDT, *Byte* 15(4):205-211, 1990.

Hortsman HM, Levine SP, Jaros LA: Keyboard emulation for access to IBM-PC-compatible computers by people with motor impairments, *Assist Technol* 1:63-70, 1989.

Johnson E, Korn P, Walker W: A primer on the Java platform and Java accessibility, *Proc CSUN Conf,* 1999 (http://www.dinf.org/csun_99/session0193.html).

Lazzaro JL: Helping the web help the disabled, *IEEE Spectrum* 36(3):54-59, 1999.

*Microsoft Windows manual for users,* Seattle, 1990, Microsoft.

Schwejda P, Vanderheiden G: Adaptive-firmware card for the Apple II, *Byte* 7(9):276-314, 1982.

Schwerdtfeger RS: Making the GUI talk, *Byte* 16(13):118-128, 1991.

Shein F et al: WIVIK: A visual keyboard for Windows 3.0, *Proc 14th Annu RESNA Conf,* pp 160-162, June 1991.

Vanderheiden GC: Cross-modal access to current and next-generation Internet—fundamental and advanced topics in Internet accessibility, *Technol Disabil* 8:115-126, 1998.

Vanderheiden GC, Chisholm W: The ongoing evolution of the WAI authoring guidelines, *Proc 99 CSUN Conf.* (http://www.dinf.org/csun_99/session0094.html).

# PART 4

# The Activities: Performance Areas

## CHAPTER 9

# Augmentative and Alternative Communication Systems

## Objectives

Upon completing this chapter you will be able to:

1. Describe the different communicative needs of persons with disabilities
2. Discuss the basic approaches to meeting these differing needs
3. Recognize the needs that individuals have for conversation, as well as graphical output such as writing, mathematics, and drawing
4. Describe the major characteristics of alternative and augmentative communication devices
5. Describe current approaches to speech output in assistive technologies
6. List and describe the major approaches to rate enhancement and vocabulary expansion
7. Describe the major assessment questions that must be asked and answered in determining the most appropriate AAC device for an individual user
8. Discuss the major goals for and the significance of training in AAC device use and communicative competence
9. Delineate the steps and procedures involved in implementing an augmentative and alternative communication device for an individual consumer

## Key Terms

| | | |
|---|---|---|
| Abbreviation Expansion | Dynamic Communication Displays | Selection Set |
| Acceleration Vocabularies | Dysarthria | Semantic Encoding |
| Apraxia | Graphics | Speech Synthesis |
| Aphasia | Icon Prediction | Text-To-Speech Programs |
| Augmentative and Alternative | Numeric Codes | Traditional Orthography |
| Communication (AAC) | Predictive Selection | Vocabulary Expansion |
| Conversation | Rate Enhancement | Word Completion |
| Coverage Vocabularies | Salient Letter Coding | Word Prediction |
| Digital Recording | | |

In this chapter we describe **augmentative and alternative communication (AAC)** systems that are designed to ameliorate the problems faced by persons who have difficulty speaking or writing because of neuromuscular disease or injury. Our emphasis is on the total process of delivering these systems to those who need them, from initial need and goal setting, through assessment and recommendation, to implementation and training. The material presented in Chapters 3, 4, and 7 is applied to AAC systems here.

### ◼ OVERVIEW

### Disabilities Affecting Speech and Language

There are many disabilities that can affect an individual's ability to speak or write. In the section on cognitive function and development in Chapter 3, we examine normal language, speech, and language development, and that information forms the basis for our current discussion. If the larynx is damaged, such as by trauma or cancer, this can result in the inability to generate the sounds necessary for speech. In this case an artificial larynx is often used to create the sounds normally produced by the vocal cords (Gunderson, 1985). Alternatively, there are many individuals who can make sounds but have insufficient control of the muscles of the chest, diaphragm, mouth, tongue, and throat to form these sounds into understandable words. **Dysarthria** is a disorder of motor speech control resulting from central or peripheral nervous system damage and is characterized by weakness, slowness, and incoordination of the muscles necessary for speech (Yorkston and Dowden, 1984). **Apraxia** refers to motor control limitations caused by a central nervous system dysfunction that prevents coordination of peripheral muscles (Miller, 1981). When the ability to write is impaired by neuromuscular disease or injury, the individual may need an augmentative device for all graphical output (e.g., writing, drawing, calculating).

We also distinguish between speech disorders such as these and language disorders. In Chapter 3 we define a language as any system of arbitrary symbols organized according to a set of rules and we define speech to be the oral expression of language. We refer to language disorder as **aphasia;** there are many types of aphasia, affecting both expression and reception of spoken and written language. Aphasia can limit the individual's language ability in several ways. Some people lose the ability to recall vocabulary (e.g., names, places, events), and others lose the ability to organize language into meaningful utterances. Aphasia may be receptive, expressive, or both. The degree to which various language functions are impaired is quite variable as well. Because aphasias of all types are *language* disorders, any AAC intervention must include ways of compensating for lost function in this area.

The major causes of the inability to speak or write are neuromuscular conditions such as cerebral palsy, degenerative diseases such as amyotrophic lateral sclerosis (ALS), traumatic brain injury (TBI), stroke, and high-level spinal cord injury. It is difficult to determine the exact number of people who have these problems, but estimates range from 0.2% to 0.6% of the total world population (Blackstone, 1990a). Although this may seem to be a small number in terms of the total population, it still encompasses many people (500,000 to 1.5 million in the United States alone). Not all the people in this population are served equally. Blackstone (1990a) conducted a survey to determine how well various populations were served. Children with cerebral palsy and good cognitive skills, children with developmental disabilities, and adults with motor neuron disease (ALS) were perceived as being well served by AAC service delivery. Children with severe retardation, who were ambulatory or had dual sensory impairments (e.g., deaf and blind), and adults with aphasia or TBI or who were older (geriatric population) were perceived as not having their AAC needs met. The reasons for this division become clear from the material presented in this chapter.

We can also categorize these disabilities by severity from mild to severe impairment, and our approach to using AAC systems varies with the severity, type, and onset of the disability. There are significant differences in our approach to those who have never spoken or used written language (congenital or very early disability) and our approach to persons who have developed language, speech, and writing and lose these skills because of disease or injury. For example, a person who is unable to speak or write from birth because of cerebral palsy must develop language concepts using augmentative or alternative communication modalities instead of via speech and writing. The experience of using AAC systems is very different for a nondisabled man who develops ALS at 46 years of age. He has learned to speak and write and has a great deal of experience with these

forms of communication. His AAC device must take into account this experience base, and it can build on his developed language skills.

## Augmentative and Alternative Communication

There are many ways of looking at AAC systems. We use *unaided communication* to describe any communication that requires only the person's own body, such as pointing, pantomime, manual signing, or finger spelling. These types of communication are used in addition to our common methods of speaking or orthography (writing). Unaided modes of communication can be significantly different in the presence of a disability. For example, Kraat (1986) reports that communication partners frequently interpret nonverbal behaviors of disabled persons as if they had been produced by a nondisabled individual. However, physical disability may affect eye gaze, facial expression, body movements, posture, traditional head nods, and pointing or reaching. These movements may not be controlled or controllable in the same way as those of the nondisabled partner. Interpretation of the meaning of these behaviors may therefore be inaccurate, and the inaccuracies may lead to communication misunderstandings. Rush (1986) gives a good example of this when he describes the difficulty his cerebral palsy causes him in delivering his line (a yell) in a play: "When a person with cerebral palsy wants to do something, he can't and when he wants not to do something, he involuntarily does it. So getting my vocal cords to cooperate with the cue was as hard as memorizing a Shakespearean play [for a nondisabled person]" (p. 21).

We use *augmentative and alternative communication* to describe any communication that requires something other than the person's own body, such as a pen or pencil, a letter or picture communication board, a typewriter, or an electronic communication device. Augmentative devices may be further delineated as electronic and manual. It is obvious that paper letter boards (an example of a manual device) differ from computers (electronic devices). It is important to remember, however, that although manual and electronic devices do differ in the complexity of the technology (low tech versus high tech; see Chapter 1), they have many similarities. Both require a symbol system and a method of selection, and both can implement communication goals. As we shall see, these similarities are more important than the differences resulting from specific device characteristics.

Interestingly, the attitudes of children who do not have disabilities toward children who do and who use AAC is not dependent on the level of technology used. Beck and Dennis (1996) found that attitudes of fifth grade boys and girls toward an AAC user were the same whether the user had an electronic AAC device or a simple paper language board. They also found that girls had a more positive attitude

---

### CASE STUDY 9-1

#### MEETING A CONGENITAL NEED FOR AAC

Joyce is 39 years old. She has cerebral palsy, and she currently lives with her parents. Her speech is dysarthric, and she is unable to use a pen or pencil for writing. Her communication systems are listed in Table 9-1. Unaided modes include head nods and eye gaze. Joyce currently uses a tread switch (see Chapter 7) mounted near her knee to control her scanning communication device, which has synthesized speech output and a small word processing program for writing. To meet Joyce's need to activate a call device for emergency help over the telephone, she uses an alarm tied into a 24-hour surveillance company and activated by a wobble switch (see Chapter 7) using her left arm. She uses her arm for the emergency call device because this movement is less limited by being supine in bed than is knee movement. Also, when she is seated in her wheelchair, arm use does not interfere with either her powered mobility or her communication, since they use other control sites.

---

### TABLE 9-1     AAC Case Study Examples

| Subject | Communication Need | Modality | Activation/Control |
|---|---|---|---|
| **Joyce** | Conversation/ writing | Unaided | Eye gaze or head nod |
| | | Electronic AAC device | Knee/tread switch |
| | Emergency call | 24-hour service | Hand/wobble switch |
| **Eileen** | Conversation | Unaided | Vocalizations, head nods, facial expression |
| | | Letter board | Eye gaze |
| | | Electronic AAC device | Optical pointer/ head movement |

---

toward the AAC user than did boys. The familiarity with children who have disabilities (i.e., whether the nondisabled students had a classmate with a disability) did not affect Beck and Dennis' results.

## Communication Needs That Can Be Served by Augmentative and Alternative Communication Systems

There are two basic communication needs that lead to the use of augmentative and alternative communication systems: **conversation** and **graphics** (Cook, 1988). These

---

### CASE STUDY 9-2

#### AAC FOLLOWING STROKE

Eileen is a 62-year-old woman who has sustained a brainstem stroke and now requires maximal assistance for daily living. Eileen's unaided communication modalities, shown in Table 9-1, include isolated words, facial expressions, yes/no responses, and inflectional vocalizations. She also has two AAC devices. The first of these is a letter board, accessed by her eye gaze, that she uses to indicate her needs and choices (Figure 9-1). All these systems have limitations. The unaided systems require significant amounts of interpretation by the partner, and the manual eye gaze device is slow because it relies on spelling and interpretation by her partner. These limitations are partially overcome by Eileen's electronic AAC device, which she accesses using head movement to make selections with a light pointer mounted on a headband on the side of her head (Figure 9-2). This device includes vocabulary storage so she can use whole words and phrases, and it provides synthesized speech output. These features allow Eileen to converse with more people, and they make it easier on the communication partner. Each of these devices contributes to the quantity and quality of her communication interactions.

---

two needs differ in many important aspects. Conversational needs are those that would typically be accomplished using speech if it were available. Examples of these needs are an informal conversation with a friend, a formal oral presentation to a group of people, a telephone conversation, and a small group discussion. *Graphical communication* describes all the things that we normally do using a pencil and paper, typewriter, computer, calculator, and other similar tools, and it includes writing, drawing, mathematics, and Internet access. In the following sections we look more closely at both conversational and graphical communication.

## Multimodal Communication

When an AAC system is required, we generally use several communication modalities and devices in order to meet a full spectrum of needs. Case studies 9-1 and 9-2 illustrate this concept.

As both these studies illustrate, having more than one communication mode available provides options for the user and for the partner. This often contributes to more effective overall communicative competence and leads to greater interaction. Thus, in general, a multimodal approach to AAC intervention is most effective.

However, in some cases a unimodal approach is more effective. Iacono, Mirenda, and Beukelman (1993) illustrate

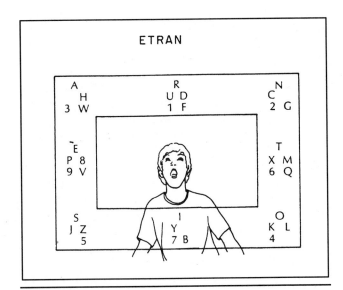

**Figure 9-1**  This communication system is based on the user and partner facing each other. Two eye movements are required. The first movement selects the group, and the second movement selects the letter. For example, to select the letter *A*, the user first looks to the upper left, then to the upper center. Eye gaze using pictures or other symbols is also common. (From Blackstone S: *Augmentative communication*, Rockville, Md, 1986, American Speech Language Hearing Association.)

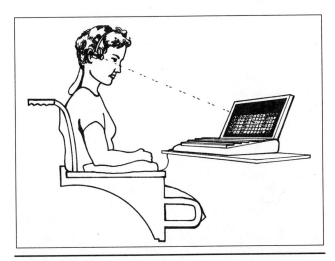

**Figure 9-2**  In this device a light is attached to the user's head. When the light beam is aimed at the panel of the device, it is detected and an entry is made. (From Blackstone S: *Augmentative communication*, Rockville, Md, 1986, American Speech Language Hearing Association.)

this point by presenting two case studies of young children (3 years, 6 months; 4 years, 6 months) with cognitive disabilities. Each individual used either (1) electronic devices coupled with manual signing (multimodal) or (2) signing alone (unimodal) to produce two-word semantic combinations. One of the children was more effective using both modes, and the other preferred to use only one mode. Iacono and co-workers discuss factors that may have influenced this outcome. One of these is the reliance of signing

on recall memory and use of an electronic device with symbols on recognition memory (see Chapter 3). Individuals with cognitive disabilities may have more difficulty with recall than with recognition, which may have made the electronic device easier to use. This may have placed different enough demands on the use of the two devices that their use together was difficult for one of the children. It was also possible that spontaneous use of the device was limited during play because it interfered with the use of toys and signing did not. Thus it is clear that, whereas multimodal communication is generally accepted as valuable, there are many considerations that must be taken into account to apply this intervention approach appropriately.

## ■ CONVERSATIONAL NEEDS SERVED BY AUGMENTATIVE COMMUNICATION SYSTEMS

In this section we focus on the needs that conversational AAC devices must meet to be successful. Much of conversational use focuses on interaction between two or more people. Light (1988) describes four types of communicative interaction: (1) expression of needs and wants, (2) information transfer, (3) social closeness, and (4) social etiquette. Before looking at general needs served by conversational systems, it is useful to consider the needs, preferences, and priorities of parents for AAC devices and services. Angelo, Kokoska, and Jones (1996) surveyed 85 mothers and 47 fathers of adolescent children. Both mothers and fathers expressed a need for more knowledge of AAC systems. Mothers also ranked social opportunities with both nondisabled children and other AAC users, integrating AAC into the community, and planning for future needs as highest priorities. Fathers focused on planning for future needs, knowing how to repair and maintain the AAC device, integration of AAC into educational settings, knowing how to program the device, and obtaining computer access via the AAC device. These results paralleled those obtained with parents of younger children (Angelo, Jones, and Kokoska, 1995).

### Conversational Communication Rates

Speech allows communication at a rapid rate, between 150 and 175 words per minute (Miller, 1981). For an individual using an augmentative communication device to generate unlimited vocabulary, some form of letter or symbol selection is required; in many cases, persons who are unable to speak use a keyboard to type their messages, which are then spoken by an AAC device. This can result in significantly lower rates of communication than for speech. For example, a trained, nondisabled typist can generate typed text during transcription at a rate of nearly 100 words per minute.

However, this is still only about two thirds of the rate of speech. If this same typist is asked to compose rather than transcribe, her rate will drop by 50% to a maximum of 50 words per minute (Foulds, 1980). The situation is even worse for many people who have disabilities and must rely on single-finger typing for conversation. Using this mode, a person with a disability may only be able to type at a maximal rate of 10 to 12 words per minute. For individuals who use scanning (see Chapter 7), the maximal rates can be as low as three to five words per minute. Although there are several methods of increasing communication rate, the great disparity in rates of communication between a speaking person and an AAC system user often results in the speaking person's dominating a conversation with a nonspeaking person. Thus one of the goals in the design of augmentative communication devices is to reduce the magnitude of this disparity in communication rates.

## User Skills Affecting Communication System Output Rate

Communication device output rate depends on many factors. Two of the most important are the user's skills and the characteristics of the AAC devices employed. Often limitations in skills can be partially compensated for by device characteristics. For example, many augmentative communication devices have special features that speed up the generation of text.

There are many skills required for effective use of an augmentative communication device. Physical skills such as gross and fine motor control are required to make selections using AAC devices. Sensory capabilities, including visual, auditory, and tactile functions, are also important in generating rapid communication rates. Many language and cognitive abilities are desirable for increasing the effectiveness of AAC device use. Other skills are so basic that they apply to all AAC device use (e.g., the use of some symbolic representation). Language and cognitive skills that are important for AAC device use in conversational interaction include morphemes, spelling, categorization (semantic, syntactical, and pragmatic), use of codes, and symbolic language representation. Not all these skills are *required* for effective AAC conversational use; however, they are all *desirable* to maximize effectiveness.

## Interaction and Rules of Conversation in AAC

For effective conversational communication to occur, it is necessary that all participants understand the rules of conversation. These rules govern turn taking, initiation of a conversation, appropriate methods of interrupting, and methods of repairing a conversation when an utterance is misinterpreted and maintaining a conversation once begun (Miller, 1981). The conversational rules that apply to two

speaking persons, and about which there is a great deal of information, need to be altered to be applied to the situation in which one partner in a conversation is speaking and the other is using an AAC device, as shown in Figure 9-3 (Kraat, 1985). Certainly the speaking partner must alter the rules in order to compensate for the differences in communication rate. However, the nonspeaking partner may also alter the ways in which she says things and even the content of what is said (Harris, 1982). For example, the most efficient type of utterance for a nonspeaking person is "telegraphic"; that is, only the key words are used and the result sounds like a telegram. For example, an AAC user may say, "What time dinner." Unfortunately, this type of utterance sounds primitive and may lead the partner to assume that the user is not capable of complex thoughts. Likewise, the nonspeaking person may avoid this type of utterance despite its high rate because he does not want to appear "stupid." Instead he may choose to say "When will we eat dinner?" and it obviously takes longer to convey this message.

The implications of AAC use on conversational interaction are not well understood, and it is difficult to define communicative competence by AAC users. In one study (Light, 1988), a group of clinicians at one center were asked to select users whom they judged as competent communicators. They identified the following factors as consistently present in those individuals: (1) possessed a positive self-image; (2) showed an interest in others and seemed to draw others into interaction; (3) participated actively in conversations with fairly symmetrical patterns of turn taking; (4) responded to partners with sharing of topics; and (5) put partners at ease so partner knew what was required and

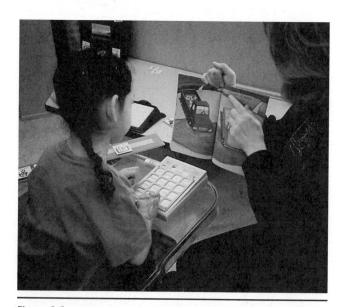

**Figure 9-3**  In conversations between speaking and AAC-using partners, the speaker may dominate the conversation unless careful selection, implementation, and training in use of the AAC system occurs.

expected. These characteristics of good communicators are only loosely related to the hard assistive technologies they use, but the soft technologies (strategies) play a major role.

We often store whole words or phrases in augmentative communication devices to allow more rapid communication than letter-by-letter selection (spelling); there are various ways of categorizing this storage. Equally important is the use of a small set of phrases or sentences that can be accessed quickly. These phrases and sentences (called "grabbers," "quickies," or similar names) can serve several types of communicative functions. For example, a conversation can be continued by selecting, "Please wait while I type my next statement." A conversation with a stranger can be initiated with the statement, "I use this as my voice. I'll type and you read the display." These utterances also are used to create greater normalcy for the user. For example, different greetings can be used to fit with a person's age, gender, and situation: "How's it going?" "Hello, how are you today?" "What's new? It's good to see you," "What's happening?" These phrases can be stored so they can be selected using only one or two movements (e.g., pointing at a picture, pressing a key or switch). By carefully choosing these quick phrases, we can make it possible for the user to express her personality: humorous, serious, reserved, outgoing, and so

on. Table 9-2 lists some categories for quick phrases and sentences and some examples of typical utterances in each category.

Another important discourse function is commenting (Buzolich, King, and Baroody, 1991). Commenting can be distinguished from topics in a conversation. Topics generally make up the information transferred between the AAC user and his partner. Comments, on the other hand, keep the conversation going. They may be nonverbal (e.g., a head nod or eye wink) or more complete (e.g., "What a great idea!" or "I don't like this"). Buzolich and her colleagues developed a training paradigm to help children who use AAC devices acquire skill in commenting. Each of their subjects was seen as capable of using communication devices for defining and talking about topics but was unable to use commenting spontaneously. Buzolich and co-workers used a criterion of the number of turn exchanges taken during a conversation in a baseline (no commenting) and maintenance (with commenting) phase of training. In a sample conversation, the number of turn exchanges in the baseline phase was four and in the maintenance phase it was seven. The children in this study were also perceived as having greater communicative skill as a result of their commenting ability, even though the content of the conversation had not changed. Other language discourse functions that need to be included in AAC systems are listed in Table 9-2. These categories should be included in all AAC systems used for conversation. Examples of differing moods, styles, and degrees of formality are also shown in Table 9-2.

The way in which vocabulary information is stored in a communication device can significantly affect overall rate of communication. In addition to the use of easily recalled codes, AAC use can be facilitated by carefully selecting storage categories. The major types of storage are syntactical (e.g., nouns, verbs, adjectives grouped together), semantic (e.g., similar meanings together, such as foods, activities), and pragmatic (vocabulary stored by discourse functions such as greetings, comments, frequency of use).

| TABLE 9-2 | Categories To Be Included in Conversational AAC Systems |
|---|---|
| **Category** | **Sample Vocabulary** |
| Initiating and interaction | Hey, I've got something to say. Check this out. Come talk to me. May I help you? |
| Greetings | Hello, I'm pleased to meet you. Where have you been? I've been waiting forever. What's happening? |
| Response to greetings | I'm fine. Great, how are you? Not so hot, and you? |
| Requests | I'd like a _____. (object, event) I'd like to go to _____. (place, event) |
| Information exchange | What time is it? I have a question. The concert begins at 8:00 PM. |
| Commenting | I agree (disagree). What a great idea! Uh-huh. OK. |
| Wrap-up/farewell | Well, gotta go. See you later Bye, nice talking to you. |
| Conversational repair | Let's start over. That's not what I meant. You misunderstood me. |

## ■ GRAPHICAL OUTPUT NEEDS SERVED BY AUGMENTATIVE COMMUNICATION SYSTEMS

There are three types of graphical communication: writing, mathematics, and drawing/plotting. Each serves a different need; therefore AAC devices designed to meet each type of need have different characteristics. In this section we discuss each of the three types of graphical communication needs listed in Table 9-3. In this chapter our emphasis is on electronic AAC devices for graphical output. In Chapter 11 we discuss devices that aid manipulation of pencils, pens, and keyboards. These often serve graphical communication needs. In Chapter 8 we discuss ways in which people who

| TABLE 9-3 | Types of Graphical Communication |
|-----------|----------------------------------|
| **Type** | **Definition** |
| Writing | All modes of communication in which a hard copy of language output is produced. Includes transcription, in which output is dictated to a partner and written by the partner. |
| Mathematics | All modes by which calculations are made, equations solved, and quantitative answers obtained. Includes calculator-like functions, mathematics worksheets, spreadsheets, and equation-solving programs. May or may not result in hard copy, depending on application. |
| Drawing/plotting | All activities in which a pictorial representation is created (drawing) or a graphical representation of a physical or mathematical relationship is generated (plotting). |

| TABLE 9-4 | Types of Writing Commonly Aided By Augmentative Communication Systems |
|-----------|------------------------------------------------------------------------|
| **Type** | **Characteristics** |
| Note taking | High rate of entry required; must be portable; shorthand can be idiosyncratic; hard copy required; accuracy less important |
| Messaging | Slower rate; shorthand must be intuitive or obvious; accuracy important; can be stationary |
| Formal writing | Generally based on stationary system; accuracy more important than speed; must have editing, saving, and printing capabilities |

have disabilities gain access to the Internet. In this chapter we discuss Internet access as an output mode for graphical communication using computers. This capability is built into some AAC devices.

## AAC Systems for Writing

The most important result accomplished by writing is communication in a hard-copy format. Thus writing does not need to be via traditional orthography (letters used to form words on a page). Symbols that are printed on paper can also be used to accomplish the hard copy result of writing. Spelling is not a prerequisite for the generation of written output, since some devices allow the selection of whole words, which are then output to a printer. Writing can be accomplished by having a nonspeaking person point to letters on a board and having an attendant write down the letters.

As shown in Table 9-4, we distinguish three types of writing: note taking, messaging, and formal writing (Cook, 1988); the requirements for each differ. *Note taking* generally requires a portable device, since notes are typically taken in such different contexts as home, library, school, job, or meetings. When taking notes, it is necessary to write at a high rate in order to keep up with the speaker, and we typically use abbreviations and other shorthand notations. Users of AAC writing devices also use abbreviations when taking notes, and stored words and phrases may be included to further increase the rate of text entry. Because the notes are generally only used by the person who takes them, the abbreviations only need to be understood by that person.

Even though the function we are replacing is writing notes on paper, it is not necessary to have a portable printer built into the device, since some devices allow storage of the notes in the device during the day. The notes can then be printed out at the end of the day at home using a page printer.

*Messaging* has many of the same requirements as note taking. However, the usual situation is that a note is made for another person to read, and the abbreviations and shorthand notations must be intuitively obvious. For example, most people would recognize *ASAP* as "as soon as possible," but they might not recognize a less common or more individualized abbreviation. An advantage of this mode of writing over note taking is that the writing rate may be slower because the person receiving the message is not present and waiting for it.

An interesting approach to messaging for individuals who have intellectual disabilities and use symbols for communication was developed by Brodin (1992). These individuals live in group homes and wish to send messages to their families, but they are unable to use voice communication over the telephone. Brodin's approach is to create rubber stamps with the appropriate symbols used by the AAC user. These stamps are used by the person to create a message on paper. This message is then faxed to the significant others as a message. The family responds by using a second set of rubber stamps with the symbols on them. In this way, communication is established between the person and the family.

The most demanding type of writing is *formal writing;* reports, school homework, writing for publication, and similar applications are included in this category. For formal writing, accuracy is of prime importance, with rate of entry becoming secondary. However, with a typing rate of three to five words per minute, input acceleration techniques are still necessary to allow an individual to keep up with the demands of work or school. Some acceleration features have been developed specifically for writing devices. For example, an autocapitalization feature speeds up writing by automatically inserting two spaces and shifting (for an uppercase letter to start the next sentence) after a period, exclamation point, or question mark is typed.

Because AAC users often have motor disabilities that result in an increased number of selection errors, it is essential that editing capabilities tailored to the needs of the user be included in a writing device (Vanderheiden, 1985). Most text editors used in AAC devices for writing include basic word processing functions (e.g., insert, delete, move text, print). All these must be available to the user regardless of what input method she is using (e.g., one-key typing, scanning, Morse code). Often we use an input-emulating interface (see Chapter 8), a portable or stationary computer, and a word processor to provide formal writing capabilities. When this approach is taken, all the features of the word processor are available to the user. For example, storage and retrieval of text files allows for work on a document in small segments of time. This is important because fatigue may preclude finishing an entire document in one sitting, and storage also allows multiple use of similar passages for different functions. For example, a college student could save a file that included all the headings and course information for laboratory reports and then fill it in with each individual report as the course progressed. Formal writing devices also require a full-page printer, so that edited text can be directly printed in a form suitable for submission.

Smith et al (1989) analyzed the formal written output of a group of adolescents who had congenital disabilities limiting their abilities to speak and were competent conversational users of AAC devices. Each of these individuals had developed language using Blissymbols (see Vanderheiden and Lloyd, 1986), and they had made the transition to traditional orthography (letters and spelling). Smith and co-workers analyzed the homework produced by these individuals. More than 80% of the homework was produced independently. The rate of production of written output was only 1.5 words per minute, reflecting the amount of planning and thinking time required, as well as the limitations imposed by physical disabilities. As expected, the majority (more than 50%) of the writing was for school assignments. The second largest category was personal correspondence, a finding that Smith and co-workers ascribed to the inability to use a telephone. Some difficulties with grammatical structure and form were observed in all the subjects, but there was great variability even in this small sample. This study, one of the few designed to study writing skills in AAC users, provides a basis from which to examine written output, and it indicates that individuals who have congenital speaking and writing difficulties because of physical limitations can develop successful writing skills.

Light and Smith (1993) compared the home literacy experiences of preschool children by surveying a group of parents of children who use AAC and a group of parents of nondisabled children. Through a series of questions, Light and Smith determined the functional context (e.g., how reading and writing occur, when they occur, communication during reading), language context (roles of parent and child,

nature and degree of participation), and cultural context (parental priorities and beliefs regarding literacy). Both groups of children were interested in literacy activities, but the AAC users had fewer opportunities to read, participated less during reading, and had less access to writing and drawing materials. Although both groups of parents gave high priority to communication, the parents of the nondisabled children gave highest priorities to making friends and literacy activities. The parents of AAC users gave second level priorities to physical needs such as mobility and feeding. Studies such as this underscore the importance of attitudes, beliefs, and accessibility to materials in the development of cognitive communication skills.

A more detailed discussion of literacy issues related to AAC is beyond the scope of this text. Blackstone (1996a,b) discusses literacy from a number of points of view and offers suggestions for other resources.

## AAC Systems for Mathematics

Imagine learning even the most basic arithmetic without being able to write the numbers down. Although it is possible to become proficient using this strategy, it is certainly more difficult than basic pencil and paper mathematics. Seven-year-old Rob has difficulty using a pencil and paper because of his cerebral palsy, but he is able to use a computer for writing by hitting the keys with one finger. He wants to learn math (at least his parents and teacher want him to), but this is very difficult using the standard keyboard and cursor movement. After he has two rows of numbers, he must move over to the far right-hand side of the first column of numbers and enter the first correct number *(7)*. Then he must backspace two times to get the cursor in the proper position for the second number *(1)*. The cursor in a graphical communication device is a flashing marker that indicates the location on the screen for the next entry. In writing English text, the cursor always moves left to right and moves down one line at the right margin. In contrast to this, for mathematics the cursor moves left to right as numbers are entered to be added, but once there is a column of numbers, the cursor moves right to left as the sum is entered. Figure 9-4, *B*, illustrates this cursor movement. Also, when learning to add or subtract, children are taught to carry or borrow by crossing out the number at the top of the adjacent column and substituting the borrowed or carried value. It is desirable for this type of cursor movement to be available in a math worksheet as well. For example, when in the math mode, the letter *C* could be pressed to indicate *carry*, causing cursor to jump to the top of the next column. All these cursor movements can be very time consuming, especially if a writing device is used and the person must tediously backspace to obtain the right to left cursor movement.

In algebra, special symbols (e.g., Greek letters) and the

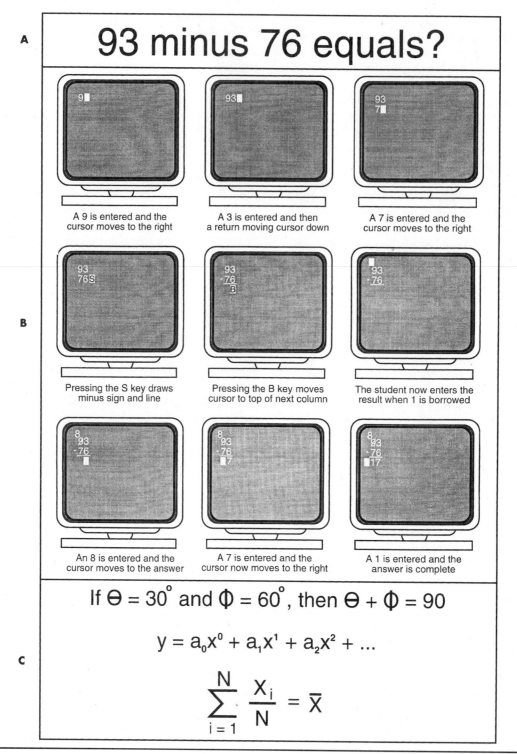

**Figure 9-4**   Math problems require different cursor movements and symbols than text entry. **A,** A math problem as it would normally be written. **B,** The sequence of cursor movement required to enter the problem, create a subtraction notation (line plus minus sign), and complete the problem (including using "borrow"). **C,** Special symbols such as these are used in higher mathematics.

use of superscripts and subscripts are also required (Figure 9-4, *C*). Higher math such as statistics or calculus adds the need to have special symbols like summation signs and integral signs and the need for formatting problems. There are devices (sometimes as programs for personal computers) that are set up specifically for these math functions.* Several commercial AAC devices also include some or all of these mathematical functions.

## AAC Systems for Drawing and Plotting

The final type of graphical output is *drawing or plotting*. We use drawings of all types to convey information, to help us clarify our thinking, and for creative expression. We may use pencils, paint and brush, drawing instruments (e.g., ruler, compass), or computer programs. Many persons who are unable to use these conventional means of drawing because of motor limitations need to accomplish drawing or plotting for graphical expression. The purpose of the drawing or plotting may be to generate scientific graphs of data, to produce formal engineering drawings, to draw chemical structures, or to produce freehand drawing for artistic expression. The following AAC device characteristics are required for all these types of drawing. First, as in the case of mathematics, cursor movements for drawing differ from those required in writing. If a computer-based drawing device is used, the cursor must be allowed to move in any of the four screen directions (up, down, left, or right) at any time. Often this movement is generated by using a mouse, and for individuals unable to accomplish this motor skill, alternative input means must be found (see Chapter 7). Second, the user must be able to move the cursor without drawing (as if the pencil were off of the paper), and he must also be able to create erasures and perform such functions as filling a specified area with a specific color. For plotting of scientific data, it is often possible merely to enter the data and then to specify the format (e.g., line graph, bar graph, pie chart), and the device scales and plots the results automatically. Drawing and plotting programs provide the capability of generating printouts in a variety of formats. It is also necessary to have storage of partial or complete drawings, so that they can be edited for other uses or worked on a little at a time. Most of these functions are available in drawing or plotting programs written for personal computers. In many cases either keyboard or mouse emulation, or both, needs to be included in a device.

---

*Mathpad for Apple Macintosh series computers, Intellitools, Novato, Calif.; Liberator, Prentke Romich Co., Wooster, Ohio; Access to Math, Don Johnston Developmental Systems, Wauconda, Ill.; Mathtool, Words Plus, Palmdale, Calif.

## ◼ CHARACTERISTICS OF AUGMENTATIVE COMMUNICATION SYSTEMS

For AAC, the activity output component of the Human Activity Assistive Technology (HAAT) model is conversational or graphical communication; this activity can take place in any of the settings shown in Figure 2-6: an individual or group home, at work or school, or in the community. Social context, also shown in Figure 2-6, plays a major role in AAC as well, and communication partners may be strangers, friends, a caregiver, a teacher, a boss, or a relative. Each of these individuals requires a different style of communication, and our design of AAC devices should accommodate as many of these as possible. In the two previous sections we described the communication needs that AAC systems must serve. Based on that background, we can now describe the characteristics of AAC devices that allow them to meet these needs.

O'Keefe, Brown, and Schuller (1998) compared the importance of AAC characteristics across five groups: AAC users, familiar partners, service providers, manufacturers, and individuals unfamiliar with AAC. They found that AAC users rated more of the 186 items included in their survey as critical than did the other four groups. The categories of conversational control and speed of communication were ranked higher by both users and familiar partners than by AAC service providers and manufacturers. Users and their communication partners also rated ease of learning a communication aid more highly than did the other groups. Studies such as this and the investigation of consumer-based criteria for AAC devices by Batavia and Hammer (1990) are important both for the future development of AAC devices and for the successful application of currently available systems.

We group the AAC device characteristics into the three major components shown in Table 9-5: (1) human/technology interface, (2) processor, and (3) activity output. The human/technology interface includes a user control interface, a selection method, a selection set, and an optional user display. The processor is further broken down into components of (1) selection technique, (2) rate enhancement and vocabulary expansion, (3) vocabulary storage, (4) text editing, and (5) output control. The activity outputs to the communication partner include visual display, speech, and printer. A control port for external devices (e.g., computers or EADLs) is sometimes included. This set of functions is based on those described by Cook (1988), Kraat and Stiver-Kogut (1991), and Vanderheiden and Lloyd (1986).

Not all the individual functions shown in Table 9-5 are included in every device. Electronic AAC devices may have differing structures that implement and group the functions in alternative ways. AAC devices based on "low technologies" include many of the functions listed in Table 9-5. For example, in Figure 9-5 the parts of a language board are labeled to correspond to the components listed in Table 9-5. The selection method is direct selection and the entire communication board is the selection set. The user selects by using her finger to point directly to the desired item. This device also allows for output control by including "control" squares such as "END OF WORD," "START OVER," and "I CAN'T SPELL IT." The functions of rate enhancement, vocabulary expansion, and vocabulary storage are all implemented through the inclusion of whole words and phrases that can be selected with one pointing motion.

High-tech approaches are almost all computer based, with the functions shown in Table 9-5 implemented in software programs. Some of these devices use special-purpose computers designed specifically for use in the communication device, whereas others use personal computers of various types (e.g., laptop computers). Different commercial devices may have different ratios of software to hardware to accomplish the same functions.

## Control Interface

The *control interface* is the hardware by which the consumer accesses the device (see Chapter 7). There are various types of interfaces based on the number of independent choices that can be made by an anatomical site or a combination of anatomical sites (e.g., hand, arm, head, chin, leg, foot). Keyboards, single or dual switches, and joysticks or multiple switch arrays are the most commonly used control interfaces for augmentative communication devices. It is often necessary for the novice user to develop motor skill with the control interface before it can be used effectively as an input to an augmentative communication device. Training programs that serve this purpose are also discussed in Chapter 7.

## Selection Method

The control interface interacts with the processors of the device through one of two basic *selection methods:* direct selection or indirect selection (e.g., scanning, directed scanning, or coded access). The basic principles of these approaches and their many variations are discussed in Chapter 7. In this section we are primarily concerned with the manner in which these selection methods interact with the

| TABLE 9-5 | Characteristics of Augmentative Communication Systems | |
|---|---|---|
| Human/Technology Interface* | Processor | Activity Output |
| Control interface | Selection technique* | To partner: |
| Selection method | Rate enhancement and | Visual |
| Selection set | vocabulary expansion: | Speech |
| User visual | Codes | Print |
| display | Prediction | To external device: |
| | Levels | Computer† |
| | Vocabulary storage | EADL‡ |
| | Output control | |

*EADL,* Electronic aid to daily living.
*See Chapter 7.
†See Chapter 8.
‡See Chapter 11.

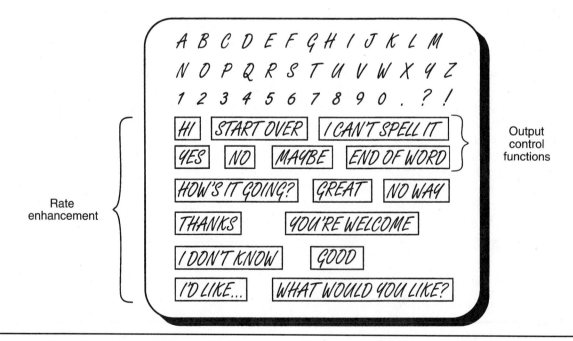

Figure 9-5  A hypothetical language board illustrating the use of different conversational categories and functions.

remainder of the augmentative communication device. The signal produced by the selection method is either a single letter or an electronic code signifying that some other vocabulary element (e.g., a word or phrase) has been selected. For example, in a row-column scanning device, the signal from the selection method is a marker that indicates which of the selection set elements has been selected. Alternatively, in a direct selection expanded keyboard device, the selection method signal may be a memory address where an entire sentence is stored. It is important to keep in mind that the selection method is merely a way of accommodating a particular set of user cognitive and motor skills and a specific control interface. A user's motor action on the control interface results in the generation of a selection code. The interpretation of this code by the control circuits and software of the processor results in the generation of an utterance.

Individuals who have visual impairments and who require scanning as a result of physical limitations may not be able to use visual scanning arrays. For these individuals we often use auditory scanning. In this approach the choices are presented in auditory form and the user selects his choice from the auditory prompts. In many commercial AAC systems there is provision for both a prompting phrase and a selected utterance. The prompting phrase is often provided via an earphone so only the user hears it.

Auditory scanning can also be used without a device. In this case a list of vocabulary items is read aloud by the communication partner. The AAC user then chooses a vocabulary item by using a predetermined signal such as a vocalization in order to identify the desired vocabulary item. Kovach and Kenyon (1998) analyze a variety of approaches to auditory scanning, summarize current research in this area, and describe considerations to be included when developing an auditory scanning system for an AAC user. There is also a Web site for auditory scanning (espse.ed.psu.edu/SPLED/McN/audtoryscanning).

## Selection Set

In the section on cognitive function and development in Chapter 3, we define a language as any system of arbitrary symbols organized according to a set of rules agreed to by the speaker and partner (Miller, 1981). To facilitate communication, an AAC system must be capable of providing a language system for the user and her communication partner. The portion of the augmentative communication device that presents the symbol system and possible vocabulary selections to the user is the **selection set**. For example, the labels on the keys of a keyboard are one type of selection set. These may be individual letters, words, phrases, or other symbols. For the language board shown in Figure 9-5, the selection set is the letters and words printed on the board.

Many types of symbol systems are used in augmentative

communication devices (Lloyd and Karlin, 1982; Vanderheiden and Lloyd, 1986). Several of these are illustrated in Figure 9-6. Perhaps the most concrete type of symbolism is the use of real objects (full size or miniature). However, to a person with cognitive disabilities, a miniature object may not appear to represent the full-size version, and care must be taken to ensure that the association is made by the user (Vanderheiden and Lloyd, 1986). There are many sets of pictures that are used as symbol systems. These vary from photographs of the item to line drawings, which are pictographic representations. Real objects and photographs have the disadvantage that many communicative concepts (e.g., good, more, go, hurt) are difficult to portray. Pictographic symbols include provisions for more abstract communicative intents and allow much greater flexibility in developing vocabulary usage. Vanderheiden and Lloyd (1986) discuss the major types of symbol systems currently in use on AAC devices. A more flexible symbol type is the use of a symbol system possessing grammar and syntax (e.g., Blissymbols). The nature of this symbol system allows the inclusion of more linguistic functions, such as categorization by parts of language. We use the term **traditional orthography** to refer to the symbolic representation based on letters and words. Some individuals have reading skills that exceed their spelling skills, and they cannot rely on spelling for communication. If the person has a large word recognition vocabulary, the selection set should be based on words with possible "carrier phrases" that are filled in with limited spelling (e.g., "I would like a drink of ____"). Spelling is the most flexible symbol system because it can be used to create a large number of different utterances, but it can also be the slowest because of letter-by-letter entry rather than selection of whole words. Many computers, printers, and keyboards accommodate languages other than English.

Traditionally, selection sets were static; that is, there was one set of elements from which the user could choose. Some devices address this problem by using **dynamic communication displays**. Dynamic displays change the displayed selection set when a new level is selected, as shown in Figure 9-7.* Because the user's selection set is on the display panel, this set can be altered easily, depending on previous choices. For example, a general selection set may consist of categories such as work, home, food, clothing, greetings, or similar classifications. If one of these is chosen, either by touching the display surface directly or by scanning, then a new selection set is displayed. For example, a variety of food-related items and activities (eat, drink, ice cream, pasta, etc.) would follow the choice of "foods" from the general selec-

---

*Dynavox, Dynavox, Pittsburgh, Pa.; Talking Screen, Words Plus, Palmdale, Calif.; Talk:About, Don Johnston Developmental Systems, Wauconda, Ill.; Speaking Dynamically, Mayer Johnston, Solana Beach, Calif., Vanguard, Prentke Romich, Wooster, Ohio; GUS!, Gus Communications, Vancouver, B.C., Canada.

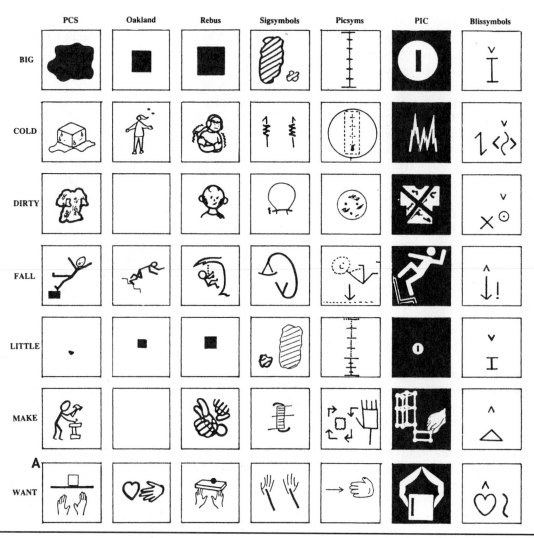

**Figure 9-6**   Examples of the variety of symbol systems that have been developed for AAC use. (From Blackstone S: *Augmentative communi-cation*, Rockville, Md, 1986, American Speech Language Hearing Association.)

tion set. The symbols on the display can be varied, and this changes the targets for the user. Because each new selection set is displayed, the user does not have to remember what is on each level. This approach, illustrated in Figure 9-8, also avoids having to squeeze several pictures into one square on a static display.

Blackstone (1994) describes a number of key features of dynamic displays. The nature of these devices allows the user to quickly change the screen and to configure the size, color, and arrangement of the symbols to match the topic. Dynamic displays also reduce memory requirements because the user is prompted by the display after each choice. There are also specific cognitive and visual perceptual demands placed on a user by dynamic displays. The constant vigilance to the screen requires a high level of visual attention and constant decision making. These may be challenging for some AAC users who have cognitive limitations. Some AAC devices that use dynamic displays are software prod-

ucts that are used with laptop computers. Others use dedicated computer-based hardware.

## Selection Technique

The selection technique is the way in which the device interprets the action of the user. In Chapter 7 we defined three scanning selection techniques: automatic, step, and inverse. Scanning AAC devices typically allow the choice of any of these three techniques to meet the consumer's needs.

## Accelerating and Extending the Basic Vocabulary

As we have described, one of the limitations of augmentative communication devices is that the rate of communication is much slower than human speech. There are several device features that directly address the speed of communication, and we use the term **rate enhancement** to

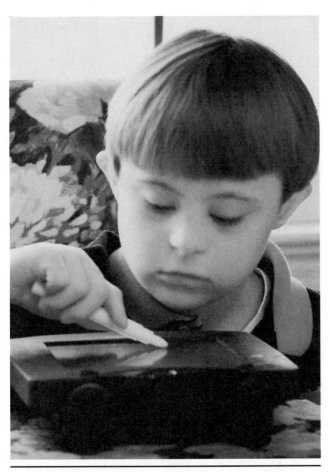

Figure 9-7    Dynamic display devices are often accessed with touch screen interfaces, making them accessible and providing a cognitively concrete user interface. (Photo courtesy Dynavox.)

describe them. A second limitation is that the vocabulary size in a device is limited to the size of the basic selection set unless we make some provision for extending it. We use the term **vocabulary expansion** to refer to all approaches that allow the user to have access to a vocabulary larger than the one provided instantly by the selection set. Rate enhancement and vocabulary expansion present different problems, but the solutions to each are similar. Some of the approaches we describe apply only to rate enhancement or vocabulary expansion, whereas others apply to both. Even when the same approach is used for both needs, its application and the strategies employed may be different for rate enhancement than for vocabulary expansion.

**Rate enhancement.** *Rate enhancement* refers to all approaches that result in the number of characters generated being greater than the number of selections the individual makes. Because an increased level of efficiency is obtained, the user has to make fewer entries and the overall rate is increased. Rate enhancement may be used with any of the selection methods; however, the goals and approaches differ

for direct selection and scanning. In direct selection the goal is to reduce the number of keystrokes while increasing the amount of information selected with each keystroke. In scanning the goal is to optimize the scanning array to reduce the time required to make a desired selection (acceleration rate). This is done by developing optimal arrangements of scanning arrays that reduce the average number of switch activations and waiting times for a selection based on frequency of character representation, not frequency of word representation. We discuss rate enhancement approaches for both direct selection and scanning in this section.

Blackstone (1990b) describes several important considerations in rate enhancement. The first of these relates to the automaticity of motor tasks in selecting vocabulary elements. Motor patterns become more automatic as they are practiced. This applies to using AAC devices, as well as to riding a bicycle or any other motor task. As the skills improve, motor and cognitive tasks become more automatic and the user becomes an "expert." As Blackstone points out, once these motor patterns are established, even small changes in the task may result in dramatic *decreases* in rate. A second consideration Blackstone presents is that faster is not always better. Some devices (e.g., those with speech synthesis output) may become less intelligible when the output is produced at a higher rate. If the rate is increased, manual signing (an unaided modality) may also become less intelligible, especially to a partner who is not proficient.

For our purposes, we can group rate enhancement techniques for direct selection into two broad categories: (1) encoding techniques and (2) prediction techniques. As we shall see, these two categories are closely related, and under some circumstances they collapse into one approach. There are several approaches in each of these categories. Vanderheiden and Lloyd (1986) distinguish three basic types of codes: memory based, chart based, and display based. A memory-based technique requires that both the user and his partner know the codes by memory or that the user have the codes memorized for entry into his device. Examples include eye movements in a given direction (e.g., looking toward the refrigerator means "let's eat"); another example is hand signs that are known by both communication partners. Memory-based codes can also be used more easily by persons who have visual limitations. Chart-based techniques are those that have an index of the codes and their corresponding vocabulary items. This can be a simple paper list attached to an electronic device or a chart on the wall (e.g., two eye blinks = "call nurse"; three eye blinks = "please turn me"; eyes up = "yes"; eyes down = "no"). Display-based codes are those that require the user to respond to the selection set to enter a code. Figure 9-9 illustrates both a chart-based and display-based approach for Morse code (Vanderheiden and Lloyd, 1986). In each device, two switches are used. The right switch produces dots and the left one produces dashes. On the display-based device, the

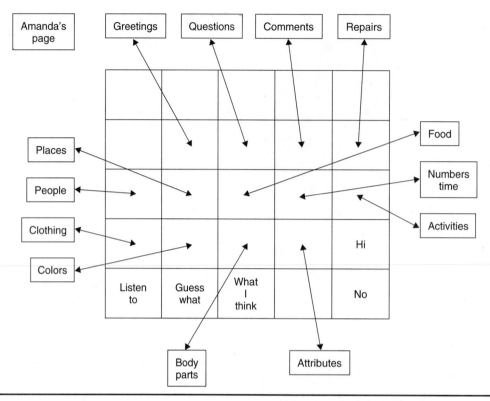

**Figure 9-8**  Dynamic display devices change the selection set presented to the user each time an entry is made.

lights move to the right when a dot is entered and to the left when a dash is entered. To select the word "tan," the person using the chart-based device in Figure 9-9, *A,* would select dash, dot-dash, dash-dot to get the three letters. This is a sequence of switch movements of left, right-left, left-right. The person using the display-based device in Figure 9-9, *B,* would cause the lights to move left for *t,* right-left for *a,* and left-right for *n.* Note that the sequence of movement is exactly the same in both cases, but the display helps the user by providing feedback (illuminated light) for each entry. A memory-based approach to Morse code requires that both user and partner know the code (e.g., eye blinks used to produce dots and dashes) or that the user memorize the switch actions required for each letter.

**Numeric codes** can be used to stand for a word, complete phrase, or sentence. The user merely enters one or more numbers, and the device outputs the complete stored vocabulary item. The main advantage is that fewer key or switch presses need to be made by the disabled user than the number of characters selected. Additional advantages are that the numerical codes can be memorized and a display is not required. The primary disadvantage of this approach is that the relationship between the code and the vocabulary is arbitrary, and it is difficult for most people to memorize more than a few hundred codes.

**Abbreviation expansion** is a technique in which a shortened form of a word or phrase (the abbreviation)

stands for the entire word or phrase (the expansion). The abbreviations are automatically expanded by the device into the desired word or phrase. Vanderheiden and Kelso (1987) describe two types of vocabulary sets for AAC devices: coverage vocabularies and acceleration vocabularies. As used by these authors, **coverage vocabularies** are intended to provide a set of topics and concepts that can be used for basic communication by a person who cannot spell. The vocabulary may consist of pictures, symbols, or words. We can meet all the basic communication needs of persons who can spell by including the alphabet in the selection set of their devices. **Acceleration vocabularies,** on the other hand, are intended to be used by spellers to increase the rate of communication, and words included in the set are chosen to serve this purpose rather than to provide basic communication ability, which is achieved by spelling. Acceleration vocabulary selection sets contain the letter codes for words, phrases, or entire sentences.

In selecting words or phrases for inclusion in acceleration vocabularies, there are several principles that we can apply (Vanderheiden and Kelso, 1987). For sentences or phrases, the most useful entries are those that are open ended and general (e.g., the carrier phrases described above). For word lists, it is tempting to consult vocabulary studies such as those discussed later in this section and include all the most frequently used words in our list. Because the first 200 words in a 1000-word list account for more than 80% of all

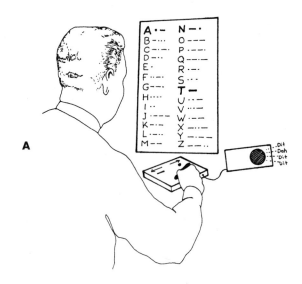

A

MORSE CODE DISPLAY AID

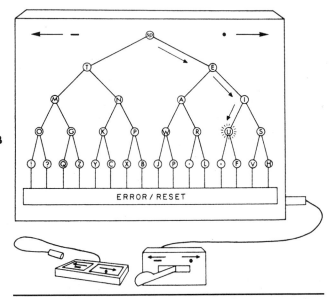

B

Figure 9-9    Encoding systems may be either **(A)** chart based or **(B)** display based. (From Blackstone S: *Augmentative communication*, Rockville, Md, 1986, American Speech Language Hearing Association.)

**BOX 9-1**    **Classification of Termination Techniques**

Variable length autoterminating
Variable length with terminating period
Variable length with terminating expand key
Variable length numeral terminating (10-branch)

---

Data from Vanderheiden GC, Kelso DP: Comparative analysis of fixed-vocabulary communication acceleration techniques, *Augment Altern Commun* 3:196-206, 1987.

There are several basic approaches to abbreviation (Bailey, 1989). *Truncation* results in a shortened form of the word, and *contraction* is formed by eliminating vowels. The word *function* becomes "funct" when truncated and "fctn" when contracted. Other techniques used with AAC devices included **salient letter coding,** in which key words are included in the abbreviation. For example, *HJ* becomes "Hi Jane." Another method is to use a categorization approach, such as *GHH*, meaning "*H*ello *h*ow are you?" (G = greeting + HH, based on first letters of key words) for a greeting or *INM* to interrupt and correct (I = interruption, NM = "That's *n*ot what I *m*eant to say") (Goosens and Kraat, 1985).

Beukelman and Yorkston (1984) evaluated five different coding strategies for abbreviations: (1) random number, (2) alphabetic numeric, (3) numerical groupings with alphabetic codes, (4) alphabetic with alphabetic word groupings, and (5) menu based (similar to number 4, but provides prompting to the user after the category is entered). The third and fourth approaches included both a category (e.g., food) and an item in that category (e.g., banana). These coding strategies were found to be more effective (measured by accurate selections/minute) than either the numeric (worst performance) or alphabetic codes alone. The menu approach yielded midrange performance.

Because all abbreviation expansion techniques used with AAC devices are intended to be expanded automatically, the method used to indicate to the device that the abbreviation the user has entered is complete is important. Vanderheiden and Kelso (1987) use the term *termination techniques* to describe this process, and they identify several types. Box 9-1 lists several types of terminating techniques. The autoterminating technique requires no action by the user to let the device know that an abbreviation has been typed, and this is its major advantage. The major disadvantage is the possibility of overlap between abbreviations and letter sequences used in spelling. For example, if the letters *th* are used for an abbreviation, then every time the user tries to spell *the* the device assumes that the first two letters are an abbreviation and expands it. This is referred to as a "collision." The period or expand key approaches are similar. In

usage, this is attractive. However, if an analysis is done on the lengths of these words, it is found that the shorter words are often near the top of the list in frequency. Therefore, Vanderheiden and Kelso suggest using the number of keystrokes combined with word length to select vocabulary. This makes a word such as *because*, which is fifty-sixth on the list, more important than the word *up*, which is much higher on the list. This is because the keystroke savings in using a code for a longer word are greater. This approach reduces the "coverage" of the word set from 80% for the first 200 words to about 56%, since the most frequently used words are short.

each case an additional key must be pressed to expand the abbreviation. This slows things down, but it places the expansion under the control of the user. These approaches also avoid collisions; they are used in several AAC devices.* A final approach listed in Box 9-1 uses a number or numbers to end the abbreviation. For example, *H1* may be "Hello, how are you?" This has the advantage of automatically expanding the abbreviations and avoiding collisions, but it may require additional keystrokes because of the numeric codes. Some commercial AAC devices allow the user to select the type of termination technique to be used, and many include an UNDO key to allow use of unexpanded abbreviation.†

All the rate enhancement methods described so far are based on text entry, and they use text characters to access codes. An alternative approach, which uses coding of words, sentences, and phrases on the basis of their meanings, is called **semantic encoding** or Minspeak‡ (Baker, 1982). The key to this approach is to substitute pictorial representations, called *icons,* for numerical or letter codes. There are several advantages obtained by doing this. First and most obvious is the ease of recall that can occur. For example, if I use a picture of an apple for "food," and a sun rising for "morning," then selecting "apple" and "sunrise" could be a code for "What's for breakfast." A second advantage of this approach is that we can allow the icons to have multiple meanings. Thus the apple symbol can take on the meaning of "eat" rather than food. Several examples of Minspeak sequences are shown in Figure 9-10. There is an inherent tradeoff between fluency (speed or rate) and flexibility (Baker, 1987). The original Minspeak system was intended to use codes for whole sentences (Baker, 1982). In this mode there was a significant increase in rate, but flexibility was sacrificed. One of the major limitations of the semantic encoding technique is that because it is based on icons instead of text, it is difficult to combine retrieval of sentences or phrases or words with spelling. In an attempt to increase the flexibility of the Minspeak concept, Baker (1986) developed an approach based on the use of syntactical labels coupled with icons. Figure 9-11 illustrates this concept. For example, the apple icon becomes "eat" when combined with the key labeled "verb" and becomes "food" when combined with the noun key.

Williams (1991), an accomplished user of numeric, abbreviation expansion, and word-based Minspeak,§ describes several advantages of this approach. In comparison to sentence-based Minspeak, he states that he (and most of the rest of us) does not think in sentences, but in words or short

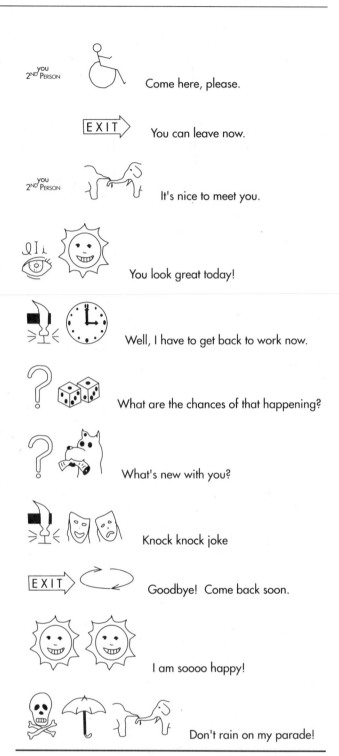

**Figure 9-10**    Examples of Minspeak symbol sequences. (From Romich B: *Liberator manual,* Wooster, Ohio, Prentke Romich.)

phrases. This makes a word-based device easier to use. Second, he indicates that of the three encoding approaches in which he has achieved skill (each after hundreds of hours of practice), the word-based Minspeak "offers powerful advantages over the rest" (p. 133). His major reasons for this is the ease with which words are recalled during use and the large vocabularies that are possible with the use of icons

---

*Words+ EZ Keys series; Toby Churchill's Lightwriter (Zygo Industries in the United States).
†Words+, Palmdale, Calif.
‡Trademark of Semantic Compaction Systems, available on the AAC devices from Prentke Romich Co., Wooster, Ohio.
§Word Strategy, Prentke Romich Co., Wooster, Ohio.

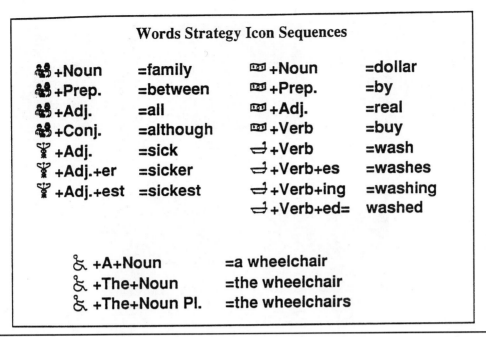

**Figure 9-11**   Symbols such as those used with Minspeak can be given syntactical meaning, as in this example from the Word Strategy application program. (From *Liberating the power of Minspeak*, Wooster, Ohio, 1991, Prentke Romich.)

rather than arbitrary codes. Williams also points out that it requires a large amount of practice and effort to become proficient with this type of device, and we must build this in to our training programs for new AAC users (see the section on implementation in this chapter). Williams also addresses the initial reluctance that many cognitively able but physically limited adults have to use pictorial representations as codes. Often parents of potential AAC device users will reject this approach because of the pictorial icons, when it could be very powerful for the device user. However, as with all the characteristics of AAC devices, no one approach serves every person's needs, and different encoding techniques are useful to different individuals.

A significant limitation of commercial AAC systems in general is that they are often delivered "empty" (i.e., there is little or no prestored vocabulary). For individuals who have large potential expressive vocabularies, this can create a daunting task of programming large amounts of information into the device before it is usable by the person. In order to overcome this deficiency, Minspeak Application Programs (MAPs), which contain vocabulary intended for different end users, were developed. For example, there is a MAP for preschool-age children, one for school-age children, and the one illustrated in Figure 9-11, called *Word Strategy*, for users who are literate.

As a further extension of this concept, the Unity MAP* was developed to address the relationship among the separate, target audience-specific MAPs. So rather than require a user to learn an entire new system as she develops her language skills, the Unity MAP provides for transition in which the later MAPs build on earlier ones by keeping icon sequences, icon locations, and stored vocabulary in advanced applications consistent with more basic applications. This approach minimizes relearning of icon sequences, takes maximal advantage of automatic motor patterns learned with basic MAPs, and allows vocabulary to be built logically and sequentially as the user progresses. To account for differences in motor skill, the Unity MAP includes 8, 32, and 128 location overlays that differ in the pointing resolution required by the user. There is as much consistency as possible among the 8, 32, and 128 overlays in order to account for motor skill development while preserving the other benefits of Unity. There are four icon overlays used. Overlay 1 uses single icons for recall of words. Overlays 2, 3, and 4 add to this basic vocabulary and include two- and three-icon sequences to retrieve stored words. Overlay 4 incorporates the written grammar labels shown in Figure 9-11, whereas overlays 1, 2, and 3 use characterized icons as grammar labels. The word lists included in Unity include the most frequently used words (see below).

Despite the advantages of recall provided by the Minspeak technique, when large numbers of sentences, words, and phrases are stored, the icon sequences can become difficult to remember. For this reason software has been developed to allow icon prediction in some Minspeak-based devices.* **Icon prediction** is a feature that aids in recalling stored sequences. It uses a light associated with each symbol in the selection set. Only those symbols that form the

*Prentke Romich Co., Wooster, Ohio.

*Prentke Romich Co., Wooster, Ohio.

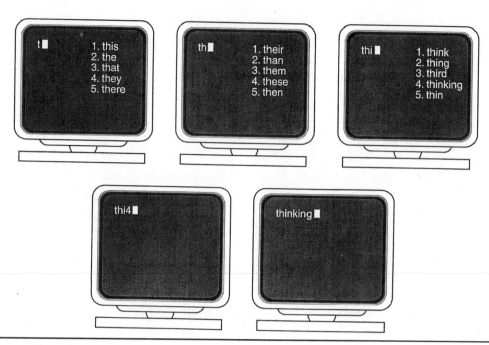

Figure 9-12    Word completion systems present a series of choices based on previous letters entered.

beginning of an icon sequence are lighted initially. Thus the user knows which symbols are possible first icons. When one of these icons is selected, only those icons light up or flash that are part of a sequence beginning with the first selected icon. This continues until a complete icon sequence has been selected. Because the device limits the number of icons that must be visually scanned for each selection, icon prediction also serves as a further rate enhancement technique. Because the allowed selection set is decreased for any given choice, icon prediction can also increase selection accuracy and reduce errors. An added feature when the selection method is scanning is **predictive selection** in which only valid icons in a sequence are scanned after the initial icon is selected. There is also a Minspeak-based device (Vanguard)* that utilizes a dynamic display to implement icon prediction and further reduce the cognitive load on the user.

By studying the frequency with which certain letters follow others in English, we can develop a computer program to automatically alter the order in which letters are presented or selected, depending on the previously chosen letters. This is called *predictive scanning*. If *t* is typed, then it is very likely that the next letter will be *h*, followed by *e*. This type of device scanning is referred to as an *anticipatory approach* because the choices offered to the user are based on previous entries and the vocabulary set from which the user selects is constantly altered based on previous entries (see Heckathorne, Voda, and Leibowitz, 1987). As Heckathorne and co-workers point out, these devices are often considered

to require large cognitive and attentional demands on the user. In assessing the success of users in an evaluation of one such device, the PACA,* these authors attribute major significance to the fact that the device is structured; that is, with practice, the users learn to expect certain arrays based on previous entries. In fact, the improvements made in the PACA after initial evaluation were mainly directed toward improving the *predictability* of vocabulary item presentations. In this case the motor response was a single switch closure, but the motor patterns associated with visual tracking and target identification improved when the device was more predictable and the users were able to learn what display characteristics to expect. This is an illustration of the value of automaticity in rate enhancement approaches (Blackstone, 1990b).

Whereas the predictive scanning method described is based on changing the selection set order to reflect previous entries, it is also possible to realize significant increases in rate by using **word prediction** or **word completion** approaches with any selection technique (Swiffin et al, 1987). Word prediction or word completion devices have several potential advantages over abbreviation expansion techniques. In these devices there is typically a window on the screen that displays the most likely words based on the letters entered. In word completion the user selects the desired word, if any, by entering its code (e.g., a number listed next to the word) or continuing to enter letters if the desired word is not displayed. The displayed words change as more letters are entered (Figure 9-12). Word prediction

*Prentke Romich, Co., Wooster, Ohio.

*Formerly produced by Zygo Industries, Portland, Ore.

CASE STUDY 9-3

WORD PREDICTION VOCABULARIES

Assume that one college student is taking a course in assistive technologies and another student is taking a course in world religions. If both students have word completion/prediction systems, compare the word lists you might expect to be used for writing homework assignments for each course. Would most words be the same or different for the two applications? How would the word lists vary in (1) an adaptive system, and (2) a nonadaptive system? What words would you start with as a basic vocabulary in each case?

devices offer a menu of words based on previous words entered, rather than on the basis of letters. For example, if the word *computer* is entered, a word completion device may list "software," "system," "program," "keyboard," and so on as choices to follow "computer." The display of alternative words eliminates the need for memorizing codes, and this is probably the most important advantage of this type of device. Word prediction (or completion) approaches require that the user attend to a list of words after each entry of a letter. This reduces the item selection rate compared with letter-by-letter typing. According to Hortsman and Levine (1996), this reduction in selection rate is due to "cognitive or perceptual load." The magnitude of the reduction in rate decreases with practice. However, Hortsman and Levine conclude that these loads can offset the benefits achieved in keystroke savings and result in an overall decrease in text generation rate.

Predictive devices may be fixed or adaptive. Fixed types have a stored word vocabulary that never changes. These are typically based on frequency of use studies. Adaptive vocabularies change the ordering of words in the list and the actual dictionary by keeping track of the words used by the person storing them. The words are always listed in frequency-of-use order on the prediction display. In an adaptive approach, this order is continually upgraded based on recent usage.

An adaptive predictive device would accommodate for this by changing the frequency rankings; the fixed vocabulary device would not do this. The tradeoff is that the fixed device is more predictable to the user, and this can help in the development of motor and cognitive patterns for retrieval. It is also important to have a prebuilt vocabulary stored when the novice begins using the device (Swiffin et al, 1987). This gives the person an instantaneous capability on which to build. Even if the vocabulary is adaptable, it should have an initial set stored.

Word completion and word prediction devices can also contribute to the development of writing skills. Newell et al

(1992) summarize a series of studies using word completion and prediction with children and adults who had poor literacy skills (e.g., spelling). The long-term use of these devices resulted in improvements in spelling and the intelligibility of written work. Because many of the participants in these studies had good word recognition and were able to identify first letters of words, they frequently had the desired word presented to them after entering the first letter. Over time they began to recognize the words and to learn to spell those used most frequently. One major limitation with standard word completion devices is that if the desired word does not appear on the first menu, then a second letter must be entered. The ability of children and adults with weak spelling skills to select the second letter correctly is much lower than the ability to identify and select the initial letter of a word. Thus if an incorrect second letter is entered, the desired word will never be presented in the choices (see Figure 9-12). Despite this limitation, Newell et al (1992) reported significant increases in spelling ability for both children and adults resulting from long-term use of word completion and prediction devices. They also described some of the features of word completion devices that make them most effective in this application.

Children who have difficulty with writing often also have problems with grammar. Morris et al (1992) added features related to syntax to a word prediction device (Syntax PAL). In addition to the basic word prediction based on frequency of use, Syntax PAL adds a syntactical parse (e.g., dividing the sentence into noun phrase or verb phrase) of the partial sentence that has been typed. This parse identifies the grammatical class of each word and presents choices based on the probability of their following the words entered. This includes the use of function words (e.g., *the, and, a, an*) and correct verb tense based on the noun chosen. Syntax PAL was used in a preliminary case study with two children. In one case the use of Syntax PAL helped to reduce omissions of function words, helped to select the correct verb tense, and reduced the overall number of grammatical errors. The other subject actually decreased her amount of writing during the trial period with Syntax PAL. Morris et al (1992) discuss both these cases in detail. Grammatical prediction applications are likely to increase as more emphasis is placed on literacy and development of writing skills.

In some current AAC technologies, both abbreviation expansion and word prediction are included. This takes advantage of the strengths of each approach. Abbreviations are more direct, since the user can merely enter the code and immediately get the desired word, and they allow complete phrases and sentences. Predictions are easier to use because they do not require memorization of codes.

Higginbotham (1992) compared keystroke savings of five rate enhancement techniques over standard letter-by-letter typing with a standard keyboard. He used written essays by nondisabled students in fourth, eighth, and twelfth grades and at college level as the test vocabulary. Several comparisons were made: (1) the number of keystrokes saved overall in a given text by using the rate enhancement technique, (2) the keystroke savings for each of the words included in the lexicon (word list) of the technique, and (3) the number of words in the text accounted for by the lexicon. The five techniques evaluated were word prediction (EZ Keys* and Predict-It†), Write 100 syllable-based writing system, iconic representations (Word Strategy‡), and abbreviation expansion. For the overall text, the number of keystrokes saved ranged from 1.59 (abbreviation expansion) to 2.33 (Write 100 and word prediction). Grade level had little effect on these results. The predictive devices accounted for the greatest number of words in the lexicon (96%), followed by abbreviation expansion (84%) and Word Strategy (79%). Word Strategy had the greatest keystroke savings for words included in its lexicon. These results need to be applied with care to conversational use of AAC devices by nonspeaking persons. The text samples (written essays prepared by nondisabled students) are not typical of AAC use. These results also apply only to direct selection approaches.

Rate enhancement in scanning differs from that for direct selection. Several approaches are possible (Lesher, Moulton, and Higginbotham, 1998). One of these is based on placement of the most frequently used characters near the beginning so they are scanned first. This is often referred to as *optimization of the row-column matrix*. Another approach is to rearrange the matrix layout after each input. This is the predictive scanning approach described earlier; variations on this approach were studied by Lesher, Moulton, and Higginbotham (1998). Finally, we can use word completion or prediction with lists of words presented based on input, as we have described for direct selection. In the case of scanning, we have options for how we present the word lists. In one case they may be offered as scanning choices before beginning the scan of the character matrix. A second choice is to start the scan with the character matrix, then scan the word list. A third approach allows the user to choose between the word list and character matrix as the first scanning choice. Each of these approaches has advantages and disadvantages. Lesher, Moulton, and Higginbotham (1998) compared 14 different approaches in order to evaluate the relative switch savings of each. They defined switch savings as the percentage saving in the technique under study when compared with a commonly used arrangement (termed the *baseline configuration*). They used *switch count* (defined as the summation of the number of switch hits and the scan times required to make the desired selection) as the measure in calculating switch savings. Using a computer analysis program that determined switch

counts for seven text samples, each technique was tested with each text sample. The baseline configuration used to calculate switch savings was a fixed array with the most frequently used characters at the beginning (Foulds, Baletsa, and Crochetiere, 1975). This array is often used on commercial AAC systems.

Lesher, Moulton, and Higginbotham (1998) found that when the matrix is reorganized in a fixed format, the choice of placement of symbols (e.g., shift, backspace, comma) and numbers was the major factor contributing to switch savings, rather than letter choices. When the matrix was changed with each input (termed a *dynamic matrix rearrangement*), they found that the greatest average switch savings occurred when the prediction was based on the previous four entries rather than with predictions based on shorter (e.g., two or three) previous entries.

Lesher, Moulton, and Higginbotham also evaluated the effect on switch savings of the inclusion of word and character lists in conjunction with the scanning matrix. The greatest savings in these character list methods was obtained when the list was presented first and then the matrix was scanned. However, the character length also affected the results.

The final general class considered by Lesher, Moulton, and Higginbotham was the inclusion of word prediction lists, rather than just characters. The results varied with the length of the word list, but they generally resulted in switch savings for all scanning methods and all word lengths. Switch savings are, in general, less for word prediction than for character prediction.

Many possible combinations of the approaches described above can also be implemented in scanning systems for AAC use. Lesher, Moulton, and Higginbotham described several others and discussed some general guidelines. It is important to remember that the results obtained by Lesher, Moulton, and Higginbotham were based on computer modeling that merely counted the number of switch activations (combined with scan times). Issues of cognitive load (such as those discussed later for word prediction) can dramatically affect these results when the approaches are applied in systems for human users. Lesher, Moulton, and Higginbotham concluded that rearrangement, character and word lists, and other optimization techniques can provide theoretical increases in switch savings of an average of 36.9% and can be as high as 52.9%.

Studies of the effectiveness of various rate enhancement techniques have generally been conducted with nondisabled users over short times. As a result of the necessity for the user of a particular technique to develop skill with the technique, these studies may be misleading when applied to actual populations of users. This learning curve can be quite long, and intermediate results are often not what we expect. In one study, persons with disabilities were trained to use either word prediction or abbreviation expansion techniques

---

*Words+, Palmdale, Calif.
†Formerly produced by Don Johnston Developmental Equipment Co, Wauconda, Ill.
‡Prentke Romich, Co., Wooster, Ohio.

(Rizer, 1991). This study showed that, with both word prediction and abbreviation expansion, the characters per minute initially *decreased* over straight letter-by-letter typing (baseline value). After 18 training sessions, the rates returned to near the baseline values. Rizer did find, however, that both total keystrokes and number of errors decreased rapidly when either of these rate enhancement techniques were used. Both these parameters have a direct bearing on fatigue and work tolerance, and improvement in these areas may be an unexpected benefit of the use of rate enhancement.

Because a major use for communication devices is to facilitate conversations, it is helpful to develop rate enhancement techniques based on conversational patterns. One such approach is called CHAT (Conversation Helped by Automatic Talk) (Alm, Newell, and Arnott, 1987). CHAT is based on the premise that each keystroke should produce a complete "speech act" (an utterance with a purpose). Alm and co-workers break a conversation into five discrete sections: (1) greetings, (2) small talk, (3) main section, (3) wrap-up remarks, and (5) farewells. Except for the main section, these parts are relatively consistent. They can be scripted in advance and are included in CHAT. An additional feature of CHAT is that it allows "grabbers or fillers" (see the section on needs served in this chapter) within each of the conversational stages. These may be comments, repair ("That's not what I meant"), or utterances that keep our turn in the conversation. Finally, CHAT allows the superimposition of mood on the other features: polite, informal, humorous, or angry. The user of CHAT is presented with the conversational sections in order. A greeting (or filler) is selected in a given mood, and then choices in small talk are presented. In each case only a single key is needed to select an entire phrase. CHAT also allows storage of names of people with whom the user is likely to communicate, and these can be inserted into the conversation as desired. Because it is a software program designed to run on any computer, it is also possible to combine CHAT with word prediction or abbreviation expansion to cover the main section of the conversation. Alm, Arnott, and Newell (1992) present the details of the CHAT software program. Approaches such as CHAT that model conversational flow and provide clues to word vocabulary choices based on context can also assist aphasic individuals (Kraat, 1990).

Another way in which the main body of the conversation can be facilitated is to recognize that many of our conversational topics are repeated (Alm, Arnott, and Newell, 1989). For example, a conversation about work or family or a joke is often repeated in different contexts and with different communication partners. One approach, developed as a companion to CHAT, is TOPIC (Text Output In Conversation) (Alm, Arnott, and Newell, 1989). TOPIC is a software program developed using a database, database management software, and an intelligent user interface.

Each "conversational contribution" is held in a database record. Individual fields in the record hold the text itself, an identifying number, subject descriptors (e.g., work, family, books, science), speech act descriptors (e.g., request for information, information, disclosure), and a frequency of use counter. The user interacts with TOPIC through a window on the screen that presents a choice of topics based on previous utterances. The choices presented take into account frequency of use, semantic information in the current utterances descriptors, and the existence of possible "scripts" (stereotypical series of utterances) that the user may want to output.

**Vocabulary expansion.** In many AAC devices it is not possible to present all the vocabulary on the selection set display at one time. We use the term *vocabulary expansion* to refer to methods by which we can increase the available vocabulary through the use of codes or levels. Many of the rate enhancement techniques described earlier also provide vocabulary expansion.

One of the simplest types of vocabulary expansion is the "translation" of vocabulary elements from one symbol system to another when the user needs one type of symbol and the receiver needs another. For example, a person who is unable to read may use a special symbol system. However, his symbols may be misinterpreted. We can increase the possibility of his partner's receiving the proper message by placing words above the symbols; the "translation" is made directly on the board as he points to the symbols. His vocabulary has been expanded because he is now able to converse with more people than he otherwise would have. If the words are in both English and Spanish, then a further translation and expansion can occur. Other examples of vocabulary expansion via translation to another form are the use of words, pictures, or symbols as input for speech output devices or text-to-speech devices (see the section on current technology in this chapter for examples of electronic devices).

Abbreviation expansion, as discussed earlier, can also serve to expand vocabulary. In the development of abbreviations for vocabulary retrieval, there are user strategies that can facilitate effectiveness (Goosens and Kraat, 1985). For example, letter codes corresponding to the first letter of the word or phrase may help the user remember the codes.

An alternative method of vocabulary expansion is the use of *levels*. In this technique, multiple language items can be stored and retrieved from one location (Kraat and Stiver-Kogut, 1991). In operation this technique is like a SHIFT key on a typewriter or computer keyboard. When the SHIFT key is pressed, each key takes on a new meaning (e.g., an uppercase letter, a # rather than a 3). In AAC devices the storage or retrieval is accomplished by selecting the level and then selecting the location. Commercially available AAC devices have from 2 to more than 50 levels.

When more than a few levels are used, it is difficult to display visually all the items represented by that location.

The Minspeak* approach provides for the equivalent of levels by using *themes*. In a theme the first one or two symbols in a set of utterances are automatically entered and do not need to be selected by the user. For example, assume that if the first symbol is an apple, we may have several stored utterances beginning with this symbol: apple + clock + night = "What time is dinner?"; apple + clock + sunrise = "What time is breakfast?"; apple + elephant + cup = "I'd like a large drink." In a one-symbol theme mode, the apple symbol would be selected once and then assumed from then on. So to select the dinner phrase, the user would just press the clock and night symbols. Likewise, to select breakfast the user would only need to enter the clock and sunrise. In a two-symbol theme mode, the user could enter apple and clock once only and then use either sunrise or night to complete the appropriate phrase. The reason that we consider this to be equivalent to levels is that the symbols for night and sunrise take on two meanings (e.g., "night" and "What time is dinner?"), just as the number 3 key takes on the # when the user presses the SHIFT key.

The majority of developments and applications in augmentative communication have been for persons who are unable to speak or write but who have language skills. Persons who suffer cerebrovascular accidents (CVAs) often experience language difficulties that we collectively call *aphasia*. One of the major problems these individuals have is vocabulary expansion.

There are several AAC approaches that have potential for use in aphasia rehabilitation (Kraat, 1990). One of the most common problems encountered is word finding. It is possible to use word prediction if the individual is able to recall first letters. This often leads to recognition of the desired word from the list presented. Unfortunately, most prediction devices present only five or six choices with each entry, and it is necessary to enter the second letter to increase the number or choices and the likelihood of finding the correct letter (see Figure 9-12). If an incorrect second letter is entered, the desired word will never be displayed. This can be a major limitation for persons who are aphasic. Colby et al (1981) developed a microcomputer-driven device that used a specially designed database containing words, their frequency of use, and features of each word. This device was specifically designed for use by persons who are aphasic. Features include words that "go with" the desired word. This can be a sound-alike relationship; a semantic (meaning) relationship; a categorization (e.g., a piece of furniture or a fruit); and initial, middle, and ending letters. Each of these has been shown to be effective for persons with certain types of aphasia. This database is adaptive, just as are current word prediction devices. A similar approach has been developed by Hunnicutt (1989).

Another AAC approach that is of use to some persons with aphasia is alternative symbol systems. Although some individuals can make use of alternative symbols, there are many factors that must be considered when applying these in aphasia rehabilitation (Kraat, 1990). Koul and Harding (1998) evaluated the ability of persons with severe aphasia to both identify and produce graphical symbols using a custom-designed software program. One commercial device designed specifically for persons with aphasia was the Lingraphica.* This device used pictographic symbols organized by semantic categories (e.g., places, foods, clothing) and included such features as synthetic speech output and animation of verbs. This device was shown to be effective for individuals with some types of aphasia (Steele and Weinrich, 1986).

Dynamic display AAC devices can also be of use to individuals with aphasia. Because the display changes each time a selection is made in dynamic display AAC devices, the user is continually prompted for each new set of choices. This reduces the memory requirements placed on the user and can aid in word or concept recall.

Fox and Fried-Oken (1996) discuss the relationship between intervention in cases of aphasia and many of the AAC topics discussed in this chapter. They relate AAC intervention to aphasia intervention and propose research questions related to effectiveness, efficiency, and generalization in AAC aphasiology research.

## Vocabulary Storage

Communication devices may use several different ways of storing the required vocabulary. Many AAC devices have a basic vocabulary consisting of those elements contained in the symbol system being used (e.g., the letters of the alphabet). Other devices depend on the user's developing a vocabulary based on the symbol system chosen (e.g., devices that use digitized speech specific to the user).

Several AAC systems utilize *application programs* or *prestored vocabularies*. No matter how powerful a rate enhancement or vocabulary expansion technique is, it can be frustrating to a user and to those working with her if the initial device is delivered "empty"; that is, if there are no vocabulary items stored in the device. In response to this, several different manufacturers include prestored vocabularies of various types. Sometimes these are application-oriented packages that are offered at extra cost. In other cases there are built-in vocabularies for all users.† Some predictive devices also have several vocabularies included, and they can be selected for a particular user.

---

*Prentke Romich Co., Wooster, Ohio.

*Formerly produced by Tolfa Corp., Palo Alto, Calif.
†For example, EZ Keys from Words+, Palmdale, Calif.

## Text Editing

Text editing functions are also available in some devices. These allow the user to make a small change in an utterance (e.g., change the spelling of a word that was not understood when spoken by a voice synthesizer) without retyping the whole utterance. Without text editing, an AAC device user must type a whole sentence, hit a "talk" key, discover that one word is wrong because one letter has been typed incorrectly, and then type the entire sentence over. In a device with text editing, this user could simply go back and fix the one letter and speak it correctly.

Correcting erroneous entries and modifying text are other forms of editing. This may take the form of simply backspacing and obliterating the letter or it may involve the movement of a cursor that marks the location in the entered text at which the correction is to be made. In some devices the user is able to insert characters, words, or whole paragraphs; to delete any of these; or to move large blocks of text to new locations, as in word processing systems.

## Output Control

The amount and quality of communicative interaction is dramatically affected by the type of output a communication device has. We distinguish two major types of outputs: transient and permanent. In augmentative communication devices, transient outputs are only present while the device is turned on (electronic device) or while the user points to a vocabulary item (manual device). Transient outputs may be visual (e.g., a light, display, or video screen) or auditory (sound or synthetic speech). In all cases the partner must be present to receive the message. This can increase the amount of interaction by making the partner an active participant in the conversation. Conversely, this type of output can impede conversational interaction if the message generation is very slow and the partner either gets bored waiting or goes on with his conversation, ignoring the user. A permanent output (most commonly printer paper) allows preparation before an utterance is to be made. It allows the user to generate the message in the absence of the partner and then print it for the partner. This has the disadvantage of limiting interactions, but it can be more comfortable for some users, since it can reduce the stress of performance. Printed output can also be used to clarify an utterance when it is not otherwise understood. With visual displays, the receiver must be able to read, recognize a symbol, or know that a picture represents a certain concept.

Proxemical factors (i.e., the physical relationship between the user and partner) are affected by the type of output mode. Visual displays (transient and printed) require that both partners look at the output rather than at each other. This can reduce the amount of information transferred by nonverbal means (e.g., facial expression, eye contact, gestures). The use of speech output allows eye contact, as well as attention to these other modes of communication. Speech output also allows the user and partner to face each other at a conversational distance, instead of being next to each other at the closer and more intimate distance required to see and read the display.

Speech output allows use with partners who cannot read (e.g., small children or cognitively impaired persons). It is also nonpermanent, so it can be used for intimate or private utterances. Speech is also the only type of output that can conveniently be used for speaking to groups (including use in classroom discussions) or speaking over the telephone (unless both the user of the device and the partner have special equipment; see Chapter 12).

Another type of output control is the use of such characters as "print" or "enter" or simple markers such as "end of word." With speech output devices, we sometimes use control characters that allow speaking only part of a text buffer or an *exception table* that allows spelling a word phonetically for correct pronunciation by a voice synthesizer (e.g., *brekfast* to speak "breakfast") and spelling correctly for display or printing.

## Speech Output

Most AAC devices and some assistive technology applications rely on *speech output*. Because speech is the auditory form of language, human users of technology rely on artificial speech output for the auditory output of language-based information. This includes all text, such as that which would normally be displayed on a screen, numbers, and simple messages indicating status (e.g., "system on," "the time is ten past three"). In assistive technologies there are many different uses for speech output. However, the three major applications are screen readers for individuals who are blind (see Chapter 8), voice output augmentative communication devices, and print-material reading machines for persons who are blind (see Chapter 12). There are two types of speech output, differing in the manner by which the speech is electronically produced. These are (1) digital recording, and (2) speech synthesis. Each of these approaches may be implemented in electronic circuits (hardware) or computer programs (software) or both, and they each have advantages and disadvantages that affect their use in assistive technologies. In this section we discuss both these types and how and where they are most frequently used. Table 9-6 lists the two approaches, their features, and typical assistive technology applications.

**Digital recording.** In **digital recording,** human speech is stored in electronic memory circuits and can be retrieved later. It takes a great deal of memory to store even a few seconds of speech. For example, 16 seconds of speech may take up to 1 megabyte (MB) of memory for storage. Even with current memory technologies, it is not practical to store enough speech to be useful in many augmentative communication applications. For example, each individual utter-

| TABLE 9-6 | Types of Speech Output Employed in Assistive Technologies | |
|---|---|---|
| Type of Speech Output | Major Features | Typical Assistive Technology Applications |
| Digital recording | Uses actual voice and can easily be child, male, female<br>Speech is limited to what is stored<br>Relatively low cost | Augmentative communication |
| Speech synthesis | Very high quality for single words or complete phrases<br>Intelligibility decreases for unlimited vocabulary with text-to-speech<br>Unlimited vocabulary with text-to-speech<br>Moderate intelligibility with letter-to-sound rules only<br>Highly intelligible with morphemic rules<br>Cost depends on text-to-speech approach | Speech output for electronic aids to daily living<br>Augmentative communication<br>Screen readers for blind users<br>Speech output for users with learning disabilities<br>Speech output for phone communication by persons who are deaf |

ance of two to four words lasts about 1 to 1.5 seconds. A typical memory capacity is 32 seconds. It is only possible to store 20 to 30 utterances. This is a very small vocabulary, and much effort has gone into extending the available capacity. For these reasons, the speech waveform is processed by a computer-based system to compress the speech and to allow it to be played back with different levels of fidelity. Digital recording of speech is limited to reproducing exactly what was spoken.

Perhaps the major advantage of digital recording of speech is that it allows any voice to be easily stored in the device and played back. For example, if the user of an augmentative communication system employing digital recording (e.g., those listed under Simple Voice Output in Table 9-8) is a young girl, we can use another young girl's voice to store the messages the user needs. Likewise, if the user is an adult male, we can have a man speak the messages to be stored. Another advantage is that in these commercial systems the speech to be stored can be entered at any time by just speaking into a built-in microphone. This flexibility in matching the type of voice to the speaker is not as flexible in most systems using speech synthesis.

**Speech synthesis.** Instead of storing the entire speech signal, we can generate the speech electronically. There are several advantages to this approach: (1) the amount of memory required is greatly reduced, (2) the speech can be created from any electronic text, and (3) the speech can be altered (e.g., pitch or rate can be changed). To synthesize the speech, a mathematical model of the human vocal system is used. One example of a vocal tract model is shown in Figure 9-13. There are two types of sounds in speech, voiced and unvoiced (a hissing sound similar to unvoiced sounds such as s or f), and both these types of speech must be included in the vocal tract model. These signals are then fed into a model of the vocal tract that is varied to produce the speech in a manner similar to the variation of the tongue, teeth, lips, and throat during human speech.

**Prosodic features.** All the speech output approaches described earlier are designed to provide the segmental aspect of speech. As discussed in Chapter 3, human speech consists of both these basic or segmental sounds and prosodic or suprasegmental features. The prosodic features are what give speech its human quality, and they are generated by changes in three parameters: (1) amplitude, (2) pitch, and (3) duration of the spoken utterance. These features allow us to stress a phrase or word, to emphasize a point, or to generate an utterance that portrays a particular mood (e.g., angry or polite or happy). These features also are responsible for the inflection changes that distinguish a yes/no question (rising pitch at the end of the sentence) from a statement (falling pitch at the end). For example, the statement, "He is going to dinner" has a falling inflection at the end. However, the inflection in the sentence, "Is he going to dinner?" rises at the end. Several commercially available speech synthesizers have a crude implementation of prosodic features that relies on changing the overall pitch, amplitude, and duration based on punctuation. Although this approach does provide some variety in the speech output, it does not contribute a great deal to the overall quality of the speech or allow for the expression of various moods.

Several investigators have developed systems that include prosodic features. Cook et al (1985) developed software for a notebook computer that allowed the user to emphasize a syllable to provide the correct pronunciation of certain words (e.g., the two pronunciations of the word *content*). They also modified the pitch, duration, and amplitude of the entire sentence pattern, depending on the end of sentence punctuation. This approach provided greater control of the prosodic features and more natural speech, but it did not allow for moods to be included.

Murray et al (1991) developed software used in conjunction with the DECTalk speech synthesizer to provide vocal emotion effects to the synthetic speech. This system, called Hamlet, simulates six discrete emotions (anger, happiness, sadness, fear, disgust, and grief). Murray and co-workers

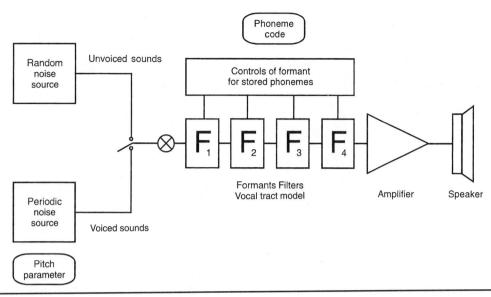

**Figure 9-13**   Speech synthesis systems are often based on a vocal tract model. Sound sources for both voiced (periodic noise) and unvoiced (random noise), as well as a computational model of the vocal tract characteristics, are included.

---

**TABLE 9-7**   **Types of Text-to-Speech Systems Employed in Assistive Technologies**

| Type of Text-to-Speech System | Major Features | Advantages and Disadvantages |
|---|---|---|
| Whole word look-up | Speech pattern for each word stored in memory<br>Look-up of words as they are typed | Requires large memory for even modest vocabulary size<br>Very high intelligibility for words stored<br>Vocabulary limited to words stored |
| Letter-to-sound conversion | Text is matched to sounds letter by letter according to a set of rules<br>Can use phonemes, allophones, or diphones<br>Limited prosodic features | Unlimited vocabulary with very low memory requirements<br>Relatively low intelligibility<br>Rules have many exceptions and overall quality depends on sophistication of rules |
| Morphonemic text-to-speech conversion | Relies on combination of stored morphs and letter-to-sound rules<br>Can use phonemes, allophones, or diphones<br>Includes prosodic features | Unlimited vocabulary with moderate memory requirements<br>Relatively high intelligibility<br>Much higher cost than letter-to-sound rules alone |

---

used voice quality (a characteristic of the DECtalk system), the pitch contour of the entire utterance, and timing (duration) to create the moods. The Hamlet module was incorporated into a predictive (PAL) and a conversational rule-based software program (CHAT) (described earlier in this chapter) to allow the user easy access to moods, as well as basic segmental features. In a listening experiment, Hamlet was found to produce recognizable moods in a series of utterances. The inclusion of prosodic features in voice synthesis systems can have a significant impact on the use of such systems in augmentative communication devices. Prosodic features can also make synthetic speech easier to listen to for long periods, such as in screen readers for persons who are blind (see Chapter 8).

**Text-to-speech programs.  Speech synthesis** systems can generate any word if the correct codes are sent to them in the correct order. The conversion of text characters into the codes required by the speech synthesizer is accomplished by software called **text-to-speech programs.** These programs analyze a word or sentence and translate it into the codes required by the speech synthesizer. When these codes are received by the speech synthesizer, they are combined into the word the user wants to say.

There are several approaches that can be taken to generate speech from text input (Allen, 1981). Table 9-7 lists the major approaches and their features. The first approach is to store all the words the user wants to say, together with their speech synthesis codes, and merely look them up and speak them. When text is typed in, for example, the program matches the text with the word stored in memory and determines how to pronounce it. This approach suffers from the major disadvantage that the user can only speak words that have been previously stored. Because there are hundreds of thousands of possible words in English (or any other language), it is not practical to store them all. A second approach is to break words into syntactically significant groups called *morphs* (see Chapter 3). The codes associated with each morph are then stored, and the computer matches the morph to the letters typed. Because approximately 8000 morphs can generate more than 95% of the words in English, this approach significantly reduces the memory requirements. However, it requires that we develop some rules to break words down into morphs and then match the morphs to the speech sounds. One of the first developments of a morphonemic text-to-speech system was the MITalk-79 system (Allen, 1981). This software included procedures that provided analysis or conversion of the text to a phonetic version suitable for speaking. To overcome some of the limitations of a strict letter-to-sound approach, the morphonemic system utilizes a large lexicon (dictionary) of stored morphemes.

A commercially available system that employs morphonemic principles of speech synthesis is the DECTalk* (Bruckert, 1984). This speech synthesizer uses a 6000-entry lexicon that contains basic pronunciation rules similar to those of MITalk-79. The emphasis of this type of system is on maximizing the use of prestored pronunciation rules and relying on letter-to-sound rules only for uncommon or user-specific words (e.g., proper names or technical terms). There are seven built-in voices and one user-definable voice. The latter allows the user to pick fundamental frequencies, speech rate, and other parameters to create any voice (e.g., Mickey Mouse or a robot). These built-in voices include children, adult females, and adult males with different features. A small (150-word) user-defined dictionary that can contain words unique to the individual user is also included. Many augmentative communication systems now include this speech output system. The DECTalk has also been used in computer screen readers for individuals who are blind (see Chapter 8) and in automated reading systems (see Chapter 12). Bruckert (1984) describes DECTalk in greater detail. A portable version, Multivoice, is also available.† DECTalk and some other commercial speech synthesizers are also available in Spanish, French, and some other European languages (e.g., German, Swedish, Italian).

Finally, we can match individual letters to speech codes and then assemble these into spoken output. This approach requires only the storage of the speech codes (from 64 to 1500, depending on the specific approach), and it therefore reduces memory requirements substantially. This method is based on a set of rules for converting English (or any other language) through text-to-speech synthesis (Elovitz et al, 1976). An example of a rule is whether the letter is at the beginning of the word, at the end, or in the middle. For example, the letter *e* is often silent in English when it occurs at the end, and the letter *p* is silent in "pneumonia." Our set of rules must take this into account. Also the pronunciation of certain letters is affected by surrounding letters. The reliance of this approach on a set of rules results in significantly more pronunciation errors than do the other methods. The most effective text-to-speech systems use a combination of all three of these methods.

**Audio considerations.** The intelligibility and sound quality of any speech synthesis system are dramatically affected by the quality of the amplifier and speaker used to provide the final speech output. Many commercial systems use low-power amplifiers and small, low-fidelity speakers. This can reduce the quality of the sound and therefore make it more difficult to understand. However, in most AAC applications the speech synthesis system must be portable. Higher power output amplifiers require larger batteries, and larger speakers that have greater fidelity are heavier than lower quality speakers. Both these factors affect weight and therefore portability. The most important rule that applies here is that "you don't get something for nothing"; higher quality in speech sound output is obtained only at the cost of increased weight and reduced portability.

**Intelligibility studies.** No matter how sophisticated the hardware or software for speech synthesis (including text-to-speech), the final determination of effectiveness is how intelligible the speech is to human listeners. Although it is true that personal preference plays a part in this determination, there are objective ways in which to evaluate the intelligibility of various speech synthesizers. Mirenda and Beukelman (1987) compared three speech synthesizers in a study involving three age groups of listeners. The synthesizers chosen are all typically used in augmentative communication systems: (1) the Echo* synthesizer used in a text-to-speech (allophone) mode, (2) the Votrax Personal Speech system,† and (3) DECTalk.‡ The synthesizers used had eight voices: (1) DECTalk male, (2) DECTalk female, (3) DECTalk child, (4) Echo with text-to-speech, (5) Echo with phonemes input directly (no text-to-speech rules), (6) Votrax with text-to-speech, (7) Votrax with phonemes input directly (no text-to-speech rules), and (8) natural female voice. Five subjects in each of three age groups (6 to 8, 10 to 12, and 26 to 40 years) were first familiarized with each synthesizer by listening to a short story. Then a series of single words and sentences was presented using each of the eight voices. The procedure employed was similar to that used in studies of intelligibility of human speech. Several

---

*Digital Equipment Corp., Maynard, Mass.
†Institute on Applied Technology, Children's Hospital, Boston, Mass.

*Echo Speech Corp., Carpinteria, Calif.
†This is a formant synthesizer with letter-to-phoneme text-to-speech rules, manufactured by Votrax, Inc., Troy, Mich.
‡Digital Equipment Corp., Maynard, Mass.

types of analysis were carried out by Mirenda and Buekelman (1987). The difference in intelligibility among pairs of synthesizers was determined for single words. There were no significant differences among the pairs of voices using the same synthesizers (e.g., the two DECTalk voices, the two versions of the Echo, or the two versions of the Votrax). The greatest intelligibility for all groups was obtained with the natural human voice, followed by the DECTalk voices. The lowest intelligibility was with the Echo and Votrax synthesizers. Based on the methods of synthesis and text-to-speech employed in each of these systems, these results are not surprising. There were differences in the results for single words and sentences and for intelligibility scores achieved by the different subject age groups.

Mirenda, Eicher, and Beukelman (1989) carried out a similar study designed to determine preferences of male and female listeners in four age groups (6 to 8 and 10 to 12 years, adolescent, and adult). These investigators used the same voices as Mirenda and Beukelman (1987) with the addition of natural adult male, child female, and child male voices. In order to determine preferences of the 40 subjects (five in each group), Mirenda and co-workers played recordings of each voice for the subjects. They then showed slides of adult and child male and female persons and asked the subject to pick a voice that would fit that person. In all cases the preference was for the appropriate natural voice (e.g., adult female voice for adult female pictured). When male speakers were shown in the slide, male subjects tended to pick voices that they judged most intelligible regardless of gender (e.g., DECTalk female over Echo male). On the other hand, the female subjects generally picked the male synthetic voices when shown slides of male speakers. For both child pictures and the adult female picture, all subjects preferred the DECTalk voices, with the Votrax second and the Echo third. In almost all cases, even the DECTalk voices were judged significantly less desirable than the natural speakers. These results from nondisabled listeners reveal important considerations in choosing a synthetic voice for a nonspeaking person. All subjects, when asked about the preference for others, chose an appropriate gender voice, but adult males were more flexible in choosing a voice for themselves, opting for intelligibility. The most important result of these two studies is that synthetic voices, even those judged to be highly intelligible in the first study (Mirenda and Beukelman, 1987), were not viewed as being acceptable (a score of three on a seven-point scale) in the later study (Mirenda, Eicher, and Beukelman, 1989).

**Implications for assessment.** As is evident from our discussion of speech synthesis, there are many approaches, and their cost, quality, and intelligibility vary widely. It is important to take these factors into account when carrying out an assessment to select an assistive technology system employing speech synthesis. It is desirable to have the person who is to use the synthesizer and all those significant others in her life listen to the proposed system. They should be asked to identify both single words and whole sentences, and they should indicate which synthesizer (and possibly which voice in that synthesizer) is most acceptable for that individual. Because voice output is a major factor in AAC devices for conversational use, this type of assessment is very important. Auditory function and perception (see Chapter 3) also play an important role in the selection of a voice output system.

### Internet Access

With the development of the Internet, significant new resources are available from the computer desktop. Among the most important is electronic mail (e-mail). This capability allows individuals to communicate quickly and easily to other individuals around the world. Because access is through a local Internet service provider, the costs are not dependent on distance. Many people who have disabilities have begun using e-mail to communicate with friends, business associates, and organizations. Many AAC devices include computer keyboard and mouse emulation (see Chapter 7). This allows an AAC user to access the Internet using his AAC device. Thus any stored vocabulary or special access methods are available for use while on-line. Because many commercial AAC systems are actually portable computers with AAC software, they can also function as Internet work stations.

Blackstone (1996c) describes some of the advantages of e-mail for individuals who have disabilities and use AAC. As she points out, e-mail allows composition at a slower speed because the partner reads it at a later time. E-mail also allows an AAC user to communicate with another person without someone else being present. Because the person's disability is not immediately visible, AAC users report that they enjoy establishing relationships with people who experience them first as a person and then learn of their disability.

A second feature of the Internet is access to information. Many companies, organizations, and individuals have Web sites that contain valuable information (see Resources, pages 495-496). By accessing this information, AAC users can learn about new technologies, conduct business independently, carry out research for academic pursuits, and book airline reservations.

The Internet also includes a variety of chat rooms where people who have common interests can exchange information in a real-time format. These chat rooms can help AAC users establish advocacy groups, share information, and engage in leisure pursuits. Listservs, which consist of a group of individuals with common interests but are more like bulletin boards, also provide rich sources of information and friendly interaction.

Blackstone also notes that the Internet provides many

## CASE STUDY 9-4

### AAC IN POST-SECONDARY EDUCATION

Heidi (Figure 9-14) is a doctoral student studying English at a major university. She has cerebral palsy, which limits her ability to speak and to use her hands for writing. She uses her computer to complete writing assignments and has written two plays (one for her master's degree thesis) and one book for teenagers who have cerebral palsy. She uses her notebook computer with a speech synthesizer for conversation and a word processor for writing. She also uses e-mail to communicate with her PhD thesis advisor, colleagues, students, and friends. This allows her to keep in touch with people without the use of the telephone, which is difficult with her AAC device. Her computer system allows her several modes of communication, as well as providing the opportunity for her to work at home much of the time and avoid the hassles of special transportation arrangements. Her e-mail contacts also prevent her from being isolated in her home environment.

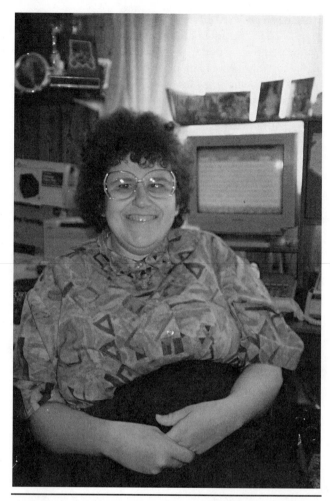

**Figure 9-14** Access to the Internet provides Heidi with the tools necessary to pursue her PhD. She contacts her professors and students via e-mail, conducts literature searches over the Internet, and participates in Web-based courses and discussion groups. This access is all obtained via the same laptop computer that she uses as an AAC device in face-to-face conversations.

opportunities for reading and writing, and this can have a positive impact on literacy skills for AAC users. In Chapter 8 we describe the major features of accessible Web pages on the Internet. Having access to the Internet has made a significant difference to many individuals who use AAC.

## EVALUATION AND ASSESSMENT FOR THE RECOMMENDATION OF AUGMENTATIVE COMMUNICATION SYSTEMS

The process of assessing persons with speaking or writing impairments for the purpose of recommending an augmentative communication system requires a systematic methodology that includes consideration of many factors. Some general approaches to this problem have been described (Beukelman and Mirenda, 1998; Coleman, Cook, and Meyers, 1980; Owens and House, 1984; Shane and Bashir, 1980), and we have described some of the essential parts of the assessment in Chapters 4 and 7. It is necessary to define the consumer's goals and needs carefully, as well as the expectations of those with whom she is likely to communicate. Once the goals and needs are clearly understood and agreed to by all team members (e.g., parent, spouse, teacher, employer, care provider, speech pathologist), we need to determine the consumer's physical, sensory, cognitive, and

language skills as they relate to augmentative communication. We can then match characteristics of AAC devices to consumer skills and goals in a systematic manner. This process generally identifies potentially useful AAC devices based on consumer goals and skills. These alternatives can then be compared to select the most appropriate system for the person. In this section we describe this process.

### Selection of a Control Interface

The first step in this process is a careful analysis of seating and positioning needs of the consumer and provision of a stable and functional seating system (see Chapter 6). Once this is accomplished, a three-step process is employed to select a control interface for a given consumer, as described in Chapter 7.

## Cognitive and Language Evaluation for Augmentative Communication

In order to recommend an augmentative communication device for a consumer, we must determine his cognitive and language abilities. Many of the assessment tests commonly used to evaluate cognitive or language ability require verbal (speech) responses. Because the consumer seeking an AAC device may lack these abilities, the tests must be modified. Also many of these tests have been normalized using a nondisabled population, and they cannot be directly applied to evaluation of persons with disabilities. Many nonspeaking persons also have physical limitations that limit their ability to point to objects in multiple choice tests. All these limitations make it necessary to modify standard cognitive and language tests or to develop new tests.

The person's age, the degree of disability, the magnitude of physical impairment, and the needs of the consumer determine the type of testing to be done. Specific assessment approaches are described by several authors (Beukelman and Mirenda, 1998; Coleman, Cook, and Meyers, 1980; Owens and House, 1984; Shane and Bashir, 1980; Yorkston and Karlin, 1986). Adaptations of test materials for use by persons with severe disabilities are described by Beukelman and Mirenda (1998) and Wasson, Tyman, and Gardiner (1983). Karlan (1982) presents a complete battery of tests and the theoretical basis for their use with persons who have severe physical and cognitive disabilities.

We typically evaluate a consumer's abilities in two basic areas: comprehension (receptive language) and production (expressive language). Both these areas present special difficulties when applied to individuals who have difficulty speaking or writing. In order to assess nonspeech language production, an augmentative communication device of some sort must be used. If the person has an AAC device (e.g., a language board), then it can be used. If no device has been used, a small communication board with a set of words, pictures, or other symbols can be presented to the consumer; she is asked to describe a picture by pointing to relevant items on the communication board. If this is not physically possible, the examiner may point to the items on the communication board sequentially; the consumer indicates the desired item by an eye gaze or head nod. This is referred to as *manual* scanning. These and other similar methods may make it possible to determine the consumer's expressive language skills.

Several specific cognitive and language skills are typically evaluated. Cognitive tasks that are directly related to the choice of an AAC device include symbol type, categorization, sequencing, matching, and sorting. Evaluation of skills in these areas may involve specially developed criterion-referenced tests (see Chapter 4).

It is often necessary to determine what types of symbols will be most useful to an AAC user. We have discussed a variety of symbol types earlier in this chapter. Regardless of the symbol type, there are several assessment protocols that can be used. Franklin, Mirenda, and Phillips (1998) evaluated the use of five symbol assessment protocols to determine their relative effectiveness. As a comparison group, Franklin et al chose preschool children (26 to 41 months). The five protocols all involved matching of a single stimulus to one item from a multiple-symbol array (single symbol to multiple symbol) or matching one of a group of symbols to a single symbol (multiple to single). There are two variations on this general task: identity matching (in which the symbols to be matched are identical) and nonidentity matching (in which the symbols to be matched are not identical, such as a picture to an object). Franklin et al also included the order of the symbols in their protocol. Lower order symbols are those that are more iconic or transparent (or intuitive). For example, colored photographs are lower order than black and white photographs. The five symbol assessment protocols used by Franklin et al were (1) single higher order to multiple lower order nonidentity matching (photograph to objects), (2) multiple higher order to single lower order nonidentity (photographs to object), (3) single lower order to multiple higher order nonidentity matching (object to photographs), (4) multiple lower order to single higher order nonidentity matching (objects to photograph), and (5) multiple higher order to verbal label nonidentity matching (photographs to verbal label).

For nondisabled preschool children, Franklin et al found no statistically significant difference in difficulty among the five symbol assessment protocols. To determine the relative difficulty for learners who have cognitive disabilities, Franklin et al evaluated the five protocols with a group of 20 subjects (10 male and 10 female) 17 of whom had severe intellectual disabilities and 3 who had diagnoses of autism with severe developmental disability. Prescreening included five criteria: ability to use speech functionally for communication, ability to attend to the assessment task, presence of an interpretable pointing response, vision and hearing within normal limits, and English as primary language at home. In addition, those children passing the prescreening criteria had two additional criteria: developmental age scores of at least 24 to 36 months and general medical/dental evaluation screenings.

The mean percentages of correct responses for this group were statistically different across the five protocols. The mean percentage of correct responses varied from 71% on protocol 5 to 83% for protocol 4. Several general conclusions were drawn from these results. Subjects with verbal label comprehension skills did better on all five protocols than those subjects without such skills. Franklin et al concluded that, for individuals who have intellectual disabilities, intersensory matching tasks (protocols 1 to 4) are more difficult than intrasensory matching tasks (protocol 5). This finding leads to the caution that the use of verbal matching tasks may introduce extraneous variables and can affect the results of the symbol assessment. They also found that a task requiring a learner to select a symbol from an array of lower level symbols and match it to a higher order symbol is easier than one requiring selection of a higher order symbol from an array and matching it to a lower symbol equivalent. Because the four protocols were not equivalent in difficulty for the group of learners who had intellectual abilities, we must use caution in symbol assessment and we may need to use multiple protocols to gain a true picture of symbol understanding. Although these results can provide some guidance in assessing potential AAC users for symbol understanding, they must be applied with caution in individual cases.

To assess sorting using pictures, six pictures belonging to two groups are presented in random order, with the groups verbally identified for the consumer. The consumer is asked to sort the pictures into one of the groups. A categorization task is similar. However, this is a higher level skill, since the groups are not identified for the consumer. Receptive language skills (e.g., recognition of words or symbols, understanding of simple commands) are also important. For a person who uses pictures as a symbol system, we can assess receptive vocabulary by orally presenting a word and asking him to select the corresponding picture from an array. The size (number of elements) of the array depends on the skill of the consumer. Another typical assessment test for receptive vocabulary is to present an array of pictures. The consumer is asked to answer questions by pointing to the appropriate pictures. Examples of questions asked include "What do you need in the rain?" (picture of an umbrella) and "What do you use to eat?" An inherent limitation of this type of evaluation is that the pictures used and the concepts presented must be familiar to the consumer. For example, a child who is fed via a tube will not have much interest in or familiarity with food items. Oral presentation of words and sentences followed by selection of the corresponding word from an array addresses word recognition. Advanced language capabilities in syntax (e.g., correct use of punctuation) and semantics are also evaluated when possible.

It is also necessary to determine whether a consumer will be able to understand and use rate enhancement methods. We want to determine whether the consumer can use numbers, abbreviations, or symbols to represent words and whether word completion can be used as a means of communication. Typically the consumer is shown the most appropriate rate enhancement methods to produce several phrases. After a demonstration, the consumer is asked to use the technique and her performance is evaluated.

Motor speech skills and pragmatic language skills are also evaluated when it is possible for the consumer to generate language output (Coleman, 1988). Dowden (1997) describes the major factors to consider and assessment approaches when the potential AAC user also has some functional speech. Social communicative skills (e.g., degree of interaction, attention to task) are generally assessed by interviews with family, caregivers, teachers, and others and through observation during an assessment. It is often helpful to create opportunities for interaction and to observe the consumer in these situations.

The assessment measures discussed here are meant to be representative rather than comprehensive. The outcomes of a cognitive and language evaluation for AAC are a symbol system usable by the consumer, the number of elements that the consumer can use at one time (array size), and the consumer's skills in categorizing, sequencing, encoding, spelling, and reading. The ability of the consumer to utilize rate enhancement and vocabulary expansion techniques should also be determined.

## Relating Consumer Goals and Skills to Device Characteristics

In Chapter 2 we describe the assessment and recommendation process in assistive technology as designing a total system for the user. This is particularly true in AAC because it is necessary to define a set of system characteristics that meets the needs of the consumer and is consistent with his skills. The most important principle involved in this process is the determination of the match between the tasks an augmentative device must accomplish for a person (embodied in the consumer's goals) and the characteristics that must be contained in the device in order for those tasks to be accomplished. This implies that each goal may be accomplished only if certain essential characteristics are included in the augmentative device. Many relationships between characteristics and goals are subtle, and generic characteristics of devices are not always equivalent to specific features of commercially available communication aids. For example, a writing device requires printed output. This is the generic characteristic of all writing aids. However, different manufacturers of aids meet this need in different ways (e.g., adding machine-size or full-page printers). The type of printer may also be important and can serve as a characteristic, but the need for printed output does not restrict one to any particular type of printer.

## Selection of Candidate Systems

A systematic method of proceeding from consumer goals to device characteristics allows us to relate these characteristics to the skills of the consumer. Finally, the characteristics may be transformed into features of available communication aids. Several decision matrix approaches have been presented for selecting devices based on consumers' goals and skills (Owens and House, 1984; Shane and Bashir, 1980). An alternative approach is to develop a set of critical questions, the answers to which narrow device choices

<table>
<tr><td>

**BOX 9-2**  **Communication Goals Presented by Consumers Seeking Augmentative Communication Systems**

**IMPROVE CONVERSATIONAL SKILLS**
In one-to-one conversation
By increasing ability to get attention
By increasing interaction with strangers or peers
By increasing rate of communication output
When using the telephone
By increasing the size of the user's vocabulary
In speaking to groups
General
In classroom or meeting situations

**IMPROVE GRAPHICAL COMMUNICATION SKILLS**
By aiding handwriting
By augmenting or replacing writing
General
Note taking
Classroom use
Meetings
Messaging
Formal writing
Editing and correcting
Homework
Business correspondence and reports
In mathematics
In drawing, plotting, graphing

Modified from Cook AM: Communication devices. In Webster JG, editor: *Encyclopedia of medical devices and instrumentation,* New York, 1988, John Wiley and Sons.

</td><td>

**BOX 9-3**  **Critical Questions Related to Selected Categories in Box 9-2**

**FOR INCREASING INTERACTION WITH STRANGERS AND PEERS**
Will the partners and consumer use the same symbol system?
What type of communication needs to take place?
Where will conversations take place (e.g., home, school, job)?
Will there be a need for a carrying case or strap (ambulatory consumer) or mounting system (wheelchair user)?
Are there any size or weight restrictions?

**FOR INCREASING RATE OF COMMUNICATION OUTPUT**
Would reorganization of the current system (e.g., categories, control characters) increase rate?
Would training and practice lead to increased rate?
Is rate enhancement usable and effective for the consumer?
Would storage of messages or permanent output increase rate?

**FOR EDITING AND CORRECTING IN FORMAL WRITING**
Would a simple "cross-out" be sufficient?
Would an error deletion (e.g., correctable typewriter) be sufficient?
Are editing features such as insert, delete, replace, and storage required, and can the consumer understand their use?

**FOR MATHEMATICAL MANIPULATION**
Is a special format or layout required?
Will built-in calculator capability be required?
If used in the classroom, what are the academic goals?
Are cursor movement and borrow-and-carry functions necessary?

Modified from Cook AM: Communication devices. In Webster JG, editor: *Encyclopedia of medical devices and instrumentation,* New York, 1988, John Wiley and Sons.

</td></tr>
</table>

(Cook, 1988). The organization of these questions is based on the needs served. First, conversational and graphical needs are separated. Then, within these two broad categories, more specific needs are defined. Samples of these goals are shown in Box 9-2 (Cook, 1988). Within each of these need areas, the specific consumer needs are evaluated. Once the type of need has been defined to this level, critical questions such as those shown in Box 9-3 regarding use of augmentative communication devices to meet these needs can be asked (Cook, 1988). These questions are answered by the consumer, caregivers, teachers, speech pathologists, and any other persons who are involved in the assessment process. The answers provide a framework for determining relevant device characteristics and designing an AAC system for that person. Box 9-3 shows typical questions used to narrow the choices in the needs categories of one-to-one conversation, increased rate, editing, and mathematical manipulation. We can define similar questions for other areas (Cook, 1984).

The answers to these questions all help in identifying the best approach for a given person's AAC device. Some questions address the type of output required, whereas others are related to the method used for rate enhancement or vocabulary expansion. Still others relate to the symbol system type, portability, input requirements, and strategies of use. Given the answers to these types of questions, we can relate them to candidate devices through the use of the characterization discussed in the section on characteristics of AAC devices in this chapter, as well as knowledge of commercially available device features. When the goals have been verified, the proposed devices are presented and related to the goals they are to meet. The consumer is then given the opportunity to use the device for a brief period.

Although it is not possible to make a final determination of the effectiveness of the device in a short trial, we can gain valuable information. For example, we may find that the consumer has no interest in the device when she sees it or that the person feels that the device is too heavy or has a strange-sounding voice. We can also determine where a training program must begin in order to develop the necessary skill for communicative competence. If there are special features that require additional skills (such as storing and retrieving information), then the consumer's ability to operate these is also assessed during this trial. In some cases it is decided that this trial is inadequate to make a final decision, and a lease of the device for a 1- to 3-month period is implemented. This allows a more thorough evaluation, and if successful it provides a stronger case for purchase.

The outcomes of this total assessment process are a set of devices that have been validated and an initial approach to the strategies necessary to use the devices effectively in various environments. One or more of these devices will then be recommended for purchase or further trial.

## ■ CURRENT TECHNOLOGICAL APPROACHES

As with most other electronic equipment, changes in the features of commercially available augmentative communication devices occur rapidly. Because most devices are computer based, their features can be easily altered by changing the software program built into the device. For this reason, we have grouped devices into broad, generic categories. The categories reflect different groupings of the characteristics discussed earlier in the section on AAC characteristics. Kraat and Stiver-Kogut (1991) have compiled a wall chart featuring most of the currently available augmentative communication devices. Mollica and Peischl (1997) describe an alternative approach to categorization of AAC devices that builds on the wall chart of Kraat and Stiver-Kogut (1991).

### Comparison of Electronic and Manual Devices

There are many similarities between manual (e.g., communication boards) and electronic communication devices. However, the differences in the characteristics of these devices create significantly divergent patterns of use, strategies for effective interaction, and user skill requirements. Superficially it is tempting to focus on the mechanics of using the device; that is, selecting vocabulary, controlling outputs, and caring for the device. Far more subtle and important for effective communicative interaction are the unique features offered by electronic devices. Goosens and Kraat (1985) discuss four advantages of electronic devices for teaching language. First, synthetic speech output is motivating to both the consumer and his partners, and it may attract attention to the device user, thereby encouraging him to initiate communication. Second, electronic communication devices provide a variety of output modes that can be used in various situations. Third, electronic devices also allow the combination of vocabulary units (words, letters, or symbols) into utterances that are presented to the partner as a whole. When using a language board (manual device), the partner must assemble the utterance either by writing it down one unit at a time or (more commonly) by verbally

repeating each unit and the utterance as it is completed. There is no completed utterance to view, hear, or print in a manual device. Additionally, when using a manual device, the partner often interprets and corrects the utterance. With an electronic device, the user may hear or see her own errors and learn to correct them. Goosens and Kraat point out that this may assist the language development of the user. Finally, electronic devices often have the capability of quickly repeating an utterance without it being reentered. This feature is useful not only to clarify utterances for the partner, but also in a language learning situation to help the user correct mistakes. Goosens and Kraat (1985) also present several case studies that illustrate the role these characteristics play in communicative interaction.

Electronic communication devices also have advantages over manual devices when used for conversation. Three that are particularly important are (1) greater storage and access to vocabulary, (2) greater communicative autonomy, and (3) increased rate of selection (Goosens and Kraat, 1985). We have discussed rate enhancement and the use of codes and other methods for increasing stored vocabulary. Communicative autonomy is gained by the variety of modes available and by increased flexibility. For example, with a language board, the user cannot communicate unless the partner is present to actively decode the utterance, whereas the electronic device does not impose these requirements. Flexibility includes the use of alternative output modes such as speech, visual display, and printer.

The added features of electronic devices also carry with them the necessity to develop a communicative style substantially different from that required for a language board or other manual devices. Goosens and Kraat (1985) also address this problem through two carefully developed case studies. They state that "the discrepancy between the efficacy of natural speech or of language boards and the efficacy of technological devices often requires that augmentative communication consumers and clinicians modify their communication goals and expectations" (p. 61). We discuss training and development of communicative competence using AAC devices in the section on implementation of augmentative communication systems.

### Configurations of Commercial AAC Devices

In order to describe existing augmentative communication devices, we have created the five categories shown in Table 9-8. These groupings allow categorization of the major commercially available augmentative communication devices, and they are based on the properties presented in the earlier section on AAC characteristics. No categorization scheme is perfect, and ours is no exception. We have opted for a few large categories based on the most essential features, rather than more restrictive groupings. The limitation of this is that there is some variability within each

**TABLE 9-8   Feature Categories Commonly Combined in Commercial AAC Systems**

| Category | Distinguishing Features | Examples (Manufacturer) |
|---|---|---|
| Simple scanners | Single-switch scanning<br>Visual light output<br>No speech output<br>two-, four-, or five-switch scan options<br>Limited vocabulary size | All-Turn-It (A)<br>Steeper (Zygo)<br>Versascan (PRC)<br>Zygo 16<br>Zygo 100 |
| Simple speech output | Digitally recording speech (or prestored speech)<br>Limited vocabulary size<br>Coverage vocabulary only<br>Scan or direct selection<br>Minimal rate enhancement or vocabulary expansion | AlphaTalker (PRC)<br>Chat Box (PRC)<br>Dynamo (DV)<br>Macaw (Zygo)<br>Messagemate (Words+)<br>Parakeet (Zygo)<br>Sidekick (PRC)<br>Speakeasy (DJ)<br>Talk-Trac (A) |
| Direct selection, spelling only | Built-in printer<br>No rate enhancement<br>Generally no speech<br>Small size and weight<br>No vocabulary expansion | Canon Communicator<br>QED Scribe<br>Secretary (Zygo) |
| Direct select with rate enhancement | Text-to-speech voice synthesis<br>Rate enhancement<br>Vocabulary expansion<br>Large vocabulary storage<br>Optional printer<br>Direct selection | Delta Talker (PRC)<br>Dynamyte (DV)<br>Dynavox (DV)<br>EZ Keys (Words+)<br>Freedom 2000 (Words+)<br>Light Writer (Zygo)<br>Tuff Talker (Words+)<br>Vantage (PRC) |
| Multiple selection method with rate enhancement | Text-to-speech voice synthesizer<br>Rate enhancement<br>Vocabulary expansion<br>Large vocabulary storage<br>Optional printer<br>Variety of control interfaces<br>Variety of selection methods | Dialect (Zygo)<br>Dynavox (DV)<br>Freedom 2000 (Words+)<br>Light Writer (Zygo)<br>Optamist (Zygo)<br>Pathfinder (PRC)<br>Scan Writer (Zygo)<br>Vanguard (PRC)<br>WSKE* (Words+) |

*A,* Ablenet; *ACS,* Adaptive Communication Systems; *DJ,* Don Johnston Developmental Systems; *DV,* Dynavox; *IC,* Innocomp; *PRC,* Prentke Romich Co.
*Includes Scanning WSKE and Morse WSKE as separate products.

category, which can lead to somewhat dissimilar devices appearing in the same grouping. For example, in the Simple Speech Output category, some devices feature 16 seconds of speech access in a direct selection mode only, whereas others have several minutes of speech in direct selection and several types of scanning with levels and rate enhancement codes. However, the format in Table 9-8 does appropriately group devices serving very distinct populations. Within each category there is still significant opportunity for decision making based on a thorough assessment of skills and needs. The commercial devices listed in each category are examples only. We have included a variety of manufacturers, models of products, and varying device features, but Table 9-8 is not inclusive.

Simple scanners, the first category in Table 9-8, are generally operated by a single switch, although some can have dual-switch scanning and others allow four- or five-switch directed scanning. Other major distinguishing features of the devices in this category are that they use a light to indicate the output selection and they do not have voice output as a standard feature. A few can have speech as an option, but it is generally obtained by interfacing with one of the devices in the second category. For example, the Zygo Steeper can utilize the Parakeet for voice output. These devices also have very limited vocabularies (32 items or less), and they have no rate enhancement or vocabulary expansion.

The devices we categorize as Simple Speech Output were all developed to provide a limited-vocabulary, easy-to-use output for very young children or individuals with limited language abilities. In general they require direct selection, but some also allow scanning. The speech is generally digital recording. Rate enhancement in this category varies from none, to levels, to simple codes or key sequences. Vocabulary storage varies from a low of 2 or 3 seconds to several minutes.

The devices in the Direct Selection, Spelling Only category are distinguished by their small size and focus on features that support writing. Some may have a built-in printer. Several devices in this category provide direct file transfer to a desktop computer, and several also have rate enhancement (generally abbreviation expansion, instant phrases, or word completion). In general they do not have speech output, although several devices in this category do have text-to-speech output and are used as both conversational and writing systems (e.g., Light Writer).

The last two categories in Table 9-8 represent the highest level of sophistication in currently available devices. They incorporate all the rate enhancement and vocabulary expansion techniques that we have discussed. Some of these devices utilize general-purpose computers such as laptops or notebooks. Others are built around hardware based on special-purpose computers specifically designed for AAC use. Vocabulary storage capacity varies from a few hundred utterances to thousands of utterances. Interaction with other devices (e.g., computers, powered wheelchairs, or EADLs) and peripherals such as printers is possible for most of the devices in this group using either serial or parallel ports (see Chapter 8). Within these two categories are devices that can meet the needs of a variety of consumers, from very young children who cannot spell to quantum physicists who make full use of sophisticated rate enhancement techniques. In some cases the same device can serve a wide range of needs because the software and vocabulary stored can be customized. In other cases the devices are relatively inflexible, but this makes them more attractive to the person who does not want to deal with a large number of choices.

Devices in the last two categories provide great flexibility in control interfaces and selection methods. Several of the direct selection types allow both standard size and expanded or contracted keyboards as control interfaces. Several devices in these two categories allow scanning with single-switch or four- or five-switch directed scanning. Some also provide both one- and two-switch Morse code, and some provide direct selection via head pointing. For direct selection via head pointing, some devices use light pointers or sensors attached to the head, whereas others use reflective systems requiring the attachment of only a reflective dot. Some light pointers can also be held in the hand.

The flexibility provided by devices in these categories is particularly useful in dealing with degenerative diseases such as ALS. Initially a person may use direct selection with his hand. As he loses this ability, direct selection using head control is feasible. However, because the device has not changed, the stored vocabulary, rate enhancement strategies, and operational characteristics of the device remain the same. If direct selection via head control becomes impossible, scanning or Morse code can be used. Once again the device is not changed, and the vocabulary, rate enhance-

## CASE STUDY 9-5

### AAC AND ALS—CHANGING NEEDS

Mr. Webster was assessed for an AAC device shortly after he began to lose the ability to speak as a result of ALS. He received a direct selection spelling device, which he accessed using his right index finger. This device was highly effective for him, and he was fond of making lists of tasks to be done around the house, planning menus, and creating shopping lists for his wife and son. This allowed him to maintain his role as head of the household. Unfortunately, Mr. Webster eventually lost the ability to use his finger to type and was again referred for an AAC assessment.

A new device was recommended and purchased for him. This device utilized single-switch scanning accessed through eyebrow movement. This system was not effective for Mr. Webster. Several factors led to the difference in results between the two systems. First, there was a 9-month period between when he was unable to use the first system and the delivery of the second system. This time without a functional communication system probably contributed to a much more dependent role in the family for Mr. Webster, and he told us that he had "nothing to say" when we asked about his nonuse of the new system. His dependent role in communication also changed his role as head of the household. The new system was also more complicated to set up and to operate. This required his wife and attendant to learn more about the system, and he had to wait for one of them to set it up for him. The effort involved on everybody's part may have been overwhelming.

ment, and operational features remain the same. This is a great advantage over having to learn a new device at each stage of the disease.

What distinguishes the last two categories is the nature of the human/technology interface. Devices in the fourth category all are based on the use of a dynamic display as a user interface. These displays, which we described earlier in this chapter, provide continuous prompting of the user and primarily require recognition memory. Devices in the last category have fixed or dynamic displays that provide a consistent user interface but that rely on recall, as well as recognition. There are a variety of ways in which each of these user interfaces is implemented on the devices listed in Table 9-8, so this allows for a variety of physical and cognitive skills on the part of users.

In summary, the categories shown in Table 9-8 are intended to provide a rough framework in which to view

AAC devices. It is important for the ATP to remain current regarding technologies. One of the easiest ways to do this is to attend conferences that feature assistive technologies. If you will be charged with making recommendations for AAC devices, it is also important to place your name on the mailing lists for the manufacturers of these devices. Most AAC manufacturers also maintain home pages on the Internet. There are several Web sites that provide links to AAC manufacturers (e.g., www. atia.org). Other information collection suggestions are discussed in Chapter 1.

## ■ IMPLEMENTATION OF AUGMENTATIVE COMMUNICATION SYSTEMS

As discussed in Chapter 4, in the total process of delivering assistive technologies, the recommendation of a communication device based on a formal assessment is only the beginning of the process. Once funding is obtained and the device is procured, implementation begins. Other steps that may be required include customization to integrate components from different manufacturers (e.g., a communication device from one manufacturer and a control interface from another), programming of a device to include vocabulary specific to the individual consumer, fitting of the device to the consumer's wheelchair, and mounting a control interface in an accessible location. It is impossible in one chapter to cover all the issues related to AAC implementation. Beukelman and Mirenda (1998); Beukelman, Yorkston, and Dowden (1984); Kraat (1985, 1986); Musselwhite and St. Louis (1982); and Riechle, York, and Sigafoos (1991) are sources rich in practical information and case studies related to AAC implementation. There are also frequent case studies presented in journals such as *Augmentative and Alternative Communication* and newsletters such as *Communication Outlook,* * *Communicating Together,*† and *Augmentative Communication News.*‡ These case studies vary from anecdotal reports written by device users or those working with them to formal case studies based on single-subject research designs. In this section we discuss the most basic considerations related to training and follow-up. It is important to note that things do not always progress smoothly through the implementation phase. Fields (1991) presents a case study indicating the steps that one family went through to implement an AAC system for their son. There is also a

*Artificial Language Laboratory, Michigan State University, East Lansing, Mich.
†P.O. Box 986, Thornhill, Ontario, Canada, L3T 4A5; (416) 771-1491.
‡One Surf Way, Monterey, Calif.

listserv for AAC users at http://listserv.temple.edu/archives/acolug.html.

## Vocabulary Selection

Once an AAC device is selected for an individual, it is necessary to create an initial vocabulary set for programming into the device. We have found that the conversational categories shown in Table 9-2 provide a useful framework for initial vocabulary selections. Each of these categories should be included in even the most basic vocabulary set. A minimal vocabulary of approximately 200 words is necessary for adult conversation using an AAC device (Beukelman and Yorkston, 1982).

Yorkston et al (1988) studied 11 vocabulary lists compiled from various sources. They found that most lists were unique because they contained mostly content words (those related to a specific topic), rather than function or structure words (e.g., articles, pronouns, conjunctions). The authors also compiled these 11 lists into one large list that can be used as a starting point for developing user vocabularies for AAC devices. Yorkston et al (1989) describe a case study that illustrates the process of selecting vocabulary for a person who cannot read and is severely physically disabled. They found that the list developed for this person contained words that were not on even the largest of the 11 lists of the earlier study. This indicates how unique the needs of each individual user are. Several techniques, including environmental surveys, communication diaries, and review of standard vocabularies, are described by Yorkston and co-workers. Beukelman, McGinnis, and Morrow (1991) describe the factors that need to be considered in selecting vocabulary for AAC devices. They also analyze the factors that differ in developing AAC vocabularies for individuals who can spell (and therefore have access to a large vocabulary with only the alphabet) and those who cannot spell (and who need a large coverage vocabulary).

Because most AAC devices are programmable, it is possible to continually add or amend vocabulary as needs change. The choice of additional vocabulary items is generally made based on needs that occur frequently; input from family, care providers, and other communication partners; and new situations that arise. In the majority of cases, vocabulary development (after the initial set is implemented) is relatively slow and occurs over a long period. Some devices (e.g., word completion or prediction systems) automatically add items to the stored vocabulary based on frequency of use.

Beukelman and his colleagues and students at the University of Nebraska at Lincoln have complied a large number of resources relating to vocabulary selection and messaging in AAC. This information can be accessed through their Web site (http://aac.unl.edu/vbstudy). Included in this resource are core vocabulary lists consisting of high-frequency words for preschool and school-age children, young adults, and older adults. They also include unabridged vocabulary lists (with use statistics) for nondisabled persons (20- to 30-year-old adults, older adults, and preschool children) and AAC users (four volumes). Vocabulary lists of small talk for children and adults, as well as context specific messages suggested by AAC specialists, are also included. This site also provides vocabulary lists for school settings (preschool activities and classroom activities). Finally, vocabulary lists for use as initial recommendations in AAC are reported, as well as references for AAC messaging and vocabulary selection. This site is a rich source of information for the ATP charged with developing vocabulary for AAC users.

## Training System Use

Figure 9-15 shows a competed installation ready for checkout for proper operation. When the installation is completed, the consumer and those working with him (e.g., care providers, family, teachers, employers, therapists, speech language pathologists) can begin the process of learning to use the device. Depending on the complexity of the device

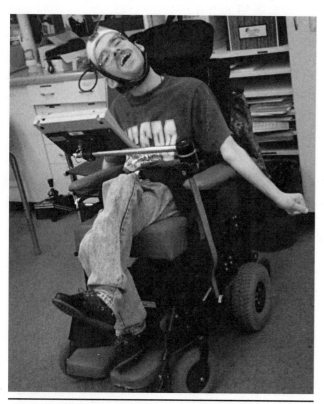

**Figure 9-15** Implementation of an AAC system includes proper mounting of the AAC device and control interface to the wheelchair if necessary. Here is a competed installation ready for checkout.

and the sophistication of the features included, this can take from a few hours to several months.

Training in communicative competence is highly dependent on the models we use for interpersonal interaction. Traditionally the models employed for both language acquisition and conversational interaction have been those developed for nondisabled children or adults. As we have discussed, the assumptions on which these models are based are probably not warranted for AAC users because significant differences exist in the interactions that these persons have compared with those of speaking persons. For example, Harris (1982) found that school-age children using augmentative communication devices had the majority of their communicative interactions with adults, whereas speaking children have the majority of their interactions with other children. Spradlin and Siegal (1982) point out the relative advantages and difficulties of training language competence in a therapy setting versus a "natural environment." These factors also affect our AAC training efforts. When we do train in a natural context (e.g., home, school, job site), there are additional problems of collecting data used to monitor progress in training. Some measures have been developed and used with adults and children (Beukelman and Yorkston, 1980). When the natural environment is a residential living facility, the training is further complicated by frequent turnover of relatively unskilled staff and multiple communication goals for the consumers (Calculator and Dollaghan, 1982; Shane, Lipshultz, and Shane, 1982). Kraat (1985) has provided a review of a large number of published and unpublished studies relating to interaction between augmented and natural speakers. Bottorf and DePape (1982) discuss the major issues and offer suggestions for developing effective interaction in individuals with severe speech impairments. Development of strategies for effectively using augmentative communication devices is more important than any other factor, and this aspect of training is the most time consuming and difficult.

Much of the use of AAC in aphasia rehabilitation involves soft technologies of training and strategies. Blackstone (1991) reviews many of the issues involved in the use of AAC in aphasia rehabilitation. She includes a discussion of public policy issues related to AAC (e.g., funding for assessment and therapy services) and a discussion of clinical studies of AAC use with aphasic individuals. One of the most important clinical results is the recognition that AAC does not necessarily mean a device, but it involves strategies, partner training, and other issues. Technologies can also aid in training of persons who have aphasia. King and Hux (1995) describe the use of a talking word processor to increase writing accuracy for an individual with aphasia. The speech feedback provided additional monitoring of the written work, which helped the person to identify and correct errors. Also, Garrett and Beukelman (1992) present a classification system for aphasic individuals that is used in planning AAC interventions. This scheme describes five types of aphasic communicators: basic choice, controlled situation, augmented, comprehensive, and specific need. For each of these categories, they identify residual skills, intervention goals, and AAC skills and suggest AAC activities for both partners and the individual with aphasia.

**Physical skill development.** We separate the physical skills required for the use of an augmentative communication device from the communication skills required. Once sufficient skills are available in both domains to allow basic communication, the further development of communicative competence can be addressed. Physical skills are obviously required to make choices from the selection (vocabulary) set included with the device, and these skills may need to be developed in order for the consumer to use the device effectively. This aspect of training is described in Chapter 7.

If the consumer has insufficient motor skill to make reliable selections but we expect him to develop the necessary motor control, it is important that this *physical competence* be developed separately from the *use of the physical skill* for communication. If we attempt to teach motor skill using the communication device, it is possible that errors in selection caused by lack of motor skill will be misinterpreted as lack of communicative skill; for example, the person may have intended to select the picture of the apple (signifying "eat"), but she missed the mark and selected the picture of the cup ("drink"). Conversely, errors caused by communication or language inability may be interpreted as motor selection difficulties. In the previous example the person may have been capable of physically choosing apple, but she chose cup because she did not understand either the question or the communication task.

To avoid confusion regarding physical and language skills, we may train a consumer to use a simple communication board to communicate basic ideas while he is also developing motor skills using the training strategies discussed in Chapter 7. If the person is to access an electronic device using scanning with a single switch, then use of the manual communication board will involve the communication partner's pointing to items on the board sequentially and waiting for the user to indicate the item of choice. Often the means of indicating in cases of severely limited motor capabilities is eye gaze. In other cases a gross head nod or arm movement is used as an indicator.

**Developing communicative competence.** Communicative competence depends on many factors (Light, 1989). The context in the HAAT model affects competence in several ways. The partner and her skill in listening, the environment of use, and cultural factors all contribute to or detract from communicative competence. The degree of competence is also variable, and complete mastery of an AAC device is not necessary to have functional communica-

tion interactions. Light (1989) describes four areas of competence required for successful use of AAC devices: (1) operational, (2) linguistic, (3) social, and (4) strategic.

Operational competence requires the physical skills described earlier, as well as an understanding of the technical operation of the AAC device. Once again, the degree of operational competence can be quite variable from very basic operation to advanced features. An AAC device is like a musical instrument that can be played by a skilled user. Operational competence includes the cognitive demands dictated by rate enhancement techniques. Training operational competence requires a systematic introduction of technical features, coupled with ample opportunities for practice in their use, as shown in Figure 9-16. The consumer's facilitators must also be trained in certain operational features of the device (e.g., battery charging, connecting control interfaces), even though they will not develop the same level of competence as the consumer.

Palin (1991) has further defined AAC operational training to include presentation of major features and basic operation. The amount of time spent on each phase varies depending on the complexity of the technology, the sophistication of those working with the person, and the person's ability to develop his skills. The first phase focuses on the major features such as making single selections from the vocabulary set. Once the consumer is able to make single

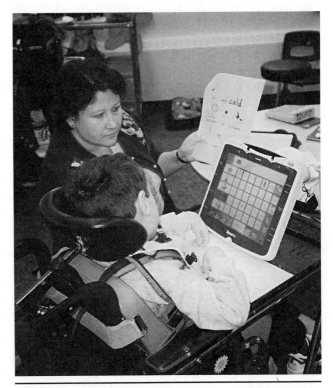

**Figure 9-16** Development of operational competence with an AAC device requires a structured training program in which the device features are carefully explained and skill in their use is developed.

selections reliably and accurately using the device, additional features (e.g., use of codes, control functions such as speak or print) may be introduced. The ability of consumers to understand the required tasks for device operation varies widely, and some consumers initially become overwhelmed by the complexity of the device. Other consumers immediately comprehend all the features and their implications. For this reason, training programs are highly individualized.

The second phase, basic operation, includes how to connect the device to the control interface, how to charge batteries, how to attach it to a wheelchair, how to add vocabulary using rate enhancement techniques (e.g., codes), and an introduction to troubleshooting in case the device fails to operate properly.

The last features to be introduced are those related to storage of new vocabulary, input acceleration techniques, and vocabulary manipulation features such as text editing and reformatting the output. Often the first two phases are accomplished in one session. However, in some cases, they may require multiple training sessions, and the process is often a lengthy one that may be integrated with the other aspects of training in communicative competence.

Linguistic competence requires that the symbol system and rules of organization be understood by the AAC device user. As Light (1989) points out, the AAC user often must be competent in two languages: the spoken language of the community and the language of her AAC device. It is likely that the user also lacks models of proficient use in the language of her device. Development of competence in this area may require many hours of practice. Often this practice is built around a functional reading task such as that shown in Figure 9-17.

In contrast to the typical "drill and practice" approach to developing vocabulary and AAC use, Mirenda and Santogrossi (1985) used a prompt-free strategy to teach a young child to use a picture-based communication board. The approach involved a four-step process, which began with a picture of a soft drink being available to the child during her regular therapy session. A drink was visible to her, as was the picture of the drink. The child was not told that touching the picture would result in her getting a drink, nor was she prompted in any way to touch the picture. If she touched the drink directly, she was told that she could have some later. If she accidentally or deliberately touched the picture, she was immediately given the drink with the explanation, "Yes, if you touch the picture, you may have the drink." Once the deliberate response had been established over several sessions, Mirenda and Santogrossi proceed to shape the pointing behavior by progressively moving the picture farther away, until it was out of sight and the child had to actively find it. As the child became proficient in this task, the number of pictures was increased to four and the process repeated for the other choices. Eventually the child

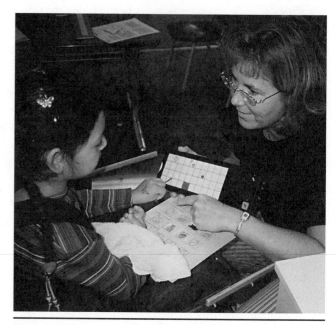

**Figure 9-17**  Development of linguistic competence is often taught in conjunction with other functional tasks such as the one shown here.

was able to generalize to a language board of 120 pictures. The advantage of this approach is that the child learns the meaning and significance of the symbolic representation by discovery rather than by drill. This leads to greater generalization and more functional use of the AAC system.

Many users of AAC devices have little or no experience in social discourse. Even individuals who have used normal language for communication and who have sustained a disease or injury are faced with a very different mode of interaction when an AAC device is used. As we have described, rules of conversation are altered, and the perception of the individual by his communication partners is different. In order to be socially competent, the user must have knowledge, judgment, and skills in both sociolinguistic (e.g., turn taking, initiating a conversation, conversational repair) and sociorelational areas (Light, 1989). The latter term describes the understanding of interaction between individuals. We described the good communication device user (Light, 1988) as having a positive self-image, interest in her partner, skill at drawing others into the conversation, ability to put a partner at ease, and active participation in the conversation. These are sociorelational skills, and the degree to which they are understood and used is one measure of social competence. These skills are best taught in the contexts in which they are to be used. One example of such training is shown in Figure 9-18, in which the child is being taught strategies for interacting with an adult partner.

Every user of an AAC device develops strategies to make that use more effective. Examples include letting the partner guess the next letter on a spelling board and using gestures

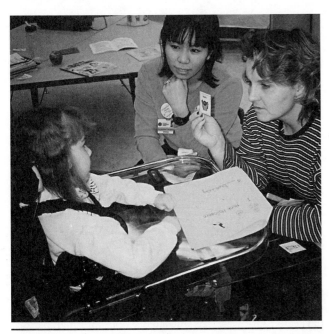

**Figure 9-18**   AAC users need to learn about conversational conventions and strategies. Training of these skills is often done in simulated situations. Here an aide is teaching the child how to use her AAC tools to interact with another adult partner.

(e.g., waving to indicate that a misunderstanding has occurred) with an electronic device. Strategic competence describes the degree to which the user of the device is able to develop adaptive strategies to make the most of the device. These may differ in different contexts. For example, a child's speech may be better understood at home than at school. He will rely on the electronic AAC device more in school, but he will also develop strategies to make maximal use of both systems. Strategies are best taught by consumers. Unfortunately, highly competent users are not always available to help a new user. The ATP needs to collect strategies from consumers and train new users in their application.

Just as the user of an AAC system must develop several types of competencies, there are many ways of carrying out the training. One approach, shown in Figure 9-18, is to simulate a situation, model the types of interaction likely to occur and have the user "practice" the strategies and skills necessary to make it a success. This can be followed by an actual situation in which the ATP accompanies the user as she encounters the situation. The ATP can then prompt the user at appropriate times, add encouragement, and help to clarify when necessary. This combination of clinic-based practice and community-based skill development is often very effective.

Training of the AAC user is only effective if communication partners are also trained. For children, the training of parents to recognize communication attempts and to understand the operational, linguistic, strategic, and social compe-

tencies is also important. Bruno and Dribbon (1998) evaluated a parent training program conducted as part of an AAC summer camp experience. Parents attended the camp with their children. The camp featured structured therapy sessions, activities with nondisabled campers, and activities planned for families. The parent training had both device and interaction training aspects. The device training was conducted by manufacturers' representatives. Parents were asked to identify targeted behaviors that they wanted the child to develop. They also observed the training sessions for their child, which included modeling of AAC system use.

Bruno and Dribbon (1998) collected data on both parent and child performance at the beginning of the camp, at the conclusion of the camp, and 6 months after the camp. Parents were asked to rate their skills in device operation and interacting with their child using AAC, as well as their child's performance in using AAC. Four conversational categories were used for the parent's evaluation of their child's performance: communication with familiar partners, communication with unfamiliar partners, communication when a context is known, and communication when the context is not known.

Parents reported making positive changes in both operational and interactional skills during the camp. This was reflected in gains made by the children in skill in the use of pragmatic functions (e.g., giving and requesting information, requesting assistance, responding and protesting) over the course of the camp. In some cases, skills in these areas remained constant at the 6-month follow-up, and in some there was a decrease. The areas of social exchange and giving of information continued to increase at the 6-month follow-up evaluation. Bruno and Dribbon argue that the identification of AAC as a secondary system was in part responsible for the parent's not providing access to the manual or high-tech AAC system for their child. Many parents report being able to understand their child well enough and believe that the AAC system is to be used to help the child interact with others. The camp training did significantly increase the degree to which parents gave their child access to the AAC system. Although the results of this camp experience are encouraging, Bruno and Dribbon do caution that parents' perceptions, on which the study is based, may not be totally objective, and the results should be applied with caution. Nevertheless, this study does point out the importance of training both the AAC user and his partners.

As can be seen from the above discussion, AAC training can be both complicated and lengthy. Beukelman and Mirenda (1998) present many useful suggestions for developing and conducting this training. Light and Binger (1998) have developed a seven-step process for developing communication competence in AAC users. Their seven steps are (1) specify the goal, do baseline observations;

(2) select vocabulary; (3) teach the facilitators how to support the AAC user in developing the target skill; (4) teach the skill to the AAC user; (5) check for generalization; (6) evaluate outcomes; and (7) complete maintenance checks. Light and Binger develop these seven steps in detail and provide data collection and assessment forms, as well as strategies for implementing this program.

## Follow-up

As discussed in Chapter 4, follow-up services are essential to ensure that assistive technology systems meet the needs of the person for whom they have been designed. In AAC service delivery, there are many aspects of each individual system (including additional people such as caregivers, teachers, employers, and family), and their effective integration often occurs gradually during the first few months of use. An effective follow-up program can ensure that this integration actually takes place.

The evaluation of communicative competence in the four domains (operational, linguistic, social, and strategic) may identify areas in which the AAC system is not adequately meeting the consumer's needs. This then leads to reevaluation of the consumer's skills and needs and may result in changes in the training or the AAC device. The ATP, in conjunction with the other members of the delivery team, must analyze the situation and make recommendations for continued intervention. In some cases the consumer may require additional training. The reevaluation may lead to new training goals in one or more of the four areas of communicative competence, and a training program will be implemented to meet these goals. In other cases the caregivers, family, or other support staff may require additional training in order to facilitate the use of the AAC device. This training can be planned and implemented to meet specific goals.

In other cases the AAC device as it is configured may be inadequate to meet the consumer's needs. It may be possible to adjust some of the features (e.g., scanning rate, stored vocabulary), or it may be necessary to consider a completely new device. The magnitude of the changes in the device dictates the amount of additional operational training required. In some cases the consumer's skills may decrease (e.g., degenerative disease) or increase (e.g., a young child who develops greater language skills). In either case a reevaluation and adjustments in the AAC system (device plus training and support) will be required. Thus, as we discuss in Chapter 4, AAC assessment and training are ongoing.

Murphy et al (1996) identified obstacles to effective AAC system use. This study, carried out in Scotland, included 93 users of AAC systems and 186 partners of these users. The partners were grouped into formal (93) and informal (93). The formal partners were speech-language pathologists (the majority), care providers in the day or living program, and teachers. Informal partners were family, friends, and others selected by the AAC users as those with whom they felt most comfortable using their AAC systems. In some cases one partner filled both the formal and informal roles. Of the total of 186 survey forms, Murphy et al received completed surveys from 89 pairs (formal and informal partners for the same user). They evaluated the results in several categories. The majority of AAC system use was in the day placement (90%), residential (70%), and leisure (60%) settings. These results were consistent across low- and high-tech systems. Comments received from respondents indicated that use was limited to organized therapy sessions in general.

Murphy et al also investigated the availability of the AAC system to the user. They found that AAC systems were only available to 48% of the users while shopping, 62% during outings such as day trips during their program, and 66% where they lived. Speech-language pathologists were the most frequent (80%) formal partners, and residential or day care staff were the most common informal partner (62%). Friends and family were both reported as the primary informal partner in less than 10% of the cases. They also evaluated "accessibility" of the AAC system, that is, the users' ability to physically access the system independently without a partner's help. They found that only 57% of the low-tech AAC users and 59.4% of the high-tech AAC system users were able to independently access their systems. Knowledge of the system sufficient to interact with the AAC user was reported in less than half of the formal partners and one third of the informal partners. This area was further evaluated by Murphy et al because of its implications for training of both the user and the partners. They found that 88% of the users received training from their formal partners. However, for the majority of the users, the training consisted of 60 minutes or less (or 40 hours per year based on sessions conducted). This is a low number compared with other types of therapy and training such as that for second language instruction (estimated by Murphy et al to be more than 200 hours per year).

An important consideration in effective use of an AAC system is the choice of vocabulary. Murphy et al also evaluated this feature in their survey. They found that basic vocabulary required for daily interactions (see Table 9-2) was not included in the AAC systems. Few users had greetings, wrap-ups, or conversational flow vocabulary (e.g., comments, repair vocabulary). Thus, for these areas, the users in this study most commonly used other modes of communication (e.g., eye gaze, gestures, facial expressions), rather than their AAC device.

These results, which match those informal observations often reported by clinicians, have significant implications for training of AAC users. The result regarding availability of AAC systems and the preponderance of formal partners also reinforces the need for inclusion of both useful vocabulary and the development of strategic competence to increase the likelihood that an AAC user will be able to independently carry out conversations in a variety of settings. Accessibility of AAC systems must also be addressed by appropriate mounting of systems on wheelchairs and training of care providers in the need to have the system available to the user at all times. The results reported by Murphy et al also emphasize the importance of multiple modes of communication by AAC users.

The most important result of the follow-up phase is to evaluate the outcomes of the AAC intervention to determine their effectiveness. This includes both the hard and soft technologies, as well as the appropriateness of the match between the originally specified needs and the resulting system. The principles of outcome measurement discussed in Chapter 4 apply to AAC system evaluation as well.

## ■ SUMMARY

Augmentative and alternative communication systems serve needs for both writing and conversation for individuals who have difficulties in these areas. Low-technology AAC systems provide quick and easy help for meeting communication needs, whereas high-technology devices offer great sophistication in available vocabulary, speed of communication, and flexibility of access. The latter features allow persons who have very limited physical skills to utilize AAC systems. AAC systems also have great flexibility in required user cognitive skills, allowing for persons with a diversity of intellectual abilities to benefit from AAC. Thoughtful assessment, careful training, and thorough follow-through are essential to effective AAC intervention.

## Study Questions

1. What are the two major communicative needs normally addressed by augmentative communication systems?
2. Distinguish between aided and unaided communication.
3. What are the major goals for augmentative communication systems designed for conversational use?
4. What needs do parents have for AAC for their nonspeaking children? Do mothers and fathers have the same needs for their children?
5. Describe differences in the conversational rules that apply between two speaking persons and those between one speaking person and one augmentative communication user.
6. What features distinguish competent augmentative communicators from those who are not successful?
7. Select three discourse functions from those listed in Table 9-2. Now pick an augmentative communication device (e.g., electronic, direct selection, with voice output; or a language board with letters and words) and develop a vocabulary and set of strategies for the implementation of each of the discourse functions that you choose.
8. What are the three types of graphical communication? List three ways in which they differ.
9. In what ways does the formal writing of adolescent AAC users differ from that of nondisabled adolescent writers?
10. Distinguish between formal writing and note taking in terms of the characteristics AAC devices must have to meet each need. What is the most important feature in each case?
11. What two factors must be included for a math worksheet to be effective for both arithmetic and higher math (e.g., algebra)?
12. List three features that a drawing system should have to be of use in creative expression.
13. How do drawing systems differ in structure and function from systems for scientific plotting?
14. Describe auditory scanning. Give an example of both a low-tech or no-tech approach and an electronic AAC approach. What are the essential features for the AAC auditory scanning device?
15. List three encoding methods used in AAC devices, and give one advantage and one disadvantage of each.
16. What are the major types of abbreviation approaches used in AAC devices, and what are the major advantages and disadvantages of each?
17. Pick three discourse functions and develop a logical coding scheme for each using (1) numeric codes, (2) abbreviation expansion, and (3) Minspeak codes.
18. Compare word completion and prediction with abbreviation expansion and Minspeak encoding.
19. What are the major approaches used to increase conversational rate when the consumer is using scanning?
20. What are dynamic displays, and what advantages do they provide?
21. List and discuss three advantages that the Internet provides for communication by AAC users.
22. What are the major advantages of conversationally based communication devices such as CHAT and TOPIC?
23. What are the four types of competencies acquired in

AAC training? Pick an AAC system for a consumer and design the training. You must make assumptions regarding the person's skills, her needs, and other people available to help facilitate the training.

24. For each of the categories of devices described in the section on current technologies, define a user profile (skills and needs) that would lead you to focus on that category in selecting a device for that person.

## References

Allen J: Linguistic-based algorithms offer practical text-to-speech systems, *Speech Technol* 1(1):12-16, 1981.

Alm N, Arnott JL, Newell AF: Database design for storing and accessing personal conversational material, *Proc 12th Ann Conf Rehabil Eng,* pp 147-148, June 1989.

Alm N, Arnott JL, Newell AF: Prediction of conversational momentum in an augmentative communication system, *Commun ACM* 35(5):46-57, 1992.

Alm N, Newell AF, Arnott JL: A communication aid which models conversational patterns, *Proc 10th Ann Conf Rehabil Eng,* pp 127-129, June 1987.

Angelo DH, Jones SD, Kokoska SM: Family perspective on augmentative and alternative communication: families of young children, *Augment Altern Commun* 11:193-201, 1995.

Angelo DH, Kokoska SM, Jones SD: Family perspective on augmentative and alternative communication: families of adolescents and young adults, *Augment Altern Commun* 12:13-20, 1996.

Bailey RW: *Human performance engineering,* Englewood Cliffs, NJ, 1989, Prentice Hall.

Baker B: Minspeak, *Byte* 7:186-202, 1982.

Baker B: Using images to generate speech, *Byte* 11(3):160-168, 1986.

Baker B: Semantic compaction for sub-sentence vocabulary units compared to other encoding and prediction systems, *Proc 10th Ann Conf Rehabil Eng,* pp 118-120, June 1987.

Batavia AI, Hammer GS: Toward the development of consumer-based criteria for the evaluation of assistive devices, *J Rehabil Res* 27(4):425-436, 1990.

Beck AR, Dennis M: Attitudes of children toward a similar-aged child who uses augmentative communication, *Augment Altern Commun* 12:78-87, 1996.

Beukelman DR, McGinnis J, Morrow D: Vocabulary selection in augmentative and alternative communication, *Augment Altern Commun* 7(3):171-185, 1991.

Beukelman DR, Mirenda P: *Augmentative and alternative communication: management of severe communication disorders in children and adults,* ed 2, Baltimore, 1998, Paul H Brookes.

Beukelman DR, Yorkston KM: Nonvocal communication: performance evaluation, *Arch Phys Med Rehabil* 61:272-275, 1980.

Beukelman DR, Yorkston KM: Communication interaction of adult communication augmentation use, *Top Lang Dis,* pp 39-53, March 1982.

Beukelman DR, Yorkston KM: Computer enhancement of message formulation and presentation for communication augmentation, *Sem Speech Lang* 5(1):1-10, 1984.

Beukelman D, Yorkston K, Dowden P: *Communication augmentation: a casebook of clinical management,* San Diego, 1984, College Hill Press.

Blackstone S: Populations and practices in AAC, *Augment Commun News* 3(4):1-3, 1990a.

Blackstone S: The role of rate in communication, *Augment Commun News* 3(5):1-3, 1990b.

Blackstone S: Persons with aphasia: what does AAC have to offer, *Augment Commun News* 4(1):1-6, 1991.

Blackstone S: Dynamic displays, *Augment Commun News* 7(2):1-6, 1994.

Blackstone S: AAC and emergent literacy, *Augment Commun News* 9(3):1-8, 1996a.

Blackstone S: What's standing in the way, *Augment Commun News* 9(4):1-8, 1996b.

Blackstone S: The Internet: what's the big deal, *Augment Commun News* 9(4):1-5, 1996c.

Bottorf L, DePape D: Initiating communication systems for severely speech impaired persons, *Top Lang Dis* 2:55-71, 1982.

Brodin J: Facsimile transmission for graphic symbol users, *Eur Rehabil* 2:87-92, 1992.

Bruckert E: A new text-to-speech product produces dynamic human-quality voice, *Speech Technol* 4(1):114-119, 1984.

Bruno J, Dribbon M: Outcomes in AAC: evaluating the effectiveness of a parent training program, *Augment Altern Commun* 14(2):59-70, 1998.

Buzolich MJ, King JS, Baroody SM: Acquisition of the commenting function among system users, *Augment Altern Commun* 7(2):88-99, 1991.

Calculator S, Dollaghan C: The use of communication boards in a residential setting, *J Speech Hear Dis* 47:281-287, 1982.

Colby KM et al: A word-finding computer program with a semantic lexical memory for patients with anomia using an intelligent speech prosthesis, *Brain Lang* 14:272-281, 1981.

Coleman CL: *Augmentative communication training modules,* Sacramento, 1988, Assistive Device Center, California State University.

Coleman CL, Cook AM, Meyers LS: Assessing non-oral clients for assistive communication devices, *J Speech Hear Dis* 45:515-526, 1980.

Cook AM: *The decision making process and selection of alternative systems.* Presented at Workshop on Transdisciplinary Teaming Skill Development in Application of Alternative Systems of Communication, Columbus, Ohio, 1984, Ohio Resource Center for Low Incidence and Severely Handicapped.

Cook AM: Communication devices. In Webster JG, editor: *Encyclopedia of Medical Devices and Instrumentation,* New York, 1988, John Wiley and Sons.

Cook AM et al: Development of a portable voice output communication system with prosodic feature control, *Proc 8th Ann Conf Rehabil Tech,* pp 314-316, June 1985.

Dowden PA: Augmentative and alternative communication decision making for children with severely unintelligible speech, *Augment Altern Commun* 13(1):48-58, 1997.

Elovitz HS et al: Automatic translation of English text to phonetics by means of letter to sound rules, *IEEE Trans Acoust Speech Signal Process* 24:446-458, 1976.

Fields C: Finding a voice for Daniel, *Team Rehabil Rep* 2(3):16-19, 1991.

Foulds RA: Communication rates for non-speech expression as a function of manual tasks and linguistic constraints, *Proc Int Conf Rehabil Eng,* pp 83-87, June 1980.

Foulds R, Baletsa G, Crochetiere W: The effectiveness of language redundancy in non-verbal communication, *Proc Conf Syst Devices Disabled,* pp 82-86, 1975.

Fox LE, Fried-Oken M: AAC aphasiology: partnership for future research, *Augment Altern Commun* 12:257-271, 1996.

Franklin K, Mirenda P, Phillips G: Comparison of five symbol assessment protocols with nondisabled preschoolers and learners with severe disabilities, *Augment Altern Commun* 14(2):63-77, 1998.

Garrett K, Beukelman D: Augmentative communication approaches for persons with severe aphasia. In Yorkston K, editor: *Augmentative communication in the medical setting,* Tucson, 1992, Communication Skill Builders.

Goosens C, Kraat A: Technology as a tool for conversation and language learning for the physically handicapped, *Top Lang Dis* 6:56-70, 1985.

Gunderson JR: Conversation aids for nonvocal physically impaired persons. In Webster JG et al, editors: *Electronic devices for rehabilitation,* New York, 1985, John Wiley and Sons.

Harris D: Communicative interaction processes involving nonvocal physically handicapped children, *Top Lang Dis* 2:21-37, 1982.

Heckathorne CW, Voda JA, Leibowitz LJ: Design rationale and evaluation of the portable anticipatory communication aid-PACA, *Augment Altern Commun* 3(4):170-180, 1987.

Higgenbotham DJ: Evaluation of keystroke savings across five assistive communication technologies, *Augment Altern Commun* 8:258-272, 1992.

Hortsman H, Levine S: Effect of word prediction features on user performance, *Augment Altern Commun* 12:155-168, 1996.

Hunnicutt S: ACCESS: A lexical access program, *Proc RESNA 12th Ann Conf,* pp 284-285, June 1989.

Iacono T, Mirenda P, Beukelman D: Comparison of unimodal and multiple modal AAC techniques for children with intellectual disabilities, *Augment Altern Commun* 9:83-94, 1993.

Karlan G: Assessment and intervention using aided non-speech communication systems with severely physically and mentally handicapped persons, *Proc 2nd Ann Conf Non-speech Commun,* pp 4-9, November 1982.

King JM, Hux K: Intervention using talking word processor software: an aphasia case study, *Augment Altern Commun* 11:187-192, 1995.

Koul RK, Harding R: Identification and production of graphic symbols by individuals with aphasia: efficacy of a software application, *Augment Altern Commun* 14:11-23, 1998.

Kovach T, Kenyon P: Auditory scanning: development and implementation of AAC systems for individuals with physical and visual impairments, *ISAAC Bull* 53:1-7, 1998.

Kraat AW: *Communication interaction between aided and natural speakers: a state of the art report,* Toronto, 1985, International Project on Communication Aids for the Severely Speech Impaired.

Kraat AW: Developing intervention goals. In Blackstone S, Bruskin D, editors: *Augmentative communication: an introduction,* Rockville, Md, 1986, American Speech-Language and Hearing Association.

Kraat AW: Augmentative and alternative communication: does it have a future in aphasia rehabilitation? *Aphasiology* 4(4):321-338, 1990.

Kraat A, Stiver-Kogut M: *Features of portable communication devices,* Wilmington, 1991, Applied Science and Engineering Laboratories, University of Delaware.

Lesher GW, Moulton BJ, Higginbotham DJ: Techniques for augmenting scanning, *Augment Altern Commun* 14(2):81-101, 1998.

Light J: Interaction involving individuals using augmentative and alternative communication systems: state of the art and future directions, *Augment Altern Commun* 4(2):66-82, 1988.

Light J: Toward a definition of communicative competence for individuals using augmentative and alternative communication systems, *Augment Altern Commun* 5(2):137-144, 1989.

Light JC, Binger C: Building communicative competence with individuals who use augmentative and alternative communication, Baltimore, 1998, Paul H Brookes.

Light J, Smith AK: Home literacy experience of preschoolers who use AAC systems and their nondisabled peers, *Augment Altern Commun* 9(1):10-25, 1993.

Lloyd LL, Karlan GR: *Nonspeech communication symbols and systems: where have we been and where are we going.* Presented at Sixth Congress of the International Association for the Scientific Study of Mental Deficiency, 1982.

Miller GA: *Language and speech,* San Francisco, 1981, Freeman.

Mirenda P, Buekelman DR: A comparison of speech synthesis intelligibility with listeners from three age groups, *Augment Altern Commun* 3(3):120-126, 1987.

Mirenda P, Eicher D, Buekelman DR: Synthetic and natural speech preferences of male and female listeners in four age groups, *J Speech Hear Res* 32:175-183, 1989.

Mirenda P, Santogrossi J: A prompt-free strategy to teach pictorial communication system use, *Augment Altern Commun* 1:143-150, 1985.

Mollica BM, Peischl D: Plain talk: a guide to sorting out AAC devices, *Team Rehabil Rep* 8(8):19-23, 1997.

Morris C et al: Syntax PAL: a system to improve the written syntax of language-impaired users, *Assist Technol* 4(2):51-59, 1992.

Murphy J et al: AAC system use: obstacles to effective use, *Eur J Dis Commun* 31:31-44, 1996.

Murray IR et al: Emotional synthetic speech in an integrated communication prosthesis, *Proc 14th Ann Conf Rehabil Eng,* pp 311-313, June 1991.

Musselwhite CR, St. Louis KW: *Communication programming for the severely handicapped: vocal and non-vocal strategies,* Houston, 1982, College Hill Press.

Newell AF et al: Effect of the "PAL" word prediction system on the quality and quantity of text generation, *Augment Altern Commun* 8(4):304-311, 1992.

O'Keefe BM, Brown L, Schuller R: Identification and ranking of communication aid features by five groups, *Augment Altern Commun* 14:37-50, 1998.

Owens RE, House LI: Decision-making processes in augmentative communication, *J Speech Hear Dis* 49:18-25, 1984.

Palin M: *Techniques for successful use of augmentative communication systems.* Presented at Demystifying Technology Workshop, CSUS Assistive Device Center, Sacramento, Calif., 1991.

Riechle J, York J, Sigafoos J: *Implementing augmentative and alternative communication,* Baltimore, 1991, Paul H Brookes.

Rizer B: *Word prediction and abbreviation expansion: benefits and considerations for people with disabilities,* doctoral dissertation, Baltimore, 1991, Maryland Rehabilitation Center.

Rush WL: *Journey out of silence,* Lincoln, Neb, 1986, Media Productions and Marketing.

Shane HC, Bashir AS: Election criteria for the adoption of an augmentative communication system: preliminary considerations, *J Speech Hear Dis* 45:408-414, 1980.

Shane HC, Lipshultz RW, Shane CL: Facilitating the communication interaction of nonspeaking persons in large residential settings, *Top Lang Dis* 2:73-84, 1982.

Smith AK et al: The form and use of written communication produced by physically disabled individuals using microcomputers, *Augment Altern Commun* 5(2):115-124, 1989.

Spradlin JE, Siegel GM: Language training in natural and clinical environments, *J Speech Hear Dis* 47(1):2-6, 1982.

Steele RD, Weinrich M: Training of severely impaired aphasics on a computerized visual communication system, *Proc RESNA 8th Ann Conf,* pp 320-322, June 1986.

Swiffin AL et al: Adaptive and predictive techniques in a communication prosthesis, *Augment Altern Commun* 3(4):181-191, 1987.

Vanderheiden GC, Kelso DP: Comparative analysis of fixed-vocabulary communication acceleration techniques, *Augment Altern Commun* 3:196-206, 1987.

Vanderheiden GC, Lloyd LL: Communication systems and their components. In Blackstone S, Bruskin D, editors *Augmentative communication: an introduction,* Rockville, Md, 1986, American Speech-Language and Hearing Association.

Vanderheiden P: Writing aids. In Webster JG et al, editors: *Electronic devices for rehabilitation,* New York, 1985, John Wiley and Sons.

Wasson P, Tyman T, Gardiner P: *Test adaption for the handicapped,* San Antonio, Tex, 1983, Education Service Center Region 20.

Williams MB: Message encoding: a comment on Light et al., *Augment Altern Commun* 7:133-134, 1991.

Yorkston KM, Dowden PA: Non-speech language and communication systems—adults. In Holland A, editor: *Recent advances: language disorder,* Baltimore, 1984, College Hill Press.

Yorkston KM, Karlan G: Assessment procedures. In Blackstone S, Bruskin D, editors: *Augmentative communication: an introduction,* Rockville, Md, 1986, American Speech-Language and Hearing Association.

Yorkston KM et al: A comparison of standard vocabulary lists, *Augment Altern Commun* 5:189-210, 1988.

Yorkston KM et al: Vocabulary selection: a case study, *Augment Altern Commun* 5:101-114, 1989.

## CHAPTER 10

# Technologies That Enable Mobility

## Chapter Outline

## Objectives

Upon completing this chapter you will be able to:

1. Discuss needs underlying evaluation of the consumer for a mobility system
2. Describe the three categories of mobility systems based on the need served by each
3. Describe the two primary structures of wheelchairs
4. Identify the major characteristics of manual wheelchairs

5. Identify the major types of powered mobility systems and their characteristics
6. Describe the implementation phase for personal mobility systems
7. Delineate a training program for the development of independent powered mobility
8. Characterize driving controls and vehicle modifications used by persons with disabilities for independent driving
9. Describe various systems used to make transportation safer for wheelchair riders

---

## Key Terms

| | | |
|---|---|---|
| Add-On Power Unit | In-Wheel Motors | Secondary Driving Controls |
| Belt Drive | Low-Shear Systems | Standard Powered Wheelchair Base |
| Chain Drive | Modular Power Base | Supporting Structure |
| Dependent Mobility | Platform Lift | Tilt-in-Space |
| Direct Drive | Power Assist | Transitional Mobility Device |
| Friction Drive | Primary Driving Controls | Under-the-Vehicle Lift |
| Geriatric Wheelchair | Propelling Structure | Wheelchair Tie-Down and Occupant |
| Hoist Lift | Reclining Back | Restraint Systems (WTORS) |
| Independent Manual Mobility | Rotary Lift | Zero-Shear Systems |
| Independent Powered Mobility | Scooter | |

---

Mobility is fundamental to each individual's quality of life and is necessary for functioning in each of the performance areas: self-care, work or school, and play or leisure. As we have described for other activity outputs, limitations to functional mobility can be either augmented or replaced with assistive technologies. The activity output of ambulation can be augmented with low-tech aids such as canes, walkers, or crutches or replaced by wheeled mobility systems of various types. In addition to the functional gain of increased independence in mobility, such other goals as positive self-image, social interaction, and health maintenance are achieved. In this chapter we focus on wheeled mobility systems to enhance an individual's mobility. This includes manual and powered wheelchairs. We also discuss technologies that allow the person to be independent in another form of mobility: driving. Our emphasis is on the total process of delivering these systems to those who need them, from initial need and goal setting, through assessment and recommendation, to implementation and training.

## ■ HISTORY OF THE WHEELCHAIR

The first wheeled vehicle was likely made more than 20,000 years ago by placing two logs under a sled. The first reference to a wheelchair in literature was in 1588 in mid-Europe (Trujillo, circa 1960). Artists' drawings in the early 1500s show persons with disabilities still being transported in litters and carts. The first wheelchairs were wooden with solid wood wheels. They were too cumbersome to be self-propelled. King Phillip V of Spain used a wheelchair in 1700. His device had wooden wheels with wooden spokes, a reclining back, and an adjustable leg rest. This design was used for more than 200 years.

Wheelchairs were not used much in the United States until the Civil War. At that time chairs similar to King Phillip's were used. These wheelchairs had cane seats and backs and wooden wheels; however, by the end of the war they had metal rims on the wheels. In the late 1870s wire-spoked wheels came into use, probably as a technology transfer from the bicycle industry. This design dominated wheelchairs until the 1930s. In 1932 Mr. H.A. Everest, a mining engineer who had sustained a spinal cord injury in a mining accident, teamed up with Mr. H.C. Jennings, a mechanical engineer. They developed the first folding wheelchair using an X-brace construction. This design was considered lightweight (less than 40 pounds) for the times and only measured 10 inches wide when folded. This allowed it to be placed behind a car seat. The collaboration between Everest and Jennings led to the formation of the E & J Wheelchair Company, still one of the largest manufacturers of wheelchairs in the United States. This design, with some modifications in materials and accessories (e.g., removable armrests, reclining features) dominated the industry for quite some time.

After World War II, wheelchair sports started as a part of the rehabilitation program at Stoke Mandeville Hospital in England. The purpose was to provide exercise and a recreational outlet for the many individuals who had been injured during the war. The success of this program spread to other countries and eventually led to the first international wheelchair sporting competition, held in 1952. Athletes with disabilities competed for the first time in the same venues as Olympic athletes in 1960 (Cooper, 1998). The popularity of wheelchair sports has grown considerably since this time and has had a significant effect on wheelchair design and performance.

Advances in medicine and medical technology also followed World War II. This led to a significant increase in the numbers of individuals with paraplegia or quadriplegia surviving an accident or a disease who before that time would have died or lived a very short life. People with mobility impairments began to participate more actively in life roles and saw to it that improvements were made in mobility technology, which allowed them to maximize their participation in everyday life activities. As wheelchair users became more active and empowered, they started modifying their own chairs to suit their needs (Cooper, 1998). These needs led to the development in the late 1970s of lighter, more maneuverable wheelchairs that could be used in racing, basketball, tennis, and other sports. These needs also led to the development of the rigid or box frame style, which provided a better ride and was stronger. Some of these individuals went on to form their own wheelchair companies and revolutionized the manual wheelchair industry. The advances made in sports and ultralight wheelchairs eventually became available in chairs for everyday use.

Powered wheelchairs are a much more recent development. Although a patent was issued in 1940, these systems did not come into common use until 1957 (Hobson, 1990). The first models were standard folding wheelchairs with automobile motors and batteries added that functioned at a single speed. Gradually engineers began to develop new designs specifically intended for powered use. The revolution in electronics and computer technology also had an impact on powered mobility systems. The use of solid state electronics for control systems increased reliability over previous electromechanical (relay) systems. Improvements in microcomputers allowed flexibility in control and provided the ability to alter the mobility system characteristics to match the users' needs more closely. These advances have made it possible for individuals who have difficulty controlling a standard joystick to operate a powered wheelchair.

Changes in wheelchair technology over the last century have allowed individuals with limitations in mobility to become more independent and to actively participate in society. Today many of these early inventions still are evident in current designs, but dramatic advances in materials, electronic controllers, and mechanical design have led to a proliferation of types, styles, and approaches to both manual and powered mobility. Changes in wheelchair technologies are expected to continue. Thus it is imperative that the assistive technology practitioner (ATP) keep current on new technologies as they become available and know how to define the user's needs and skills so that a match can be made to the appropriate technology.

## ■ MOBILITY NEEDS SERVED BY WHEELCHAIRS

There has been a significant increase in the number of individuals using mobility systems. Improvements in medical technology have led to an increase in the survival rate for individuals who experience a traumatic injury or disease and an increase in individual life expectancy. Not only is the number of people with mobility impairments increasing, but the population of those with mobility impairments is also changing. The continued aging of the population will be reflected in the number of persons living with mobility impairments. Many mobility impairments are related to aging and age-related disorders such as arthritis. In addition, attitudes toward people with disabilities have changed, resulting in greater acknowledgment of their abilities and increased opportunities.

After evaluating a number of data sources, Jones and Sanford (1996) concluded that the most accurate estimate of the number of persons with mobility impairments is derived from the Assistive Devices Supplement of the National Health Interview Survey (NHIS) conducted by the National Center for Health Statistics. Using information from the most recent survey, conducted in 1990, Jones and Sanford (1996) reported that approximately 6.5 million people in the United States have mobility impairments and use an assistive device such as a leg or foot brace, cane, crutches, wheelchair, or scooter. Of those 6.5 million people, approximately 1.5 million reported using some type of wheelchair (manual, electric, or scooter). Restrictions to mobility occur in many forms and to various degrees.

### Disorders Resulting in Mobility Impairments

There are many causes of mobility impairment. Disorders that result in mobility impairment may be neurological, musculoskeletal, or cognitive in nature. Bear in mind that not all individuals with a given diagnosis experience a similar impairment in mobility. The onset of the disorder, whether it was acquired or congenital, also affects the individual's mobility needs.

Data from the Assistive Devices Supplement (Table 10-1) present by diagnosis those respondents who reported use of an assistive device for mobility (Jones and Sanford, 1996). Forty-four percent of all mobility device users have a disability related to arthritis, making this the largest single diagnostic group. Some of the symptoms commonly seen in individuals with arthritis include painful, swollen, and stiff joints; muscle wasting around the affected joints; and, in

**TABLE 10-1**   Diagnostic Data from the Assistive Devices Supplement

| Diagnosis | n | % of Total | Total in U.S. Population |
|---|---|---|---|
| Arthritic disorders | 1,375 | 43.54 | 2,891,163 |
| Stroke | 187 | 5.92 | 393,198 |
| CNS disorders | | | |
|    Cerebral palsy | 114 | 3.61 | 239,704 |
|    Multiple sclerosis | 53 | 1.68 | 111,441 |
|    Parkinson's disease | 31 | 0.98 | 65,183 |
|    Other CNS disorders | 136 | 4.31 | 285,962 |
| Musculoskeletal disorders | | | |
|    Acquired limb deformities | 213 | 6.74 | 447,867 |
|    Bone fractures | 84 | 2.66 | 176,624 |
|    Dislocations, sprains, etc. | 24 | 0.76 | 50,464 |
|    Other musculoskeletal | 193 | 6.11 | 405,814 |
| Diabetes mellitus | 21 | 0.66 | 44,156 |
| Late effects of injury, trauma, toxins, etc. | 163 | 5.16 | 342,734 |
| Other undiagnosed symptoms | 132 | 4.18 | 277,552 |
| All other causes | 333 | 10.54 | 700,187 |
| Unknown | 115 | 3.64 | 241,806 |

Modified from Jones ML, Sanford JA: People with mobility impairments in the United States today and in 2010, *Assist Technol* 8:43-53, 1996.
*CNS*, Central nervous system.

**BOX 10-1**   Scope of Mobility Limitations

**Full ambulator:** no mobility impairment
**Marginal ambulator:** can walk short distances; may need wheelchair at times, particularly outside the home
**Manual wheelchair user:** has some method of propelling a manual wheelchair, whether it is with both upper extremities, both lower extremities, or one upper and one lower extremity
**Marginal manual wheelchair user:** may have upper extremity injury caused by overuse, or manual wheelchair mobility may not be the most efficient means of mobility for the person; manual wheelchair is used part of the time and powered wheelchair part of the time
**Totally/severely mobility-impaired user:** unable to propel self independently in a manual wheelchair; dependent mobility base, or powered mobility base the only option for independent mobility

later stages, joint contractures resulting in range-of-motion limitations. Other disorders that affect the musculoskeletal system and may result in mobility impairments include ankylosing spondylitis, osteogenesis imperfecta, osteoporosis, Paget's disease, and scoliosis.

Neurological disorders that may result in mobility impairment include cerebral palsy, cerebral vascular accident, Guillain-Barré syndrome, Huntington's chorea, traumatic brain injury, muscular dystrophy, Parkinson's disease, poliomyelitis, spinal cord injury, stroke, spina bifida, and multiple sclerosis. Symptoms commonly seen in these neurological disorders are muscle weakness or paralysis, sensory deficits, and abnormal muscle tone. All these disorders can lead to limitations with joint range of motion, postural control, and mobility. The individual may also have cognitive and behavioral problems as a result of the disorder. For the most part, individuals with neurological disorders tend to be under the age of 60 and eventually become full-time wheelchair users (Ham, Aldersea, and Porter, 1998).

Disorders that affect an individual's cognitive functioning and ability to learn, such as Alzheimer's disease and mental retardation, can also be the cause of mobility impairments. Whereas the onset of mental retardation is at birth, the onset of Alzheimer's disease is later in life. Consequently, there are unique aspects to each of these disorders that need to be considered by the ATP; some of these are discussed in this section.

## Functional Limitations of Mobility

Limitations to mobility can also be viewed as functional limitations of an individual rather than as conditions related to specific diagnoses (Warren, 1990). The degree of limitation in mobility varies across a broad scope, as shown in Box 10-1. At one end of the range are individuals who are considered *marginal ambulators*. At the opposite end of the range are those individuals who have severe mobility limitations and are dependent in manual mobility, with powered mobility being their only option for independence.

Warren (1990) describes marginal ambulators as able to move independently in their environment but functional only at a slow rate or for short distances. Persons who have marginal ambulating skills can benefit from part-time use of a powered wheelchair such as a scooter. This allows them to walk inside the home using a walker or cane and use a scooter outside the home to augment ambulation. Later in this chapter we discuss this further.

Next are individuals who are exclusively users of manual wheelchairs. Either they are dependent in the use of a manual wheelchair or they propel a manual wheelchair using one of three methods: (1) using both upper extremities, (2) using both lower extremities, or (3) using an upper and lower extremity on the same side of the body (e.g., a person who has had a stroke). There are also *marginal manual wheelchair users,* who are able to propel a wheelchair manually but have upper body weakness, respiratory problems, or postural asymmetry as a result of pushing (Warren, 1990). Marginal manual wheelchair users may also include individuals who formerly used a manual wheelchair for their mobility needs and have sustained an overuse injury from propelling the chair. The shoulder is the most common site of musculoskeletal injuries in manual wheelchair users (Cooper, 1998). Propelling a wheelchair for any length of time depletes the energy of these individuals and compromises their productivity in other areas of life. Marginal manual wheelchair users can benefit from powered mobility on a full-time or part-time basis.

At the extreme end of the range are those individuals who have a severe mobility limitation; their only means of being independent in mobility is through the full-time use of a powered mobility system. These individuals typically have a manual wheelchair that someone pushes them in as a back-up chair. Warren (1990) and Trefler et al (1993) describe various situations in which powered mobility should be considered.

Individuals with severely limited motor control, who without equipment would be physically unable to move around in their environment, are the ones traditionally considered for powered mobility and for whom the benefits are clear. With the provision of powered mobility, these individuals can independently participate in work, school, and recreational activities. The control interfaces (see Chapter 7) that are available today make it possible for someone with only one or two movements to operate a powered wheelchair; however, perceptual, cognitive, and behavioral impairments may prevent individuals from using a powered wheelchair even if they have the necessary motor skills. All the factors that we describe for the recommendation of manual mobility systems also pertain to recommendation of powered mobility systems. Careful evaluation of seating and positioning needs (see Chapter 6) and selection of a suitable control interface (see Chapter 7) are of primary importance. The person needs to be able to operate the powered wheelchair safely, and this should be evaluated before recommending any system. Integration of other devices, such as an augmentative communication system (Chapter 9), with the chosen powered wheelchair and control interface also needs to be carefully considered.

## Mobility Issues Across the Lifespan

Mobility needs differ across the lifespan, with children having much different mobility needs than adults. Although there are many lifespan issues to consider, we focus on two issues that warrant special attention: (1) powered mobility for young children and (2) mobility for older adults.

The use of powered mobility by young children is an area that has received a great deal of attention in the last decade. In the past, powered mobility was deemed inappropriate for young children for a number of reasons. These concerns were related to the ability of children to operate a powered wheelchair safely, the initial cost of the wheelchair and cost of replacing it as the child grows, and possible detrimental affects on physical development if the child depends on a powered system instead of his own locomotion (Kermoian, 1998). Recent studies have demonstrated

that children as young as 18 to 24 months can safely operate powered vehicles, which often resemble a child's toy (Butler, 1986; Magnuson, 1995; Trefler and Cook, 1986). Powered vehicles allow disabled children to experience movement and control and can facilitate their social, cognitive, perceptual, and functional development (Butler, 1997; Trefler, Kozole, and Snell, 1986).

Like other areas of assistive technology use, it is suggested that a child be given access to multiple modes of locomotion and be allowed to select the one that is most convenient and most efficient for the given activity (Butler, 1997). By augmenting a child's self-locomotion with wheeled mobility devices, normal childhood development can be simulated. There are an increasing number of powered mobility devices available that can be used to augment a young child's mobility. A **transitional mobility device** can provide the young child with the means for independent locomotion without the complexity and expense of a powered wheelchair. Transitional mobility devices include motorized toy cars and powered standing frames. Frequently, parents who resist standard powered mobility devices for their child are more accepting of motorized toy cars that facilitate play with their peers (Deitz, 1998). Deitz (1998) discusses the many factors that should be considered in the design and evaluation of mobility devices that facilitate self-locomotion in young children.

At the opposite end of the lifespan is a population that also deserves special attention when it comes to designing and recommending assistive technologies for mobility impairment: the older adult. Older adults represent a large proportion of individuals who use mobility devices. As the number of people in this group increases, so will the people with mobility impairments. Wheelchair users over the age of 60 tend to have limited mobility associated with the aging process, osteoarthritis, and cardiorespiratory disease and typically are occasional wheelchair users (Ham, Aldersea, and Porter, 1998).

Some needs that are specific to the older adult wheelchair user have been identified in the literature. The older adult wheelchair user often depends on another person to push the wheelchair. Therefore a mobility device that can be used easily by an attendant is important (Ham, Aldersea, and Porter, 1998; Trefler et al, 1993). Comfort, safety, and security have been identified as important needs related to seating and mobility for residents of long-term care facilities (Lacoste et al, 1998). Safety and security were deemed important for the user of the wheelchair, as well as for the care provider. For instance, it is important that the care provider be able to transfer a person in and out of the wheelchair safely. Both the user and the care provider will be more inclined to utilize a wheelchair that is comfortable, safe, secure, and "attendant friendly." Because the ultimate goal of wheeled mobility is to allow individuals to participate in their environment, taking these factors into consideration will ensure that the older adult with a mobility limitation is not prohibited from being a part of society.

Each person needs to be evaluated in view of her diagnosis, functional limitations, and lifespan to determine the type of mobility device that will best serve her needs. Through an evaluation we determine which basic type of mobility system the user needs and then identify desired characteristics and features.

## ■ EVALUATION FOR WHEELED MOBILITY

Box 10-2 identifies the factors that should be considered when selecting a mobility base for a consumer. It is important to know what the person's disability is so that its impact on the person's level of functioning can be ascertained. The person's prognosis and prior experiences with assisted mobility influence wheelchair selection. It is important to know whether the disability is temporary or permanent and whether the person's condition is expected to improve, progressively deteriorate, or remain stable. For example, an individual who has recently had a stroke may be expected to regain functional ambulation but for the short term requires a system for mobility. In this situation a rental of a wheelchair would be warranted. On the other hand, an individual with amyotrophic lateral sclerosis (ALS) is expected to lose functional abilities and requires a mobility system that will accommodate this deterioration in functional status. An individual with a complete spinal cord injury at the C6 level will not typically demonstrate changes in mobility after injury and permanently requires a mobility system.

There are several areas that are addressed regarding the consumer's mobility needs and preferences. How active the individual is and what types of *activities* he will be participating in from the wheelchair is information that needs to be gathered by the ATP (e.g., will he use it for recreational or sporting activities?). It is also important to know in what *contexts* the mobility system will be used. Will the mobility system be used at home, work, school, or in the community? How accessible are these environments? Width of doorways, floor surfaces, bathroom layout, and access to the structure (e.g., ramp, stairs) all need to be considered. Will it be used outdoors, indoors, or both? What modes of transportation will be used (van, car, bus, airplane), and are there special needs related to transportation? For example, the person may drive a car and need to have the wheelchair fold and fit behind the driver's seat. Is the user able to maintain and repair the wheelchair or have access to someone who can? The user's preferences for color and style also need to be considered. Wheelchair users consider the wheelchair an extension of their body, and therefore the wheelchair should reflect their personality. Each person will have

---

| BOX 10-2 | Factors to Consider When Selecting a Wheelchair |
|---|---|

1. Consumer profile: disability, date of onset, prognosis, size, and weight
2. Consumer needs: activities, contexts of use (e.g. accessibility, indoor/outdoor), preferences, transportation, reliability, durability, cost
3. Physical and sensory skills: range of motion, motor control, strength, vision, perception
4. Functional skills: transfers and ability to propel (manual or powered)

---

different needs and preferences when it comes to wheeled mobility. A young woman who works all day and participates in wheelchair sports will have much different mobility needs and preferences than an older woman who is retired and is less active.

The individual's physical and sensory skills are evaluated for range of motion, strength, motor control, skin integrity, vision, and perception. This also includes determining the user's optimal control site and interface for propelling the wheelchair. All these factors are discussed in Chapters 4, 6, and 7. Information on the person's weight and size, including measurements of specific dimensions (see Figure 7-2), is gathered in order to determine the size and capacity of the wheelchair. A very large person will need a heavy-duty wheelchair. If the consumer is a child and is expected to grow, that needs to be reflected in the decision making as well.

The person's functional abilities are also evaluated. This includes determining her ability to propel the wheelchair and to transfer to and from different surfaces. The type and features of a mobility system are determined by the individual's ability to propel either a manual or powered system. One approach to determining the user's level of skill in propelling a wheelchair is the use of a checklist such as that presented by Behrman (1990). This checklist is organized in a hierarchy from tasks that are easiest (e.g., moving on a level surface) to those that are more difficult (e.g., uneven terrain, inclines, and curbs). By observing the person's level of performance, we can identify equipment and strategies that may assist her in completing these tasks. For example, if a person has difficulty propelling over uneven terrain, tires that minimize rolling resistance can be recommended. A similar approach (Behrman, 1990) is taken to identify the level of skill an individual has in transferring. This checklist (shown in Table 10-2) starts with level surfaces and progresses to floor-to-wheelchair transfers. It is important to make note of equipment options and needs during transfers and mobility. For example, if a person needs to get the wheelchair very close to the surface she is transferring to, removable leg rests and armrests are required.

From the information gathered, goals for the mobility

## TABLE 10-2    Transfers

| | I | D | Comments* |
|---|---|---|---|
| **Bed** | | | |
| Level Surface | ___ | ___ | _____ |
| Uneven Surface | ___ | ___ | _____ |
| Car | ___ | ___ | _____ |
| Truck/Van | ___ | ___ | _____ |
| **Loading Wheelchair** | | | |
| Car | ___ | ___ | _____ |
| Truck/Van | ___ | ___ | _____ |
| Tub | ___ | ___ | _____ |
| Shower/Commode Chair | ___ | ___ | _____ |
| Commode | ___ | ___ | _____ |
| Wheelchair to and from sofa | ___ | ___ | _____ |
| Wheelchair to and from floor | ___ | ___ | _____ |

Modified from Behrman AL: Factors in functional assessment, *J Rehabil Res Dev Clin Suppl* (2): 17-30, 1990.
*I*, Independent; *D*, Dependent.
*Include specific requirements for successful accomplishment of the transfer relative to the wheelchair requirements, e.g., chair must be folded to a maximal rim-to-rim width of 13" to fit behind the driver's car seat.

base can be developed and potential characteristics identified. Wheeled technologies having features that match these goals and characteristics can be selected and evaluated by the consumer. Behrman (1990) gives examples of case studies with sample goals and device characteristics to meet those goals.

## ■ CHARACTERISTICS AND CURRENT TECHNOLOGIES OF WHEELED MOBILITY SYSTEMS

In this section we discuss the major characteristics of manual and powered mobility systems. Modern mobility systems are more flexible and more capable of being adapted to a variety of functional tasks. This may include height adjustment, recline, axle position adjustment, and combinations of all of these. The selection of a wheelchair is based on the evaluation discussed in the previous section and is a process of matching characteristics to the consumer's needs and skills.

To meet the varied needs of individuals with mobility impairments, there are three broad categories of wheeled mobility systems: dependent mobility, independent manual mobility, and independent powered mobility. **Dependent mobility** systems are propelled by an attendant and include strollers, geriatric wheelchairs, and transport chairs. A dependent mobility system is chosen when (1) the individual is not at all capable of independently propelling a wheelchair (likely because of cognitive, perceptual, or behavioral defi-

cits) or (2) a secondary system is needed that is lightweight and easily transported. An **independent manual mobility** system is for those individuals who have the ability to propel a wheelchair manually. These bases have two large wheels in the back and two smaller front wheels that allow the user to propel independently. **Independent powered mobility** systems are required when the user has difficulty propelling a manual wheelchair. These are motorized wheelchairs that are driven by the user. Within each of these categories there are many commercial options available to meet the needs of the individual user. In this section we discuss the characteristics of mobility systems, starting with the wheelchair's two basic structures: a supporting structure and a propelling structure.

### Supporting Structure

The **supporting structure** of the wheelchair consists of the frame and attachments to it. Specialized seating and positioning (see Chapter 6) is often considered part of the supporting structure. Accessories to the frame (e.g., armrests, footrests) are also a part of the supporting structure. In some wheelchairs these accessories are manufactured as part of the frame. Some supporting structures are unique in that they are adjustable to allow for changes in the orientation of the user in space. This includes systems that tilt, those that change the seat-to-back angle, and those that provide support in a standing position.

**Frame types.** Wheelchair frames are often classified by the materials used in their construction (Ragnarsson, 1990). *Standard* or *conventional* wheelchairs have the features shown in Figure 10-1. Those made of cold-rolled steel weigh between 40 and 65 pounds. Conventional wheelchairs made of stainless steel or aluminum are called *lightweight* wheelchairs. These weigh between 26 and 40 pounds. *Heavy-duty* wheelchairs have frames that have been strengthened to support very large individuals. Conventional wheelchairs typically use a crossbar folding construction that allows them to be collapsed for transportation. The frame includes the seat rails (to which the seat or positioning system is attached), the back posts, and the hardware for attaching the wheels. These wheelchairs may vary in seat height from the floor, and those with lower seats are often referred to as *hemiheight* wheelchairs. This designation comes from the frequent application of these wheelchairs to mobility for persons who have had a stroke and who use one foot and one arm to push the wheelchair. The lower height makes it possible for these individuals to reach the floor with a foot and control the direction of the wheelchair.

Armrests on conventional wheelchairs may be manufactured as a fixed part of the frame, flip back out of the way, or be completely removable. Nonremovable armrests decrease the width of the wheelchair slightly, and they do not get lost

## CASE STUDY 10-1

### WHEELCHAIR ASSESSMENT

Matthew is a 5-year-old boy who just started kindergarten. He has severe cerebral palsy. His teacher referred him to you for a wheelchair and seating evaluation. He currently does not have a wheelchair. At home Matthew is either carried from place to place, placed in a high-density foam positioning seat, or stands in his vertical stander. Outside the home he is pushed in an umbrella baby stroller. The parents have agreed to go along with the evaluation, although they are hesitant about getting a wheelchair for Matthew at this time. They are still hoping he will walk and feel that putting him in a wheelchair will hinder his progress in ambulating. They are also afraid that he will be kept in the wheelchair for long periods without a change in his position.

Your evaluation findings indicate that Matthew has mixed tone. At rest his tone is low. When excited or when completing an activity, his tone increases. His head control is fair. He is unable to sit independently. He has a slight startle reflex to loud noises. Matthew has some right hand function, as evidenced by his ability to play computer games using a four-position switch array. Matthew is nonverbal and communicates with facial expressions, gestures, sounds, yes/no signals, and a picture board. His functional vision appears to be intact.

Matthew lives with his parents and a younger sister in a single-story house. The flooring in the main living area of the home is linoleum with area rugs. The bedrooms are carpeted with a low shag carpet. Doorways inside the home are all wheelchair accessible. The front doorway to the home is wide enough for a wheelchair but has two steps leading up to it. The family has two midsize sedans and cannot afford to purchase a wheelchair van at this time.

### QUESTIONS:

1. Is there other information that you need about Matthew before making a recommendation for a mobility system? If so, what is that?
2. Given the information that you know about Matthew at this time, what types of mobility systems would you potentially consider for Matthew? What might be some features needed in a mobility system for Matthew?

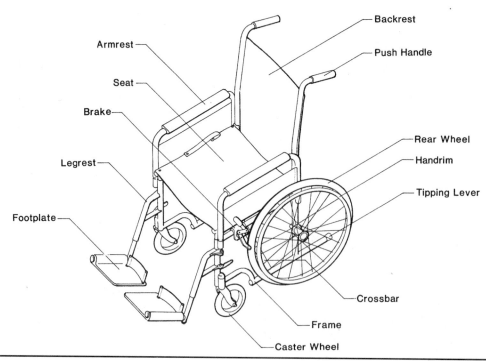

Figure 10-1 A conventional wheelchair showing the major parts of the supporting and propelling structures. (From Ragnarsson KT: Prescription considerations and a comparison of conventional and lightweight wheelchairs, *J Rehabil Res Dev Clin Suppl* [2]:8-16, 1990.)

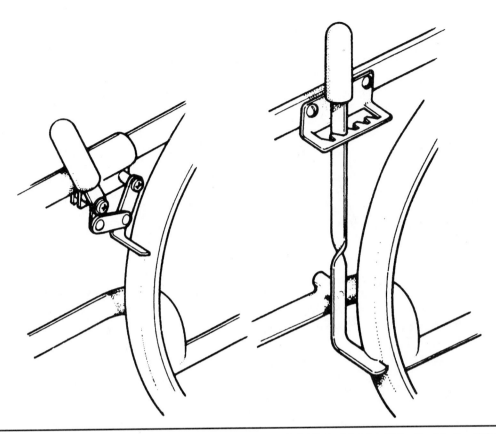

Figure 10-2    Two styles of wheel locks or brakes for wheelchairs. (From Wilson B, McFarland S: *J Rehabil Res Dev Clin Suppl* [2]:104-106, 1990.)

because they cannot be removed. In general it is advantageous to have armrests that flip back or are removable in order to facilitate transfers and other activities. Two lengths of armrests are available. Desk-length armrests are shorter in the front to allow the consumer to move close to a desk or table. Full-length armrests, which provide more support, extend to the front of the seat rails. Armrests may be fixed or adjustable in height. Armrests that are height adjustable can be moved up or down to accommodate the length of the user's trunk and provide the proper amount of support for the arms. A clothing guard on the armrests prevents clothing and body parts from rubbing against the wheels. In some cases, armrests are attached directly to the seating system (see Chapter 6).

Leg rests and footplates support the legs and feet. Taken together, these two components are often called the *front rigging* of the wheelchair. Leg rests may be fixed (built into the frame) or removable (swing away). Styles that swing away make it easier to transfer in and out of the wheelchair. Footplates are attached to the leg rests, and the height of each footplate is often adjustable to accommodate the consumer's leg length. The angle of the footplate can also be adjusted to accommodate ankle flexion or extension. It is critical that the leg rests and footplates be properly adjusted because they provide much needed support for the individual's lower extremities (see Chapter 6). Heel loops can be

attached to the back of the footplate to prevent the foot from sliding out (see Figure 10-1). In some cases foot straps, which extend over the top of the foot, are added for additional stability, or an H-strap may be added to the leg rests to prevent the lower leg from slipping back.

Other components included in conventional wheelchairs are *brakes* (often called *wheel locks*), push handles, *antitip devices*, and headrests. Two types of brakes are shown in Figure 10-2. Brake handle extensions are available for individuals who cannot reach the standard brake or who cannot exert sufficient force to set the brake. Push handles allow a care provider to push the wheelchair from behind. Antitip devices add stability to the wheelchair and can be attached to either the front or the rear of the frame. Depending on the placement of these devices, they prevent forward or backward tipping of the wheelchair when weight is shifted. They are particularly important in reclining and tilt-in-space systems. They can be fixed, removable, or adjustable. The advantage of removable or adjustable styles is that they can be moved out of the way to clear obstacles, such as curbs or uneven terrain. Headrests are also included in the supporting structure; they are described in Chapter 6.

The *ultralight* frame style, shown in Figure 10-3, is typically made of aluminum alloys, titanium, or composite materials and weighs about 25 pounds (Ragnarsson, 1990). A variety of colors are available from most manufacturers.

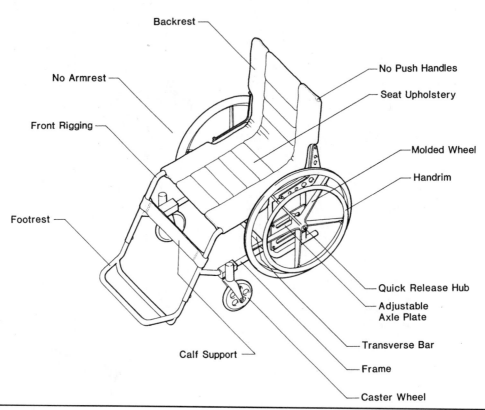

**Figure 10-3**   An ultralight wheelchair showing the major parts of the supporting and propelling structures. (From Ragnarsson KT: Prescription considerations and a comparison of conventional and lightweight wheelchairs, *J Rehabil Res Dev Clin Suppl* [2]:8-16, 1990.)

The composite materials have several advantages over steel or aluminum (Briskorn, 1994). Composite materials can be molded, which allows for more attractive designs than those based on tubes welded together. Composites are also durable, and their properties can be tailored to achieve desired shapes, strengths, and stiffness. Because shock and vibration are not transmitted as well by composite materials as they are by metals, there is decreased vibration felt by the consumer in a wheelchair made of composite materials. The major disadvantage is much higher cost; however, as volume of production rises and advances in other areas (e.g., bicycle fabrication) are applied, prices are expected to decrease. Briskorn (1994) discusses the pros and cons of composite materials as they are used in wheelchair design.

Frames may be either folding or rigid, and there are three common frame styles (Cooper, 1998). Rigid frames are available in a box, cantilever, and T or I frame style. Typically the box frame construction (see Figure 10-3) has a rectangular shape that provides a strong and durable base to which the seat and wheels are attached. Lighter weight designs are accomplished by replacing the box with a single bar extending between the wheels, forming a cantilever structure. Upright tubes from this main support are used to attach the seat and back. The footrests are extensions of the seat rails. As shown in Figure 10-4, the T construction uses a bar similar to the cantilever design but has a single bar attached

to the center of the cantilever that connects to a single front caster. This forms a T shape under the seat. If two front casters are used, then the T becomes an I shape. For transportation, the wheels on all these chairs are removed, and in some cases the back folds down. The choice between rigid or box frame and folding frame styles involves a number of considerations that are weighed during the assessment (Cooper, 1998). These include the consumer's needs, functional ability, method of transfer, and level of activity.

As shown in Figure 10-3, ultralight wheelchairs often have leg rests and footplates (sometimes called footrests) that are fabricated as part of the basic frame. In some cases a strap may be added to the leg rests to support the calves. Ultralight wheelchairs do not generally have armrests or push handles.

Highly maneuverable, ultralight wheelchairs are favored by active riders with good upper body strength and stability. They are often used in wheelchair athletics. Several manufacturers make sports wheelchairs (Table 10-3). These are specially designed for the sport of interest (i.e., a basketball chair is different from a tennis chair, which is different from a marathon chair). An alternative is to use a regular ultralight wheelchair with modification for the particular sport. For example, large wheels and small push rims could be used for marathon racing. Pfaff (1994) describes a number of examples of the use of wheelchairs in sports.

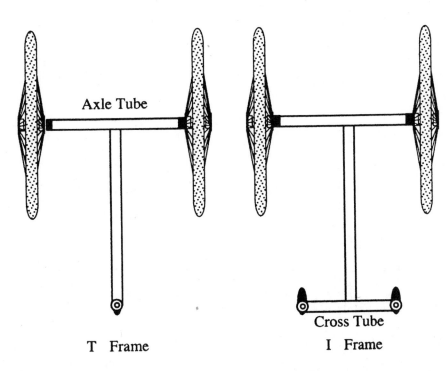

**Figure 10-4**    T and I frame styles. (From Cooper RA: *Wheelchair selection and configuration,* New York, 1998, Demos Medical Publishing.)

Powered wheelchair frames are often made of heavier and stronger materials than manual chairs. The conventional type of frame is frequently used as the supporting structure in powered wheelchairs. Other types of powered wheelchairs (modular bases and scooters) have unique supporting structures because of the design of the propelling structure. These are discussed in the following sections.

The standard seat and back in both conventional and ultralight wheelchairs are made of hammock-style upholstery attached to the frame. The major advantage of this type of seat and back is ease of transportation because they can fold and the upholstery is lightweight. However, for many individuals, this type of seating does not provide adequate support. In Chapter 6 we discuss the implications of hammock-type seating on posture and sitting stability.

**Frames for recline and tilt-in-space.** Often the consumer's position relative to gravity needs to be changed on a regular basis. Two specialized frames are used to accomplish this: recline and tilt-in-space. A **reclining back** refers to systems that allow a change in the seat-to-back angle of the wheelchair. **Tilt-in-space,** also called orientation-in-space or rotation-in-space, refers to systems in which all seating angles (seat to back, seat to calf, calf to foot) are preset to consumer's needs and the entire seating system is tilted back as one piece (Pfaff, 1993b). Each of these options has desirable characteristics, and each has its limitations. Manual and powered versions are available for both reclining and tilt-in-space systems.

As we discuss in Chapter 6, tissue breakdown caused by prolonged pressure is a major problem for individuals who have lost sensation as a result of spinal cord injury. When the back of the wheelchair is reclined, the consumer is repositioned and the pressure is redistributed. In other cases, recline may be used to modify the effects of the force of gravity. For example, a consumer who has difficulty controlling head position when upright may find it easier if the back is reclined (Fields, 1991a). Reclining also can accommodate cases in which more than 90 degrees of hip flexion is required. Finally, reclining can provide a more comfortable rest position without the need to transfer out of the wheelchair, although this does not completely eliminate the need for transferring an individual during the day.

The greatest problem with reclining systems is the shear forces that occur on the back and buttocks during recline (Minkle, 1992). As the back of the wheelchair is reclined, the user's body is displaced along the seating surface as much as 11 centimeters (Cooper, 1998). This displacement generates shear forces (see Chapter 6). Two approaches are used to reduce this effect: low shear and zero shear (Fields, 1992a). **Low-shear systems** place the point at which the back hinges to the seat a few inches above the point at which the seat and back meet (Figure 10-5). Because this location corresponds more closely to the rotation point of the consumer's back, there is less movement of tissue across the seating surface. In **zero-shear systems** the seat back is attached to sliding mounts that move the seat back down as it is reclined. This minimizes the movement of the seat across the body surface. As Fields (1992a) points out, shear forces cannot be reduced to zero because there is still a slight amount of movement of the back relative to the skin and because shear can also result from clothing moving across the skin. The main drawback of zero-shear systems is their higher cost. Some zero-shear systems are built into the

**TABLE 10-3**   **Major Wheelchair Manufacturers**

| Manufacturer | Types of Wheelchairs | Web Address |
|---|---|---|
| Alber<br>  In the United States: Frank<br>  Mobility Systems, Inc.<br>  742-695-7822 | Stair-climbing wheelchair; add-on power unit | www.ulrich-alber.de/index_e.htm |
| Altimate Medical, Inc.<br>  507-697-6393 | Standing systems | www.easystand.com |
| Amigo Mobility<br>  800-692-6446 | Scooters | www.myamigo.com |
| Bruno Independent Living Aids<br>  800-882-8183 | Adult and pediatric scooters; sedan and van wheelchair lifts | www.bruno.com |
| Columbia Medical<br>  800-454-6612 | Dependent mobility bases | www.columbiamedical.com/ |
| Convaid, Inc.<br>  888-266-8243 | Dependent mobility bases; transport chairs | www.convaid.com |
| ConvaQuip<br>  800-637-8436 | Wheelchairs for heavy people | www.convaquip.com |
| Etac | Independent manual wheelchairs for children and adults | www.etac.se/english/on-line/wheelchairs/ |
| Everest and Jennings<br>  800-235-4661 | Dependent and independent manual; powered wheelchairs; sports wheelchairs; adults and pediatric chairs | www.everestjennings.com |
| Freedom Designs, Inc.<br>  800-331-8551 | Pediatric wheelchairs; tilt-in-space wheelchairs | www.freedomdesigns.com |
| Global Power Systems<br>  800-554-8044 | Pediatric powered wheelchairs, head control interface | www.globalpowersystems.com |
| Gendron<br>  800-537-2521 | Add-on power unit, bariatric manual and power wheelchairs; scooters | www.gendroninc.com |
| Gunnell, Inc.<br>  800-551-0055 | Custom wheelchairs | www.gunnell-inc.com |
| Innovative Products, Inc.<br>  800-950-5185 | Pediatric powered mobility | www.iphope.com |
| Invacare<br>  800-333-6900 | Manual, power, and sports wheelchairs | www.invacare.com |
| Levo USA<br>  888-LEVO-USA | Manual and powered stand-up wheelchairs | www.levo.ch/ |
| LifeStand<br>  800-782-6324 | Manual and powered stand-up wheelchairs | www.vivre-debout.com |
| MacLaren<br>  877-442-4622 | Dependent mobility bases | www.majorstrollers.com |
| Mulholland<br>  800-543-4769 | A variety of standing aids; pediatric wheeled bases and tilt-in-space bases | www.mulhollandinc.com/ |
| Otto Bock<br>  800-984-8901 | Adult and pediatric manual and powered wheelchairs; heavy-duty wheelchairs | www.ottobockus.com/products |
| PDG<br>  888-858-4422 | Wheelchairs for individuals with special needs, such as bariatric chairs, high agitation, and manual tilt-in-space wheelchairs | www.prodgroup.com |
| Permobil of America, Inc<br>  800-892-8998 | Stand-up powered wheelchairs; powered wheelchair with elevating seat; sports wheelchairs, lightweight manual wheelchairs | www.coloursbypermobil.com |
| Pride Mobility Products Corp.<br>  800-800-8586 | Scooters and midwheel-drive powered bases | www.pridehealth.com/ |
| Pro Activ<br>  +49 7427 9489-0 | Ultralight wheelchairs; adult and pediatric wheelchairs | |
| Redman Power Chair<br>  800-727-6684 | Stand-up powered wheelchair and powered recline; add-on power unit | www.redmanpowerchair.com |
| RunAbout, Inc.<br>  800-832-2376 | Dependent mobility bases | |
| Snug Seat<br>  800-336-7684 | Specialty bases for children and adults, car seats, dependent and independent mobility bases | www.snugseat.com |
| Stand Aid of Iowa, Inc.<br>  800-831-8580 | Add-on power unit; standing systems | www.stand-aid.com |

| TABLE 10-3 | Major Wheelchair Manufacturers—cont'd | |
|---|---|---|
| **Manufacturer** | **Types of Wheelchairs** | **Web Address** |
| Sunrise Medical<br>800-388-5278 | Dependent and independent manual bases; sports wheelchairs; lightweight manual wheelchairs; powered wheelchairs; add-on power unit; adult and pediatric wheelchairs | www.sunrisemedical.com/<br>category_index.html |
| Teftec<br>888-234-1433 | All-terrain powered wheelchair | www.teftec.com |
| Theradyne<br>800-328-4014 | Dependent and independent manual wheelchairs; stand-up wheelchairs; power wheelchairs | www.theradyne.com |
| TiSport Chairs<br>800-545-2266 | Titanium wheelchairs | www.tisport.net |
| TumbleForms<br>866-529-8407 | Standers; dependent mobility bases; tilt-in-space bases; car seats | www.tumbleforms.com |

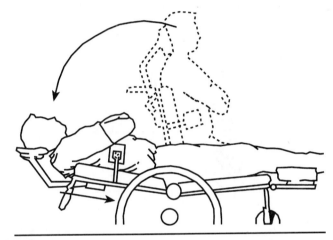

Figure 10-5   Low-shear systems place the pivot point for the back above the point at which the seat and back meet. (From Fields CD: Finding comfort in recliners: looking at power, *Team Rehabil Rep* 3[1]:34-36, 1992a.)

wheelchair design, and other systems are added on to the standard wheelchair base.

Manual recliners are available in two basic types. *Incremental* designs have a series of small steps into which the reclining mechanism locks as it is reclined. This establishes preset angles of recline. Systems with *infinite* adjustment can stop and lock into any angle during recline. Powered recliners give the consumer more independence. There are several control methods available (Minkle, 1992). The simplest control mechanism is a toggle switch for each function. One switch reclines the back and the other switch moves it up. If the consumer has more limited motor control, two functions can be included in a single switch. The first time the switch is activated, the back reclines as long as the switch is pressed. The next time the switch is pressed the back is brought up. It is also possible to have a separate control for the leg rests and back or to have both of these coupled to the same control interface. In some systems a switch is used to change the wheelchair controller from drive to recline functions using

the same control interface. Minkle (1992) lists eight factors to consider when choosing a power recline system: consumer's ability to adjust position independently, need for independent movement of components (e.g., leg rests and back), method of control, finished seat height from floor, battery access, stability of the wheelchair, turning radius, and cost. Fields (1991a, 1992a) describes commercially available options in both powered and manual versions.

Tilt-in-space frames use different types of pivoting systems (Fields, 1991b). These are distinguished by the location of the point of rotation of the seating system relative to the base, as shown in Figure 10-5. *Rear pivot* systems (Figure 10-6, *A*) have the point of location located near the rear of the seat. When this type is tilted, the consumer's knees are raised above the center of gravity (see Chapter 6 for a discussion of center of gravity). *Forward pivot* systems (Figure 10-6, *B*) rotate around a point located under the front of the seating surface. When this type is tilted, the user's buttocks are lowered to achieve the desired tilt angle. *Center pivot* systems (Figure 10-6, *C*) provide a counterbalancing effect between the front and rear frames as the system is tilted. This balance makes tilting easier than it is for either the front or the rear pivot. The fourth type, *floating pivot* (Figure 10-6, *D*), uses plunger attachments at both the front and back of the seat to achieve greater stability while allowing adjustment of the tilt angle. The tilting components are attached to the frame in a V shape, with the tops attached to the front and back and the base of the V attached to the frame. As the seat tilts forward, the front plunger is compressed and the rear plunger extends. The opposite occurs when the seat is tilted backward. Both powered and manual tilt options are available. Powered systems place the tilting function under the control of the consumer, while manual tilt requires the assistance of a care provider. Some wheeled bases can be purchased with built-in tilt-in-space. Add-on tilting systems that attach to a variety of bases are also available. Fields (1991b) describes an array of commercial options for tilt-in-space.

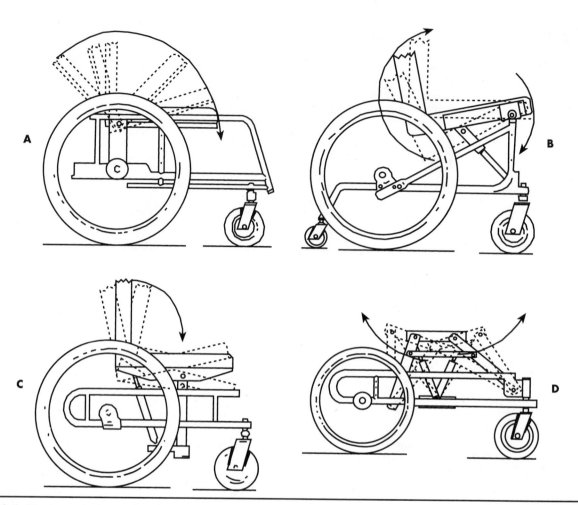

Figure 10-6   Pivoting mechanisms used in tilt-in-space systems. **A,** Rear pivot. **B,** Forward pivot. **C,** Center pivot. **D,** Floating pivot. (From Fields CD: Getting centered with tilt-in-space, *Team Rehabil Rep* 2[5]:22-27, 1991.)

There are several mechanisms used for stabilizing tilting systems (Jones and Kanyer, 1992). The first of these is the *pin-in-hole* mechanism, in which a pin is placed in one of a series of holes that correspond to the pivot of the system. This is the simplest and least costly approach. It has a finite set of tilt angles, since the pins must match preset holes. Major disadvantages are the elongation of the holes over time, leading to a looseness and perception of instability, and difficulty in inserting and removing pins that become bent with use. The second type is a *mechanical lock and cable release* mechanism. In this type a mechanical lock that controls the expansion of a spring to grip a rod holds the tilt angle. As the spring is expanded, the rod is free to move. This type is infinitely adjustable, but the rod and spring mechanisms must be kept clean and free of dirt and dust to avoid slippage. Often this type of mechanism is counterbalanced with a gas cylinder. *Gas springs* are cylinders that keep a piston in an extended position. Gas cylinders may be either locking or free travel. The locking variety has an infinitely adjustable tilt angle.

Pfaff (1993a) lists several reasons for using tilt-in-space

systems. They are indicated if the consumer has poor upright tolerance and needs frequent changes in position. Reasons for these include a fixed kyphosis, poor postural control, low or high muscle tone, limited hip flexion, or a need for pressure relief (these conditions are described in Chapter 6). Tilt-in-space is also used when a functional position is difficult for the consumer to maintain for long periods. The system can be tilted to the more functional position during periods of activity, and it can be tilted back for rest periods. When a person is transferring into a wheelchair, tilt-in-space can also be used to facilitate proper positioning. This is especially helpful with individuals who have increased tone. When tilting the system back after transfer, gravity helps to obtain proper position. Then the entire system can be tilted up for use. The ability to adjust the position in space without affecting the preset seat-to-back angles allows tilt-in-space systems to provide dynamic (i.e., changing) positioning.

There are several disadvantages of tilt-in-space systems (Fields, 1991b). First, most systems add seat height and length to the overall seating system. This can be enough to make transportation in a van difficult. The additional height also may limit the consumer's access to table surfaces. Second, because the center of gravity is raised in some approaches, the total system is less stable. Even if the system is stable, additional height may give the consumer a perception of less stability, and this needs to be evaluated. Finally, transfers may be more difficult because of the added height and access to the consumer may be hindered by the added components.

Special concerns that need to be addressed for use of tilt-in-space systems in different contexts are discussed by Fields (1992b). These include the access to desks and work surfaces described above; the turning radius of the wheelchair while in full tilt, ensuring that the system is stable and will not tip; and transportation issues. The space required for tilting must also be considered in relation to the consumer's work or school environment.

**Frames for standing.** We normally think of mobility in terms of wheelchairs; that is, the user is seated. There are, however, many advantages to placing an individual in a standing position (Walter and Dunn, 1998; Woo, 1992). Among the positive effects of standing are physiological improvement in bladder and bowel function, prevention of decubitus ulcers (see Chapter 6), reduction in muscle contractures and osteoporosis, and improved circulation. In addition, there are psychological benefits from being able to interact face to face with other people. There are several types of standing systems, and their function and benefits vary. Standing frames and stand-up wheelchairs are two different types of supporting structures that allow the individual to stand.

Standing frames are categorized as prone standers, supine standers, vertical standers, and units that allow sit-to-stand movements (Woo, 1992). Prone standers, such as the one shown in Figure 10-7, are the most common type. They provide support on the anterior side of the body. Weight bearing on the long bones and lower extremity joints is a major benefit. Often a lap tray is added to the stander. This serves two purposes. First, it provides a supporting surface for the upper extremities as the user leans on it. Second, it provides a work surface for activities such as writing, playing with toys, or using a communication device. Prone standers are generally tilted forward to use gravity for keeping the body upright in the stander. Some types have fixed angles and others are adjustable. Adjustment for growth is incorporated into some designs. Both stationary and mobile versions are available, and some of the mobile types have large wheels with hand rims that the user can push to move from place to place. A mobile standing frame affords mobility exclusively in the standing position. This type of standing frame does not give the individual the option of moving into a seated position, as does the stand-up wheelchair discussed below.

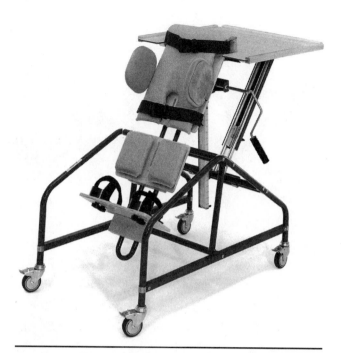

Figure 10-7    Large prone stander. (Photo courtesy Rifton.)

*Supine standers* are less common, and there are fewer options. This type of stander provides support for the posterior surfaces of the body. Because the user is leaned back, hand use is less functional. This type of stander is useful for persons who do not have good head control, since the stander supports the head and neck. *Vertical standers* provide for complete weight bearing on the lower extremities. People who have good upper body strength can use stationary models. Mobile versions are often sit-to-stand wheelchairs that allow changes in position from sitting to standing throughout the day. The change from sitting to standing and vice versa can be either powered or manual. When in a vertical position, these units generally function like a prone stander.

Although *stand-up wheelchairs* have been around for some time, it is only recently that they have become more sought after by the consumer. Many tasks of daily living, such as cooking, are simplified with the use of a stand-up wheelchair. Additionally, the use of a stand-up wheelchair may make it possible to avoid having to make modifications to a home or work setting. For example, a person cooking dinner while using a stand-up wheelchair is able to reach items in upper cabinets and reach the surface of cabinets and stoves without requiring modifications.

Stand-up wheelchairs (Figure 10-8) are available in three basic configurations: manual driven with a manual lifting mechanism, manual driven with a power lifting mechanism, and power driven with a power lifting mechanism. Stand-up wheelchairs with manual lifting mechanisms consist of a hydraulic system that uses either a pump or a lever to raise the person to the standing position. With a powered system,

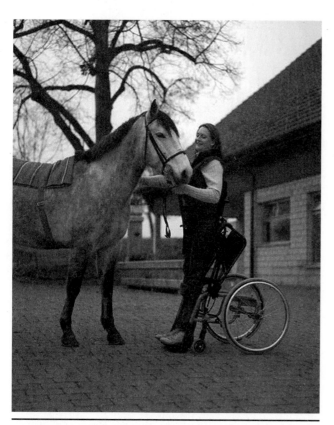

Figure 10-8    Stand-up wheelchair. (Photo courtesy Levo AG.)

the person activates a button to move into the upright position. When standing, the person is supported with padded bars at the knees and torso. Stability in the upright position is a concern with stand-up wheelchairs, and for that reason not all stand-up wheelchairs are mobile while in the upright position. Those that are designed to be mobile in the stand-up positioning have a wider-than-normal base of support.

Although there are significant benefits to be gained from the use of standing frames and stand-up wheelchairs, their cost and size often limit usefulness, especially in a home environment. Selection must be based on a systematic evaluation, and the requirements of the individual consumer for a standing system are determined during the needs assessment. Woo (1992) describes the essential elements of an assessment for a stander. Hunt (1993) describes a case study in which the needs of a consumer with quadriplegia resulting from a C3-C4 spinal cord injury were met by a powered mobile stander. She also describes how to select a stander and the process of matching standing system features to consumer needs. Fitting a consumer to a stand-up wheelchair poses some unique challenges in that the individual will be changing positions from sitting to standing; these dynamic positioning needs should be taken into consideration. Cooper (1998) offers some suggestions for fitting an individual for a stand-up wheelchair.

**Frames that provide variable seat height.** Another available option on powered wheelchair frames is a seat that can be lowered or raised.* The person remains in a seated position, and when the mechanism is activated, the wheelchair seat raises and lowers within a given range. The mechanism to change the height of the wheelchair seat may be operated manually or with power. A seat that lowers near the floor is particularly useful for small children. Being at floor level allows the child to play on the floor and interact at a level with children his age. There are also benefits to raising the height of a seat. As with a stand-up wheelchair, a seat elevator is useful because it raises the person up and can make it easier for the individual to participate in certain self-care, work, and educational activities.

**Frames that accommodate growth.** For children, a major requirement of the supporting structure of the wheelchair is that it accommodate growth. Economic factors, as well as the inconvenience of prescribing and purchasing an entire new wheelchair every year or two, dictate this. Years ago wheelchairs were available only in a few sizes, and children were given the smallest of these. If the wheelchair was too large, inserts (often pillows) were added. Today the situation is much better, and many manufacturers have systems that are adjustable in width, seat depth, back height, and wheel size. There are also adjustments for armrest height and the height of the footplate on the leg rest (to accommodate changing leg lengths).

The need to accommodate growth has a major impact on the supporting structure of the wheelchair; three primary approaches are commonly used. The first of these is to design the supporting structure so that it can be adjusted directly. This is generally accomplished by using tubing that is cut for the smallest width desired. The main frame members are cut in half and a sleeve is placed over them. Each half of the tube is inserted into the sleeve and the sleeve is tightened to hold them in place. As the child grows, the wheelchair is widened by pulling the tubes apart and retightening the sleeve, effectively lengthening the tube. This allows adjustment of several inches in each direction. A second approach, sometimes combined with the first, is to provide different lengths of frame tubing, which are replaced as the child grows. In this case the whole frame is modular, and it is adjusted by changing frame and cross-brace components. In some cases the tubes are again placed inside sleeves; the sleeves accommodate adjustments of a few inches, whereas different size tube sets are used for greater changes. The third approach is to use a full-size frame and use adjustable components attached to the frame to reduce the size of the sitting area. For example, side supports can be added that adjust in or out to accommodate growth. Likewise, the seating surface has

*For example, Permobile (www.coloursbymobil.com).

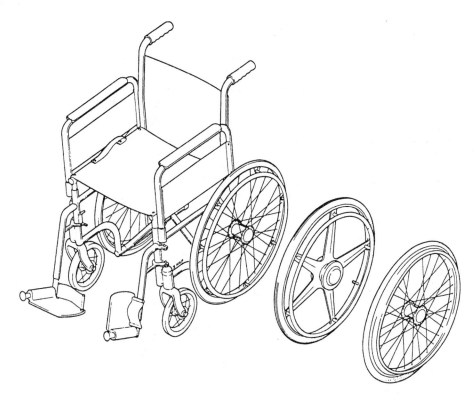

Figure 10-9   Types of rear wheels: wire and molded. Also shown is a wheel with hand rims built in to the wheel. (From Wilson B, McFarland S: *J Rehabil Res Dev Clin Suppl* [2]:104-116, 1990.)

adjustable components that change the seat depth and width. This approach generally has a greater range of adjustment than the others. Adjustable supporting structures are available for both powered and manual wheelchairs. Versions that include recline or tilting mechanisms are also available.

## Propelling Structure: Manual

For manual or *body-powered* wheelchairs, the **propelling structure** consists of two main parts: (1) wheels (including tires and casters) and (2) an interface that the consumer uses to move the wheelchair (Ragnarsson, 1990). We discuss each of these components in this section.

**Tires.** Two types of tires are used on wheelchairs: pneumatic and airless (Fields, 1991c). *Pneumatic tires* generally have an inner tube, which is placed inside a tire shell. When a tire is punctured, the inner tube can be repaired. Pneumatic tires are easier to push, provide a smoother ride, and are more maneuverable. They are also the lightest of the tires and add the least weight to the overall wheelchair. The major disadvantages of pneumatic tires are that they can be punctured and are generally more difficult to maintain because the inflation must be checked frequently.

There are three types of *airless tires:* semipneumatic, foam, and solid (Fields, 1991c). Manufacturers sometimes refer to these as flat-free or puncture-proof tires. *Semipneumatics* have a solid rubber or plastic construction with a

metal ring running through the center. These are the closest to pneumatic tire performance. They also have low rolling resistance and offer some shock absorption. *Foam-filled tires* are pneumatic tire inserts filled with foam instead of air. These have better performance than solid rubber tires but not as good as pneumatic types. *Solid tires* are the most durable and are generally less expensive, but they are heavier and have higher rolling resistance. None of the airless tires are subject to flats. Fields (1992c) discusses choices among these tire types based on consumer need, context of use, and availability of maintenance and repair capability.

**Wheels.** Rear wheels are of two basic types, shown in Figure 10-9 (Fields, 1992d). Wire wheels have spokes that attach the rim to the hub. Molded types are made of solid or composite materials. These wheels used to be made of magnesium and are often referred to as "mag wheels." Current models are more likely to be made of aluminum, nylon, and plastic composite materials. Mag wheels require less maintenance, whereas spoked wheels are lighter in weight and preferred by active wheelchair users (Cooper, 1998). Wheels range in size from 18 to 26 inches in diameter. Power wheelchairs typically have 18-inch wheels, and conventional manual types have 24-inch wheels.

The degree to which the wheel is able to roll smoothly without shimmy is referred to as its *trueness* (Fields, 1992d). The trueness of wire wheels is related to the even adjustment of the tension on the spokes, and this must be checked at least yearly for normal use. Molded wheels are trued

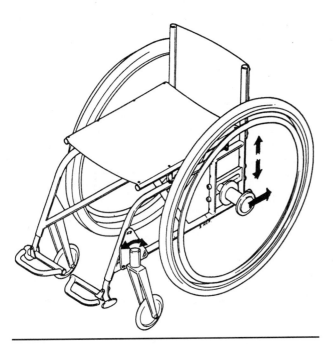

Figure 10-10    Adjustability of rear wheel position available in ultralight wheelchairs. (From Wilson B, McFarland S: *J Rehab Res Devel* [Clin Suppl 2], pp 104-116, 1990.)

during manufacture and should remain true unless they are subjected to high temperatures or impacts. Wheel alignment also affects the ease with which the chair can be propelled. *Alignment* refers to the degree to which the two wheels are parallel to each other. If they are not parallel and at equal distance from each other, there is greater rolling resistance for the wheelchair.

In ultralight designs the axle has multiple positions to allow variation in propelling action (Figure 10-10) (Ragnarsson, 1990). If the axle is moved forward, there is a shorter wheel base and the chair is easier to maneuver. However, this position also makes the wheelchair more susceptible to tipping backward. Moving the axle back leads to greater stability. Moving the axle up lowers the seat and thus the center of gravity. This increases stability, and the propulsion with each stroke is stronger. In some cases the axles are mounted so that the top of the wheel tilts inward toward the frame; this is called *camber*. This creates a larger base at ground level and brings the wheel closer to the user for more effective propulsion. A quick-release feature (see Figure 10-3) makes it possible to remove the wheel easily for transportation.

**Casters.**   The front wheels on wheelchairs are referred to as *casters*. They range in diameter from 2¾ to 8¼ inches (Fields, 1992c). Both airless and pneumatic types are available. Pneumatic caster tires give a smoother ride, but they require more maintenance. For ultralight wheelchairs, the front casters are normally made of polyurethane (Ragnarsson, 1990). One of the major problems with casters is

shimmy (Fields, 1992c). This is the rapid vibration that is often experienced when pushing a shopping cart. Smaller casters tend to have less shimmy than larger ones, but larger casters offer a smoother ride and are less likely to be caught on uneven surfaces. The major factors resulting in shimmy are the position of the caster fork and stem, the shape of the wheel, and the tension in the caster axle and swivel mechanism where they attach to the frame. Caster float occurs when one of the casters does not touch the floor when the wheelchair is on level ground (Cooper, 1998). This can result in reduced stability and performance. Excessive wear on one caster or unequal camber in the rear wheels will bring about caster float. Replacing the caster, adjusting the rear wheel camber, or lowering the caster that floats with a spacer can eliminate the problem (Cooper, 1998).

**The human/technology interface.**   The human/technology interface for a manual wheelchair is most commonly a ring attached to the wheel, called a *push rim* or *hand rim*. Conventional wheelchair hand rims are made of chrome-plated cold-rolled steel. Lightweight and ultralight wheelchair push rims are made of aluminum and often have a vinyl coating over them. The size of the push rim affects propulsion. Smaller push rims are like a high gear on a bicycle; they require more force to get started, but they are easier to maintain at speed once rolling. Large push rims are like a low gear: easy to start but more work to maintain at higher speeds. For individuals who have difficulty gripping push rims, knobs or extensions can be added (Figure 10-11). Some wheelchair users wear gloves to get a better grip and to protect their hands.

If an individual has the use of only one arm and hand, two hand rims are put on the intact side and a linkage is attached between the inner push rim and the opposite wheel, as shown in Figure 10-12 (Wilson and McFarland, 1990). By grasping both push rims, the user can move forward. Turning is possible using one push rim at a time. Lever drives are also available in which the user pulls and pushes by grasping a lever, rather than by grasping and pushing on the hand rim. These are called *one-arm drive wheelchairs*. These mechanisms require a fair amount of user coordination and strength, and the consumer should be evaluated with each method to determine its viability.

## Propelling Structure: Powered

The **propelling structure** of powered wheelchairs have more variability than do manual systems. The major components are a wheeled mobility base with a power drive to the wheels, a control interface that the consumer uses to direct the movement of the wheelchair, an electronic controller, and powered accessories (e.g., recline, ventilator). In this section we discuss current approaches.

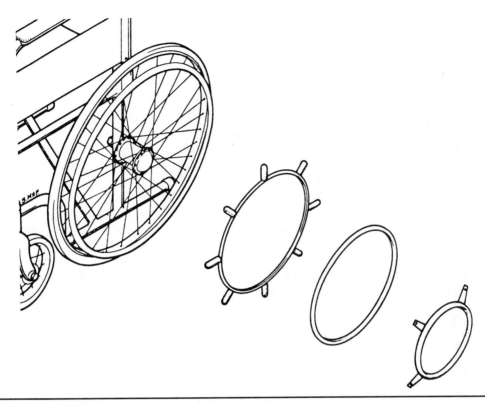

Figure 10-11    Examples of hand rims. (From Wilson B, McFarland S: *J Rehabil Res Dev Clin Suppl* [2]:104-116, 1990.)

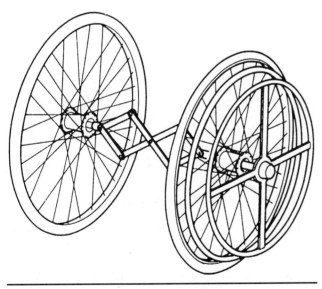

Figure 10-12    One-hand drive mechanism. (From Wilson B, McFarland S: *J Rehabil Res Dev Clin Suppl* [2]:104-116, 1990.)

**Types of drives.** Powered wheelchairs provide propulsion by linking the output of an electric motor to the wheels. In most cases the drive motor is attached to the rear wheels. In some designs (e.g., some scooters; see the section on bases for independent powered mobility), however, the drive is supplied to the front wheel or wheels. Recently, powered wheelchair manufacturers have added chairs with

midwheel-drive systems to their product lines. Chairs with rear- and front-wheel drive typically provide good stability. Midwheel-drive chairs have a shorter turning radius and are more responsive but may be less stable. Many midwheel-drive chairs have an antitip device placed in the front, which adds to the length of the chair. Selection of a drive for a powered wheelchair depends on the consumer's needs and abilities, the environment the wheelchair will be used in, and transportation and positioning needs (Segedy, 1998).

**Friction drive** systems apply a driving force through a roller attached to the motor, which is pressed against the tire. This is often used in add-on power units (see the section on bases for independent powered mobility). The main disadvantage is that water or grease on the tire results in slippage of the drive. This type of drive is also subject to slippage when the required torque is high (e.g., when climbing a ramp or hill).

Older wheelchairs used either a **belt drive** or **chain drive** to connect the wheel axle to the motor pulley. In the case of a chain drive the motor and wheel axle are coupled through a drive chain with gears at each end. These drive systems have been replaced by **direct drive** systems. In this case the motor is directly coupled to the wheels through a gearbox. This type of drive does not slip, and it has high starting torque and high-speed characteristics. The only drawback is that this type of system is often heavier than others.

Direct drive systems also often provide dynamic or active braking of the wheelchair by providing a voltage that stops the motor. This offers more control than the common situation of letting the chair coast to a stop after the voltage is turned off to the motor. Most motors used are direct current types in which the speed is proportional to the voltage applied and the torque is proportional to the applied current. Cooper (1998) describes in detail the engineering considerations in wheelchair drive systems.

### Control interfaces for powered mobility systems.

There are a number of ways in which a powered wheelchair can be controlled. The most natural interface for powered wheelchair control is the four-direction joystick. This is a direct selection method for mobility, since each of the four headings of movement can be directly chosen using the joystick. Proportional or continuous control joysticks (see Chapter 7) are the most commonly used because greater deflection of the joystick results in greater speed. Joysticks can be positioned to be used with the hand, chin, foot, or head. When a chin joystick is used, an additional switch (often activated by a shoulder shrug) can be used to control a powered arm that moves the joystick into position for use and swings it out of the way for eating, talking, or mouthstick use. Joysticks also can be used with different tops other than the standard ball. For example, a U-shaped cuff that supports the person's hand on the sides may enhance his control of the joystick. Other variations include smaller or larger balls, a T-bar, and an extended joystick. Remote joysticks, wherein the joystick is separate from the control box, are available if positioning and mounting of the joystick are a problem.

There are also proportional control interfaces designed for use specifically by the head. One such interface,* embedded in a headrest, utilizes a remote, electronic, two-dimensional position-sensing device to generate wheelchair control commands. Nothing is physically attached to the user. A low-level, high-frequency electrical field provides the invisible contact between the user and the wheelchair. To operate the wheelchair, the user selects the desired drive code by tapping a touch switch concealed in the headrest with the back of her head; for example, three taps activate the switch for forward drive motion and two taps indicate reverse motion. The driver then moves the wheelchair by tilting the head in space in the desired direction of travel. The degree of head tilt directly controls the speed of the wheelchair, similar to a standard proportional joystick; that is, the farther the head moves away from the vertical reference point, the faster the chair goes. In this regard the head itself actually acts as the joystick. To reduce motion to zero, the head is returned to the vertical position. One tap to the head switch stops the chair completely. In this stop position the user is free to move her head without generating wheelchair motion.

Another type of proportional head control interface* requires that the user have contact with the headrest. This type of control interface consists of a proportional actuator, a movable padded headrest, and a control switch. The controller converts movement of the headrest into directional commands. Power is applied by pushing the head backward, and side projections are used for lateral control of the wheelchair. Two additional switches are provided: one to turn all power on and off and one to change to the reverse mode function. Backward head motion of approximately 1.5 inches is needed for operation from stop to full speed. Angular head motion of 15 degrees to the right and to the left is needed for turning the wheelchair 90 degrees to each side. With the advent of electronic controllers (see next section), different parameters of proportional controls can be adjusted to match the skills of the user.

For individuals who lack the fine motor control for continuous joysticks, a four-position switched or discrete joystick is often used. In this case the controller features (see next section) are different to allow for functional control of the wheelchair. In lieu of the discrete joystick, any array of four switches can also be used by any of the control sites. Often a fifth switch is added to toggle between different functions. For example, the fifth switch could be for a power recline or to change the control interface for use with communication or environmental control.

One switch array that is often used in powered mobility is the sip-and-puff array. The user activates the array through a straw placed near the mouth. These switches provide two signals, one for a soft blowing action (called *puff*) and the other for a slight sucking action (called *sip*). Two of these switches are generally used, one for each drive motor. In its simplest form, puffing causes the motor to move forward and sipping causes it to move in reverse. Thus sipping on both switches moves the wheelchair backward, puffing on both moves it forward, and puffing on only one causes a turning action. Another approach to sip-and-puff control is switches that sense the amount of sip or puff and in this case act like a continuous control interface. A hard puff, for example, generates a larger signal and a faster speed than a soft puff.

Indirect selection using scanning is also available for consumers who can only use a single switch. In this case there are four lights, one for each direction, arranged in a cross pattern. The lights scan around the pattern until the user presses his switch. The wheelchair then moves in the direction selected. Other functions (e.g., high-low range) are also scanned. Single-switch scanning is time-consuming, as well as cognitively demanding, and should be

---

*Peachtree Head Control-2 (www.concentric.net/~Matrix), Global Power Systems, Inc., Hamilton, Ind.

*Proportional Head Control (Model 3500), Dufco Electronics, Inc (A Division of Sunrise Medical), Fresno, Calif. (www.sunrisemedical.com); RIM Head Control (www.everestjennings.com).

considered for powered wheelchair control only after other options have been excluded.

For general principles regarding evaluation and selection of a control interface, refer to Chapter 7. Joysticks, switch arrays, single switches, and mounting of control interfaces are also discussed further in Chapter 7. The unique aspect of selecting a control interface for a powered mobility system is that the user will be moving while using the interface, and any changes noted in the individual's position with exertion or movement of the wheelchair may affect control of the interface. It is critical to avoid an increase in tone that could cause the user to fall out of the wheelchair. The electronic controller of most powered wheelchairs includes the capability of varying parameters such as acceleration, braking, turning speed, compensation for tremor, and force generated by the wheels (see next section). Thus the evaluation of a user for a powered mobility system should take into consideration the selection and variability of these parameters to meet the specific needs of the user.

**Controllers.**  A *powered wheelchair controller* connects the control interface to the drive system. This is the processor in the assistive technology component of our Human Activity Assistive Technology (HAAT) model. In its simplest form, the controller converts the control interface action into a voltage signal that is applied to the drive motors. In a standard rear-wheel drive wheelchair, the controller drives both motors forward for forward movement and for turns drives one motor forward and one backward (e.g., for a left turn, the right motor is driven forward and the left motor is driven backward). To move backward, both motors are driven in reverse. All controllers have an adjustment of the maximal voltage that can be supplied to the motor, and many include both a high and low setting that is changed with a toggle switch. This allows one speed setting for those times when maneuvering around obstacles (e.g., in an office) is necessary and one for cruising along a hallway or sidewalk. Some controllers also allow adjustment of the torque. This adjustment changes the amount of current supplied to the motor, rather than changing the voltage (which would result in a change of speed). As we have discussed, this parameter is related to how much torque the motors can generate. If the current is higher, the torque will be higher. Often this adjustment is included in a two-range system referred to as *indoor-outdoor*. In this case the torque limit can be set for each situation, and then the user can switch between them as needed. Because increased current results in faster battery drain, it is better to use the smallest amount of current necessary. Increasing the torque can also be useful when traveling over thick carpets, as opposed to a smooth floor, or going up a ramp.

In a proportional drive system the controller determines the amount of voltage to supply to the motor by the amount of deflection in the joystick, and this voltage is directly related to motor speed. In a switched control system this type of proportionality is not obtained from the control interface. To allow the wheelchair to accelerate gradually (as the user with a proportional control would do), the controller provides a gradual acceleration when any direction is selected. In most controllers the rate of acceleration can be adjusted to meet the consumer's needs. For example, an expert powered wheelchair user could have the acceleration set on the high end so that the chair is highly responsive, whereas a novice user could set the rate of acceleration slower to allow for a slower start. The rate of deceleration (braking) can also be adjusted. Deceleration is the swiftness with which the wheelchair comes to a stop once the control interface is deactivated. With these two features on a controller, it is possible to set one rate for acceleration and a different rate for braking.

Controllers also provide either momentary or latched switch control. In *momentary control* the motors are activated only while the switch is pressed. This provides the greatest control for the user. Some consumers are unable to maintain switch activation, but they can press and release quickly. In this case *latched control* is used. In this mode, when the switch is pressed once, the motors turn on and remain on. When the switch is pressed again, the motors turn off. It is important that the consumer be able to activate the switch reliably and rapidly when it is in the latched mode, so as to stop quickly when necessary. This feature is often used with sip-and-puff switches. It allows the user to give a hard puff once to latch the control for the wheelchair to move either forward or backward and then use soft sips and puffs to turn left or right (Taylor and Kreutz, 1997).

Most powered wheelchair controllers are based on microcomputers. This gives them much more flexibility and adjustability. Forward and reverse maximal speeds can be independently adjusted. On some devices the ratio of forward to reverse speed is selected. It is more difficult to control the wheelchair when turning than when going straight, and the controller feature that allows turning speed to be set independently of (or as a function of) forward speed is useful.

Some consumers have difficulty controlling their movements because of tremor. This can make the use of a joystick or other wheelchair control interface difficult. To accommodate this, an averaging feature is incorporated into some controllers. The averaging system effectively damps out the tremor by ignoring small rapid movements and responding to larger, slower ones (Aylor et al, 1979). The disadvantage of this approach is that the system can become sluggish, resulting in reduced capability to respond to obstacles quickly. This feature is sometimes referred to as the *sensitivity* or *tremor dampening* of the controller.

Another adjustment allowed by the controller is the ability to alter the degree of range of motion required for an individual to operate a control interface. This is called the *short throw adjustment* and is most commonly used with joysticks. This feature is useful for consumers who have limited range of motion at the control site that is being used.

Computer-based controllers allow the storage of a set of values for parameters like those described earlier. These parameters can then be recalled for use in a particular situation (e.g., outdoors on a hill or indoors on a smooth floor). A therapist working with a consumer to gradually develop driving skills can also store the setups and recall them when needed. In training or assessment settings where several consumers may use one powered wheelchair, there can be different configurations stored for each consumer. Most powered wheelchair controllers also have provision for the attachment of an "attendant control," which is very useful for training. This control can override the user's control interface in an emergency situation. We discuss training of powered mobility skills in more detail later in this chapter.

Another feature of many controllers is the ability to operate different functions of the wheelchair or other devices with the same control interface. Generally an output from the controller is connected to the external device (e.g., an augmentative communication system or electronic aid to daily living [EADL]). These outputs may be called *auxiliary* or *ECU* on different commercial wheelchair controllers. Using a switch, the user is able to transfer the output of the controller from the motors to the external device. The control interface is then able to control the external device directly. A visual display identifies which function is being used. For example, if a joystick were being used for mobility, then switching to communication would allow directed scanning (see Chapter 7) to be used for selections on an augmentative communication device. A switch would allow the user to change between these two operations.

**Batteries.** The power for a powered wheelchair is supplied by a pair of batteries that are mounted under the seat of the chair. The batteries used are rechargeable lead-acid types. The name comes from the suspension of lead plates in a solution of sulfuric acid. There are two plates. The positive terminal is called the cathode and the negative plate is the anode; the size of the plates determines how much current can be drawn from the plate. When the wheelchair controller and motors are attached to the battery and turned on, current is drawn out of the battery. This causes current to flow from the negative terminal to the positive terminal. Inside the battery, chemicals from the acid solution are deposited on the plates. When a majority of the chemicals have moved out of the solution, the battery is discharged. Applying an external current to the battery terminals using a battery charger reverses the process and causes the deposited materials to move back into solution. This recharges the battery.

Batteries differ in several ways. Automobile batteries require a high current for a short period to start the car.

Wheelchair batteries, on the other hand, require smaller amounts of current for a longer time. This difference is reflected in the use of *deep-cycle* lead-acid batteries for power wheelchairs. These have thicker plates, which allow them to provide current for longer periods. The chemicals inside the battery may be in a liquid form, called a *wet cell*, or in a semisolid form, called a *gel*. Wet-cell batteries are less expensive and last longer; however, the fluid is subject to spilling and evaporation. Replacement of the fluid with distilled water is required at regular intervals. Gel (often called *sealed*) batteries will not spill, and this makes them more desirable for transportation. Some public carriers (e.g., airlines) require that gel batteries be used. Gel types also require less maintenance.

Battery power between charges is determined by the capacity measured in ampere-hours. At room temperature, wheelchair batteries commonly have 30 to 90 ampere-hours capacity at 12 volts (Cooper, 1998). The type of motors, environmental conditions (e.g., extremes of temperature), and amount of regular maintenance can all affect battery life and performance. Different batteries require different types of chargers, and it is imperative that the correct battery charger be used. The technology for wheelchair batteries has changed very little over the years. Smaller, lighter-weight batteries with an increase in capacity would help to decrease the weight of powered wheelchairs and increase the distance that the user can travel on one charge.

**Ventilators.** Frequently consumers who require powered mobility depend on ventilators for respiratory support. In most cases a humidifier is also required. These components are heavy and bulky, and accommodating them on a wheelchair frame is difficult. If the consumer also needs tilt or recline features, the problems are compounded. The options for including a ventilator and humidifier on a powered wheelchair are discussed by Laurence (1992). The components required are an additional battery, the ventilator, and the humidifier. The ventilator is normally mounted on a plate under the rear of the wheelchair frame. This can be difficult if the wheelchair batteries and motors take up so much space that there is inadequate room. Placement is determined by the space available; by the need to situate the air intake system away from dangerous sources, such as battery fumes and mud puddles; and by any restrictions on the ventilator function (e.g., orientation for mounting and distance from the consumer).

There are two options for battery power. These are an external power source and use of the wheelchair batteries through a separate DC-DC converter. The former approach is favored because power failure to the ventilator is life threatening. Swing-away mountings allow the humidifier to be in one position for service and another for use. If a tilt system is used, additional compensation must be made for this function and there may not be room under the seat when the seating system is tilted back. Laurence (1992) presents several examples of ventilator and humidifier mounting.

## Specialized Bases for Dependent Mobility

Having described the major wheelchair characteristics, we can now look at dependent mobility bases that have unique structural and propelling characteristics. Because an attendant or care provider is responsible for pushing the consumer in a dependent-mobility wheelchair, special attention is given to making this as easy as possible. Items normally required for independent manual mobility (e.g., large rear wheels with push rims) are often omitted in these systems. Bases for dependent mobility are commonly lighter in weight and lower priced than wheelchairs for independent manual mobility (Trefler et al, 1993). We discuss several alternatives for dependent mobility in this section.

**Stroller bases.** *Strollers,* similar to those used for transporting very young children, are typically of two types: (1) umbrella folding with a sling seat and (2) full-sized units with solid seats (Trefler et al, 1993). Although originally designed for children, there are now strollers that accommodate consumers who weigh up to 200 pounds. The umbrella type generally does not provide good sitting support, but it folds easily for storage in a vehicle. Consumers who use strollers should not be transported in the stroller unless it has been crash tested (Kemper, 1993). The lightweight construction of some units makes the attachment of solid seating systems difficult; however, on other units it is possible to attach seating components. Some of these seating components can be removed from the stroller base and used as car seats.

In recent years, funding constraints related to the purchase of manual wheelchairs and the ability of strollers to accommodate growth have made them popular choices, especially for children (Kemper, 1993). As a result, more solidly built stroller bases that can accommodate specialized seating systems (see Chapter 6) are available from several manufacturers. In some cases these systems have provision for growth. The most common approach is to use a frame large enough to accommodate a few years' growth and then add components that keep the child in a stable and functional position.

Another attraction of stroller bases is that they resemble standard strollers in appearance. This can be appealing to parents, but the child's need for independent mobility must be constantly reevaluated as she grows. A feature that appeals to parents is the ease with which they can be transported. The small wheels and short wheelbase of most strollers makes them easily maneuverable by an attendant. One disadvantage of the stroller is that the child is often in a reclined position, and this may limit his ability to carry out functional tasks. Strollers are sometimes purchased as a second wheelchair to facilitate transportation, with a standard wheelchair used for functional tasks. Lange and Longo (1999) compare a number of commercially available stroller bases.

**Modified conventional wheelchairs.** An alternative to the stroller base for dependent mobility is the modification of conventional wheelchairs (Trefler et al, 1993). The most common modification is the removal of the large rear wheel and substitution with small (8- to 10-inch) wheels and tires. These are easier to maneuver by an attendant pushing the chair and are more compact and lightweight than conventional versions. They are designed to be used by more than one person and are often used in airports and hospitals. Modified bases also fold to smaller sizes for easier storage.

**Geriatric wheelchairs.** **Geriatric wheelchairs,** also referred to as "Geri" chairs, are a type of dependent manual wheelchair especially designed for elderly persons. The primary purpose of these chairs is to provide comfort to the user while minimizing independent mobility. Typically they have small wheels and an easychair-type seat (Figure 10-13) that can be placed in a reclining position. Often a lap tray is placed over the armrests of the chair. These features make it difficult for the user to move the chair or get out of it. In institutions such as long-term care facilities, this makes it easier for the care staff to manage patients who have a tendency to wander or fall. Lately manufacturers have started producing models of these chairs that have a rocking

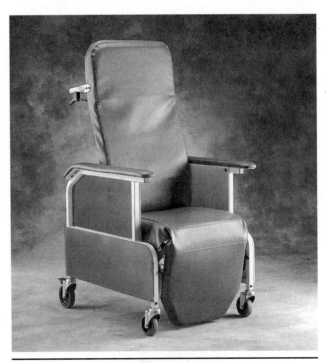

**Figure 10-13** Geriatric reclining wheelchair. (Photo courtesy Invacare.)

| TABLE 10-4 | Characteristics of Powered Mobility Systems | |
|---|---|---|
| Type of Base | Technical Features | Functional Features |
| Light-duty base | Usually reinforced manual wheelchair bases with motors and batteries | Meant for very light use, such as indoors or outdoors over even, paved surfaces |
| Light-duty electronics | Basic programmability of electronics; usually no specialty controls; no EADL/alternate ports; usually only proportional joystick | Meant for users with static conditions, who can use a joystick positioned outboard of armrest for the life of the chair |
| | | Not meant for users who need EADL or alternate controls |
| Medium-duty base | Base designed for more challenging terrain | Meant for users who need to go over rougher terrain, such as grass, broken sidewalks, etc. |
| | | Used with more sedentary user, such as elderly individual who needs mobility around home or other indoor areas |
| Medium-duty electronics | Electronics able to handle alternate controls; can also add EADL and alternate ports | Flexibility in electronics allow use by those who need input device other than standard joystick or who need access to other functions, such as tilt/recline or EADL, through wheelchair electronics |
| | | User may have limited upper extremity range of motion or only have breath control; may also have degenerative disease, such as ALS |
| Heavy-duty base | Base designed for most challenging terrain and hills | Meant for user who needs long distance, rugged mobility, such as college student in San Francisco |
| | Also able to handle weights up to 350 lb with special motor/frame packages | |
| Heavy-duty electronics | Electronics may have top-of-the-line options, such as multiple "channels" for programming characteristics of driving and chair speeds | May be appropriate for users who function in multiple indoor and outdoor environments |

Modified from Susan Johnson Taylor, *Justifying powered mobility*, www.rehabcentral.com, 1999.

feature.* For those individuals with Alzheimer's disease or dementia, the opportunity to rock the chair channels their energy and can provide a calming effect.

**Transport wheelchairs.** Another special design for dependent manual mobility is the *transport wheelchair*. These chairs can be collapsed into small sizes, and they are often designed for use in limited spaces such as airline aisles (Trefler et al, 1993). The Air Carrier Access Act, which took effect in April 1992, contains regulations for the use of wheelchairs on commercial airline flights (Wermers, 1991). Among other regulations (e.g., accessibility of airport terminals), the act also specifies on-board accessibility requirements for accommodation of wheelchairs. A number of special-purpose wheelchairs designed specifically for use on aircraft are commercially available. Wermers (1991) describes several of these. The major features are narrow width for use in the aircraft aisle, folding design for stowage, light weight, and provision for stabilizing the rider in the wheelchair during movement.

Some wheelchairs† are designed to disassemble, fold, and fit into a pack measuring 6.6 × 13.7 × 23 inches (17 × 35 × 58 cm) and weighing 26 pounds (12 kg) for transpor-

tation. Once in their pack, they are small enough to carry on an airplane. These chairs are narrower than a standard chair and make moving through crowded areas, such as an airport, easier.

## Systems for Independent Powered Mobility

The technology for powered mobility systems has changed significantly over the last several years, giving the consumer and the ATP innumerable options to choose from. There are five major approaches to powered mobility: standard powered wheelchairs, modular powered bases, scooters, add-ons, and powered assist units. When considering each major approach, we can further characterize powered mobility systems according to their functional use and the technical features of the wheelchair, as shown in Table 10-4. Bases for powered mobility systems can be characterized as light duty, medium duty, and heavy duty. *Light-duty bases* are intended to be used primarily inside. *Medium-duty bases* are meant to function inside, as well as outside over rough terrain such as grass or uneven pavement. *Heavy-duty bases* are those that can be employed by an active user for long distances and in rugged environments. The electronics on powered wheelchair bases can also be characterized as light, medium, or heavy duty. Powered wheelchair systems with light-duty electronics have only a basic programmability, whereas heavy-duty electronics have numerous programming op-

---

*For example, Rock 'N Go, Homecrest Industries (www.homecrest. com); Rx Rocker, Newbury Park, Calif.

†For example, ProActive Traveler, +49 7427 9480-0.

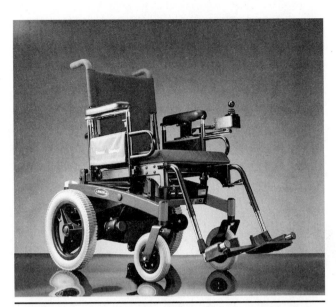

Figure 10-14    A standard powered wheelchair. (Photo courtesy Everest & Jennings.)

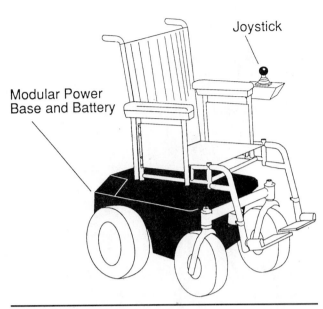

Figure 10-15    A modular power base. (From Church G, Glennen S: *The handbook of assistive technology,* San Diego, 1991, Singular Publishing Group.)

tions. In this section we discuss the major approaches to powered mobility. Table 10-3 lists some of the main manufacturers of powered wheelchairs and their Web sites.

**Standard powered wheelchairs.** The structures of **standard powered wheelchair bases** are similar in design to the conventional wheelchair frame, with large rear wheels and small front casters (Figure 10-14). The frame of the standard powered wheelchair is stronger to support the weight of the motors and the batteries. Any type of seating system can be interfaced to a standard powered wheelchair, and tilt-in-space and reclining systems are also available for these systems. Standard powered wheelchairs most commonly use direct drive. As we have described, the standard powered wheelchair is commonly controlled with a proportional joystick; however, the joystick can be replaced with a variety of other control interfaces (see Chapter 7).

Standard powered wheelchairs do best indoors or on level, smooth outdoor terrain. Although most standard powered wheelchair bases require the use of a van for transportation, there are some models that are lighter in weight and have batteries and a removable drive system, so that the wheelchair can be folded and placed in the trunk of a car. These lighter-weight chairs are primarily intended for use indoors. Tie-downs for securing the wheelchair in the van are discussed in the section on safe transportation.

There are many manufacturers of standard powered wheelchairs, and each typically has available a range of powered wheelchairs with various features. Powered wheelchairs at the lower end of the price range have fewer control options and accessories, whereas those chairs with sophisti-

cated controllers that allow for adjustment of multiple parameters are priced higher.

**Modular powered bases.** Whereas standard powered wheelchairs use the same frame design as conventional manual wheelchairs, the **modular power base** is designed specifically to maximize power. This includes attaching the motors directly to the wheels (direct drive), using small heavy-duty wheels, and eliminating the cross-brace folding structure to increase strength and maneuverability. Figure 10-15 illustrates a modular power base. Different types of seating systems can be interfaced to the power base, including reclining and tilt-in-space frames. Because of the modularity of the seat and the base, the seating system can be easily changed without replacing the propelling structure if this is made necessary by a change in the user's physical status.

Modular power bases are also stable and powerful. This makes them particularly useful for individuals who frequently travel outside over rough or uneven terrain. The biggest disadvantage of these bases is their weight. This makes it difficult for them to be pushed by an attendant and to be transported. A van is required for transportation.

A significantly different approach to powered mobility is incorporated in the INDEPENDENCE 3000 IBOT Transporter,* shown in Figure 10-16. In this approach an electronic balance system is used. This allows the mobility system to be customized for a user's size, weight, and center of gravity. Using a complex set of gyroscopes and computer-

---

*Independence Technology (www.independencenow.com).

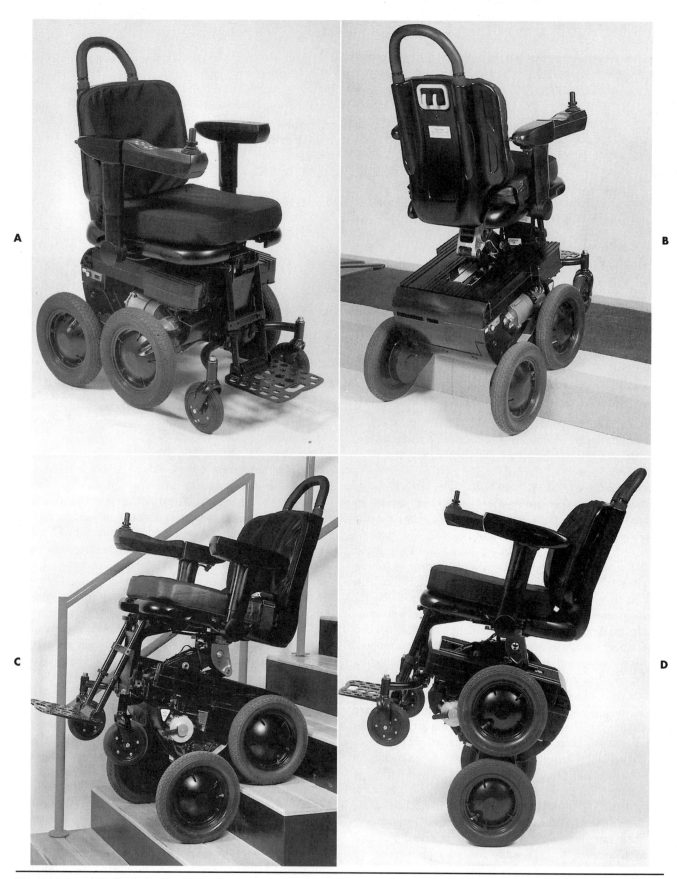

**Figure 10-16** INDEPENDENCE 3000 IBOT Transporter.
**A** and **B,** Four-wheel function. **C,** Stair function. **D,** Balance function. At this writing, according to the manufacturer, "This medical device had not been approved for use in this function. It is currently being tested for safety and efficacy of operation in these functions. This is an investigational medical device and is not yet available for commercial distribution." (Photos courtesy Independence Technology.)

controlled electronics, the INDEPENDENCE 3000 constantly adjusts its position to ensure that the user remains balanced and stable regardless of the terrain, movements of the user, or functions of the device. There are five functions for the device: standard, four-wheel, stair, balance, and remote. In its standard function the INDEPENDENCE 3000 uses two powered rear wheels, as in a standard wheelchair. In its four-wheel function (Figure 10-16, *A* and *B*), the INDEPENDENCE 3000 can navigate uneven surfaces, travel through sand and gravel, and climb over street curbs. In each of these activities the user is kept in a horizontal position and is balanced and stable. This function significantly expands the recreational options for users, since they can visit the beach, go over hiking trails, and cross grass fields. Uneven pavement, cobblestone sidewalks, and other similar obstacles can also be navigated using the INDEPENDENCE 3000 in four-wheel function. In the stair function (Figure 10-16, *C*) the INDEPENDENCE 3000 is able to go up or down flights of stairs, although users must have sufficient upper extremity strength to stabilize themselves using handrails. If the user lacks this capability, a trained assistant can provide the necessary help for stair climbing. The most unique feature of the INDEPENDENCE 3000 is its balance function (Figure 10-16, *D*). In this function the INDEPENDENCE 3000 utilizes its control system to balance the system on two wheels. This has several advantages. First, the user is raised to eye level, a significant factor for many individuals with mobility needs. Second, the balance function allows the user to reach objects on shelves, to reach the back of counters, and to generally function in a manner closer to that of standing. While in balance function, the INDEPENDENCE 3000 can be controlled by the joystick interface, just like a powered wheelchair. Finally, remote function allows the user to transfer out of the INDEPENDENCE 3000, fold down the seat, and unlatch the control interface (joystick, keypad, and display). The INDEPENDENCE 3000 is tethered to the control via a cable and can be "driven" slowly. This allows the user to drive the INDEPENDENCE 3000 into the rear of a van (up a ramp with up to a 25-degree slope) for transportation. The INDEPENDENCE 3000 uses several independent gyroscopes, redundant computers, and multiple sensors to continuously adjust the system to accommodate the user's characteristics and environmental obstacles during system operation. To maintain balance and stability, the INDEPENDENCE 3000 constantly adjusts wheel and frame positions to compensate for changes in pitch, wheel velocity, wheel position, seat height (the seat height is adjustable and can be raised during operation), and other parameters through a complex system of hardware and software components. The user interface is a joystick for driving and a series of buttons used to select functions. Feedback regarding the function, battery charge, and other features is provided via a liquid crystal display.

**Scooters. Scooter** wheelchairs (Figure 10-17) are the most unique of all the powered systems. This uniqueness arises from its structure and its application. Individuals who are marginal ambulators and need mobility to conserve energy most often use the scooter. For this reason, it is most commonly used by the consumer outside the home. Grocery stores and shopping malls often provide scooters for customers who may need them. The propelling structure of the scooter includes the drive train, the tires, the tiller, and the battery. There are a number of models available, in either three- or four-wheel versions, with front-wheel drive or rear-wheel drive. Scooters with front-wheel drive do better on level terrain and are more maneuverable. For this reason, they perform better in small spaces. In rear-wheel drive scooters, the rider's weight is positioned over the motor, so there is better traction and more power. The bases of rear-wheel drive scooters are wider and longer than the other powered chairs. These scooters are better able to handle inclines and uneven or rough terrain and therefore are preferable for outdoor use.

A tiller-type control is used to steer the wheelchair, and acceleration is accomplished by either grasping a lever on the tiller with the fingers or pressing with the thumb. When the accelerator is released, the scooter eases to a stop. On some scooters the height and angle of the tiller is adjustable. Depending on the model, scooters can have either proportional (variable-speed) control or switched (constant-speed) control. There is a separate control setting for adjusting the speed of the scooter. Some scooters have a dial that provides a range of settings, whereas others have a toggle switch for high and low.

The seat of the scooter is mounted to a single post coming up from the base. Typically the seat is a bucket type that has few options for seat width, depth, or back height (Toonstra and Barnicle, 1993). The seats come in padded or unpadded versions, and several types of armrest styles (fixed, flip-up, or none) are available. In the past, if a person needed a specialized seating or positioning system, it was not possible to interface it to a scooter. There are now some scooters that can accommodate specialized seating equipment. On most scooters there is a mechanism that releases the seat so it can swivel to the side and then locks it in place again. This feature is helpful for transfers in and out of the seat and for accessing a table surface.

Some of the advantages of scooters are that they are lighter in weight, can be disassembled for transportation in a car, are easy to maneuver, are less costly than other powered wheelchairs, and are more acceptable than other types of powered wheelchairs. The primary disadvantage of scooters is that they do not provide flexibility in control interfaces. The consumer needs to have a fair amount of trunk and upper extremity control to operate the tiller of the scooter. Scooters also have very little flexibility in terms of speed, braking, or turning control. Finally, the seat of a scooter

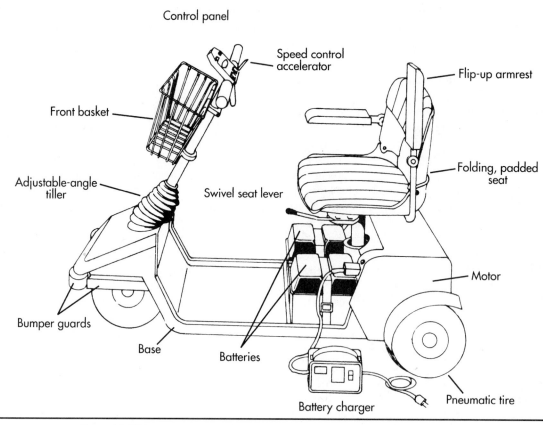

Control panel

Speed control accelerator

Flip-up armrest

Front basket

Folding, padded seat

Adjustable-angle tiller

Swivel seat lever

Motor

Bumper guards

Base

Batteries

Pneumatic tire

Battery charger

Figure 10-17    An electrically powered scooter. (Courtesy National Rehabilitation Hospital.)

typically does not provide adequate postural support, and many types of seating systems needed by individuals with postural control problems cannot be interfaced to a scooter.

**Add-on power units and power assist mechanisms.** A conventional manual wheelchair can be converted to power with an **add-on power unit** (Figure 10-18). All these units use friction drive, and their top speed is usually around 4 mph. Some of these units allow for interfacing of different control interfaces, but overall adjustments for control are limited. The add-on power unit and batteries can be removed from the base and the wheelchair folded as usual. For this reason, they are a viable option if it is necessary to transport the wheelchair and a van is not available. These systems are also recommended in situations where the person has a new manual wheelchair and funding is not available to purchase a powered wheelchair. The drawbacks with these systems are that manual wheelchairs were not designed to go at speeds higher than someone can manually propel them and adding power to the base may subject the frame to excess stress (Bergen, Presperin, and Tallman, 1990). The friction of the unit on the tires also causes the tires to wear out faster than normal. For these reasons, most manufacturers void the warranty of the wheelchair frame if an add-on power unit is used. Some companies offer a package of a frame and removable power unit

that allows the systems to be used as a manual base and the warranty to remain intact.*

An alternative to an add-on power unit is an **in-wheel motor** that is added on to manual wheelchairs (Figure 10-19). Electrical motors are integrated into the hub of the wheels. By necessity, the hub of a wheel with an in-wheel motor is much larger than that of a standard manual wheelchair. However, most manual wheelchairs with quick-release wheels can be interchanged with wheels that have in-wheel motors. The in-wheel motors can also be easily removed and the chair folded as usual for transportation. A battery pack attaches to the frame of the wheelchair, usually under the seat. A control interface such as a joystick is used to control the motors.

Another type of unit that utilizes the in-wheel motors is **power assist** for manual wheelchairs.† The wheels of a manual wheelchair are interchanged with the in-wheel motors. A power-assist unit supplies power to the manual wheelchair as needed by the user. When the user applies force above a preset level to the push rims, such as when going up an incline, the motors engage and help to propel the wheelchair. The power-assist unit also helps with brak-

---

*For example, the Quickie P200, Quickie Designs Inc. (www.sunrisemedical.com/category_index.html).
†E-motion by Alber (www.ulrich-alber.de).

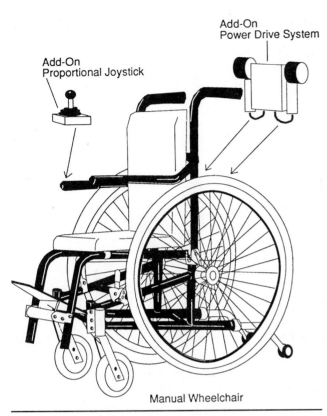

Figure 10-18   An add-on power unit can be attached to a standard manual wheelchair. (From Church G, Glennen S: *The handbook of assistive technology*, San Diego, 1991, Singular Publishing Group.)

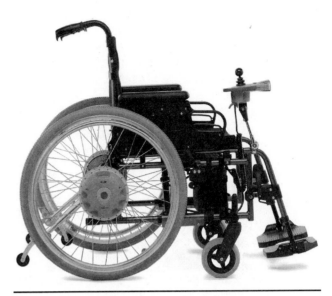

Figure 10-19   In-wheel motor retrofitted to a manual wheelchair. (Photo courtesy Alber.)

ing if needed. The user is able to select with a push of a button the level of support that the power assist provides and can set the level of support differently for the right and left arm if needed. The unit can also be turned off, which allows the manual wheelchair to function in the usual manner.

There are also power-assist units designed to be used by a person attending someone in a wheelchair.* The power assist in this case is a separate drive unit with wheels and batteries mounted under the seat of the manual wheelchair. A control interface for the attendant to use is mounted on the handgrip of the wheelchair. The unit assists the attendant pushing the wheelchair by providing power when needed, such as when going up an incline or for braking when descending a slope.

## Wheelchair Standards

As discussed in Chapter 1, *standards* can be used to provide manufacturing guidance to ensure product quality. One area of assistive technologies in which standards have been developed is for wheelchairs. There is an International Standards Organization (ISO) set of standards for wheelchair performance (www.iso.ch/welcome.html). These voluntary standards define standardized test methods and

methods for disclosing information (Bryant, 1991). A joint committee of the American National Standards Institute (ANSI) and Rehabilitation Engineering Society of North America (RESNA) developed them over a 10-year period. Purchasers can use these standards to compare different brands. The 22 standards are listed in Box 10-3. As shown, certain parts apply only to powered wheelchairs, some apply to both manual and powered wheelchairs, and some provide information regarding test procedures and information disclosure. The most important feature of the wheelchair standards is that they provide objective data for comparison (Pfaff, 1993a). This is a major improvement over the times when the ATP had only manufacturers' literature on which to base decisions.

Pfaff (1993b) discusses the application of these standards to lightweight wheelchairs. For example, one concern with lightweight wheelchairs is the degree to which they are likely to tip over backward. This is addressed in Standard 7176-01: Determination of Static Stability, which specifies how "tippiness" is to be disclosed and measured. The ATP can then determine which models under consideration will meet the needs of the consumer based on upper body strength and stability. Similarly, Standard 7176-05: Determination of Overall Dimensions, Weight and Turning Space gives dimensions of the narrowest corridor in which the wheelchair can make a three-point turn. This standard also includes data regarding the wheelchair's ability to fit in an automobile trunk. Similar considerations can be applied from other standards, depending on the type of wheelchair under consideration. In this way the standards become buyer's guides.

Although these standards are voluntary, there are strong motivations for manufacturers to adhere to them. For example, the Department of Veterans Affairs (VA) has purchasing requirements for wheelchairs. As the largest

---

*Viamobil by Alber (www.ulrich-alber.de).

**BOX 10-3**　Current ISO Standards for Wheelchairs (Approved and in Development)

| | |
|---|---|
| 7176-00 | Nomenclature, terms, and definitions |
| 7176-01 | Determination of static stability |
| 7176-02 | Determination of dynamic stability of electric wheelchairs |
| 7176-03 | Determination of efficiency of brakes |
| 7176-04 | Determination of estimated range of electric wheelchairs |
| 7176-05 | Determination of overall dimensions, weight, and turning space |
| 7176-06 | Determination of maximum speed, acceleration, and retardation for electric wheelchairs |
| 7176-07 | Determination of seating and dimensions |
| 7176-08 | Static, impact, and fatigue strength testing |
| 7176-09 | Climatic tests for electric wheelchairs |
| 7176-10 | Determination of obstacle climbing ability of electric wheelchairs |
| 7176-11 | Wheelchair test dummies |
| 7176-13 | Determination of the coefficient of friction of test surfaces |
| 7176-14 | Testing of power and control systems for electric wheelchairs |
| 7176-15 | Requirements for information disclosures, documentation, and labeling |
| 7176-16 | Determination of flammability |
| 7176-17 | Serial interface compatibility (multiple master multiple slave) |
| 7176-18 | Stair traversing wheelchair testing |
| 7176-19 | Wheelchair tie-downs and occupant restraints |
| 7176-20 | Determination of the performance of stand-up wheelchairs |
| 7176-21 | Electromagnetic compatibility for electric wheelchairs |
| 7176-22 | Wheelchair set-up procedures for testing |

**BOX 10-4**　Checklist for Wheelchair Fitting Process

Seating position
Position of control interface
Transfer method
Indoors: size, obstacles, doorways, turning circle
Outdoors: curbs, soft grass, rough ground, inclines
Distance required to travel
Maneuverability in community
Lights, horn
Care provider's training
Assembly and disassembly
Charging method
Battery life and maintenance
Transport in personal and public vehicles
Storage
Maintenance and repair

Modified from Ham R, Aldersea P, Porter D: *Wheelchair users and postural seating: a clinical approach,* New York, 1998, Churchill Livingstone, p 238.

need to be part of the system. The same holds true in order to maximize the performance of consumers who use mobility systems.

## Fitting of Mobility Systems

It is advisable that a fitting appointment be held with the consumer and caregiver. The purpose of this appointment is to make any adjustments needed to the wheelchair and to try the chair and determine whether it meets the original objectives outlined during the assessment. During the initial fitting, time should also be spent demonstrating to the user and the caregiver important features of the chair and going through instructions for maintenance. Box 10-4 shows a checklist of items to be covered during the fitting process for either a manual or powered wheelchair. Depending on the complexity of the wheelchair and whether seating components are involved, more than one fitting appointment may be necessary.

Because today's wheelchairs are often multifunctional, a number of components on the wheelchair are adjustable. Some adjustments and settings are made in the factory before shipping, but typically the provider of the wheelchair will need to make modifications to fit the chair to the user once it arrives from the factory. Adjustments to the wheelchair that can make a difference in user comfort, safety, and performance include axle position, wheel camber, wheel alignment, and center of gravity. Appropriate adjustment of the seat angle, back height and angle, and height and angle of leg rests and footrests are also critical to user performance. Cooper (1998) and Ham, Aldersea, and Porter (1998) describe in detail how to make each of these adjustments. Any adjustments to the chair should be made

purchaser of wheelchairs in the United States, the VA could significantly impact compliance with the standards shown in Box 10-3 by adopting them by reference, rather than developing their own standards. If all wheelchairs purchased by the VA must meet these standards, then all manufacturers will be strongly motivated to comply. In fact, most manufacturers of wheelchairs produced in the United States do conform to the requirements of the ANSI/RESNA standards. There are also equivalent Canadian and ISO standards to which these standards have been closely harmonized in order to minimize problems with importing and exporting of wheelchairs.

## ■ IMPLEMENTATION AND TRAINING FOR MANUAL AND POWERED MOBILITY

As we have emphasized throughout this text, the assistive technology system includes much more than a piece of equipment. For the consumer to be satisfied and successful with an assistive device, proper implementation and training

## Box 10-5  Checklist for Basic Wheelchair Maintenance

| Upon Receipt | Weekly | Monthly | Periodically | |
|:---:|:---:|:---:|:---:|---|
| | | | | **GENERAL** |
| • | | | • | Wheelchair opens and folds easily |
| • | • | | • | Wheelchair rolls straight with no excess drag or pull |
| • | | • | • | Footrests flip up/down easily |
| • | | | • | Legrests swing away and latch easily |
| • | | | • | Backrest folds and latches easily |
| • | | | • | Armrests easy to move and latch |
| • | | | • | All nuts and bolts are snug |
| | | | | **WHEELS** |
| • | | | • | Axle threads in easily or slides in and latches properly |
| • | • | | | No squeaking, binding, or excessive side motion while turning |
| • | • | | • | All spokes and nipples are tight and not bent or nicked |
| • | • | | | Tire pressure is correct and equal on both sides |
| • | | • | | No cracks, looseness, bulges in tires |
| | | | | **CASTERS** |
| • | | • | | No cracks, looseness, or bulges in caster tires |
| • | • | | | No wobbling of caster wheel |
| • | • | | | No excessive play in the caster spindle |
| • | • | | | Caster housing is aligned vertically |
| | | | | **WHEEL LOCKS** |
| • | | • | | Do not interfere with tire when rolling |
| • | • | | | Easily activated and released by operator |
| • | • | | | Hold tires firmly in place while activated |
| | | | | **ELECTRICAL SYSTEM** |
| • | | | • | Wires show no cracks, splits, or breaks |
| • | • | | | Indicators and horn work properly |
| • | • | | | Controls work smoothly and repeatably |
| • | | • | | Battery cases are clean and free from fluids |
| • | | | • | Motor runs smoothly and quietly |
| | | | | **UPHOLSTERY** |
| • | | | • | No tears, rips, burn marks, or excessive fraying |
| • | | • | | No excessive stretching (e.g., hammocking) |
| • | • | | | Upholstery is clean |

From Cooper RA: *Wheelchair selection and configuration*, New York, 1998, Demos Medical Publishing.

carefully and with the user's safety in mind. After adjustment are made, the user should be cautious in trying out the wheelchair until she gets acclimated to the changes.

## Maintenance and Repair of Personal Mobility Systems

Wheelchairs are designed to be low maintenance, and there are few items on a wheelchair, particularly a manual wheelchair, that require maintenance by the user (Cooper, 1998). The user is responsible for keeping the chair clean, the tires properly inflated, and seeing that the wheelchair is inspected on a regular basis. The user of a powered wheelchair needs to ensure that the correct battery for the wheelchair is used and that it is properly charged. A checklist of items that wheelchair users should monitor or have monitored regularly is shown in Box 10-5. The user manual for the wheelchair will also specify a schedule for periodic inspection and maintenance. A reputable assistive technology supplier (ATS) should complete any maintenance that needs to be done on the wheelchair.

## Developing Mobility Skills for Manual and Powered Systems

Training in mobility skills can occur before and after the delivery of the final chair to the consumer. In situations where it is undetermined which chair is most suitable for the consumer or if the consumer will be able to operate the wheelchair, a trial period takes place. During the trial period the person is loaned or leased a wheelchair, either manual or powered. This allows the consumer to test the chair and determine if it is appropriate to meet his needs. Often, particularly with powered mobility, this trial involves a period of training to determine if the person can develop the skills to use the wheelchair. For example, powered mobility may be identified as a goal but the individual may not yet have the skills required to control a powered wheelchair safely. If there is any question, it is best to delay making an expensive equipment purchase and risking the safety of the user and others. It is important that the potential user develop these skills through a training program before permanently acquiring the device. Implementation does not always end with the consumer's acquiring the device. In many cases, further training sessions are necessary. When developing either manual or powered mobility skills, it is important to set specific, measurable objectives for training.

For manual mobility, basic skills include maneuvering the wheelchair indoors on a level surface, in and around tight spaces, and over surfaces such as carpet, tile, or linoleum. For the active user of a manual wheelchair, preparation in advanced wheelchair mobility skills is suggested. These include the ability to negotiate rough, uneven terrain; propel up and down ramps and curbs independently; and execute "wheelies." The Manual Wheelchair Training Guide (Axelson et al, 1998) provides information on basic wheelchair setup and maneuvering the wheelchair in indoor and outdoor environments.

As with the skills required for driving an automobile, successful powered mobility use requires training and practice. This applies to everyone who uses a powered wheelchair. A systematic approach that develops these skills and progresses in small increments is most likely to be successful. As with manual mobility, the training in powered mobility skills should progress from basic skills to more complex skills and situations. Many training programs have been developed and are in use today (see Reppert, 1992). Some schools purchase a powered wheelchair that can be used with various control interfaces and seating systems. It is then possible to use the wheelchair with different children for training as needed. For young children, it is recommended that training be fun, starting with a toy cart and moving to a wheelchair base as appropriate (Barnes, 1991). Many children's games can be adapted to develop skills needed in powered mobility training, such as "red light, green light" for learning how to stop on command. Computer activities can also apply to the development of powered mobility skills; we discuss these in Chapter 7.

The development of powered mobility skills in young children can be described as progressing in three stages: stage I, exploratory; stage II, directive; and stage III, purposeful (Janeschild, 1997). In stage I, the exploratory stage, the child is encouraged to explore mobility in an environment that is safe and motivating. The goal is for the child to explore and learn how to control the mobility device. The trainer gives verbal feedback as it relates to what the child is doing at the moment and only to reinforce simple mobility concepts; for example, "You are moving *closer* to your mommy." The purpose of this stage is to minimize the amount of verbal direction given to the child and maximize the child's interest in interacting with the environment. During stage II, the directive stage, the goal is for the child to utilize the mobility device to move in the general area of a target. In the purposeful stage (stage III) the skills learned by the child are applied to home and school contexts in which more constraints are placed on the situation. Janeschild (1997) presents a tool for documenting the child's progress through the three stages.

## ■ EVALUATION AND TECHNOLOGIES FOR TRANSPORTATION AND DRIVING

Transportation for getting to school, work, and recreational activities is another area of mobility that contributes to an individual's independence. Transportation can be either public or personal. Being able to drive and get places without having to rely on public transportation provides a greater degree of independence for an individual with a disability. With the adapted equipment and programs that specialize in driver evaluation and training now available, many individuals with disabilities, even those with very limited motor control, are able to drive. The National Highway Traffic Safety Administration (NHTSA) estimates that, based on 1995 data, 383,000 registered vehicles in the United States have been modified with adaptive equipment to be used by or to transport persons with disabilities (NHTSA, 1997). As the population ages and as more individuals with disabilities become employed as a result of Americans with Disabilities Act (ADA), it is expected that the number of vehicles with adaptive equipment will increase. For more information on the use of adapted equipment in motor vehicles, see the NHTSA's Web site at www.nhtsa.dot.gov/adaptivemotor.html.

When considering personal transportation and driving for an individual with a disability, a number of areas need to be taken into account. During personal transportation, the safety of the individual accessing and being transported in a vehicle is often overlooked, and driving is a complex task that requires a high level of abilities and skills in all situations. A complete evaluation of the individual's needs and skills is essential for both driving and transportation.

### Evaluation and Training for Driving

Through careful evaluation, training, and the appropriate vehicle modifications, many individuals with disabilities learn to operate a vehicle safely and independently. Evalua-

## CASE STUDY 10-2

### DRIVING EVALUATION

Sandra was 35 years old when she had a cerebrovascular accident (CVA), affecting the right side of her brain. She has just completed a year of rehabilitation and has improved significantly. However, she continues to have left visual neglect and is unable to use her left upper extremity for functional activities. Sandra is ready to go back to work, and her vocational rehabilitation counselor has referred her to you for a driving evaluation. She still has the car that she drove before her CVA.

**QUESTIONS:**

1. How would you evaluate Sandra for driving? Identify a list of questions that you would want to ask Sandra and areas that you would want to evaluate.
2. Given the information you have about Sandra, what types of assistive technology might enable her to drive?

tion is carried out to determine not only the individual's physical ability but also her cognitive and perceptual ability to drive. In relationship to driving, it is particularly important to evaluate the cognitive and perceptual skills of individuals who have sustained a head injury or cerebrovascular accident. Some of these individuals may require few, if any, modifications to operate the vehicle but may require intensive training to overcome perceptual and cognitive deficits. Individuals with motor impairments may have difficulty driving because of limitations in range of motion, strength, coordination, endurance, or absence of a limb. For these individuals, the skills that they have need to be determined and matched to the appropriate vehicle modifications.

With the aging of our population, a growing area of concern is the older adult driver. It is estimated that by 2020 there will be 38 million drivers over the age of 70 on roads in the United States alone, compared with 13 million today (www.drivers.com/Top_Older_Drivers.html). Older adult drivers may have functional limitations caused by the aging process itself or by common conditions such as a stroke, dementia, arthritis, eye disease, and Parkinson's disease that affect their ability to drive safely. An evaluation can determine whether an older driver is safe enough to still drive, could benefit from some type of remedial training, or is no longer deemed safe to drive and should have his driver's license revoked.

There are many different driving evaluation and training programs described in the rehabilitation literature (Jones, Giddens, and Croft, 1983; Latson, 1987; Quigley and DeLisa, 1983). One of the most comprehensive approaches

is the model used at Louisiana Tech University, which has three major components: driver assessment, adaptive device prescription, and education and training (Hale and Shipp, 1987). We use the flowchart presented by Hale and Shipp (shown in Figure 10-20) as a framework to describe the process from the initial screening through driver education, and we supplement this with information from other sources. Individuals referred for driving evaluations undergo a careful screening and must meet state licensing criteria before being seen for an evaluation. The evaluation begins with a thorough needs identification.

The needs identification should include discussions with the consumer regarding the type of vehicle (van or sedan) she has or is interested in purchasing, how she will access the vehicle, and her need for wheelchair tie-downs or occupant restraints. It is important to remember when conducting a driving evaluation that it may not always be possible to realize the needs of the consumer. In driving evaluations, one of the questions that should be determined is whether the consumer is able to drive independently without compromising his safety and the safety of society at large (Gianutsos et al, 1992).

After the needs assessment, an initial skills evaluation is conducted in the clinical setting to determine the level of basic skills and abilities of the consumer. This is often referred to as the *predriving evaluation* and includes (1) evaluation of visual-perceptual skills (e.g., visual acuity, tracking, peripheral fields, depth perception, color perception, figure-ground perception, night-glare vision); (2) hearing; (3) reaction time; (4) cognitive skills (e.g., emotional control, left-right discrimination, attention, memory, distractibility, ability to follow directions, safety awareness, recognition of deficits); and (5) physical skills (active range of motion, strength, coordination, endurance, ability to transfer).

The evaluation of these consumer skills is not necessarily predictive of the consumer's ability to drive (Gianutsos et al, 1992). As a result, a number of protocols have been developed in attempts to create situations that more closely approximate the tasks associated with driving and that can be measured objectively. These are conducted before actually going out on the road, which allows the ATP to assess driving skills while minimizing risk. These protocols are also helpful in identifying and evaluating characteristics of adapted driving devices that may be useful to the consumer.

Computers and computer-assisted driver assessment systems (CADAS) are one way such protocols are implemented. There are several types of computer-assisted driver assessment systems available. One system is the Driving Advisement Program.* This is a series of computer programs for evaluating cognitive competence for safely operating a motor vehicle. The Driving Advisement Program includes steering and foot pedal modules, an input adapter,

---

*Life Science Associates, Bayport, N.Y.

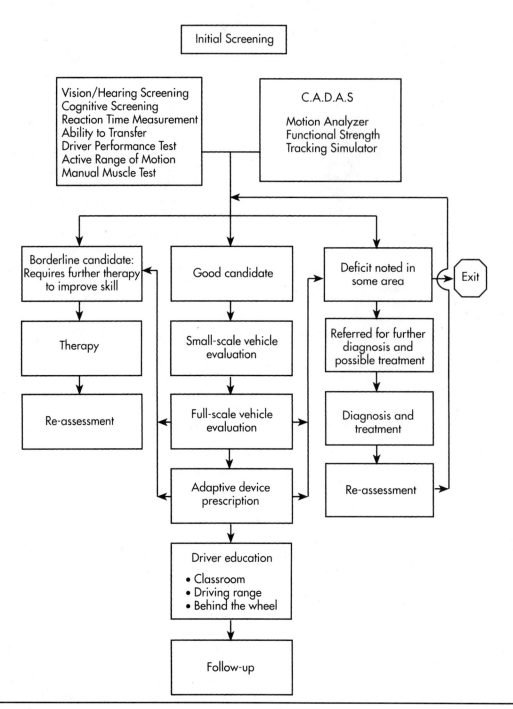

**Figure 10-20**   A framework for driver evaluation. (From Hale PN, Shipp M: Driver assessment, education and training for the disabled, *Proc 10th Annu RESNA Conf,* pp 65-67, June 1987.)

and software that measures reaction time, perceptual motor tracking, decision making, and self-assessment of driving readiness. Other CADAS include driving simulators, such as the Doron L-300 R/A[1] shown in Figure 10-21, that create a substitute for on-street driving. With a driving

simulator, the ATP can observe the individual "driving" a car in different traffic situations and environmental conditions. Driving simulators typically consist of a driver's console and an evaluator's console. The driver's console includes a driver's seat, all the controls necessary to drive an automobile, and a display that shows the simulated road and conditions. From the evaluator's console, the ATP can

*www.doronprecision.com.

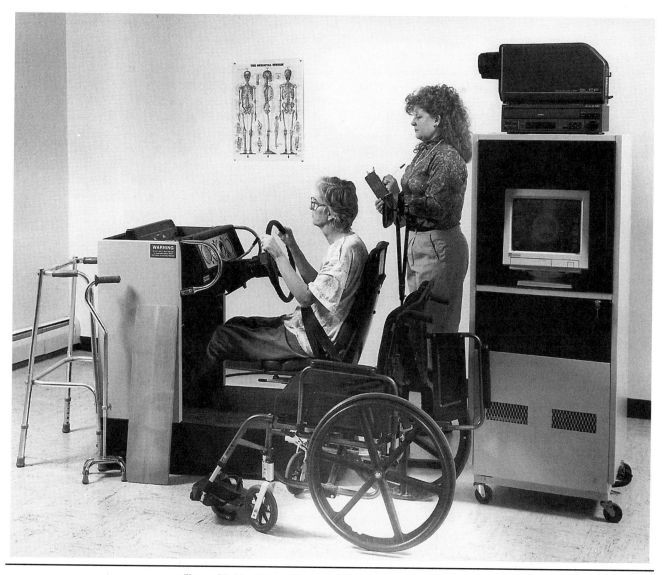

Figure 10-21    Driving simulator. (Photo courtesy Doron Precision.)

observe the reactions of the consumer in different situations and control the sequence of operation. Data regarding the traffic situations and the corresponding actions of the driver are collected and interpreted. Most systems can be modified for hand controls and wheelchair accessibility. Driving simulators are not only used for evaluation but also for driver training. The simulator can help the driver develop the ability to recognize, analyze, and respond correctly to traffic situations.

For people who are successful with simulation, an *on-the-road evaluation* is the next step. In some cases this starts with a small-scale vehicle evaluation. The vehicle typically used is a modified golf cart with the appropriate adapted controls. It is used to determine the person's ability to control a vehicle at reduced speed and in a safe environment. In other cases

the on-the-road evaluation starts with a full-scale vehicle on the streets of a quiet residential area or a large, vacant parking lot and progresses to more complex routes and traffic situations. This provides information on the consumer's ability to handle herself in graded traffic situations. The driver's performance on the road can be objectively evaluated using a checklist with a rating scale to measure specific functional tasks such as turning, backing up, and smoothness of braking and acceleration (Valois and Hittenberger, 1990). Although several formal tests that provide objective measures have been developed, they have not been standardized for any particular population of disabled individuals.

Based on the results of the evaluation, a recommendation for driving is made. The outcome of the evaluation can be one of the following: (1) the individual does not have the skills required for safe driving, (2) the individual has the basic skills and continues with the driver training program, or (3) a specific deficit is noted and further therapy or treatment is indicated. The individual is reassessed on completion of therapy or treatment (Hale and Shipp, 1987).

Driver education and training gives the opportunity for the consumer to learn driving skills and can take place on several levels. This training can include classroom activities, simulated or controlled driving practice, and on-the-road instruction. Classroom training is competency based and focuses on topics such as emergency driving procedures, defensive driving techniques, purchase of a vehicle, vehicle maintenance, accident responsibilities, and traffic laws (Enders and Hall, 1990). Simulated or controlled driving activities (driving range) give the consumer practice in maneuvering a vehicle while using the adapted controls recommended for him. Instruction behind the wheel provides practice and training for the driver on the road and builds confidence. At the end of this phase, an on-road performance test is administered to determine whether the individual is qualified to drive independently. For further information on driver evaluation and training, refer to the Association for Driver Rehabilitation Specialists (www.driver-ed.org).

In addition to the skills evaluation we have described, the ATP should also consider with the consumer vehicle selection, access to the vehicle, transportation of a wheelchair if applicable, and modifications that may be needed for operation of a vehicle.

## Vehicle Selection

When selecting a vehicle, it is first determined whether the consumer needs a sedan or a van. This determination is based on a needs identification, the functional skills of the individual, and cost of the vehicle and vehicle modifications. Generally sedans are preferred by individuals who do not depend on a wheelchair or who are able to transfer to and from the car seat without difficulty. Two-door sedans provide a wider door opening and allow easier access to the back seat for stowing a wheelchair or ambulation aid. Dimensions and characteristics of vehicles can vary. The user should test the vehicle before purchasing it to ensure that she can access it without difficulty (see the Association for Driver Rehabilitation Specialists, www.driver-ed.org).

Full-size vans or minivans are used by individuals who cannot transfer to a car or who use a powered wheelchair that cannot be folded for transportation in a sedan. There are pros and cons to both full-size vans and minivans. Regardless of the type of van selected, extensive modifications will be necessary. The advantage of minivans is that they are smaller and more maneuverable than a full-size van. The disadvantage is that the roof will need to be raised or the floor lowered in order to accommodate a person in a

wheelchair. The smaller minivan, especially once adapted, also will not have as much room to carry other passengers as would a full-size van. Because of its larger size, it is likely that modifications to the floor or roof of a full-size van will not be needed. Any modifications to the van will depend on the height of the person in his wheelchair. If modifications are necessary, they will not need to be as extensive as those required for a minivan.

The consumer may purchase a van and have it modified by a local dealer or purchase it directly from a manufacturer who does the conversion. Original equipment manufacturers (OEM) such as GM, Chrysler, and Ford sell sedans and vans that meet safety standards set by the NHSTA. Modifications made after purchase of the vehicles do not have to meet these standards (Sprigle, Thacker, and Shaw, 1993). A set of standards and guidelines for the design and testing of vehicle modifications have been developed by the Society of Automotive Engineers (SAE; www.sae.org) in an effort to protect consumers using modified vans. It is important that a reputable and qualified company performs all modifications. The National Mobility Equipment Dealers Association is made up of independent dealers of adaptive equipment and vehicle modifications for disabled people. A list of the members of the association can be found at the association's Web site, www.nmeda.org.

Important features to have on any vehicle being driven by a person with a disability are automatic transmission, power steering, cruise control, power brakes, and power windows and door locks. Power windows and door locks make it easier for the person with a disability to operate them. The cost of the vehicle, as well as costs to modify it, also need to be considered during the selection process. A van is much more costly to modify than a sedan (Peterson, 1996). Funding from Vocational Rehabilitation may be available for an individual who is employed or seeking employment, but any vehicle selected needs to be properly justified. Several automobile manufacturers offer a rebate program for consumers who need to make modifications to a new vehicle.

## Vehicle Access

Access to the vehicle includes locking and unlocking the doors, opening and closing the doors, getting in and out, and stowing and retrieving the wheelchair. If an individual is to be totally independent in driving a sedan, she needs to be able to independently transfer in and out of the car and get the wheelchair in and out of the car. There are a number of ways of assisting the user with these tasks. Transfers to and from the car can be simplified with the use of sliding boards, straps, and bars. Bench seats are easier to transfer to than bucket seats, and the type of covering on the seat (e.g., fabric versus leather or vinyl) can also make a difference. If it is not possible for the individual to load the wheelchair manually into the car, there are powered wheelchair-loading

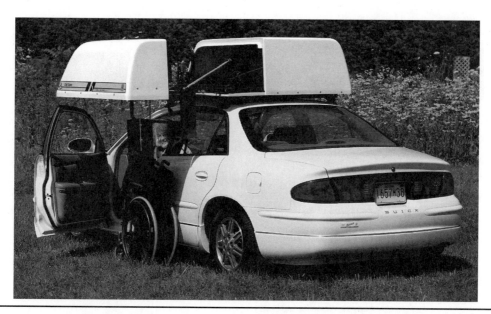

Figure 10-22   Wheelchair loading device for a sedan. (Photo courtesy Braun Corp.)

devices that can assist with this function. These devices pick up and store a manual wheelchair in the back seat, in the trunk, or in a carrier attached to the roof or back of the car. Figure 10-22 shows an example of a loading device that folds and stores a conventional wheelchair inside a cover that is mounted on top of the car. The other advantage of this type of loading device is that the wheelchair does not take up room in the trunk or back seat.

If an individual is not able to transfer independently to a car and stow his wheelchair, a van is necessary. To get in and out of the van, a ramp or lift is needed. Perr (1993) describes four types of powered wheelchair lifts: (1) platform or folding lifts, (2) under-the-vehicle lifts, (3) rotary lifts, and (4) hoist lifts. All four types are shown in Figure 10-23.

**Platform lifts** are the most common. They fold out from a frame that is attached to the opening of the van and lower to the ground. When stowed, they rest on either the inside or the outside of the van door in the upright position. The biggest disadvantage of the platform lift is that it blocks the van doorway when not in use. Some styles split or fold in half when stowed so that the doorway is not blocked.

As the name implies, **under-the-vehicle lifts** are installed under the van and extend out when activated. This type of lift does not block the doorway of the van. **Rotary lifts** have a post installed inside the van that supports a platform. Once the individual is on the platform, it rises up to a couple inches above the height of the van floor and rotates on the post into the van. The platform takes up floor space when not in use, which can cause a problem for maneuvering inside the van. There is no platform on the **hoist lift.** Instead, the wheelchair is attached with straps to an arm. The arm swings out from the door and lowers the wheelchair to the ground.

For individuals who operate their own vans, the wheelchair lift needs to be completely automatic. Powered lifts are operated by a switch, which can be selected to suit the user's abilities and control the up-down, door opening and closing, and folding functions of the lift. It is recommended that there be a means to operate the lift manually in case of a malfunction in the powered mechanism. There are also lifts that are semiautomatic. The raising and lowering functions of these lifts are powered, whereas the folding function is done manually.

A more affordable option to a powered lift is a manually operated ramp, which can be mounted to the floor of the van or fold up and be portable. These ramps are made of aluminum. Ramps that are mounted to the van typically fold up and into the van with the assistance of a spring, so that one person can manage it. Because they do not take up as much room as a powered lift, ramps are more often used with minivans. With a manually operated ramp, the consumer also does not have to worry about a power or mechanical failure of the lift.

There are a number of things that need to be considered when selecting a ramp or lift for an individual. The size of the person's wheelchair, the context in which it will be used, other uses of the van and by whom, the person's ability to use the ramp or lift, and cost all need to be taken into consideration.

In addition to installing a ramp or lift, other modifications that allow a person in a wheelchair to access a van may be required. If there is inadequate head clearance for the person to get into or sit in the van, likely the case with minivans, it may be necessary to raise the roof of the van or lower the floor. Besides being costly, these modifications alter the van's center of gravity and structural integrity

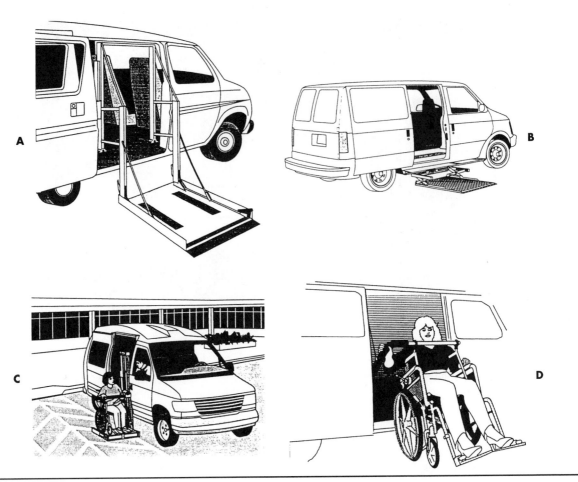

**Figure 10-23**    Different types of lifts used to provide wheelchair access to vans. **A,** Platform lift. **B,** Under-vehicle lift. **C,** Rotary lift. **D,** Hoist lift. (From Perr A: Van lifts, *Team Rehabil Rep* 4[4]:51-52, 1993.)

(Babirad, 1989). The person's wheelchair and seating system should be carefully evaluated first to see whether alterations to them could eliminate the need to make structural modifications to the van.

Once inside the van, the person may remain in the wheelchair or transfer to either the driver's or passenger's seat. In either situation, certain modifications are needed. A seat that swivels around and locks in place allows the individual to transfer safely from the wheelchair and swivel the seat back to the front. This requires adequate room between the seat and the engine cover for the individual to move her legs while swiveling the seat. In this situation the person will likely use the standard seat belts provided with the vehicle. If the individual will be driving or riding as a passenger in the wheelchair, tie-downs for the wheelchair and restraints for the occupant are needed.

### Safe Transportation of Wheelchair Riders

Originally wheelchairs were not designed with vehicle transportation and crashworthiness in mind. With personal and public transportation being more accessible to wheelchair users, it is important that this type of transportation be made as safe as possible. Two elements need to be taken into account in order to safeguard wheelchair users during transportation: the wheelchair tie-down with an occupant restraint system and the wheelchair and its seating system. Protection of an occupant in a vehicle is only effective when all these elements function together as a system.

**Wheelchair tie-down and occupant restraint systems.** The person with a disability is best protected from injury if he transfers to the vehicle seat and uses the standard OEM's restraint system (J2249 Guideline, version June 9, 1999, www.rerc.upmc.edu/STDsdev/SAE/unitindex). However, for many individuals with disabilities, transferring to the seat of a vehicle is not possible or practical. For these individuals, the wheelchair functions as the vehicle seat. Once the person is inside a personal or public vehicle, as either a passenger or a driver, both she and the wheelchair need to be properly restrained for safety. Surprisingly, many individuals drive or ride in their wheelchair in vans without using wheelchair tie-downs or occupant restraints. In one survey of consumers (Morris, Sprigle, and Karg, 1992), 86% of those responding used wheelchair tie-downs and only 54% used occupant restraints.

It is important to view **wheelchair tie-down and occupant restraint systems (WTORS)** as separate parts of a total system designed to protect the passenger or driver who uses a wheelchair (Thacker and Shaw, 1994). The wheelchair restraint system should be separate from the occupant restraint. In a collision the individual may be injured by impact with the wheelchair or seating system, he may be thrown from the wheelchair, or the wheelchair and the occupant may move together if not properly restrained. The WTORS is intended to address all these possibilities.

*Tie-downs* secure the wheelchair to the vehicle floor. There are two types of tie-downs that have been crash tested: four-point strap and docking or "trailer hitch" types (Thacker and Shaw, 1994). Other, non-crash-tested types are T-bar and rim-locking types. The four-belt type of tie-down, the most commonly used system, secures the wheelchair at each corner of the frame. In front the belts are attached to the frame (not the leg rests) just above the front caster pivot. In the rear the attachment is to the frame at seat level. The strapping system and buckles are similar to those used in the aircraft industry for securing cargo. The major advantage of belt systems is low cost and their ability to secure most types of wheelchair frames. Their disadvantage is that use is time consuming and cumbersome and cannot be done independently by the wheelchair rider.

The docking systems operate like trailer hitches. There is a bracket attached to the wheelchair frame that mates with one mounted to the van floor. The major advantages are quick and easy connection and independent use by the wheelchair rider. The disadvantage is that they require adding hardware to the wheelchair (which adds weight), and they are two to five times as expensive as belt systems.

The T-bar systems mount a plate to the wheelchair and a hook on the van floor. A threaded rod with a hook is inserted through the plate. When in the van, the hook end of the rod and the hook on the floor are connected and the rod is tightened. Rim lock systems attach to the rim of the rear wheels and to the floor. T-bar and rim lock tie-down systems have not been crash tested (Thacker and Shaw, 1994).

The Rehabilitation Engineering Research Center (RERC) on Wheeled Technology at the University of Pittsburgh is in the process of developing a universal interface device for the docking of wheelchairs in a vehicle. One of the most important features of a universal wheelchair docking system is that it allow the wheelchair user total independence. The four-point strap tie-downs described earlier require the operator of the vehicle or an attendant to fasten and unfasten the wheelchair securement device. Further information on a universal interface for

---

**BOX 10-6    Principal Elements of SAE Recommended Practice J2249**

1. Upper as well as lower torso restraint be provided.
2. Restraint forces be applied to the bony regions of the body and not the soft tissues.
3. Postural supports not be relied upon as occupant restraints.
4. The occupant face forward in the vehicle.
5. Adequate clear space be provided around the occupants seated in wheelchairs.

From J2249 Guideline, version June 9, 1999, www.rerc.pitt.edu/STDsdev/SAE/unitindex.

---

wheelchair docking can be found at the RERC on Wheelchair Technology Web site (www.rerc.pitt.edu).

For occupant restraint, variations of seat and shoulder belts used in passenger cars can be coupled with the four-belt and docking tie-downs to form a complete WTORS. The occupant restraint can be attached either directly to the van floor or to a point that is common to the tie-down attachment point. It is less likely that the wheelchair and occupant will move different distances during a collision if the occupant restraint is attached to the latter point. If they are not attached at the same point, it is likely that the wheelchair will move farther, forcing the occupant into the restraint and causing injury (Thacker and Shaw, 1994).

SAE Recommended Practice J2249, "Wheelchair Tie-downs and Occupant Restraints for Use in Motor Vehicles," was developed in recognition of the need to improve after-market equipment used to secure wheelchairs and restrain wheelchair occupants during motor vehicle transportation (J2249 Guideline, version June 9, 1999, www.wheelchairstandards.pitt.edu/SAE/unitindexSAE). Principal elements of this recommended practice are listed in Box 10-6. Although these recommended practices are voluntary, most manufacturers of wheelchair tie-down and occupant restraint devices are generating and testing products according to the recommended practice. Consumers, third-party payers, state agencies, and transportation groups can help by insisting on purchasing and installing only those devices that conform to the recommended practice. Similar standards for wheelchair transportation exist or are being developed for Canada (Z605), Australia (AS-2942), and other parts of the world (ISO 10542, Parts 1 to 5). More information can be found on standards for wheelchair transportation at the Web site for the University of Pittsburgh's RERC at www.rerc.pitt.edu/.

Thacker and Shaw (1994) list four tips for selecting a WTORS: (1) select a crash-tested system, (2) select a system compatible with the wheelchair, (3) select a system that is easy to use so it will be used, and (4) install the system properly.

**Wheelchairs for use as seats in motor vehicles.**
Occupant safety in a motor vehicle involves more than just the vehicle and the occupant restraint system. The design and construction of the vehicle seat plays a key role. The vehicle seat must provide support for the occupant under the load of an impact and subsequent rebound so that it does not contribute to occupant injury during an accident. Based on this rationale, the Subcommittee on Wheelchairs and Transportation (SOWHAT) was established to develop a voluntary standard for wheelchairs that can be used safely as seats in transport vehicles. A final draft of the standard (ANSI/RESNA WC-19) has been published and is in the process of being reviewed and voted on by various parties.

The proposed ANSI/RESNA WC-19 standard specifies general design requirements, test procedures, and performance requirements for manual and powered wheelchairs that offer suitable and safe forward-facing seating for passengers with a disability during normal transportation and in the case of a frontal impact. Box 10-7 summarizes the key aspects of this ANSI/RESNA standard. A comparable Canadian standard (Z604) was completed in 1996 and is currently being upgraded to be compatible with the ANSI/RESNA standard. A similar ISO standard (ISO 7176/19) is in the process of being developed.

## Modifications for Driving

The driver with a disability needs to be carefully evaluated for any modifications that are being considered. The assessment of an individual for driving modifications progresses in a logical manner, starting with an assessment of her ability to operate the primary controls, followed by an assessment of the use of the secondary controls. Once modifications are recommended, only a reputable dealer should install them.

**Primary driving controls.** The **primary driving controls** are those that are used to stop (brakes), go (accelerator), and steer. The degree of adaptation of the primary controls will depend on the physical limitations of the individual. In some cases all that is needed is power steering, power brakes, and an automatic transmission. For the individual with a disability affecting one or both of the lower extremities, it is necessary to augment or replace the acceleration and braking functions typically used by the feet. If reaching the pedals is a problem, they can be built up with extensions. If only the right leg is impaired (as a result of a CVA, for example) the accelerator and brake can be repositioned to the other side and the person trained to use the left leg. If both legs are impaired, the vehicle can be modified so these functions can be performed with the upper extremities using hand controls.

Hand controls for accelerator and brake consist of a mechanical linkage connected to each pedal, a control handle, and associated connecting hardware. There are three common design approaches: push-pull, push-twist, and push-right-angle-pull (Lillie, 1996; Peterson, 1996). In each case the first designation (e.g., push) refers to activation of the brake and the second (e.g., pull or twist) is used for activation of the accelerator. Using a push control (Figure 10-24, *A*), the consumer activates the brakes by pushing on a lever in a direction directly away from him, parallel to the steering column. Acceleration is accomplished either by pulling back on the control, rotating it, or pulling downward at a right angle to the steering column. The weight of the user's hand is sufficient to maintain a constant velocity. When the accelerator control is released, it returns to the off position. These controls are easily attached to almost any vehicle by the connecting hardware, which clamps a rod to each pedal and stabilizes them by attachment of a mounting bracket to the steering column. The connecting rods are adjustable in length to accommodate different vehicles. They are normally operated with the left hand, and the right hand is used for steering; however, right-hand mounting systems are also available from a variety of manufacturers.

For persons with weak upper extremities (e.g., high-level spinal cord injury), additional assistance is required. There are two basic approaches: (1) mechanical assist and (2) power assist. Mechanical assist systems use one of the approaches described above, but they provide a lever arm that affords a mechanical advantage (Figure 10-24, *B*). Instead of connecting the hand control directly to the accelerator and brake pedals, there is a mechanical linkage that magnifies the force applied by the user. Typically this is

---

**BOX 10-7    Summary of ANSI/RESNA WC-19 Standard**

The ANSI/RESNA WC-19 standard:

Specifies general design requirements, test procedures, and performance requirements related to frontal impact performance for manual and powered wheelchairs

Applies to passengers in paratransit, transit, school bus, over-the-road coaches, and personally licensed vehicles

Applies to securement of wheelchairs by four-point strap-type tie-down systems that are occupied by children and adults

Applies to a wide range of wheelchairs, including manual, powerbase, three-wheeled scooters, tilt-in-space wheelchairs, and specialized mobile seating bases with removable seating inserts

Specifies strength and geometric requirements for wheelchair securement points and occupant restraint anchorage points on the wheelchair

Provides requirements and information for wheelchair accessory components, seat inserts, and postural support devices with their regard to design and use in motor vehicles

Applies primarily to wheelchairs that are retrofitted for use as a motor vehicle seat by the addition of after-market add-on components

a long arm, attached to the floor, that is pulled back for acceleration and pushed forward for braking. The arm is also linked to the pedals through connecting hardware. Power-assisted devices use either hydraulic or pneumatic assist (similar to power brakes or steering) or electronic powered systems. Electronic powered systems add servomotors that apply force to the brake and accelerator system. An electronically assisted brake and accelerator control is shown in Figure 10-24, *C*. One of the most recent developments is the use of a joystick that the driver pushes back for acceleration and pushes forward for braking.

There are a number of options to consider for steering for drivers who use one arm, use a prosthetic arm, or have impaired arm and hand function. For a driver who uses one hand to steer, a steering device allows the driver to maintain control of the wheel at all times (Lillie, 1996). Steering

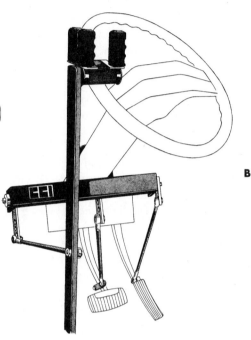

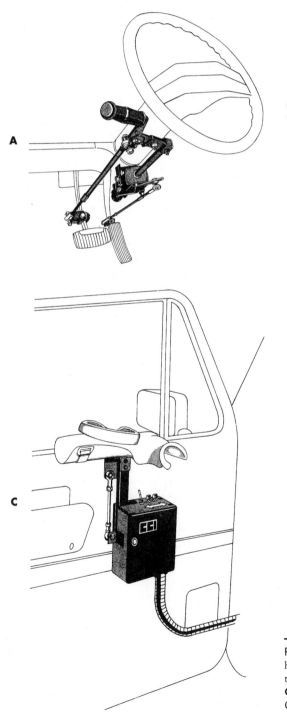

Figure 10-24    Hand control for braking and acceleration. **A**, A push-twist hand control. Pushing down applies the brakes, and twisting the lever to the left accelerates the vehicle. **B**, A mechanically assisted manual system. **C**, An electrically assisted controller and interface. (Courtesy Creative Controls, Inc.)

devices attach directly to the steering wheel or to a bar that stretches across the inside diameter of the wheel and is attached to each side of the steering wheel. Steering devices (shown clockwise in Figure 10-25) include palm grip, tri-pin, fork-grip or V-grip, spinner knob, and amputee ring (for use with prosthetic hooks). Each steering device is intended to meet a specific user need. Additional modifications for steering may include a reduced-effort or zero-effort steering mechanism, a steering wheel of reduced diameter, height and angle adjustments to the steering column, and reduced gain (the number of turns of the steering wheel required to pivot the wheels from fully left to fully right). Reduced- or low-effort steering systems reduce the effort required for steering a vehicle by 40%, whereas zero-effort systems are able to reduce the effort required by 70% (Peterson, 1996). As described above, a joystick can also be used for steering, whereby moving the joystick left or right steers the vehicle.

**Secondary driving controls.** In addition to the controls necessary to maneuver the vehicle, **secondary driving controls** are needed for safe operation of a vehicle. These include turn signals, parking brakes, lights, horn, turning on the ignition, temperature control (heat and air conditioning), and windshield wipers. Surveys to prioritize secondary controls identified the horn and turn signal as the two most important (Roush and Koppa, 1992). The knobs for operating secondary controls may not be within reach of the driver or may be of such a shape that the driver cannot operate

them (Enders and Hall, 1990). These knobs can be adapted by adding extensions or a differently shaped control or by relocating them so the driver can use them. A control panel that contains all these functions can also replace the standard controls. This panel is a special-purpose membrane keyboard that interfaces through a microcomputer to activate the secondary functions. It is mounted to either side of the steering wheel in a location that is within reach of the driver.

## ■ SUMMARY

Mobility is very important for participation in self-care, home, work, school, and leisure activities. Mobility needs for individuals with disabilities vary depending on the age and the disability status of the user. In this chapter we describe the general characteristics of personal mobility systems and the various types of mobility devices available to meet individual needs of the user. Personal mobility devices fall under the categories of independent manual, dependent manual, and powered mobility. Transportation and driving is another area considered for individuals with mobility impairments. An evaluation of this area includes the type of vehicle that suits the person's needs (sedan, full-size, or minivan), entry into and exit out of the vehicle, and wheelchair tie-downs or occupant restraints for safety during transportation. The individual also needs to be evaluated for his ability to drive and the need for vehicle modifications and primary and secondary driving controls.

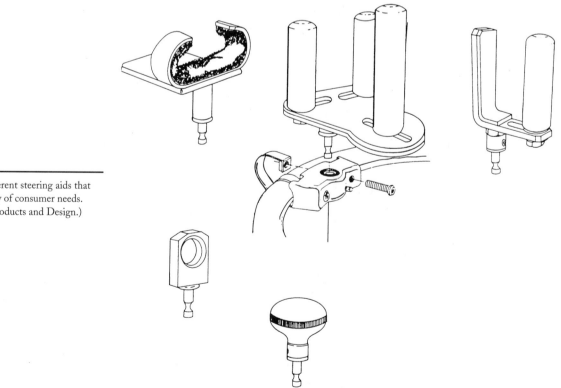

**Figure 10-25** Different steering aids that accommodate a variety of consumer needs. (Courtesy Mobility Products and Design.)

## Study Questions

1. Based on consumer needs, what are the three categories of mobility bases?
2. What factors are considered as part of a wheelchair evaluation?
3. In what situations may powered mobility be considered?
4. What are the two major structures of a wheelchair?
5. List three differences between conventional and ultra-light wheelchairs.
6. Discuss the relative advantages and disadvantages of the folding and box or rigid frame designs for wheelchairs.
7. Describe the advantages and disadvantages of reclining systems. What design features are included to minimize the disadvantages?
8. What are the four types of pivoting mechanisms used in tilt-in-space systems? What are the advantages and disadvantages of each?
9. What are the major reasons for using tilt-in-space? Compare these systems with recliners. When is each indicated?
10. What are the ways in which pediatric wheelchairs can accommodate growth?
11. List the four types of standing systems and give an advantage and disadvantage of each. What are the major benefits of these systems?
12. Describe the major considerations in choosing manual wheelchair tires, wheels, and casters. List the major options available for each.
13. What are the types of drives used in power wheelchairs? How do they differ?
14. What types of control interface are typically used for powered wheelchairs?
15. Delineate the major functions of a wheelchair controller. What additional features do computer-controlled units provide?
16. What special considerations are important in considering the inclusion of ventilators on a wheelchair?
17. What types of batteries are used in powered wheelchairs? How do they differ from automobile batteries? What is the difference between wet cell and gel batteries?
18. Why are wheelchair standards important? Name three major elements covered in the wheelchair standards.
19. Describe what should happen during the implementation phase for a powered mobility device.
20. List the major steps in a driver evaluation. What is the role of simulation in these evaluations?
21. What are the major modifications necessary for an individual to drive an automobile? to drive a van?
22. What measures should be taken to ensure safety of a wheelchair passenger during transportation in a motor vehicle?
23. Describe the design principles employed in restraint to ensure occupant safety in a vehicle.
24. List the major types of van lifts for wheelchairs. What are the advantages and disadvantages of each?
25. What are primary and secondary vehicle controls?
26. How are primary mechanical hand controls designed and operated? What are the major types?

## References

Aylor J et al: Versatile wheelchair control system, *Med Biol Eng Comput* 17:110-114, 1979.

Axelson P et al: The manual wheelchair training guide, Santa Cruz, Calif, 1998, Pax Press.

Babirad J: Considerations in seating and positioning severely disabled drivers, *Assist Technol* 1:31-37, 1989.

Barnes KH: Training young children for powered mobility, *Developmental Disabilities Special Interest Section Newsletter* 14(2), 1991.

Behrman AL: Factors in functional assessment, *J Rehabil Res Dev Clin Suppl* (2):17-30, 1990.

Bergen AF, Presperin J, Tallman T: *Positioning for function: wheelchairs and other assistive technologies*, Vallhalla, NY, 1990, Valhalla Rehabilitation Publications.

Briskorn CN: Composing the composite, *Team Rehabil Rep* 5(2):35-39, 1994.

Bryant L: Wheelchair standards ready to roll, *Team Rehabil Rep* 2(3):44-45, 1991.

Butler C: Effects of powered wheelchair mobility on self-initiative behaviors to two- and three-year-old children with neuromusculoskeletal disorders. In Trefler E, Kozole K, Snell E, editors: *Selected readings on powered mobility for children and adults with severe physical disabilities*, Washington, DC, 1986, RESNA Press.

Butler C: Wheelchair toddlers. In Furumasu J, editor: *Pediatric powered mobility: developmental perspectives, technical issues, clinical approaches*, Arlington, Va, 1997, RESNA Press.

Cooper RA: *Wheelchair selection and configuration*, New York, 1998, Demos Medical Publishing.

Deitz JC: Pediatric augmented mobility. In Gray DB, Quatrano LA, Lieberman ML, editors: *Designing and using assistive technology: the human perspective*, Baltimore, 1998, Paul H Brookes.

Enders A, Hall M, editors: *Assistive technology sourcebook*, Washington, DC, 1990, RESNA Press.

Fields CD: Finding comfort in recliners: sorting through the options, *Team Rehabil Rep* 2(6):27-28, 60, 1991a.

Fields CD: Getting centered with tilt-in-space, *Team Rehabil Rep* 2(5):22-27, 1991b.

Fields CD: Groundwork: tires, *Team Rehabil Rep* 2(6):23-24, 1991c.

Fields CD: Finding comfort in recliners: looking at power, *Team Rehabil Rep* 3(1):34-36, 1992a.

Fields CD: Living with tilt-in-space, *Team Rehabil Rep* 3(4):25-27, 1992b.

Fields CD: Groundwork: casters, *Team Rehabil Rep* 3(2):22-23, 33, 1992c.

Fields CD: Groundwork: wheels of fortune, *Team Rehabil Rep* 3(1):28-31, 1992d.

Gianutsos R et al: The driving advisement system: a computer-augmented quasi-simulation of the cognitive prerequisites for resumption of driving after brain injury, *Assist Technol* 4:70-86, 1992.

Hale PN, Shipp M: Driver assessment, education and training for the disabled, *Proc 10th Annu RESNA Conf,* pp 65-67, June 1987.

Ham R, Aldersea P, Porter D: *Wheelchair users and postural seating: a clinical approach,* New York, 1998, Churchill Livingstone.

Hobson DA: Seating and mobility for the severely disabled. In Smith RV, Leslie JH, editors: *Rehabilitation engineering,* Boca Raton, Fla, 1990, CRC Press.

Hunt JT: Standing tall, *Team Rehabil Rep* 4(6):17-20, 1993.

Janeschild M: Early power mobility: evaluation and training guidelines. In Furumasu J, editor: *Pediatric powered mobility: developmental perspectives, technical issues, clinical approaches,* Arlington, Va, 1997, RESNA Press.

Jones CK, Kanyer B: Review of tilt systems, *Proc 8th Int Seat Symp,* pp 85-87, February 1992.

Jones ML, Sanford JA: People with mobility impairments in the United States today and in 2010, *Assist Technol* 8(1):43-53, 1996.

Jones R, Giddens H, Croft D: Assessment and training of brain-damaged drivers, *Am J Occup Ther* 37(11):754-760, 1983.

Kemper K: Strollers: a growing alternative, *Team Rehabil Rep* 4(2):15-19, 1993.

Kermoian R: Locomotor experience facilitates psychological functioning: implications for assistive mobility for young children. In Gray DB, Quatrano LA, Lieberman ML, editors: *Designing and using assistive technology,* Baltimore, 1998, Paul H Brookes.

Lacoste M et al: Identifying elderly wheelchair users' needs: results of a focus group, *Proc RESNA '98 Annu Conf,* pp 158-160, June 1998.

Lange M, Longo M: Dependent mobility systems: annual comparison chart, *Team Rehabil Rep* 10(11):19-23, 1999.

Latson LF: Overview of disabled drivers' evaluation process. In Strano CM, editor: *Physical Disabilities Special Interest Section Newsletter* 10:4, 1987.

Laurence SS: Integrating ventilators with powered mobility, *Team Rehab Rep* 3(7):17-19, 1992.

Lillie SM: Driving with a physical dysfunction. In Pedretti LW, editor: *Occupational therapy: practice skills for physical dysfunction,* St. Louis, 1996, Mosby.

Magnuson S: Annotated bibliography: powered mobility for young children with physical disabilities, *Phys Occup Ther Pediatr* 15:71, 1995.

Minkle J: The power of mobility and recline, *Team Rehabil Rep* 3(6):18-20, 1992.

Morris BO, Sprigle SH, Karg PE: Assessment of transportation technology: survey of consumers. *Proc RESNA Int '92 Conf,* pp 348-350, June 1992.

National Highway Traffic Safety Administration (NHTSA): *Estimating the number of vehicles adapted for use by persons with disabilities,* www.nhtsa.dot.gov/adaptivemotor.html, December 1997, US Department of Transportation.

Perr A: Van lifts, *Team Rehabil Rep* 4(4):49-53, 1993.

Peterson, WA: Transportation. In Galvin JC, Scherer MJ, editors: *Evaluating, selecting and using appropriate assistive technology,* Gaithersburg, Md, 1996, Aspen Publishers.

Pfaff K: Lightweight standards, *Team Rehabil Rep* 4(6):37-39, 1993a.

Pfaff K: Recline and tilt: making the right match, *Team Rehabil Rep* 4(7):23-27, 1993b.

Pfaff K: Sporting wheels, *Team Rehab Rep* 5(5):31-34, 1994.

Quigley FL, DeLisa JA: Assessing the driving potential of cerebral vascular accident patients, *Am J Occup Ther* 37(7):474-478, 1983.

Ragnarsson KT: Prescription considerations and a comparison of conventional and lightweight wheelchairs, *J Rehabil Res Dev Clin Suppl* (2):8-16, 1990.

Reppert P: School zone, *Team Rehabil Rep* 3(8):14-20, 1992.

Roush L, Koppa R: A survey of activation importance of individual secondary controls in modified vehicles, *Assist Technol* 4:66-69, 1992.

Segedy A: A base hit, *Team Rehabil Rep* 9(10):37-38, 1998.

Sprigle S, Thacker J, Shaw G: Setting standards, *Team Rehabil Rep* 4(1):14-19, 1993.

Taylor SJ, Kreutz D: Powered and manual wheelchair mobility. In Angelo J: *Assistive technology for rehabilitation therapists,* Philadelphia, 1997, FA Davis.

Thacker J, Shaw G: Safe and secure, *Team Rehabil Rep* 5(2):26-30, 1994.

Toonstra M, Barnicle K: Focus on scooters, *Team Rehabil Rep* 4(1):24-26, 1993.

Trefler E et al: *Seating and mobility for persons with physical disabilities,* Tucson, Ariz, 1993, Therapy Skill Builders.

Trefler E, Cook H: Powered mobility for children. In Trefler E, Kozole K, Snell E, editors: *Selected readings on powered mobility for children and adults with severe physical disabilities,* Washington, DC, 1986, RESNA Press.

Trefler E, Kozole K, Snell E, editors: *Selected readings on powered mobility for children and adults with severe physical disabilities,* Washington, DC, 1986, RESNA Press.

Trujillo EF: *History of the wheelchair,* ca. 1960, California Wheelchair Athletic Club.

Valois T, Hittenberger L: Traumatic brain injury: who determines safe driving? In Clark D, editor: *Technology review '90: perspectives on occupational therapy practice,* Rockville, Md, 1990, American Occupational Therapy Association.

Walter J, Dunn R: Taking a stand, *Team Rehabil Rep* 9(1):31-34, 1998.

Warren CG: Powered mobility and its implications, *J Rehabil Res Dev Clin Suppl* (2):74-85, 1990.

Wermers J: The sky is not the limit, *Team Rehabil Rep* 2(6):30-31, 1991.

Wilson B, McFarland SR: Types of wheelchairs, *J Rehabil Res Dev Clin Suppl* (2):104-116, 1990.

Woo A: Standing options, *Team Rehabil Report* 3(8):39-44, 1992.

## CHAPTER 11

# Technologies That Aid Manipulation and Control of the Environment

## Objectives

Upon completing this chapter you will be able to:

1. List functional manipulative tasks that can be aided by assistive technologies
2. Describe the operation of electrically powered feeding aids
3. List the features and design properties of electronic page turners
4. List the functions carried out by environmental control systems
5. Describe the basic components of environmental control systems and how they are implemented
6. Discuss the uses of robotic devices in aiding manipulation by persons with disabilities

---

## Key Terms

| | | |
|---|---|---|
| Alternative | General-Purpose Manipulation Devices | Reachers |
| Augmentative | Head Pointers | Remote Control |
| Desktop Robots | Infrared (IR) Transmission | Robotic Systems |
| Electrically Powered Feeders | Mobile Assistive Robots | Special-Purpose Manipulation Devices |
| Electrically Powered Page Turners | Mouthsticks | Telephone Controllers |
| Electronic Aid to Daily Living (EADL) | Programmable Controllers | Trainable Controllers |
| Environmental Control Units (ECUs) | Radio Frequency Transmission | Ultrasonic Transmission |

---

One of the activity outputs described in Chapter 2 (see Figure 2-7) is manipulation. At the most basic level, *manipulation* refers to those activities that we normally accomplish using the upper extremities, particularly the fingers and hand. In using assistive devices, especially those that are electronically controlled, there are many types of "manipulation" required. For example, keys must be pressed for computer entry, joysticks controlled for powered mobility, and switches activated for communication devices. We have discussed this type of manipulation in previous chapters, and we exclude it from the general discussion of manipulation in this chapter. For our purposes in this chapter, manipulation is taken to be the end goal of the person's actions. For example, activities such as hand writing, food preparation, eating, and appliance control depend on manipulation of physical objects, and these types of activities are our focus.

Figure 11-1 is a characterization of assistive technology devices used for manipulation. As in many other areas of assistive technology application, we can provide manipulative aids that are either **alternative** (a different method of doing the same task) or **augmentative** (assistance in doing the task in the same manner as it is normally done). For manipulation, we can also distinguish devices as being either *specific purpose* or *general purpose*. **Special-purpose manipulation devices** are designed for only one task, whereas

**general-purpose manipulation devices** serve two or more manipulative activities. For example, an augmentative, specific-purpose approach to eating may include a modified fork with an enlarged handle. An alternative, special-purpose apparatus for eating is an electromechanical device that lifts food off the plate and up to mouth level when a switch is pressed. A robotic arm is a general-purpose alternative manipulative aid. It can be used for eating, but it also has application in work site manipulation and many other areas. A hand splint that allows gripping of any utensil serves as a general-purpose augmentative aid, since it can be used to hold a fork for eating or a pen for writing. In this chapter we discuss all four categories of manipulation assistive technologies shown in Figure 11-1.

## ◼ LOW-TECHNOLOGY AIDS FOR MANIPULATION

In Chapter 1 we define low-technology aids as inexpensive, simple to make, and easy to obtain. Many manipulative aids fall into the low-technology category. We group these aids into general- and special-purpose devices. Within special-purpose devices, we categorize devices according to the major performance areas of the Human Activity Assistive Technology (HAAT) model: self-care, work or school, and play or leisure. All the examples used in this section are available from mail-order catalogs.* Many of these devices are also available at drugstores and other local sources.

### General-Purpose Aids

To be classified as general purpose, a manipulation aid must serve more than one need. We include three general purpose aids: mouthsticks, head pointers, and reachers. The first two

| | |
|---|---|
| Alternative Specific Purpose | Augmentative Specific Purpose |
| Alternative General Purpose | Augmentative General Purpose |

**Figure 11-1**  Assistive technologies for manipulation can be categorized in two dimensions: general purpose versus specific and alternative versus augmentative.

---

*Suppliers of the aids described in this section include Cleo, Inc., Cleveland, Ohio; Independent Living Aids, Plainview, N.Y.; Maddak, Inc, Pequannock, N.J.; Maxiaids, Farmingdale, N.Y.; Sammons Preston, Bolingbrook, Ill.; Smith and Nephew Rehabilitation Products, Milwaukee, Wisc.

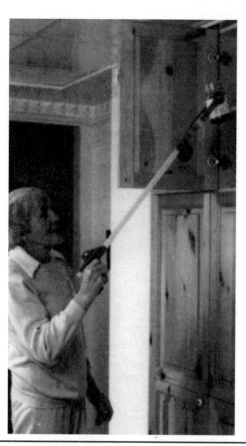

**Figure 11-2**   Mechanical reachers are general purpose devices. (Courtesy TASH, Ajax, Ont., Canada.)

control the jaws of the reacher in order to grasp an object. The grasp required to activate the grip may be of several types: squeeze with the whole hand, pistol grip with all the fingers, or trigger with the index finger. Overall length varies from 24 to 36 inches, and some models fold for ease of carrying. The gripper portion of the reacher may be circular for ease of gripping cans or pincherlike for picking up smaller objects. Rubber or other nonslip materials are often used for reacher grippers. Reachers can be used to manipulate many objects, including food (e.g., cans, packages), cooking utensils (e.g., pans, pots, plates, dishes), office objects (e.g., paper, books, magazines), and recreational or leisure objects (e.g., books, tapes, CDs).

Chen et al (1998) conducted a study of the effectiveness of reachers in meeting the needs of a population of older (over 60) subjects. The characteristics found to be most important were adjustable length, one-handed use, a locking system for the grip to hold objects, support for the forearm, light weight, and a lever trigger action in the grip. Chen et al (1998) also list 38 tasks for which their population uses reachers. These include food preparation, self-care, appliance control, and gardening. Chen et al (1998) also discuss the relative ease of use of reachers for a variety of tasks.

## Special-Purpose Aids

Because special-purpose, low-tech aids are designed for one or two tasks only, they serve those tasks very well. However, because they are so specialized, it may be necessary to have several of these available to meet the demands of self-care, work, and leisure.

Most special-purpose adaptations of products involve one of four things: (1) lengthening a handle or reducing the reach required, (2) modifying the handle of a utensil for easier grasping or manipulation, (3) converting two-handed tasks to one-handed ones, and (4) amplifying the force that a consumer can generate with her hands. A variety of modified handles are shown in Figure 11-3. These include enlarged grips for easier grasping, cuffs that hold a utensil and circle the fingers, angled handles for ease of scooping (for people with limited wrist movement), swivel handles that allow the end to be oriented differently for different positions in space (e.g., on a table or near the mouth), and handles requiring limited grasp (often called "quad handles").

**Self-care.**   Self-care includes aids for assistance in several areas: food consumption, food preparation, dressing, and hygiene. Examples of food preparation adaptations include one-handed holders for can and jar opening, brushes with suction cups for one-handed scrubbing of vegetables, bowls with suction cup bottoms for stability while stirring with one hand, bowl and pan holders (some of which tilt for pouring), and cutting boards that stabilize food during

of these are often used as control enhancers in conjunction with control interfaces. In Chapter 7, head pointers and mouthsticks are discussed in detail, including their use as control enhancers for activating control interfaces. Both **mouthsticks** and **head pointers** are also used for direct manipulation. Turning pages is often accomplished with a mouthstick or head pointer used in conjunction with a book or magazine mounted on a simple stand. A ballpoint pen tip or a pencil can also be attached to a mouthstick for writing. Additional attachments include a pincher that is opened or closed by tongue action and a suction cup end that can be used to grip objects (e.g., a page) by sucking on the end of the mouthstick. Many tasks require sliding objects (e.g., paper, pens) around on a desk or table. Both mouthsticks and head pointers can be used for this task. Mouthsticks or head pointers can also be used for such functions as dialing a telephone, typing, and turning lights on and off.

Many individuals need to extend their physical range. Often the need for extended range is a result of being seated in a wheelchair and wanting to reach an object on a counter or in a cabinet. In other cases it is a need to reach an object on the floor when bending is difficult or stability is poor. In all these cases, **reachers** can be useful. As shown in Figure 11-2, a reacher consists of a handle grip that is used to

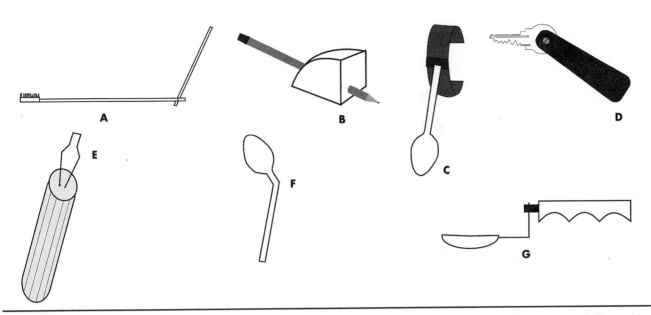

**Figure 11-3**    Types of handles used on low-tech manipulative aids. **A,** Brush with extended handle. **B,** Enlarged grip for pencil or pen. **C,** Spoon with cuff. **D,** Key holder with quad grip. **E,** Buttoner with enlarged handle. **F,** Spoon with bent handle for scooping. **G,** Spoon with swivel handle.

cutting. Modified handles are available for knives and serving spoons, as well as for other utensils.

Food consumption aids include a variety of utensils with modified handles (knives, forks, spoons, and combinations called "sporks"). Modifications to plates include suction cups for stability, enlarged rims that make it easier to scoop food onto a utensil, and removable rims that attach to any plate. Drinking aids include cups with caps and "snorkel" lids through which fluid can be sucked; nose cutouts that allow drinking to occur without tipping the head back; double-handled cups for two-handed use; and cups modified at the bottom with a quad grasp to allow lifting and tipping with limited hand function.

Dressing aids designed to compensate for poor fine motor control include adapted button hooks for single-handed buttoning and zipper pulls. These are available with enlarged, suction, and quad grip handles. For limited reach, there are aids for pulling on socks and pantyhose, long-handled shoe horn, and trouser pulls. A variety of dressing aids are shown in Figure 11-4.

Areas of hygiene that can be aided by special-purpose devices include: hair combing and brushing, tooth brushing, shaving, bathing, and toileting. Hairbrushes and combs may have any or all of the following adaptations: modified handles of all types, extended handle lengths, and angled ends (where the comb or brush attaches). Modified toothbrushes have enlarged, quad, and offset handles. Toothpaste and shaving cream containers can be adapted with a simple device that allows one-handed dispensing of the product. For shaving, there are holders with adapted handles for both electric and manual razors. For bathing, there are long-handled sponges, curved handle brushes for washing the back, and holders for sponges or washcloths that accommodate limited grasping ability.

Other self-care items are intended for use in the home. For example, there are gripping cuffs that are used with brooms and mops, extended handles on household items such as dustpans and dusters, and key holders.

**Work and school.** Throughout this book we have described assistive technologies that aid consumers in accomplishing work- and school-related tasks (e.g., computers, augmentative communication devices). In this section we discuss low-tech aids that specifically help work and school in the areas of writing and reading.

Handwriting is a major need in work and school environments. Special-purpose manipulative aids that assist handwriting focus on one of two problems: holding the pen or pencil and holding the paper. Some consumers lack the ability to grip a standard pen or pencil. Low-tech approaches to this problem include modified grippers that attach to the hand and clamp to the pen or pencil; wire, wooden, or plastic holders that support the pen or pencil off the paper and allow it to slide across the paper; weighted pens (with variable amounts of weight) that help reduce problems associated with tremor; and pens with enlarged bodies to make them easier to grasp. There are several different designs for holding paper in place for one-handed writing. Generally the paper is held to a plate using either clips or a magnet (in this case the plate is steel). Desks can also be modified using a rotating "lazy Susan" approach in which the top of the desk is rotated to bring items within reach. File folders are often modified for easier grasping by putting hooks or loops on them. The loop or hook protrudes

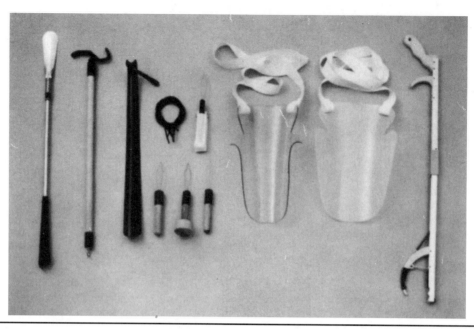

**Figure 11-4**　A variety of dressing aids. *Left to right:* Long-handled shoe horn, dressing stick, plastic shoehorn, elastic shoe laces, button hooks (4), stocking aids (2), and reacher. (Courtesy TASH, Ajax, Ont., Canada.)

above the folder so that it can be grasped more easily. High-tech aids for writing are discussed in Chapter 9, and additional work-related assistive technology applications are described in Chapter 14.

There are also low-tech reading aids. Book holders provide support for the reading material so the consumer does not have to hold it. Page turning is done either by hand or with a head pointer or mouthstick. In the next section we discuss electrically powered page turners that aid reading.

**Play and leisure.** As with other types of manipulative aids, lack of grasping ability in recreational or leisure aids is generally accommodated for by altering the type of handle. Recreation and leisure examples include cameras with modified shutter release, modified grip scissors, modified handles on garden tools, and modified grasping cuffs for pool cues, racquets, or paddles. A person with limited manipulation strength can fly a kite by adding special wrist or hand cuffs for holding the string. An adapted pinball machine that allows control via a variety of control interfaces is commercially available.* The paddles can be controlled by puff-and-sip or any other switches. This makes it possible for a consumer to compete in a fast-paced, interesting game.

One example of a holder is a gooseneck arm attached at one end to a table clamp. At the other end is a bracket that holds an embroidery frame. Using this device, an individual can embroider, crochet, or mend using only one hand. Other examples of devices designed for one-handed assistance are playing card holders, knitting needle holders, and

card shufflers. For individuals with limited two-hand function, there are handheld playing card holders.

Devices that aid lack of reaching ability include a mobile bridge for holding the end of a pool cue off the table (a small bracket with wheels to allow positioning of the pool cue) and ramps for use while bowling (the ball is placed at the top of the ramp and the user releases it after aiming the ramp toward the pins). Lange (1998) describes a variety of options for reading when manipulation of the material is difficult.

## ■ SPECIAL-PURPOSE ELECTROMECHANICAL AIDS FOR MANIPULATION

There are two primary manipulative tasks for which electromechanical devices have been specifically designed and for which there are commercially available products: (1) feeding and (2) page turning. We discuss these special-purpose alternative manipulation devices in this section.

### Electrically Powered Feeders

One area of human activity in which independence is highly desirable is eating. Anyone who has been unable to feed himself (even for a brief period) knows the frustration of looking at one type of food on the plate and being fed another (e.g., expecting peas and getting potatoes). Being fed by another person can also create a feeling of dependency, and lack of independence in eating is often equated with childlike behavior. None of these stereotypes is accurate, and most persons who are fed by an attendant maintain

---

*Silverthorn Group, Brinklow, Md.

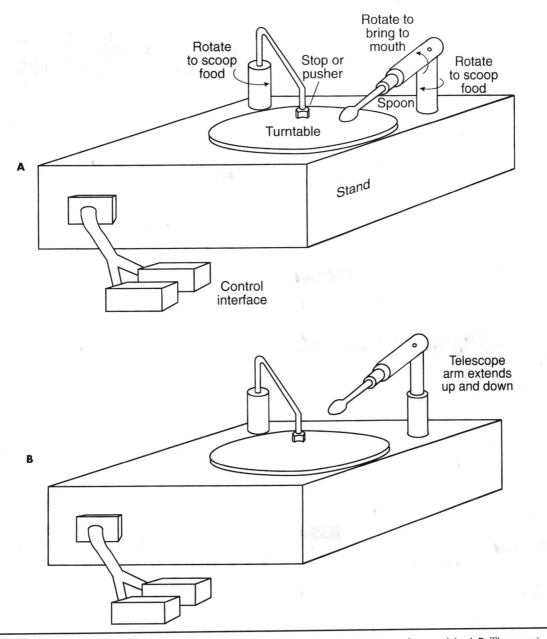

Figure 11-5   Two types of electromechanical feeders. **A,** The spoon is attached to a lever arm that is moved to mouth level. **B,** The spoon is attached to a telescoping arm that moves it to mouth level.

control over the situation through direction of the attendant's actions. Nevertheless, many people would prefer to feed themselves if it were possible. Electromechanical feeders make this an option even for individuals who have very little motor control.

Use of an automatic feeder requires that the individual be able to control two separate functions. The first of these is location of the particular type of food that is to be eaten, and the second is picking up the food and moving it to mouth level. Currently available feeders require that the human operator be able to take food off a spoon, chew it, and swallow it safely. These requirements eliminate a large number of persons, but there are many who only lack the

ability to pick up the food and get it to their mouths. It is this group for whom feeders are most beneficial.

Generic electromechanical feeders are shown in Figure 11-5. The first task of feeders, that of locating the desired type of food, is typically accomplished by placing the plate on a turntable whose rotation is under the control of the user. The user is able to stop the rotation when the desired food is properly positioned. The second action, moving the food to mouth level, is typically accomplished by a spoon attached to an arm whose height above the plate is variable. Two types of arms are used: (1) two-piece articulating and (2) telescoping. The articulating arm is capable of carrying greater weights and can position the spoon in more locations. The telescoping arm collapses into a smaller stored length and can be easier for transportation. Picking up the food is a process of scooping the food onto the spoon. One of two approaches can be used: moving the spoon against a fixed stop or moving a pusher against a fixed spoon (see Figure 11-5). For either of these approaches, both the spoon and the plate can be removed and washed with other dishes.

In order to control the feeder, the user must activate either one or two switches. The two-switch approach typically has one switch for plate rotation and one to scrape the food onto the spoon and raise and lower the spoon. In the one-switch version, activating the switch one time causes the plate to rotate; a second activation causes a complete cycle of pushing food onto the spoon and raising it to mouth level. Any single or dual switch described in Chapter 7 can be used.

The most commonly available feeder is the Winsford Feeder,* which is also marketed by several mail order equipment companies.† This feeder has rechargeable batteries that are used to power it at many different settings. It has an adjustable height base that can accommodate varying spoon height requirements. A two-switch mode of operation is used, with one switch rotating the plate and the other scooping the food onto the spoon and elevating it to mouth level. A chin-activated dual switch is mounted on a long, solid wire. When it is pushed in one direction, plate rotation occurs, and when it is pushed in the opposite direction, food is pushed onto the spoon and elevated to mouth level. A two-position rocking switch is also commonly used with the Winsford Feeder. Other dual switches or two single switches may be adapted to work with this feeder. There is also a carrying case available for transportation of the feeder.

Another commercially available feeder is the Beeson Automaddak Feeder.‡ This feeder is powered by a 110-volt line. It is operated by two switches, one for plate rotation and the other for spoon control. In contrast to the Winsford Feeder, each switch must be held down to continue action; that is, the spoon elevation stops if the spoon switch is released.

A robotic system specially designed for feeding is the Handy 1 (Topping, 1996). The Handy 1 uses a series of seven columns or compartments on a tray. When it is activated, the Handy 1 scans through the tray, illuminating a light behind each column in succession. The user activates a single switch to choose the column, and the food in that column is bought to the mouth. An eighth light allows the user to access a cup for drinking at any time during the meal. More than 100 individuals have benefited from the use of the Handy 1 on a regular basis (Topping, 1996).

Harwin, Rahman, and Foulds (1995) compare the

Handy 1 and Winsford Feeder. They point out that the Winsford Feeder has only two degrees of freedom, whereas the Handy 1 has five. This increases the flexibility of the Handy 1 in dealing with the task of feeding, and it also allows it to perform some other tasks of daily living (e.g., self-care). The interface requirements of the Handy 1 are also more flexible than those for the Winsford Feeder. For example, the location where the food is to be transferred into the person's mouth can be changed. However, the Winsford Feeder is considerably less expensive than the Handy 1. This illustrates the tradeoff between flexibility and complexity (and hence cost) discussed earlier.

All these feeders require that the food be prepared in bite-sized portions for the user. It is also sometimes difficult to eat certain foods such as soups and those composed of small pieces (e.g., rice, peas). Because of the necessity for assistance from a human aide or attendant, independence is reduced. However, the user is able to complete the eating activity independently, and this can save attendant time (and cost), as well as improve the user's sense of independence and control. Recall that the HAAT model discussed in Chapter 2 includes both an activity (in this case eating) and a context (defining the environment where the activity takes place). Each of the three types of context shown in Figure 2-6 affects the use of feeders. The physical context (heat, light, sound, moisture) can affect both the user and the assistive technology (electromechanical feeder). The feeder may be used in any of the settings shown in Figure 2-6 (e.g., home, school, work, community). Some devices are battery operated and portable, allowing a variety of settings to be used. The primary safety considerations with feeders are mechanical injury from the spoon hitting the face and embarrassment caused by food falling off the spoon or plate. These devices can be messy to use and difficult to transport, and this may cause some people to restrict their use to home and to rely on a human attendant in the community.

Even though they serve a restricted need and can be used by only a specific segment of persons with disabilities, **electrically powered feeders** can play an important role in increasing independence for persons whose motor limitations prevent them from using standard eating utensils.

## Electrically Powered Page Turners

Access to books, magazines, and other reading material is important for the acquisition of information for school, work, or leisure. There are many individuals with disabilities who are able to read, but who cannot physically manipulate the pages of the reading material. There are several approaches that can be used to assist these individuals. A book holder and mouthstick (see the section on low-tech aids in this chapter) allow independence in page turning for some persons. The major limitation of this approach is the

---

*Winsford Products, Pennington, N.J.
†For example, Sammons Preston, Bolingbrook, Ill.
‡Maddak, Inc., Pequannock, N.J.

requirement that the book be set up by an aide and properly positioned for both visual and physical access. This method also requires a high degree of head control and the ability to hold a mouthstick. A mechanical head pointer eliminates the last requirement, but there are still limitations of access.

Talking books, such as those made available for the blind, can also provide an alternative to physically manipulating pages. These are discussed in Chapter 12. Using a simple environmental control unit, a person with physical limitations can control the tape recorder and obtain access to the talking book at her own speed. Another approach is the use of books on computer disks. These can be loaded into a word processor, and the person needing access can use standard computer adaptations to turn the pages, scan through the material, find key words, and so on. This approach is also used by persons who have low vision or are blind, and we discuss it in Chapter 12. Both talking books

and computer-based reading suffer from the limitation that not all reading material is available in these formats.

An alternative to all these methods is the use of a human attendant to turn the pages. Because the turning of a page occurs every few minutes, this is not practical for any large amount of reading. The limitations in all these approaches have led to the development of **electrically powered page turners.**

From a manipulative point of view, page turning requires two primary actions: (1) separating the page to be turned from the other pages and (2) physically moving the page from one side to the other (forward or backward). Additional useful but not essential features include scanning a number of pages, turning to a specific page, and locating a bookmark and turning to that page. Currently available page turners employ one of two methods to accomplish the first task of separating pages. Some devices use a vacuum pump

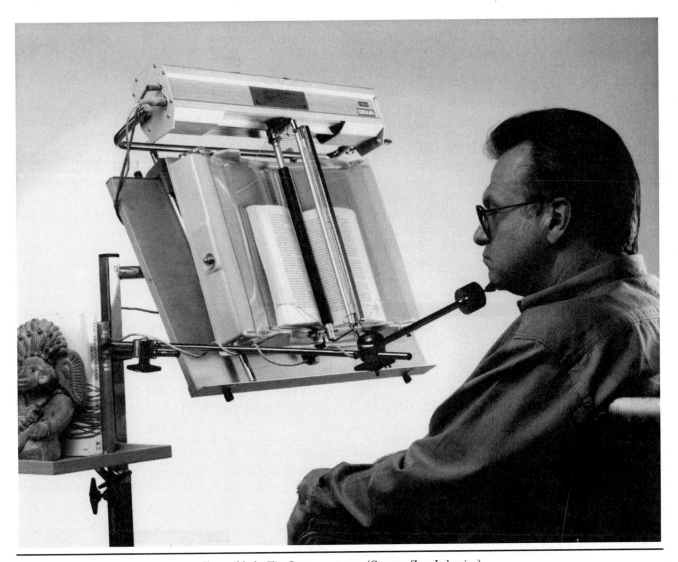

Figure 11-6    The Gewa page turner. (Courtesy Zygo Industries.)

that sucks the first page up and holds it away from the remaining pages. Other devices use a sticky roller that is placed on top of the page. When it rotates, the roller causes one page to be separated from the others. The roller may employ putty, rubber gum (like a pencil eraser), or double-sided tape. This function is the most difficult for page turners, and its success for any page turner is a major indicator of the quality of the unit. Because reading materials differ widely in size, binding (e.g., uniform, spiral, loose leaf), and paper types (e.g., rough, slick, newsprint), it is important to evaluate any individual page turner with reading materials that vary in size, paper type, and binding style.

Once the page to be turned is successfully isolated, the page turner must move it to the opposite side of the book or magazine. The Gewa page turner* (Figure 11-6) uses a rotating roller to separate pages from each other and then moves the entire roller from one side of the book or magazine to the other after the page has been separated. The standard control for the Gewa is a four-direction joystick. Two joystick directions cause roller rotation either clockwise or counterclockwise, and the other two cause the roller to move forward or backward. Any other four-switch control interface can also be used. An additional accessory for the Gewa is a scanning selection method in which a single switch is used to select one of the four control functions as they are presented in sequence. The display of functions consists of small LED indicators, each labeled function corresponding to one joystick direction.

Other page turners have different mechanisms. The Touch Turner† uses a rubber-coated wheel to separate the pages, and then a rotating semicircular disk pushes the separated page from one side to the other. As the disk rotates, the page is moved forward or backward, depending on the direction of rotation of the disk. The Touch Turner has both one-direction and two-direction models for standard books and a special model for paperback books and magazines. Vacuum-based systems often move the vacuum unit from side to side. The Deluxe Automatic Page Turner‡ uses a silicon-tipped arm that moves across the page to separate it and move it to the left. A thin wire loop follows behind the arm to hold the page in place.

## ■ ELECTRONIC AIDS TO DAILY LIVING

Many objects that need to be manipulated are electrically powered devices such as appliances (e.g., television, room lights, fans, kitchen appliances such as blenders or food processors) and others that can be modified by adding electrically powered control to them (e.g., door openers, drapery controls). The majority of these electrical appliances and controls are powered from standard house wiring (110-volt AC in North America). The assistive devices used to control them are called **environmental control units (ECUs)**.

It has recently been proposed that the term **electronic aid to daily living (EADL)** be substituted for *ECU* (MacNeil, 1998). The EADL terminology more accurately reflects the functional result of the device (daily living tasks), rather than emphasizing the things to be controlled, as in the term *ECU*. *Environmental control* also is used to refer to heating and cooling systems for buildings, which adds to the confusion of the ECU terminology. Finally, it is argued that the use of the term *EADL system* will bring greater recognition to those practitioners who recommend and select them for consumers, resulting in increased funding levels for the devices. We have chosen to use the EADL terminology because it is becoming more widely used.

Figure 11-7 shows the major parts of an EADL. The user interacts with the EADL through a control interface (see Chapter 7). Feedback to the user is provided through a display that reflects the action being controlled (e.g., which appliance is to be activated, status of the system). The control interface and user display constitute the *human/ technology interface,* and they are connected to the rest of the system and to each other by a block labeled *selection method.* Likewise, the appliances to be controlled are connected to the selection method through an *output distribution block.* The selection method and output distribution functions together make up the *processor.* In some cases the human/ technology interface and the selection method are provided through an augmentative and alternative communication (AAC) device (see Chapter 9) or a computer (see Chapter 8) via a serial input. This can reduce the number of devices and also provides an identical user interface for both AAC and EADL functions. Some AAC devices also include the output distribution component. This component is connected to either a remote (wireless) linkage or a hard-wired connection or both; it produces an *activity output* by turning on and controlling the appliances. MacNeil (1998) also lists a variety of EADLs in chart form.

Some devices or appliances require on-off control. Normally this is achieved by a switch that is pressed to activate the device. An example of this type of control is that used in many remote garage door openers. These devices are often used by persons with disabilities to open other doors (e.g., house or apartment). This may require either that the switch on the garage door opener be adapted or that the entire function be incorporated into the EADL. There are two switch outputs available on most EADLs: (1) momentary and (2) latched. A momentary switch closure is active only as long as the switch is pressed. In the case of the ECU, this

---

*In North America, distributed by Zygo Industries, Portland, Ore.
†Touch Turner Company, Everett, Wash.
‡Sammons Preston, Bolingbrook, Ill.

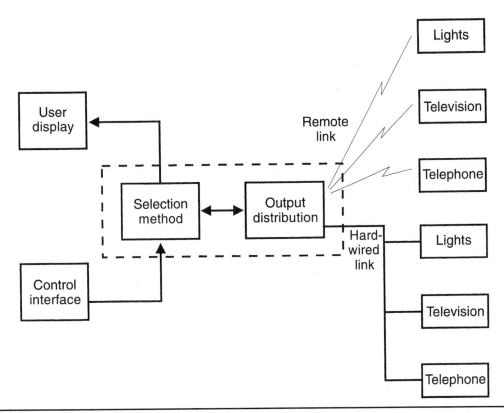

**Figure 11-7** The major parts of an electronic aid to daily living. The *control interface* and *user display* constitute the human/technology interface. The components within the dotted box are the processor. The appliances listed on the right side of the figure are the activity output.

output remains active only as long as the control interface is activated (e.g., a switch is pressed). The momentary output mode is useful for continuous functions such as closing draperies. The output can be sustained as long as the person desires it to be (e.g., to open drapes half way). In the latched mode a switch closure is turned on by the first activation and off by the next activation, and it toggles between these two states with each activation. This can be useful when turning on an appliance such as a light or radio.

## Selection Methods

In Chapter 7 we define several selection methods used for control of assistive technology devices. These include direct selection, scanning, directed scanning, and coded access. Each of these can be used in EADLs. Direct selection occurs when the user of the system can choose any output directly. For example, an EADL for controlling a room light, a fan, and a radio on-off control may have one control interface (possibly a key on a small keyboard or speech recognition) for each of the three functions (Figure 11-8). If the same three-unit system is to be operated via scanning access, then the keyboard can be replaced by a scanning panel and each of the three items to be controlled can have a light corresponding to it. When the light of the device to be

activated comes on, the user activates a control interface to select that item. Finally, a code such as Morse code (see Chapter 7) can be used for one of the four output devices. The user then enters a series of dots and dashes corresponding to the numerical code required to activate the desired appliance. Each of these selection systems is used in current EADLs, and some EADLs have multiple options available. We discuss specific selection methods in the remainder of this section. Choice of a control interface for use with an ECU is based on the considerations presented in Chapter 7. Some control interfaces (e.g., speech recognition,* single switch) are commonly used with EADLs.

## Control Functions Implemented by EADLs

In Chapter 7 we define the input domain for the control interface as either discrete or continuous. The most common type used in EADLs is *discrete control*, in which a device is either turned on or off or set to a specific value by activation of the EADL. Examples of on/off control include

---

*For example, Simplicity Voice/Plus and All in one Plus, Quartet Technology, Inc., Tyngsboro, Mass.; Butler in a Box, AVSI, Los Alamitos, Calif.; Nemo, Madenta, Edmonton, Canada; Sicare Pilot, TASH, Ajax, Ont., Canada.

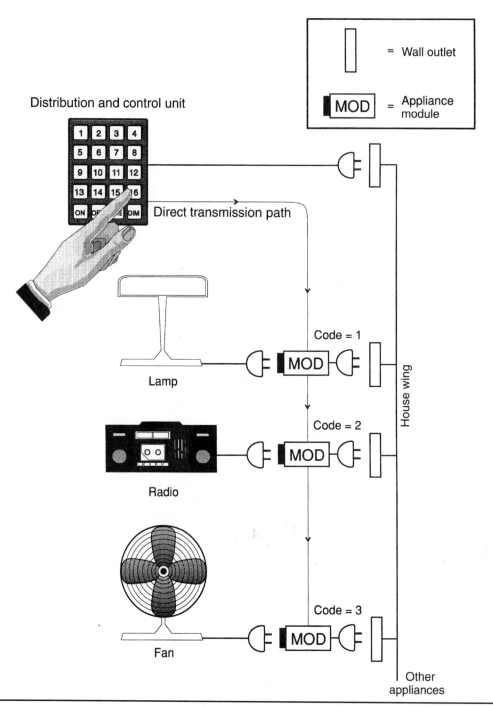

**Figure 11-8** A direct-selection EADL. Each appliance has a numeric code, and the keypad is used to select the appropriate module. Control functions such as ON, OFF, and DIM are also activated by pressing the proper key on the keypad. This figure also illustrates the use of house wiring for distribution of the control signals to the appliance modules.

lights, television, or radio controls and starting or stopping a blender. Other EADL applications require setting a value. For example, a telephone dialer may have several stored numbers that need to be selected. Each number is a discrete entry, and its selection produces a different result. Television channel selection is another example of discrete control. The other type of control function, employed in EADLs, is continuous. *Continuous control* results in successively greater or smaller degrees of output. Examples of EADL continuous control are opening and closing draperies, controlling volume on a television or radio, and dimming or brightening lights.

## Transmission Methods

All EADL systems must transmit a signal to the appliance to be controlled. There are several methods used for this transmission. Although it is theoretically possible to connect all the appliances to be controlled directly to the rest of the EADL via wires, this is not practical. Direct wiring requires that the controlled devices to be physically close together or necessitates the installation of special wiring just for the EADL. More cost-effective and practical methods utilize some form of remote control. We use the term **remote control** to mean the absence of a physical attachment among the various components shown in Figure 11-7. In general the link between the output distribution and the devices to be controlled is remote. However, it is also possible to have remote links between the control interface and the processor.

**House wiring.** One way to interconnect appliances and the output distribution function is to use the house AC wiring as a communication channel. Digital control signals are transmitted over the house wiring from the distribution control device to individual appliance modules, which are plugged into the standard electrical outlet (see Ciarcia, 1980, for a description of the operational details of these units). Figure 11-8 shows how this approach works. The distribution and control unit is also plugged into a wall outlet. This unit has a transmitter that sends out two codes over the house wiring. The first code identifies the device to be controlled, and the second selects the function to be performed (e.g., turn on or off, dim or brighten a light). Each appliance to be controlled is plugged into a module, which is then plugged into the wall. Each module contains a receiver that can interpret the codes sent out by the distribution and control unit. Most commercial systems have selector switches on the appliance modules to allow them to be set for a code from 0 to 15. In addition, both the distribution and control unit and the appliance modules can have one of 16 different "house" codes that allow two or more such systems to operate on the same wiring system. The combination of house codes and device numbers yields 256 possible controlled devices (16 × 16). Although this may seem like a large number, it can be useful to have more than a few choices, especially when the control is via computer-based software rather than manual selection of keys on the distribution and control unit. This type of appliance control was designed for use by the general population, and it is common and inexpensive. Devices are available at many consumer electronic stores.* For individuals who are able to press the buttons on the control unit, this type of device can become a relatively complete EADL. However, only binary control functions are available, and such functions as channel selection (quantitative) or volume control (discrete)

require more specialized systems. The major advantage of house wiring transmission is the lack of installation costs, since existing wiring is used (Mills, 1987). Disadvantages include (1) the lack of privacy, (2) possible interference between systems on the same electrical power system (e.g., in an apartment building), (3) the inability to use transmission when multiple circuits are used for the wiring system and, (4) the lack of portability. Multiple circuits are often used in house and commercial wiring. Each circuit has a separate circuit breaker, and they are physically separate from each other. This means that a module connected to one circuit does not receive the control signals from a transmitter connected to a different circuit.

**Ultrasound transmission.** A second type of transmission employed between the control and distribution unit and the appliances to be controlled is ultrasonic. This type of transmission uses sound waves that are too high in frequency to be heard by the human ear. In general, that is any signal over 20,000 Hz, but in practice, signals of approximately 40,000 Hz are used. These signals are transmitted through the air to a receiver located up to several hundred feet from the transmitter. Because ultrasound waves are mechanical energy, they can be blocked by solid objects (including human tissue), and it is important to have a clear path between the transmitter and the receiver. **Ultrasonic transmission** devices* often consist of a transmitter unit, which is either handheld or mounted on a wheelchair, and a set of receivers, one for each appliance to be controlled (Figure 11-9). A latched mode is typically employed. Various selection methods, including scanning and coded access, are available for these devices. The principle of operation is slightly different from house wiring-based systems. Each receiver has a code, and the transmitter sends a signal that corresponds to this code. When the transmitted code is received, the receiver is latched, which turns the appliance either on or off, depending on its state when the signal is received. Each appliance must have its own code, and most ultrasonic devices have a limited number of channels (generally four or eight).

Ultrasonic transmission is also used for some remote television controls. In this application, transmission of various codes is used for all basic television functions, such as on/off, channel change, volume control, and picture adjustments. Another use of ultrasound transmission is illustrated in Figure 11-10. In this case the coupling between the control interface and the distribution and control unit is via ultrasonic transmission. This remote coupling enables the user to be more mobile than when the control interface is hard wired to the distribution and control unit.

The major advantage of ultrasonic transmission is that it

---

*For example, the X-10 Powerhouse System, Northvale, N.J.

*For example, the Ultra Four, TASH, Ajax, Ont., Canada (www. tashinc.com).

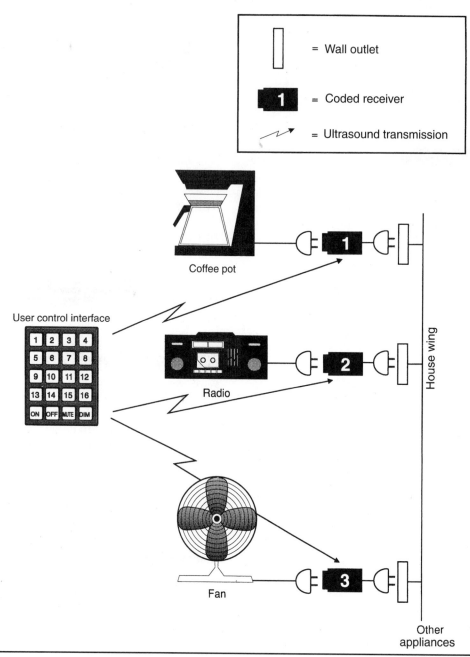

Figure 11-9    An EADL system employing ultrasound transmission to discrete modules. Each module receives its signal directly from the transmitter.

is highly portable, since it is easy to unplug the receiver modules and move them to a new location. The major disadvantages are the necessity to have the transmitter and receiver in the same room and to avoid obstacles between the transmitter and receiver that might block the signal.

**Infrared transmission.** Another mode is based on the use of invisible **infrared (IR) transmission** as the medium. This method is the most common in the control of home electronics (e.g., television set, cable television, VCR, CD player, audio cassette player). Infrared remote controls

are used for binary (latched and momentary), discrete, continuous, and quantitative types of control. The VCR functions of FAST FORWARD, SEARCH, and so on can also be controlled with an IR remote controller. Generally each remote device has a set of unique codes, and a remote unit manufactured by one company cannot be used with a television set manufactured by someone else. This means that several remote controllers may be necessary to manage TV, cable, and other devices, unless a "universal remote" is programmed to control all these appliances.

Infrared remote control is also used in EADLs. The

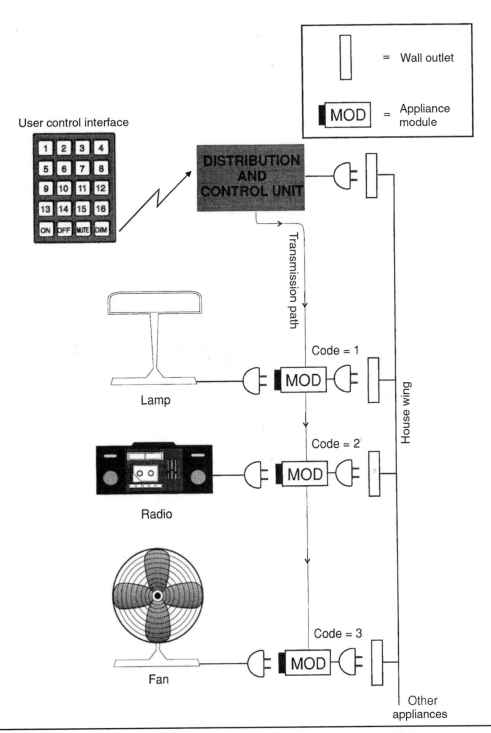

**Figure 11-10**   An EADL that employs ultrasound or infrared transmission from the control interface to the distribution and control unit. As in Figure 11-8, house wiring is used for transmission from the distribution and control unit to the appliance modules.

remote link between the control interface and the distribution and control unit in Figure 11-10 is often implemented using IR instead of ultrasound. In this case the control scheme is the same as that described above for other IR remote controls. Sometimes the link between the control and distribution unit and the remote appliances is also implemented using IR transmission. The engineering, design, and construction of IR controllers is described by Ciarcia (1987b).

The major advantages of the IR devices are no installation costs (as compared with hard wiring) and ease of portability. A major disadvantages is that the signal can be blocked by many materials, so a direct line of sight between the transmitter and receiver is required (Mills, 1987). This means that the transmitter and receiver must be in the same room. Because the receiver must be connected to the controlled appliances (possibly through the house wiring), the line-of-sight requirement limits the range of application (e.g., outside, inside, different rooms). Because the IR devices are light sensitive, they often do not work well in bright sunlight. Recall that the HAAT model includes a consideration of the physical context (see Chapter 2, Figure 2-6) in which a given activity is taking place. In this case the EADL is typically used in an interior location where light, heat, and sound can be controlled. However, interference from other appliances or interference caused by transmission from the EADL can affect the performance of these systems.

**Radio frequency transmission.** A final transmission approach is the use of radio frequency (RF) waves as the link between the distribution and control unit and the control interface, the controlled appliances, or both. The most common examples of this type of remote control are garage door openers and portable telephones. The term *RF transmission* is used because the signals are in the same range as broadcast FM radio. **Radio frequency transmission** is used as the link between the control interface and the processor.

The major advantage of RF transmission is that it is not blocked by common household materials (it can be blocked by metal that is connected to the ground), and transmission can be over a relatively long distance throughout a house and yard). Because it is less restricted, it has the major

disadvantages of interference and lack of privacy (Mills, 1987). The interference problem is generally approached by reducing the distance between the transmitter and the receiver and by having several transmission channels available. The user can switch between channels (or the device will automatically scan) to find the strongest signal. Privacy is generally addressed by allowing the user to select a transmission code (often with a bank of small switches) and then matching the transmitter and receiver codes.

## Trainable or Programmable Devices

Remote devices that utilize either ultrasound, IR, or RF typically are designed for operation with only one appliance (e.g., TV, VCR). If an individual owns several remotely controlled devices, this can lead to "controller clutter," with a separate control required for each device. To reduce this problem, several manufacturers produce remote control units that can be adapted to work with any appliance. Some of these are called **trainable controllers**. These devices operate by storing the control code for any specific appliance function (e.g., on/off). As shown in Figure 11-11, *A*, the storage is often accomplished by pointing the trainable controller at the controller for the specific appliance and sending the specific function code (TV ON in Figure 11-11). The trainable device then stores this code for future use. When the stored code is sent to the appliance, it is received and used as if it had been sent by the appliance's own controller. This is illustrated in Figure 11-11, *B*. In this manner, all the functions of the individual appliance con-

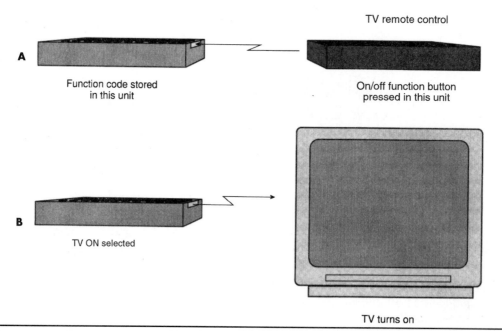

Figure 11-11    A trainable infrared controller. The trainable or programmable controller is shown on the left. **A,** Training is accomplished by aiming the device-specific control at the trainable controller and pressing the desired button (in this case, TV ON). **B,** The trained unit can then be used with the appliance to accomplish the desired function.

trollers can be stored in one master controller and the user need only activate this one device. Most of these controllers have two modes: train and operate. Figure 11-12 shows a programmable EADL unit mounted to a wheelchair and used for controlling appliances such as the television. Some controllers have codes for many appliances permanently stored in them. The user selects a code corresponding to his appliance (e.g., a television set made by a specific manufacturer) Ciarcia (1987a) describes the technical operation of trainable devices for IR controllers. These devices, like the individual appliance units, are designed using special-purpose microcomputers. In the training mode the EADL device is aimed at the individual appliance, the function to be stored is pressed on the individual control, and the code is stored. This process is repeated for all functions and for all individual controllers. These devices are relatively small, lightweight, and battery powered, and they can be hand carried or mounted to a wheelchair.

An alternative approach is based on the storage, in the controller, of codes that are appropriate to a range of appliances. The user selects her appliance and looks up the controller code in a table. Once this code is entered into the controller, it is able to control the appliance. We refer to these as **programmable controllers.**

Trainable or programmable controllers designed for the general home electronics market can be of benefit to persons with disabilities who are able to press the small keys associated with these devices. For those persons who cannot use standard controllers, there are specially adapted train-able or programmable units that provide both direct selection and scanning selection.* Control interfaces include expanded keyboards or a built-in keyboard or single switches for scanning access. In the latter case, one of two methods is typically used: (1) small lights that are located next to each button are sequentially illuminated or (2) alphanumeric labels or numeric codes for each function are sequentially displayed. For each of these approaches, the user presses the switch when the desired choice is presented.

As shown in Figure 11-11, most of the trainable or programmable EADL devices can be interfaced to other electronic devices (e.g., AAC devices, computers, powered wheelchair controllers) via a serial port (see Chapter 8). To control the EADL, a code must be sent from the communication device or computer to the controller, and all specific functions and separate appliance codes must be stored in the communication device or computer. Several manufacturers† include control software for EADL in their communication software programs. When the EADL is controlled by a computer or communication device, the software program

---

*For example, Gewa Link, Zygo Industries, Portland, Ore.; Relax II and MiniRelax, TASH, Inc., Ajax, Ont., Canada; Scanning Director II, APT/DU IT, Shreve, Ohio; Simplicity Switch & All-in-One, Quartet Technology, Inc., Tyngsboro, Mass.; Universal IR Remote, Baylor Biomedical Services, Dallas, Tex.; U-Control, Words Plus, Palmdale, Calif.
†For example, Words+, Palmdale, Calif.; Dynavox, Pittsburgh, Pa., Prentke Romich, Wooster, Ohio.

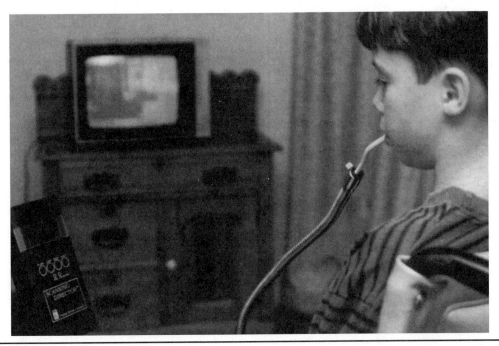

Figure 11-12    A trainable infrared EADL with scanning access. The EADL is shown mounted to a wheelchair. It is positioned so there is a line-of-sight link to the television for use of IR control. (Courtesy APT Technology, Inc., DU-IT CSG, Inc., Shreve, Ohio.)

generates the control signals and sends them through the serial port to the EADL.

## Telephone Control

Persons with physical disabilities of the upper extremities often have difficulty in carrying out the tasks associated with telephone use. These include lifting the handset, dialing, holding the handset while talking, and replacing the handset to its cradle. Telephones differ greatly in design (e.g., portable, speaker, rotary or touch-tone dial), but all require that the listed tasks be performed. As in many other areas of assistive technology, there are a variety of ways to accomplish the same tasks. Mouthsticks or head pointers (see the section on low-tech aids earlier in this chapter) can be used to press a button to open a line on a speaker phone (equivalent to lifting the hand set), dial by pressing buttons, and hang up at the end of a conversation. There are also simple holders that position a handset for hands-free operation and mechanical switches with long handles that control the switch hook for answering a call or hanging up after a call. Finally, telephone companies provide operator-assisted calling for persons with disabilities, so it is only necessary to press O for operator, who then dials the call for the consumer. Our emphasis in this section, however, is on electronic telephone access systems, which are often integrated into EADLs.

Because modern telephones are actually sophisticated electronic devices, automation via electronic **telephone controllers** is relatively easy, and there are a variety of commercial products available to accomplish telephone access for persons with disabilities.* Many of the general-purpose EADLs have telephone functions built in.† The functional components of a telephone controller are shown in Figure 11-13. Individual devices may group these components differently. Telephone controllers for a person with disabilities are built around standard telephone electronics. In some cases the controller is connected into the standard telephone, whereas in others the telephone is bypassed and the controller plugs directly into the telephone line. In any case, several of the important functions are common to consumer telephones. For example, the use of stored numbers (automatic dialing) and redial can save a great deal of

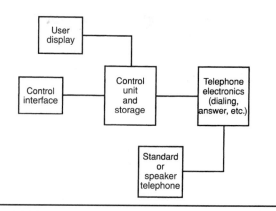

**Figure 11-13** Functional components of an automatic telephone dialer. The *control interface* and *user display* constitute the human/technology interface, the *control unit and storage* and *telephone electronics* are the processor, and the *telephone* constitutes the activity output.

time when the user must use scanning to select numbers. Another useful feature of currently available adapted telephones is that the user can answer electronically rather than physically picking up the handset. This is done as an additional choice on a scanning menu or a direct selection on an EADL telephone control panel.

Other parts of the telephone controller shown in Figure 11-13 are necessary only for persons who require single-switch access to the system (e.g., the user display). The control interface is connected to a control unit that also interfaces with a display and with the telephone electronics. Although systems vary in their design, a typical approach is for the device to present digits sequentially on the display. When the digit to be dialed is presented, the user presses his switch to select the number and the scan begins at zero. In this way, any phone number can be entered. Once the number is entered, it is sent to the telephone electronics for automatic dialing. Many persons with disabilities respond slowly, and each switch press may take several seconds. If we assume that it takes 2 seconds to respond, then we must display each number for at least 3 seconds, and we may require scanning through 10 numbers (30 seconds) just to get to the desired number. If all the desired numbers were large (e.g., 7, 8, 9), it could take almost 5 minutes (300 seconds) to dial one long-distance (11-digit) number. For this reason, all practical systems use stored numbers and automatic dialing. They also allow numbers to be entered and either stored or dialed using scanning. Redial also can speed things up, and this feature is normally included as well. Another unique feature in most telephone dialers designed for persons with disabilities is the inclusion of a HELP (e.g., a neighbor) or EMERGENCY (911) phone number that can be dialed quickly.

There are several modes of operation in automatic telephone dialers. First, the user must chose among dial, answer, or hang up. If dial is chosen, then the user must

---

*For example, E.A.S.I. Dialer, TASH, Ajax, Ont., Canada; EZ Phone, APT/DU IT, Shreve, Ohio; IR Speakerphone, Baylor Biomedical, Dallas, Tex.; Gewa IR Controlled Telephone, Zygo Industries, Portland, Ore.

†For example, Scanning Director II, APT/DU-IT, Shreve, Ohio; Ezra, KY Enterprises, Long Beach, Calif.; EZ Control, Regenesis, North Vancouver, B.C., Canada; Simplicity Switch, Quartet Technology, Inc., Tyngsboro, Mass.; Proxi and Nemo, Madenta, Edmonton, Apounds., Canada; Imperium 200H, Teledyne Brown, Huntsville, Ala.; Sicare Pilot, TASH, Ajax, Ont., Canada.

decide whether to access a stored number, redial, call for help, or dial an unstored number. For single-switch devices, this decision is generally made in one of two ways: (1) the system sequentially presents the choices to the user and the user waits until the desired choice is presented before pressing her switch, or (2) a second switch is available that accesses the operational modes only (e.g., dial, answer, store) and the other switch is used for selecting numbers. In either method, if HELP is selected, it is automatically dialed with no further entry. Some units merely reserve the first place in the stored number directory for HELP, whereas others use a special selection scheme for it (e.g., a long switch press). The next choice is generally redial. If redial is not chosen, then stored numbers are presented, usually by a code. Most systems have a capacity of 50 to 100 stored numbers. The user merely waits until the code for the number of the person he wants to call is presented and then presses the switch. At this point everything else is automatic. If the user wishes to enter a new number, either to be dialed or to be stored, he waits until that choice is presented and then activates the switch. Once in this mode, the method discussed above is used to enter the number, and the user then tells the controller whether to enter it into memory or to dial it.

Because the telephone controller obtains access to the telephone lines in the course of its normal operation, it is relatively easy to include other telephone-based functions in the adapted controller's operation. For example, apartment buildings often use the telephone system for the intercom and front door latch, and the adapted telephone dialer can access these by including additional codes selected by the user.

When a computer is used as part of an EADL, the telephone dialing functions can be implemented using software programs coupled with an electronic telephone interface that connects to the telephone line. These software and electronics are common for use in modems for communication between computers (e.g., for Internet access), and they have been adapted for some EADL systems.

## Configuring Electronic Aids to Daily Living

Having looked at the components that normally make up EADLs, we now move to a discussion of how EADLs get selected and configured to meet the specific needs of a person with a disability. The first step in this process is to carry out an assessment of the person's needs and skills.

**Assessment for EADL use.** As we discuss in Chapter 4, the initial assessment step is to determine the consumer's needs carefully, especially in the context of daily living demands (e.g., home, employment). Retrospective studies of EADL use show that such factors as employment status,

lifestyle (passive versus active), and gender all play a role in the effectiveness of EADL systems (Efthimiou et al, 1981; Sell et al, 1979). Bentham, Bereton, and Sapacz (1992) discuss major considerations to be included in a careful needs assessment for EADL selection. These studies emphasize the need for a careful analysis of factors in addition to physical and cognitive ability, such as ease of use, displays, home modifications required, and equipment standardization. We discuss several of these later in this chapter.

Holme et al (1997) conducted a survey of occupational therapists (OTs) working in spinal cord injury and disease centers. The purpose of the survey was to determine the use of EADLs by persons who have had spinal cord injuries, reasons for recommendations of EADLs (or not) by OTs, and the skills required to assess consumers for use of EADLs and recommend appropriate devices. They found that 84% of the OTs working in these centers used EADLs with their clients as part of the in-patient rehabilitation process. Consumers who had injuries at the C4 or higher level were generally viewed as able to benefit from EADLs. The top four reasons for recommending an EADL were (1) empowerment of the client, (2) improvement in the client's quality of life, (3) increased access to call systems, and (4) decreased need for attendant care. Holme et al (1997) also found that more than 50% of the EADLs recommended and purchased for clients were still in use. They also identified the major reasons for *not* recommending an EADL: (1) lack of funding (64% of respondents), (2) high cost of EADLs (47%), (3) unavailability of EADLs for trial, and (4) lack of EADL knowledge by the OT responsible for the client's rehabilitation. The major reason that clients did not use EADLs recommended for them was a preference for having another person provide the necessary assistance. Holme et al (1997) concluded that more frequent recommendation of EADLs by OTs is dependent on two factors: (1) outcome studies that identify the effectiveness of EADLs and their cost effectiveness and (2) inclusion of knowledge and skills related to EADLs in OT training.

Dickey and Shealey (1987) describe an evaluation process that follows the needs assessment and leads to the selection of EADLs. The first step in this evaluation is to determine the person's physical abilities (see Chapter 4) and her ability to use a control interface (see Chapter 7). If she is also using an augmentative communication device (see Chapter 9) or a powered wheelchair (see Chapter 10), then EADL functions may be included in one of these other devices and a separate control interface may not be necessary.

The next step in Dickey and Shealey's (1987) evaluation process is to determine the consumer's cognitive status. This includes such things as motor-planning skills, short-term and long-term memory, and problem-solving skills. These abilities are all important in understanding and effectively using an EADL. In determining the feasibility of using an

### DEVICES TO BE CONTROLLED / ENVIRONMENT(S)

**Home, Worksite, or School Environmental Assessment**

**Living, Work, or School Situation**
Living: alone, with family/roommate/attendant, group living
Work/School: type of facility, # people sharing room(s)

**Daily Routine Within Environment(s)** - How is time spent

**Devices to be Controlled** (type, number, how devices operated)

| | | |
|---|---|---|
| ___ Telephone | ___ * TV | ___ ~ Electric Bed |
| ___ Lights | ___ * VCR | ___ ~ Window Opener |
| ___ Call Bell | ___ * Stereo | ___ ~ Drapes/Curtains |
| ___ Alarm System | ___ *^ Compact Disk | ___ ~ Door Opener |
| ___ Air Conditioner |     Player | ___ DoorLock/Unlock |
| ___ Fan | ___ ^ Tape Recorder | ___ Page Turner |
| ___ Intercom | ___ ^ Tape Player | |
| ___ Radio | Other _____ | |
| ___ Computer | _____ | |

~ Items often require momentary mode
* Items often require infrared
^ Insertion?

**Where Devices Are**
rooms, centers of activity within rooms, devices in room,
number & type of outlets (2 or 3 prong receptacles)

| Room | Devices | #Outlets |
|---|---|---|
| _____ | _____ | ___ |
| _____ | _____ | ___ |
| _____ | _____ | ___ |

**Layout of Building & Rooms**
building / room considerations _____
doors opened or closed _____

**Access to EADL Needed from Different Places or Positions**
power wheelchair _____
manual wheelchair _____
other chair/ position_____
bed _____

**Other Equipment EADL to be Compatible With**
wheelchair_____
computer _____
communication device _____
other _____

**Access to Devices for Other People** _____

**Figure 11-14**  An evaluation form used for assessing environmental needs and goals. (From Barker P, Gross K, Henderson K: Control of the environment, *Proc '91 RESNA Pacific Reg Conf,* 1991.)

EADL, Dickey and Shealey (1987) suggest that the consumer's ability to learn new tasks and his most complementary method of integrating new skills with old activities should be determined. These two areas can have a significant impact on the effectiveness of an EADL. Motivation and functional capabilities must also be assessed. In the retrospective studies, motivation was found to be a major factor, and it was closely coupled to lifestyle and employment status. Dickey and Shealey (1987) also suggest that the specific tasks to be accomplished be identified both in an interview and via a home visit. Some tasks can be easily accomplished using an EADL, whereas others require different manipulation aids; a careful environmental survey can determine which tasks fall into each category. It is also important at this stage to ensure that the consumer's expectations are realistic. The consumer's daily routine, the accessibility of her residence, the attendant care available, and the existence of other assistive technologies also affect the recommendation of an EADL. Finally, available funding to acquire the EADL plays a role in the selection of a system, and it may be necessary to set priorities among needs and tasks to allow for unknown funding amounts.

Figure 11-14 illustrates an assessment form used in EADL evaluations (Barker, Gross, and Henderson, 1991). This form or an equivalent can be used to summarize the evaluation results, including the needs and EADL configuration, for an individual consumer.

The outcomes of an EADL assessment include (1) identification of control sites and control interfaces, (2) determination of cognitive abilities related to understanding EADL operation, (3) listing of EADL functions desired (in priority order), (4) evaluation of the consumer's motivation to use electronic environmental control, and (5) a listing of other electronic devices that the consumer uses. The listing of functions may include such things as lighting, TV, and drapery control. The listing of other electronic devices should include both consumer electronic devices, such as TV, VCR, computer, and speaker telephone (all with brand names and model numbers), and assistive technologies, such as communication devices and powered wheelchairs. Armed with this information, it is then possible to work with the consumer to select an EADL that meets his needs.

**Single-device binary control EADLs.** Electonic aids to daily living that control only one appliance can be useful in developing motor control, as well as cognitive concepts such as cause and effect.* In Chapter 7 we describe a motor training program that utilizes these types of EADLs. Most of these have both momentary and latched modes, and they include a timer to activate the appliance for a preset number of seconds. These devices can be used when only a single device control can be understood by the user (e.g., in the case of developmental disability) or when only one device is required (e.g., a radio or light). The cost is low (less than $200), and there can be a significant increase in independence. The use of single-function EADLs often leads to the use of multiple-function EADLs or electronic communication devices (see Chapter 9). This progression is described in Chapter 7.

**Matching the characteristics of multiple-function EADLs to the needs of the user.** When planning an EADL to meet specific needs, it is useful to group the tasks (determined during the assessment described earlier) into the five categories shown in Table 11-1. This grouping, based on the common ways of implementing specific functions, is the first step in specifying an EADL. After completing the assessment form, shown in Figure 11-14, the ATP will know the type of appliances that need to be controlled. The EADL functions required can be identified in the left-hand column of Table 11-1. The corresponding information in the right-hand column identifies the methods available for EADL implementation. This allows options to be considered.

| TABLE 11-1   Functions Performed by EADLs | |
| --- | --- |
| Functions | Methods of Implementation |
| Binary latched control of AC appliances (e.g., lights, radio, on-off only) | House wiring transmission Direct ultrasound control |
| Discrete or continuous appliance (e.g., TV, VCR, CD, cassette tape control) | IR remote transmission Ultrasound remote transmission |
| Momentary control of appliances (e.g., door opener, drapery control) | RF remote transmission |
| Telephone control | Hard-wired switch control |
| Switch control (any device requiring one or two switches) | Hard wiring IR link to switch box Ultrasound link to switch box |

The first group in Table 11-1 is binary (on/off) latched (stays on or off until the next activation) control of appliances that operate from standard household wall current. As we have described, there are two basic ways that current EADLs control such appliances: (1) by plugging them into receivers that plug into the house wiring and transmitting control signals over the house wiring and (2) by direct ultrasonic transmission to a receiver into which the appliance is plugged. The most common commercially available components for use with house wiring transmission are the X-10 modules and controllers.* These modules are incorporated into many EADLs. The major direct ultrasound receiver-based control device is the Ultra 4.† If this is the only requirement the consumer has, then the EADL is simple and inexpensive.

The second category in Table 11-1 is appliances that require discrete or continuous control, such as television channel selection or volume control. The most common EADL control method for discrete or continuous appliances is IR remote transmission, and several EADLs utilize integrated trainable or programmable IR controllers. This allows several (e.g., TV, VCR, CD, audio tape) to be incorporated into one package controlled by the EADL. Each of these devices must have its own IR control to be incorporated into the trainable or programmable controller. If the consumer does not have a remote-controlled TV, there are stand-alone TV controllers with IR remote transmitters that connect to a standard TV set. This provides adapted discrete and continuous control over TV functions. The options available to the ATP depend on what appliances the consumer has and whether they have IR remote control. If IR remote devices are available, then the choice is to use an EADL with a trainable or programmable IR device. If the consumer has needs for continuous or discrete

---

*For example, the Ablenet Power Link, Ablenet, Minneapolis, Minn.

*X-10 Powerhouse, Inc., Northvale, N.J.
†TASH, Inc., Ajax, Ont., Canada.

control but does not have IR-controlled appliances, then the ATP should consider EADLs with built-in discrete or continuous control. This may require modification of the appliance or purchase of a stand-alone IR controller.

If the consumer wants to control items such as draperies, then momentary control (i.e., the appliance is turned on for a variable period of time and then turned off) is required. For example, a drapery motor or bed elevation control may be turned on long enough to move the curtain or the bed to the proper position, and then the motor must be turned off. A latched control generally presents problems in this scenario. Very short activation times are not possible with latched control, especially if the user has delays in muscle motor response. In some cases the range of movement for the task is always the same (e.g., when opening a door), and we can use a device that is started by the user and automatically stopped at the end of the task by the device (e.g., when the door is fully open or fully closed). This type of control is often implemented using RF transmission. Hard-wired switch control can also be used for these functions. Common examples are the enlarged switches often placed near doors for persons with disabilities or the active floor mats or light sensors used to trigger the opening of these doors.

Telephone control is listed separately in Table 11-1 because the functions performed are different from other EADL tasks. Generally telephone controllers use switches connected directly to them (hard wired). Because the telephone must also be connected to the wall, this can limit the freedom of movement of the consumer. She must move to the telephone dialer to use it and then reach the switch. This can be difficult, and integrating all EADL functions is often desirable. If the consumer is also going to use IR continuous or discrete control, the ATP should consider the use of an IR-controlled telephone.* This allows the consumer to control the telephone in the same way as she controls the TV, VCR, and so on.

The final category in Table 11-1 is for devices that require one- or two-switch control. Other examples of appliances requiring switch control are call signals and drapery and door controls. The simplest method to implement this type of control is hard wiring of the switch to the EADL component. However, this approach has two major disadvantages: (1) the user is forced to go to the device to be controlled and use the switch at that location, so flexibility in movement is limited; and (2) it is difficult to integrate the switch control with other EADL functions into a total package controlled by only one control interface. If a consumer must use different switches for different devices, then independence can be reduced. If the individual does not have good motor control and requires careful positioning of the control interface for successful use, the problem is even more difficult.

One way to integrate switch control with other EADL functions is to use a component that can detect IR or ultrasound signals and generate a switch-type output. This type of output is sometimes referred to as *relay output*. For example, if the consumer is using a trainable or programmable IR EADL controller for TV, VCR, and telephone use and needs to control a drapery motor as well, a two-output IR trainable switch box (as shown in Figure 11-15) can be used. The IR EADL can provide the equivalent of a switch output directly, and the consumer does not need to have two additional switches to control the drapes (e.g., one switch to open them and one switch to close them). Some EADLs have built-in switched or relay outputs.*

Not all remote control utilizes IR transmission. Binary latched control of electrical appliances is often implemented by either ultrasound or RF transmission, and trainable or programmable IR controllers are not usable for these functions. Two basic approaches are used to integrate binary appliance control and remote IR controllers. The first of these, shown in Figure 11-15, has a control and distribution unit that employs IR transmission. The transmitted codes are used to select an appliance (the number of appliances can vary from 4 to 256) and the function to be accomplished (on/off or dim/brighten for lights only). The trainable or programmable IR device is programmed to recognize these codes, and the remote unit treats the appliance control and dual-switch receiver as IR-controlled devices.

The second approach to integration of discrete or continuous IR control with binary latched appliance control, shown in Figure 11-16, is to incorporate ultrasound and RF control into the trainable or programmable device together with IR transmission. In this case there is no need for a separate IR transmission distribution and control unit, since the ultrasound and RF transmission is built into the trainable or programmable remote controller. This combines the trainability of the IR unit for TV, VCR, and so on with the simplicity of direct ultrasound or RF transmission for binary control of appliances. This allows more flexibility in the choice of individual environmental control components, and it allows us to focus on the needs of the EADL user rather than on the devices that may be available.

**Hospital-based EADLs.** Individuals who suffer a high-level spinal cord injury are hospitalized immediately after the injury and remain hospitalized for many months. During this time, they have needs for environmental control that are similar to those for home use, but their needs also differ in important ways. Jones et al (1980) list four advantages of using hospital-based EADLs: (1) increased independence, (2) increase in motivation for self-rehabilitation, (3) reduction in anxiety from helplessness, and (4) increased nursing time available for more essential services (p. 607). As Efthimiou et al (1981) have found, an important factor in increased postdischarge use of EADLs is experience

---

*For example, Baylor Biomedical, Dallas, Tex.

*For example, U-Control, Words Plus, Palmdale, Calif.; Kincontrol, TASH, Ajax, Ont., Canada.

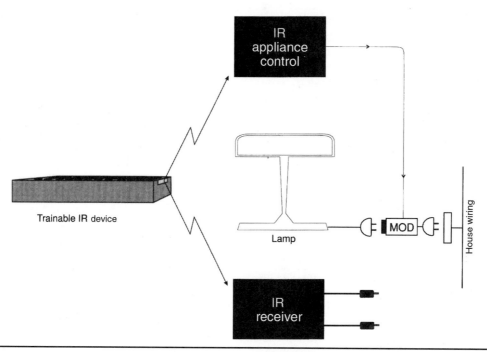

Figure 11-15    One approach to the integration of appliance control and single-switch or dual-switch control is to use an IR receiver that provides one- or two-switch closure outputs when activated. The two jacks shown in the lower right of the figure can be connected just as any switch would be.

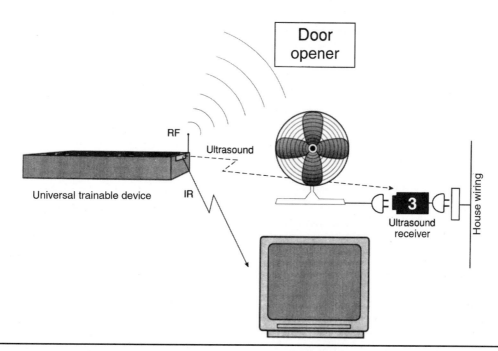

Figure 11-16    A universal trainable remote that provides control for ultrasound, RF, and IR EADL modules.

during the acute and subacute hospital-based rehabilitation phase. This is an additional advantage of hospital-based EADLs.

To achieve these advantages, it is necessary to include features not commonly found in home-based EADLs. The first of these is inclusion of access to the nurse call system of the hospital. This requires that the EADL have an interface to standard hospital nurse call systems. A variety of control interfaces must be available for the patient to use in accessing this function. As Jones et al (1980) point out, it is often necessary to have one control interface usable during the initial, acute phase of injury (approximately 6 weeks after initial admission). Because of spinal shock, the patient often has greater paralysis during this phase than in later stages, and efforts to use residual limb movement will be compromised. They recommend using above-the-neck movements to activate the control interface during this phase. Respiration may also be more significantly compromised during the acute phase, and this limits the use of puff-and-sip control interfaces. Finally, cervical traction may limit head movements during the acute phase. (Removal of the head traction apparatus often signals the transition from acute to subacute rehabilitation.) Based on these considerations, Jones et al (1980) have found that chin-controlled switches are the most generally useful during the acute phase of rehabilitation.

During the acute phase of rehabilitation, the patient is normally restricted to bed. EADL functions that are useful include television control (on/off, volume, and channel change), electric bed control, and appliance control (radio, lamp, fan). Although available on most hospital-based EADLs,* telephone control is not frequently used during the acute phase of rehabilitation.

During the subacute phase of hospital-based rehabilitation, the patient generally has greater control because of the removal of the head traction apparatus, reduction of spinal cord swelling, and an increase in respiratory capability. These changes allow for more options in control interface selection. The patient also has greater interest in his surroundings, and telephone, television, and appliance control become more important to him. EADL designed for hospital use generally do not have a wide range of options. For example, they may allow only one or two appliances to be controlled or they may have a small number of stored phone numbers (e.g., five). These design considerations reflect the unique requirements of the hospital situation. Other special features include very simple operation; large displays that are lighted for use in dim intensive care units; special electric bed and nurse control interfacing; and flexibility in the number of options and capabilities, depending on the needs of the user. Jones et al (1980) present design details for one computer-controlled hospital-based EADL.

## Studies of EADL Users

Several studies have been conducted to determine the preferred features and factors influencing successful application of EADLs. Most of the studies were conducted before some of the current features (e.g., trainable or programmable IR controllers) became available, but they still reflect basic preferences of users.

Symington et al (1986) studied the effect of EADL availability on attendant care in an institutional setting. Using a paired questionnaire for EADL users and nursing attendants in an institutional setting, they evaluated attitudes and perceptions of both users and staff regarding self-worth, independence, and usage of EADLs. The survey was administered before EADL system delivery and after EADL system use. For the users of devices, only one area (irritability) showed a statistically significant decline after EADL delivery. Perceptions of self-worth and independence increased, and users generally felt that they were less frustrated, had greater privacy, and needed to "bother" staff less frequently. The staff felt that the users had greater independence and that the staff was relieved of "extra duties" and saved time. An electromechanical counter recorded EADL usage, but no data were reported on frequency of use or usage patterns.

Woods and Jones (1990) reported on 10 years of experience with EADLs in institutional settings. They reported that EADL use can increase the independence of patients in such a setting. However, they also stressed the importance of training in proper use.

Mann (1992) studied the use of EADLs by elderly nursing home residents. In this study, residents were divided into control and experimental groups. The experimental group received EADLs for use in their rooms to control lights and radios. They also received training in the use of these devices. Those in the control group did not have EADLs. Mann found that independent use of radios by the experimental group occurred at three times the rate of the control group at the end of the study. These results indicated that elderly nursing home residents will increase their environmental interaction if they have access to EADLs.

Studies have also been conducted on EADL use in community settings. Sell et al (1979) studied eight different EADLs over a 44-month period. Their subjects were persons with high-level (C4 or higher) spinal cord injuries who used the EADLs in their homes. Both groups were physically able to access the EADL functions. Features of EADLs that were judged valuable included visual and auditory selection displays, overall size and appearance (fitting into a home), ability to make confidential telephone calls using an automatic telephone dialer, direct access to telephone dialing (rather than using the operator), and reliability. Reliability was judged by the absence of failures of the device or of operational errors by the user.

Efthimiou et al (1981) studied the impact of EADLs on the postdischarge lives of persons with spinal cord injuries. Identified factors related to EADL use included gender (74% of men chose to use EADLs, whereas only 14% of the women did); exposure to an EADL during the in-hospital rehabilitation process; and availability of EADL systems (including funding) after discharge. They also looked at scales of activity and correlated these with EADL use. One substudy included 13 EADL users and 7 nonusers, all men. All the users were employed, compared with only 54% of the nonusers. Another difference between the user and

---

*For example, the HECS-1 from APT/DU-IT, Shreve, Ohio.

nonuser groups was that users more frequently participated in educational activities, phone calls, and travel, whereas nonusers spent more time in passive recreational activities. Users more frequently employed assistive devices in general, and they performed more tasks independently than did the nonusers. In this study, use or nonuse was unrelated to adjustment to the disability and personality type. The major reasons given for not using an EADL were lack of space and an inaccessible home.

McDonald, Boyle, and Schumann (1989) studied EADL use by persons who had incurred high-level spinal cord injuries. In contrast to earlier studies that had used very small samples, McDonald, Boyle, and Schumann (1989) had 29 subjects accessed through the manufacturers who had provided their EADLs. More than 90% of their sample of EADL users found them to be helpful and more than 70% felt that EADLs increased their independence. The group of users also indicated that the EADL positively affected their disposition (67%) or was neutral in this regard (33%). The needs for EADL use were ranked in order of importance: communication, security/health, recreation, household tasks, employment, and education. EADL functions judged important (in rank order) were telephone,

television, room lights, emergency signal, door, and computer. The 29 respondents also indicated that they were comfortable and felt secure for longer periods alone when an EADL was available.

In contrast to these studies of EADLs that reported only general opinion and did not objectively measure actual usage, Von Maltzahn, Daphtary, and Roa (1995) monitored usage of EADLs in home settings. They used a data logger that kept track of time and type of activation over a 16-week period and found that the greatest usage was in the evening and the largest activity was in television control. The small sample of subjects (5) did show great variability as well, with a factor of almost 30 times between the greatest and least number of uses of the EADL per week. Von Maltzahn, Daphtary, and Roa (1995) also used an end-of-study questionnaire to determine perceptions and attitudes of the users and their care providers. Once again the importance of training was cited, and both users and caregivers indicated that there was greater user independence and fewer demands made on the caregivers. These researchers attempted to monitor staff assistance provided, but they were unable to do so. This was due to data collection methods that were too time consuming for staff to implement.

---

### Case Study 11-1

#### EADLs for Increased Independence

Joyce is 39. She has cerebral palsy, and she has just moved into an apartment with an attendant. She is unable to speak, and she uses a communication device based on a laptop computer. Joyce controls her scanning communication device with a tread switch mounted near her knee. The communication device consists of a software program* running on a laptop computer. The communication and environmental control aspects of Joyce's system were integrated by using an IR trainable or programmable remote device interfaced to the serial port of the laptop computer.† The remote device is activated by the scanning communication software computer program, and it controls a TV and VCR directly. A two-channel IR receiver with switch output is used to control an automatic telephone dialer.‡ The telephone controller also allows control of four ultrasound receivers (Ultra Four), which Joyce has connected to two lamps and to a drapery control to open her curtains automatically. All the EADL functions are controlled by selecting the device from a menu and then sending a command through the IR remote unit to activate it (turn on the switch to the telephone dialer, change TV channels, and so on).

*Scanning WSKE, Words Plus, Lancaster, Calif.
† Relax II, TASH, Inc., Ajax, Ont., Canada.
‡E.A.S.I. Dialer, TASH, Inc., Ajax, Ont., Canada.

---

### Case Study 11-2

#### EADLs Following a Stroke

Eileen, who is 62 years old, suffered a brainstem stroke and requires maximal assistance for daily living. She sits in a reclining chair at home for the majority of the day. Eileen is able to use head movement to make communication selections using a light pointer mounted on a headband to control a communication device.*

Eileen also needs a simple EADL that can control the TV (turn it on, select channels, and control volume), a lamp, and a call signal to use when her husband is out of the room. She controls a scanning trainable IR remote† using a single switch mounted next to her head. This directly accesses the required TV functions. For the call system, an IR-sensitive switch is used to control an X-10 module. The module can be plugged in anywhere in the house, and her husband carries it with him when he goes outside or into a remote part of the house. In this way Eileen can summon him at any time if necessary. She can activate the switch using her head movement, without having to have the light pointer taken off. This makes her communication function independent of her EADL function, and it offers a contrast to Joyce's preference of having them integrated.

*Vantage, Prentke Romich, Wooster, Ohio.
†Relax II, TASH, Inc., Ajax, Ont., Canada.

*Control 1, formerly available from Prentke Romich, Wooster, Ohio.

## Examples of EADL Application

To illustrate the process of configuring EADLs for specific needs, we describe several case examples. Each of these cases is based on an actual situation faced by a person with a disability (Cook and Hussey, 1992). Gross (1992) presents a detailed case study of EADL use by a person with a high-level spinal cord injury. She also describes a process for analyzing needs and converting them into EADL specifications.

## ▓ ROBOTIC AIDS TO MANIPULATION

Because *robots* or **robotic systems** are intended to assist with manipulation, they are a natural alternative manipulation device for persons who have disabilities. There are, however, some significant differences between the use of robots by persons with disabilities and their use industrially. Industrial robots often have the role of *replacing* the human operator for reasons of strength, safety, or precision. In production line environments (e.g., automobile manufacturing), it is often necessary to lift large or heavy objects and position them for attachment to other parts. Robots are stronger than humans and are not subject to fatigue after hours of service. Many work environments are hazardous (e.g., those involving radiation or very high or low temperatures). To ensure safety to the operator, handling of objects in these environments is done by a robotic manipulator controlled by the human operator. At the opposite extreme from heavy object positioning is the repeated assembly of small parts (e.g., electronics assembly). Robots can be programmed to carry out the exact same task over and over without fatigue or loss of accuracy. In each of these cases the human is an ancillary part of the total system. In contrast, in assistive robotics the human operator is at the center of the process. Instead of replacing her, the goal is to enhance her ability to manipulate objects and to function independently. This makes issues of safety more important for assistive robots. To ensure safety, forces are kept within 1 or 2 pounds (2 to 5 kg) and velocities are less than 10 cm/sec (Seamone and Schmeisser, 1985). Assistive robots perform many functions, in contrast to the relatively limited repertoire of an industrial robot. Although some tasks (e.g., feeding) are repeated, the assistive robot must be able to carry out totally unplanned movements spontaneously. In this section we discuss the development and application of assistive robots. In contrast to technologies discussed in other sections of this chapter, assistive robots are still largely in the research and development stage, and application of these systems is not yet widespread.

Stanger and Cawley (1996) evaluated the incidence of 12 disabling conditions associated with reduction of upper limb function. These were cerebral palsy, arthrogryposis, spinal muscular atrophy, muscular dystrophies, rheumatoid arthritis, juvenile rheumatoid arthritis, multiple sclerosis, amyotrophic lateral sclerosis, poliomyelitis, spinal cord injury, head injury, and locked-in syndrome. Based on the incidence of these conditions, they estimated that approximately 150,000 persons in the United States have limitations of upper extremity function and could benefit from a robotic aid.

## History of Powered Manipulators

Early rehabilitative manipulators were powered orthoses. An orthosis is an external brace that supports a body part. By adding motors to the joints (i.e., wrist, elbow, and shoulder) of an upper extremity orthosis, Correl and Wijnschenk (1964) developed one of the first rehabilitative manipulators. This system had four degrees of freedom (independent movements) and was controlled by a minicomputer. Another orthotic approach was the Rancho Arm (Corker, Lyman, and Sheredos, 1979). This system also used an external upper extremity splint, but it had seven degrees of freedom. This allowed control of the shoulder (abduction-adduction and flexion-extension), elbow (flexion-extension), wrist (pronation-supination, radial and ulnar deviation, flexion-extension), and fingers (grasp-release). Each degree of freedom was controlled by a bi-directional tongue-activated switch. This single-joint control made it difficult to carry out complex movements. To understand this, place a pencil or pen on the table. Now reach for it and pick it up, but only move in one of the degrees of freedom (i.e., one joint) listed above at a time. This type of movement takes great concentration. Now, reach for the pen or pencil as you normally would. This is called *end-point positioning,* and it is much easier to accomplish, but it makes the control system and robot much more complicated. The difficulties associated with controlling individual joints was a major downfall of early rehabilitation manipulators, and most current assistive robots use end-point positioning.

In the late 1970s and early 1980s, stand-alone assistive robots began to be developed. These devices were generally table mounted, but some were mounted to wheelchair frames or lap trays. These robots were more versatile, since they did not have to support and move the user's limb, but they created new challenges because they were not attached to the body. The user had to develop a new coordinate system for controlling the robot, one related to the workspace of the robot rather than to his own body. The rapid development of microcomputers allowed miniaturization of the controllers while adding more sophistication. These systems also were capable of being "trained" to carry out repeated tasks. These advances made everyday use of assistive robots more feasible.

In the remainder of this section we discuss currently available assistive robots and their application. We discuss three types of applications: (1) fixed workstations, which are built around assistive robots; (2) mobile robots for use in work, home, and school settings; and (3) robots developed and used to meet the educational goals of children. Each of these systems is a **general-purpose manipulation device,** as opposed to **special-purpose manipulation devices** such as the feeders and page turners described earlier. In some cases there is a blurring between these two categories. For example, we describe the Handy 1 (Topping, 1996) under Electrically Powered Feeders, but it is actually a special-purpose robotic arm.

## Robotic Workstations

A *workstation* can be defined as an area dedicated to the performance of a specific job or activity. Examples of activities are design (e.g., a computer workstation for engineering students), reading (e.g., a library-based workstation), and clerical tasks (e.g., a workstation for word processing, telephone answering, and manipulation of files). These workstations involve manipulation of papers, books, and other devices. When the user of the workstation has difficulty with upper extremity function and manipulation, **desktop robots** can play a major role in creating full access to the

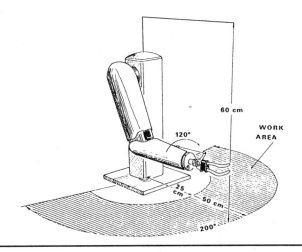

**Figure 11-17**    The coordinate system and working envelope of the APL RAWT system. (From Seamone W, Schmeisser G: Early clinical evaluation of a robot arm/worktable system for spinal-cord-injured persons, *J Rehabil Res Dev* 22:38-57, 1985.)

workstation. Because the workstation is fixed in one location, the design of the robotic system can focus on manipulation of objects only, rather than movement to the object and then manipulation of it. We describe two robotic workstations that have been evaluated in the workplace. Both these systems were developed by the Veterans Administration.

**Applied Physics Laboratory Robot Arm Worktable system.** The Applied Physics Laboratory Robot Arm Worktable (APL RAWT) system is built around a powered upper extremity prosthesis that has four degrees of freedom: (1) shoulder flexion-extension, (2) elbow flexion-extension, (3) wrist pronation-supination, and (4) hand grasping (Seamone and Schmeisser, 1985). In the workstation the prosthetic arm is mounted on a turntable, which allows a fifth degree of freedom comparable to internal-external shoulder rotation. Finally the entire arm and turntable assembly is mounted in a track that allows it to be moved from front to back of the work surface. This results in a total of six degrees of freedom for the arm. The movements of this arm are shown in Figure 11-17, together with the total size of the reachable workspace. There are three motors for the six degrees of freedom. One DC motor controls elbow flexion-extension, wrist pronation-supination, or shoulder flexion-extension, depending on the commands sent. The second motor controls turntable rotation or hand grasping. Any joint not being activated is kept in place with a solenoid lock. This allows one motor to serve several functions at different times, but it prevents multiple joint movements simultaneously. The third motor is a geared servomotor used for positioning the arm in the front-to-back track.

The APL RAWT was designed for use by persons with high-level spinal cord injuries (SCI). This limited the choice of control sites to the head, neck, and voice. Chin control was chosen over other control modes (e.g., speech recognition or sip-and-puff) because of its compatibility with powered wheelchair control. Because many persons with SCI have experience using chin control for wheelchairs, training in the use of the RAWT would be decreased. Lateral movement of the modified chin control allows wheelchair steering. Reverse is activated by a microswitch located on the chin control lever. When the user approaches the RAWT in her wheelchair, contact is made between the RAWT and the wheelchair by an optical (IR) link. The user lifts the chin control briefly and control is transferred from the wheelchair to the RAWT. The user controls the RAWT with the chin joystick (left/right, in/out) and two additional switches (up/down).

---

### BOX 11-1    Prestored Task Trajectories in the APL RAWT System

1. Move mouthstick into position
2. Pick up telephone and place it into position for use
3. Hang up telephone
4. Pick up tissue
5. Move keyboard forward
6. Remove paper from printer
7. Place floppy disk into computer disk drive
8. Pick up magazine from storage rack and place on reading stand
9. Return book to storage location
10. Eat sandwich from plate
11. Eat with a spoon in plate
12. Eat from a bowl

---

Modified from Seamone W, Schmeisser G: Early clinical evaluation of a robot arm/worktable system for spinal-cord-injured persons, *J Rehabil Res Dev* 22(1):38-57, 1985.

---

Two basic modes of control are provided. First, the user may activate any one degree of freedom and control the arm in that axis. As we have discussed, this can be tedious and difficult, but it is sometimes necessary for precise movements. The second and most common method of control is to select one of the prestored specific tasks. Examples of some of these tasks are given in Box 11-1. As is shown in the box, the APL RAWT combines the high technology of the robot with the low technology of a mouthstick for some tasks. For example, the robot can bring the mouthstick holder into position for the user and then bring the telephone into position. The user can dial the telephone using the mouthstick. Likewise, a book or magazine can be positioned in a reading stand by the robotic arm and the mouthstick can be used to turn pages. To select a prestored task, the user activates a menu of choices using the chin joystick, and then he can search through a list of tasks on the display screen to select the one he wants. Once the task is chosen, the arm automatically executes it. For some tasks such as feeding, there are intermediate points at which the user must reactivate the control. For example, a spoon of food is brought to mouth level and the arm is stopped. The user takes the food off of the spoon and then initiates a new cycle. Tasks such as self-feeding require the use of additional components, such as adapted bowls and utensils.

A block diagram of the total APL RAWT system is shown in Figure 11-18. The entire system is controlled by a special-purpose computer microprocessor. A keyboard is provided for programming new movements and general interaction with the system. It can be used by either the consumer or an attendant or therapist. Function keys on the keyboard specify robot motions. Prestored movements can be edited by use of the keyboard. This increases the flexibility because a new movement task can be created by editing an existing task that is similar.

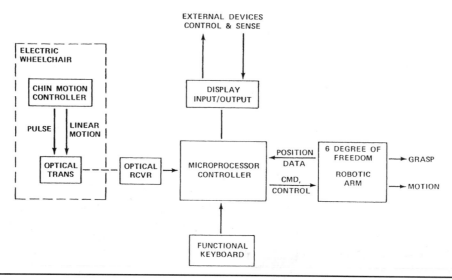

Figure 11-18   Block diagram showing the component parts of the APL RAWT system. (From Seamone W, Schmeisser G: Early clinical evaluation of a robot arm/worktable system for spinal-cord-injured persons, *J Rehabil Res Dev* 22:38-57, 1985.)

The APL RAWT was clinically evaluated at three VA centers. A total of 20 evaluators with high-level SCIs participated in clinical trials. The RAWT was typically set up in the evaluator's residence. Often this was the evaluator's home, but for some evaluators the residence was a VA medical center, nursing home, or state institution. The most popular features were self-feeding and computer and telephone use. Inadequacies of the chin controller were the most frequently cited negative feature. Seamone and Schmeisser (1985) discuss the evaluation of the APL RWAT in detail. The overall impression of the system was that it had the potential to be very effective for individuals with SCIs, but it needed further development and refinement.

**Desktop Vocational Assistant Robot.** The Desktop Vocational Assistant Robot (DeVAR-IV) system is built around an industrial-grade, low-payload robotic arm (PUMA-260*) mounted on an overhead track (Figure 11-19) (Hammel, Van der Loos, and Perkash, 1992). This system has a primary goal of vocational assistance. DeVAR-III used a table-mounted PUMA arm, and the emphasis was on completion of tasks of daily living (Hammel et al, 1989). The DeVAR *human/technology interface* includes speech recognition (Votan VPC-2100†) and multiaxis joystick control, coupled with a color monitor and voice synthesis. The voice synthesis is for user feedback (e.g., to confirm a task selection) and for warning messages. The

*AEG-Westinghouse, Pittsburgh, Pa.
†Votan, Inc., Freemont, Calif.

monitor displays command prompts and robot status during task completion. The *processor* is a dedicated computer with appropriate software. A task-oriented programming language (VAL-II) is used. Using this language, routines can be developed for specific tasks. Example tasks for self-feeding are listed in Table 11-2 (Hammel et al, 1989). Once a task is initiated, commands are issued by the user for specific functions within the task. Examples of these are shown in Table 11-3 for the task of eating soup listed in Table 11-2. Note that some commands (e.g., SOUP) have different meanings at different times during the task. Other commands (e.g., USE) are repeated many times to recycle through a subtask under the user's control. The user can also pilot the arm by using basic commands such as RIGHT, LEFT, BACKWARD, FORWARD, UP, DOWN, STOP, GO, OPEN, and CLOSE (gripper). As shown in Table 11-3, these direction commands can also be used within a prestored task. All the commands are spoken by the user and entered by the voice recognition system. The user must train the speech recognizer (see Chapter 7) to recognize her speech. For a typical vocabulary of about 60 commands, this takes approximately 10 minutes (Hammel et al, 1989). Similar tasks and command sequences can be developed for other applications (e.g., vocational work site tasks).

Outputs include environmental control (via an X-10 system), as well as the robotic arm. Examples of tasks that various versions of DeVAR have performed are listed in Box 11-2 (Hammel et al, 1989). The use of an industrial-grade robotic arm has the benefit of providing more precise control, proven safety features and reliability, and greater payloads, but the cost is significantly higher than robotic

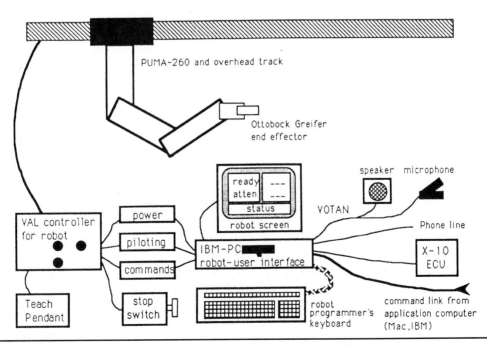

Figure 11-19   Basic components of the Desktop Vocational Assistant Robot (DeVAR). (From Hammel JM et al: Clinical evaluation of a desktop robotic assistant, *J Rehabil Res Dev* 26[3]:1-16, 1989.)

## TABLE 11-2    Desktop Vocational Assistant Robot Tasks and Their Commands

| Task | Command |
| --- | --- |
| Prepare a bowl of soup | SOUP |
| Eat the soup with standard spoon | SPOON |
| Brush teeth with electric toothbrush | TOOTHBRUSH |
| Wash and dry face with adapted washcloth | WASH |
| Shave face with electric shaver | SHAVE |

Modified from Hammel J et al: Clinical evaluation of a desktop robotic assistant, *J Rehabil Res Dev* 26(3):1-16, 1989.

## TABLE 11-3    Desktop Vocational Assistant Robot Commands Used To Prepare and Eat Soup

| Command | Action |
| --- | --- |
| SOUP | Robot takes soup out of refrigerator, puts in microwave, closes door, sets time, heats soup. |
| SOUP | Robot brings soup from microwave to table. |
| SPOON | Robot gets spoon from tool holder and brings to neutral point in front of user. User says direction commands to bring spoon near mouth (UP, DOWN, LEFT, RIGHT, BACKWARD, FORWARD). Robot remembers this point and returns to it each time. |
| USE | Robot scoops a spoonful of soup and brings to user's mouth. User says USE for each mouthful until finished eating. |
| BACK | Robot returns soup to refrigerator to finish later. |
| CLEAN | Robot puts bowl in dirty dish container to be cleaned. |

Modified from Hammel J et al: Clinical evaluation of a desktop robotic assistant, *J Rehabil Res Dev* 26(3):1-16, 1989.

## BOX 11-2    Tasks Performed by the Desktop Vocational Assistant Robot

**MEAL PREPARATION AND FEEDING**
Prepare meal
Open or close microwave
Manipulate bowls
Set timer
Pour liquids
Set timer
Beat eggs
Toss salad
Cook and serve soup
Heat and serve dinner
Serve pudding, fruit
Bake cake
Use standard utensils
Get drinks
Mix drinks

**VOCATIONAL**
Write with pen
Retrieve books
Set up books
Retrieve mouthstick
Type on keyboard
Adjust keyboard
Operate telephone
Turn pages
Insert floppy disk
Insert audio tapes
Open or close drawers
Operate printer
Manipulate printouts

**HYGIENE**
Wash or dry face
Brush teeth
Shave face
Comb or brush hair

**RECREATIONAL**
Arrange flowers
Paint
Play video game
Play board game
Light candle

Modified from Hammel J et al: Clinical evaluation of a desktop robotic assistant, *J Rehabil Res Dev* 26(3):1-16, 1989.

manipulators designed for educational or assistive uses. The gripper is a modified Otto Bock prosthetic hand.*

Two versions of the DeVAR have been field tested. DeVAR-III was evaluated by Hammel et al (1989). Twenty-four male evaluators were either inpatients or outpatients of the Palo Alto Veterans Administration SCI Center. Twenty-one of the evaluators had SCIs at the C4 or higher level, and all had little or no functional upper extremity movement. Each subject was given training by both an occupational therapist and an engineer. The speech recognition system was trained to recognize 60 command words. Both preprogrammed movements (e.g., those in Table 11-3) and directional movements were used by the participants. Pretests and posttests were administered using voice commands on the computer to evaluate the user's perception of the usefulness of the robotic system. Partici-

pants indicated a high degree of satisfaction with the performance of the robot in the tasks shown in Table 11-3. They also expressed a preference for the robot over attendant care for these tasks. The major concerns expressed were about reliability, the amount of space the robot occupied, and safety with children. Overall pretest ratings were lower than posttest ratings, reflecting a lack of knowledge of how well the robot would perform and a degree of skepticism in

*Otto Bock, Minneapolis, Minn.

the pretest. Hammel et al (1989) discuss the evaluation results in more detail.

DeVAR-IV, the version developed for a work environment, has also been evaluated (Hammel, Van der Loos, and Perkash, 1992). A single-subject research design was used with two components (R = robot assistance; A = attendant assistance). The workstation used by the evaluator also included a speech recognition keyboard and mouse-emulating device for access to his computer workstation (see Chapter 7). The evaluator was a 50-year-old man with a C4-C5 SCI. He was employed full time as a database programmer for a utility company. He used the DeVAR-IV system for his normal office activities and for some daily living tasks (e.g., serving lunch, emptying his leg bag, dispensing medications). The DeVAR-IV system was installed in his office for 6 months before data collection. This ensured that the evaluator was fully trained in and comfortable with the use of DeVAR-IV. During the first phase of data collection, the robot was used for six 10-hour days (corresponding to his normal workday of 10 hours). During the second phase (A) the robot was turned off and the attendant performed its tasks. All sessions were videotaped and observed by two project staff members. The evaluator expressed a preference for the robot over attendant assistance for all activities except feeding. When the robot was used, attendant assistance could be replaced for two 5-hour periods during the workday. Complete replacement was not possible because of required setup tasks (e.g., meal preparation for feeding by the robot). The replacement of personal assistant care is a major factor in determining the economic feasibility of the robot system. Hammel, Van der Loos, and Perkash (1992) show a projection (based on $7 per hour attendant care and a $50,000 robot) that makes the robot less expensive after a period of 5.5 years. Installation, training, and ongoing maintenance costs for the robot are included in their analysis.

Birch et al (1996) carried out a study to determine actual costs if using a robotic assistant as compared with using a personal assistant for office-related tasks. They used a simulated office environment and standardized tasks. They found that, although the robotic assistant did reduce assistant time and therefore cost, it also resulted in decreased productivity by the user. They attributed this reduction in productivity to waiting times necessitated by robotic movements, which were slower than the corresponding human attendant actions.

## Mobile Assistive Robots

Because we rarely do all our manipulation from a fixed location, **mobile assistive robots** have been developed. These fall into one of two general classes: (1) wheelchair mounted and (2) mounted on a mobile base that is

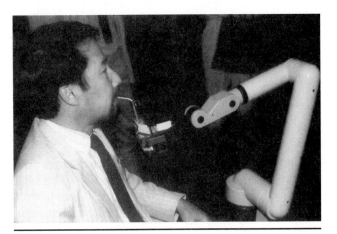

Figure 11-20   The Manus wheelchair-mounted robotic arm. (Courtesy CW Heckathorne, Northwestern University Rehabilitation Engineering Research Center, Chicago, Ill.)

controllable by the user. The major limitation of the first approach is that the most functional robot arms are relatively large. This large size, coupled with the other apparatus that must be attached to the wheelchair, makes attachment of the arm to the wheelchair impractical in many cases. Recent miniaturization of these arms has solved this problem.* The separate mobile base approach solves these problems, and it is practical in the home or at the work site. However, this approach also has disadvantages. The mobile robot requires that the user add "steering" to the required control commands. Because the user of a robot most likely has a restricted set of control signals available, the addition of these steering commands may be impossible. It is also difficult to transport the mobile base from one location to another. It is like having two powered wheelchairs to transport. Thus the most practical application of mobile robots is within one location. This location can, of course, include all rooms in a house or any location within a school, factory, or office.

In this section we describe two examples of mobile robots. One is based on a commercial educational robot, and the other has been developed specifically for assistive technology applications.

**Manus wheelchair-mounted robotic arm.** The Manus manipulator, pictured in Figure 11-20, is a robotic arm mounted to a wheelchair (Verburg et al, 1996). It was designed to serve as a general-purpose manipulative aid for people who have severe upper extremity limitations. The robotic arm has eight degrees of freedom, can lift a 1.5-kg (3.3-pound) weight when the arm is fully extended, and can

*The Helping Hand, Kinetic Rehabilitation Instruments, Inc., Hanover, Mass.

exert a gripping force of 20 N. The arm weighs 20 kg (9.09 pounds). Verburg et al (1996) describe the development of the Manus system, including several clinical and community-based trials that were employed to gain user feedback. Clinical trials of early versions of the Manus arm identified two major problems: (1) the limited interface options; (2) the fact that when the Manus arm was mounted to the wheelchair, the weight and width of it were increased too much.

Since these trials, several generations of this arm have been developed and multiple user interfaces have been tried. These include a multidimensional joystick, head control using either a joystick or the frontalis muscle electromyograph (EMG), enlarged keyboard, and foot control. There has also been work to integrate the Manus control into the wheelchair control system. The later was strongly recommended by user trials and provides a major improvement in integration of functions for the user. These changes have addressed the first of the early clinical trial concerns. A new mounting system, which includes moving the Manus out of the way when other activities are to be carried out, has addressed the second concern.

A technology assessment to determine the requirements for prescription and funding of the Manus system was carried out in the Netherlands from 1992 to 1993. This review included criteria for both the user skills required and the development of a set of prescription indicators. The report recommended that potential users should have minimal or no hand function or limited coordination of the upper extremities, inability to lift their arms against gravity, limited reach, use of an electric wheelchair, inability to feed or drink independently, and inability to manipulate objects. Indicator diagnoses included spinal cord injury, multiple sclerosis, rheumatoid arthritis, progressive dystrophies, and severe spasticity (e.g., cerebral palsy). User activities that were determined to be important for use of a Manus system included the need to engage in activities at different locations, an inability to function without assistance for large parts of the day, a living setting in which absence of a system like Manus would constitute an unacceptable load for family, and the ability to begin or resume work or school if a Manus were available. Motivational and cognitive criteria included general motivation to use Manus, ability to understand and remember the technical commands, and general familiarity with computers. The technology assessment also recommended that a three-month trial period in the community occur before final prescription approval. Criteria for evaluating the outcomes of the trial to determine whether final funding would be approved included whether the Manus was being used in the locations and for the purposes specified in the evaluation, whether the Manus had increased the user's independence, and how the Manus had affected the roles of aides and family members (e.g., increased or decreased time required for assistance and by how

much). Based on this technological assessment, the Manus was approved for funding in several European countries.

Use of the Manus system was also evaluated by 14 individuals in six European countries (the Netherlands, Germany, Norway, France, Italy, and Switzerland) (Oderud, 1997). These community-based evaluations demonstrated that the Manus manipulator was frequently used at home for activities of daily living (e.g., fetching objects, eating and drinking, preparing food in a microwave oven). Limitations in this home environment included the added size and weight of the wheelchair when the Manus was mounted to it (despite its redesign) and the need for training of the user and significant others. In these studies the Manus was not frequently used for vocational tasks. The major limitation in this context was that the Manus could not be preprogrammed for repetitive tasks, which added to the cognitive load of the user in the work environment, where speed of task performance was more critical.

There are still relatively few (less than 100) Manus systems in daily use by persons with disabilities. Cost, lack of understanding of the potential value of robotics, minimal infrastructure for marketing and support, and the need for training of users and professionals are the most often cited reasons for this slow growth in consumer base for this technology (Verburg et al, 1996; Oderud, 1997).

The Raptor robotic arm (Applied Research Corp.)* is the first such assistive technology device to be approved by the U.S. Food and Drug Administration. The Raptor is similar to the Manus in function, attaching to the wheelchair frame. A joystick, keypad, or sip-and-puff switch can control it. The Raptor has a 48-inch extension and can lift up to 4 pounds. The intended user population is the same as for the Manus.

**Mobile Vocational Assistant Robot.** The Mobile Vocational Assistant Robot (MoVAR) represents a specially configured robotic system developed for assistive applications. Many of the components of DeVAR are included in MoVAR (Van der Loos, Michalowski, and Leifer, 1988). These include the PUMA-260 robotic arm, a speech recognition control interface (Votan), a multiaxis joystick control, a task-oriented programming language (VAL-II), and a host-computer menu command interface. To meet the goals of mobility, two major additional components are added to the system. The first of these is a mobile base that is specially designed to allow easy movement in any direction in a small space. Specially designed and built wheels allow this flexibility in movement. Second, an expanded sensing system is added. A small camera is mounted on the robotic arm. This camera image is displayed directly to the user, and its image is used in modeling the environment for task-level

---

*Rehabilitaton Technologies Division, Applied Technologies Corp., Farifield, N.J. (www.appliedresource.com/RTD).

programming. Touch-sensitive bumpers that can determine whether to stop (e.g., at a wall) or to push harder (e.g., to open a door) are also included in the MoVAR. The MoVAR is about the same size as a powered wheelchair. The systems described in this section are examples chosen because of their design goals and their clinical evaluations. Several other robot systems are under development.

## Use of Robotics in Education

All the robot applications just described are intended for either personal (home) or vocational use. Robots have also been applied in educational settings. This setting places additional constraints on the robot system. First, the user may be very young, which necessitates simplified, age-appropriate control schemes and user interfaces. Second, the robot is intended to be used in a school, which places additional importance on safety because school children cannot be expected to exercise the same caution as adults.

For young children, manipulative tasks contribute to the development of cognitive and language skills (see Chapter 3). Robotic devices that aid manipulation can help young children with limited physical capabilities to develop these cognitive and language skills, as well as directly aiding manipulation. Cook, Liu, and Hoseit (1990) carried out a study to determine whether very young children would interact with a small computer-controlled robotic arm. Six disabled and three normal children, all less than 38 months old, were used in the study.

The system consisted of a microcomputer for control and data collection, a small robotic arm (about half the adult human scale), and a guidance unit used to train the arm to make specific movements (Cook et al, 1988). The arm can rotate around its base; flex and extend at the elbow and shoulder; extend, flex, supinate, and pronate the wrist; and open and close the gripper. The guidance unit used a joystick to train the arm by moving the joystick in the desired direction of arm movement. This made it intuitively simple for a teacher, therapist, or parent to train a specific movement that was of interest to the child. Three phases were used: (1) training the arm for a specific movement, (2) playback of the movement by the child using a single switch, and (3) monitoring the child's behavior during arm movement. Training of the arm was done by either using the guidance unit or by entering a series of text commands to train the arm. Using the guidance unit, the teacher, therapist, or parent moves the arm through the desired movement using the joystick, and the movement is stored for later playback. In the text training mode, commands such as 100 FORWARD (move the arm forward 1 inch) were typed and combined to form a complete task (e.g., bringing a cracker within reach of the child or dumping the contents of a cup).

In a typical task a child used the robot arm as a tool by pressing the switch only when it was necessary to bring an object closer to him or to uncover a hidden object (e.g., by tipping a cup containing an unknown object), and he did not press the switch when he could reach the object. This tool use is unique to a robotic arm as compared with toys or computer graphics used as contingent results, and it provides additional information over these simpler modes of interaction regarding the child's skills. Fifty percent of the disabled children and 100% of the normal children interacted with the arm and used it as a tool to obtain objects out of reach. All the disabled children with a cognitive developmental age of 7 to 9 months and older did interact with the arm, whereas those below this developmental level did not. Gross and fine motor skill levels were less related to success in using the robotic arm than were the levels in cognitive and language areas. This study showed that very young children will use a robotic arm to accomplish tasks that are of interest to them.

To facilitate the development of more complex tasks, it is necessary to move beyond single-switch playback for a movement. Cook et al (1988) developed a hierarchy of robotic movements that sequentially increased the complexity of the tasks the child needs to accomplish. These are related to the cognitive developmental levels described in Chapter 3. The child progresses from understanding simple playback of complete movements, to segments of movements, to complete control of the end point. Nof, Karlan, and Widmer (1988) used a two-level system for developing a child's interaction with a robotic arm. At the first level, the arm functions to carry out complete tasks. Sublevels included by Nof, Karlan, and Widmer were one- and two-step sequences, each used to carry out the same task. At the second level, the robotic arm allows the child to control component actions and incorporate these into more complex sequences.

Cook, Howrey, Gu, and Meng (2000) used a robotic arm to determine whether children (age 4 to 7) who have severe physical disabilities would be able to understand a sequence of motor actions and to use them to find buried objects of interest. Three specific robotic arm movements, each executed by a single switch press, were programmed. Dry macaroni in a tub was used to provide both sensory and motor interactions for the child. The tasks used included the following: (1) macaroni was dumped from a glass held by the robotic arm (one switch); (2) the child controlled the arm to dig an object out of the macaroni and then dump the macaroni and the object (two switches); and (3) the child caused the arm to move laterally to a location where an object had been buried, dig the object out of the macaroni, and dump the macaroni into the tub (three switches). The buried object was a plastic egg containing another object of interest to the child (e.g., finger puppet, small rubber stamp).

Cook, Howery, and Gu (1999) reported that children generally attended to tasks for significantly longer periods with the robot than with other activities (e.g., computer graphics programs). After one or two trials, all the children understood that hitting switch number 1 dumped the cup and its contents.

Adding a second switch with a different function led to some initial confusion for the child. After one or two physical prompts, each child learned to DIG (switch 2) and then DUMP (switch 1) with only verbal prompts. When the third switch (MOVE) was added (task 3), the children required differing levels of prompting to understand its function. When the third switch was added to the first two, the child required both verbal and physical prompts in order to carry out the third part of the sequence (MOVE). Children took more trials to understand this task, and each trial required more prompting.

Although all children could correctly sequence the actions to complete the entire task in multiple action tasks, the number of sessions and trials to reach this level varied. Children were much more motivated to learn how to use the robot and they kept their attention focused for longer periods, in contrast to simple toys, which do not generally allow the child to move beyond cause and effect relationships, and computer programs, which are not as concrete in relation to object manipulation and sequencing of tasks. Children were able to put two operations together to complete a task. The robot arm also gave the children the opportunity to interact with the investigators by "handing" objects to them and choosing which objects to be buried.

For school-age children, the robotic tasks become more functional. Howell, Damarin, and Post (1987) developed a robotic system for use in elementary schools. They used a small robot, a five-position slot switch, and a computer to control the arm. They defined four levels of control: (1) demonstration of the arm to the student, (2) performance of well-defined and prestored tasks, (3) unstructured movement controlled by the student, and (4) student programming and storage of movements for later playback. To accomplish these tasks, Howell, Hay, and Rakocy (1989) identified special software and hardware considerations. These include easy physical and cognitive access and fast interactional speed; understandable, powerful, and complete learner control features; and the definition of the robot motions useful in the classroom. They discuss possible solutions to each of these. This robotic system was applied to science instruction at the elementary school level (Howell, Mayton, and Baker, 1989). Two phases of field study were carried out: (1) a training component, in which the student became familiar with the use of the robotic system, and (2) an instructional component, in which the robot was used to complete science experiments. Important issues raised by this preliminary study were (1) the need for the robot to be transparent to the user (so that the student can focus on the learning task, rather than

robot control), (2) training methodology, and (3) curricular applications.

Another system for classroom use was developed in Great Britain (Harwin, Ginige, and Jackson, 1988). This system differed from other educational applications in the inclusion of a vision system based on a television camera and image recognition software. This allowed the system to be used for more sophisticated tasks such as finding and stacking blocks. Three tasks were used with this system: (1) stacking and knocking down blocks with two switches (yes/no), (2) sorting articles by shape or color with four switches (one for each feature) or two switches (yes/no), and (3) a stacking game with five switches (left, middle, right, pick up, release). Children with motor disabilities who used this system enjoyed it and were able to successfully complete the tasks described. By using the robotic arm, they could accomplish otherwise impossible tasks.

All the assistive robotic systems described in this section are still largely experimental. As technologies improve and costs come down, we will see more routine use of these systems in the home, school, and work site.

## ■ SUMMARY

Assistive technologies designed to aid manipulation help consumers in accomplishing tasks for which they normally use their upper extremities. Some manipulative aids are general purpose, meaning they serve multiple functions, and some are special purpose, designed for one task. In some cases the manipulative aid assists with normal hand function (e.g., hand-writing aids); we refer to these as *augmentative*. In other cases an *alternative* method is used (e.g., a robotic arm for moving items on a desk). In addition, special-purpose and general-purpose devices may be either high or low tech.

Low-tech general-purpose manipulation aids include mouthsticks, head pointers, and reachers. Special-purpose devices are available to meet needs in the general performance areas of self-care, work or school, and recreation or leisure.

Commercially available special-purpose electrically powered devices serve two primary functions: self-feeding and page turning. These may be controlled by many different control interfaces and selection methods. There are two types of general-purpose electrically powered devices: EADLs and robotic systems. Electronic aids to daily living include appliance control; telephone access; TV, VCR, and CD control; and remote access to doors, drapes, and windows. Robots are used to meet manipulative needs in the home, at work, and in the classroom. Both EADLs and assistive robots are controlled by computers, and each may be accessed by a variety of control interfaces and selection methods.

## Study Questions

1. List and describe the four categories of aided manipulation.
2. Give an example of a special-purpose low-tech manipulation aid for each of the three major performance areas.
3. What are the primary types of self-care adaptations provided by low-tech manipulation aids?
4. What are the primary types of work or school adaptations provided by low-tech manipulation aids?
5. What are the primary types of recreation and leisure adaptations provided by low-tech manipulation aids?
6. What are the functions provided by electrically powered feeders?
7. What are the two major approaches used in electrically powered page turners?
8. What are the functions provided by electrically powered page turners?
9. What, if any, are the advantages of using the term *electronic aids to daily living* rather than *environmental control units*?
10. What are the four control functions implemented in EADLs? Describe the differences between them and give an EADL example of each.
11. Discuss the relative advantages and disadvantages of the two modes of binary latched AC appliance control.
12. What are the four major transmission modes used in EADL systems?
13. How does a trainable or programmable IR controller work, and what are the major advantages of these types of device?
14. What is the difference between a trainable and a programmable IR controller?
15. Describe the functions of an automatic telephone dialer.
16. How do hospital EADLs differ from those used in the home?
17. List the major assessment questions to be answered when determining the best EADL for a specific user.
18. What are the most significant factors that contribute to use or nonuse of EADLs by persons with spinal cord injuries?
19. Compare the APL RAWT and the DeVAR desktop robot systems in terms of goals, basic design approach, robot arm used, control interface selected, cost, and degree of technological sophistication.
20. Describe the key design features of the Manus mobile robotic arm.
21. How do the Manus design features contribute or detract from its effectiveness and consumer satisfaction?
22. What are the key factors considered when determining if a Manus robotic arm is suitable for a consumer's needs and goals? Do you agree with these? Why or why not?
23. Describe the major differences between desktop and mobile robots from the point of view of both the required design and the user interaction with the robot.
24. How do educational applications of robotic systems differ from vocational or daily living applications?
25. How can robotic systems be used to evaluate and perhaps enhance cognitive and language functioning in young children?

## References

Barker P, Gross K, Henderson K: Control of the environment, *Proc '91 RESNA Pacific Reg Conf,* 1991.

Bentham JS, Bereton DS, Sapacz RA: The selection of environmental control systems, *Proc RESNA 13th Ann Conf,* pp 108-109, June 1992.

Birch GE et al: An assessment methodology and its application to a robotic vocational assistive device, *Tech Disabil* 5:151-165, 1996.

Chen LP et al: An evaluation of reachers for use by older persons, *Assist Technol* 10:113-125, 1998.

Ciarcia S: Plug-in remote control system, *Radio Electronics,* pp 47-51, September 1980.

Ciarcia S: Build a trainable infrared master controller, *Byte* 12(3):113-123, 1987a.

Ciarcia S: Build an infrared controller, *Byte* 12(2):101-109, 1987b.

Cook AM, Howery K, Gu J, Meng M: Robot Enhanced Interaction and Learning for Children with Profound Physical Disabilities, *Technology and Disability* 13(1):1-8, 2000.

Cook AM, Hussey SM: Meeting multiple needs with separate but equal interfaces, *Proc RESNA Conf,* pp 290-292, June 1992.

Cook AM, Liu KM, Hoseit P: Robotic arm use by very young motorically disabled children, *Assist Technol* 2:51-57, 1990.

Cook AM et al: Using a robotic arm system to facilitate learning in very young disabled children, *IEEE Trans Biomed Eng* 35(2):132-137, 1988.

Corell RW, Wijnschenk MJ: *Design and development of the Case research arm-aid,* Report No. EDC-4-64-4, Cleveland, 1964, Case Institute of Technology.

Corker K, Lyman JH, Sheredos S: A preliminary evaluation of remote medical manipulators, *Bull Prosthet Res* 16(2)107-134, 1979.

Dickey R, Shealey SH: Using technology to control the environment, *Am J Occup Ther* 41(11):717-721, 1987.

Efthimiou J et al: Electronic assistive devices: their impact on the quality of life of high level quadriplegic persons, *Arch Phys Med Rehabil* 62:131- 134, 1981.

Gross K: Controlling the environment, *Team Rehabil Rep* 3(6):14-16, 1992.

Hammel JM, Van der Loos HFM, Perkash I: Evaluation of a vocational robot with a quadriplegic employee, *Arch Phys Med Rehabil* 73:683-693, 1992.

Hammel J et al: Clinical evaluation of a desktop robotic assistant, *J Rehabil Res Dev* 26(3):1-16, 1989.

Harwin WS, Ginige A, Jackson RD: A robot workstation for use in education of the physically handicapped, *IEEE Trans Biomed Eng* 35:127-131, 1988.

Harwin WS, Rahman T, Foulds RA: A review of design issues in rehabilitation robotics with reference to North American projects, *IEEE Trans Rehabil Eng* 3:3-11, 1995.

Holme AS et al: The use of environmental control units by occupational therapists in spinal cord injury and disease, *Am J Occup Ther* 51:42-48, 1997.

Howell RD, Damarin SK, Post EP: The use of robotic manipulators as cognitive and physical prosthetic aids, *Proc 10th RESNA Conf*, pp 770-772, June 1987.

Howell RD, Hay K, Rakocy L: Hardware and software considerations in the design of a prototype educational robotic manipulator, *Proc 12th RESNA Conf*, pp 113-114, June 1989.

Howell RD, Mayton G, Baker P: Education and research issues in designing robotically-aided science education environments, *Proc 12th RESNA Conf*, 109-110, June 1989.

Jones RD et al: Microprocessor-based multi-patient environmental-control system for spinal injuries unit, *Med Biol Eng Comput* 18:607-616, 1980.

Lange M: Alternative reading options, *OT Pract*, pp 43-44, November, 1998.

MacNeil V: Electronic aids to daily living, *Team Rehabil Rep* 9(3):53-56, 1998.

Mann WC: Use of environmental control devices by elderly nursing home patients, *Assist Technol* 4:60-65, 1992.

McDonald DW, Boyle MA, Schumann TL: Environmental control unit utilization by high-level spinal cord injured patients, *Arch Phys Med Rehabil* 62:131-134, 1989.

Mills R: Impact of standards on future environmental control systems, *Proc 10th RESNA Conf*, pp 690-682, June 1987.

Nof SY, Karlan GR, Widmer, NS: Development of a prototype interactive robotic device for use by multiply handicapped children, *Proc Int Conf Assoc Adv Rehabil Technol (ICAART)*, pp 456-457, June 1988.

Oderud T: Experiences from the evaluation of a Manus wheelchair-mounted manipulator. In Anogianakis G, Bühler C, Soede M (eds): *Advancement in assistive technology*, Amsterdam, 1997, IOS Press.

Seamone W, Schmeisser G: Early clinical evaluation of a robot arm/worktable system for spinal-cord-injured persons, *J Rehabil Res Dev* 22(1):38-57, 1985.

Sell GH et al: Environmental and typewriter control systems for high-level quadriplegic patients: evaluation and prescription, *Arch Phys Med Rehabil* 60:246-252, 1979.

Stanger CA, Cawley MF: Demographics of rehabilitation robotics users, *Technol Disabil* 5:125-137, 1996.

Symington DC et al: Environmental control systems in chronic care hospitals and nursing homes, *Arch Phys Med Rehabil* 67:322-325, 1986.

Topping M: The Handy 1, a robotic aid to independence for severely disabled people, *Technology Disabil* 5:233-234, 1996.

Van der Loos HFM, Michalowski SJ, Leifer LJ: Development of an omnidirectional mobile vocational assistant robot, *Proc Int Conf Assoc Adv Rehabil Technol (ICAART)*, pp 468-469, 1988.

Verburg G et al: Manus: the evolution of an assistive technology, *Technol Disabil* 5:217-228, 1996.

Von Maltzahn WW, Daphtary M, Roa RL: Usage patterns of environmental control units by severely disabled individuals in their homes, *IEEE Trans Rehabil Eng* 3(2):222-227, 1995.

Woods BM, Jones RD: Environmental control systems in a spinal injuries unit: a review of 10 years experience, *Int Disabil Stud* 12:137-140, 1990.

## CHAPTER 12

# Sensory Aids for Persons with Visual or Auditory Impairments

---

## Learning Objectives

Upon completing this chapter you will be able to:

1. Describe the major approaches to sensory substitution, including the advantages and disadvantages of each
2. Describe device use for reading and mobility by persons who have visual impairment
3. Describe the design and specification of hearing aids
4. Describe adaptations of common devices for use by a person who is hard of hearing or deaf
5. Discuss the major approaches used to provide input for individuals who have both visual and auditory impairments

---

## Key Terms

Alternative Sensory System
Alerting Devices
Assistive Listening Devices
Braille
Clear-Path Indicator
Closed Captioning
Closed Circuit Television (CCTV)
Cochlear Implants

Digital Audio-Based Information
 System (DAISY) Consortium
Digital Talking Books (DTBs)
Electronic Travel Aid (ETA)
Environmental Sensor
Hearing Aids
Human/Technology Interface
Information Processor

Magnification Aids
Optical Aids
Optical Character Recognition
Orientation and Mobility
Reading Aid
Refreshable Braille Display
User Display

---

When an individual has a sensory impairment, assistive technologies can provide assistance in the input of information. In this chapter we emphasize approaches that are used to either aid or replace seeing and hearing. This chapter is restricted to sensory aids that are intended for *general use*. In Chapter 8 we discuss assistive technologies that are used specifically for providing visual access to computers. Assessment considerations for sensory function are described in Chapters 3 and 4. We begin this chapter by looking at the fundamental principles associated with sensory aids.

### ■ FUNDAMENTAL APPROACHES TO SENSORY AIDS

In Chapters 2 and 3 we describe the human component of the Human Activity Assistive Technology (HAAT) model in some detail. Two primary intrinsic enablers of the human in this model are sensing and perception. If there are impairments in either of these functions, it is necessary to utilize sensory aids. When we design or apply sensory aids, the level of impairment becomes a critical issue. If there is sufficient residual function in the primary sensory system being aided, we augment the input to make it useful to the person. For example, a hearing aid amplifies (augments) the level of auditory information. On the other hand, if there is insufficient residual sensory capability, then the sensory aid must use an alternative sensory pathway. For example, braille (tactile pathway) can be used for reading when vision is not functional. We describe both augmentation and replacement in this section.

Figure 12-1 shows the major components of a sensory aid based on the parts of the assistive technology component of the HAAT model. The *environmental interface* detects the sensory data that the human cannot obtain via her own sensory system. This is typically a camera for visual data, a microphone for auditory data, and pressure sensors

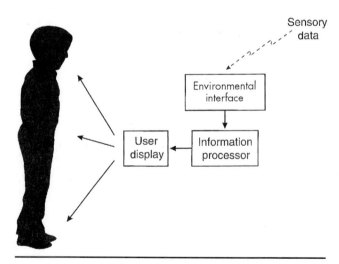

Figure 12-1   The major components of all sensory aids.

for tactile data. The environmental interface signal is fed to an **information processor,** the function of which depends on the type of aid. For sensory aids that use the same sensory pathway, the information processor primarily amplifies the signal. Examples include closed circuit television for visual input and hearing aids for auditory input. In other cases the information processor may be more complicated. For example, in an auditory substitution reading device, the information processor may take visual information from the sensor, convert it to speech, and then send it to the user as auditory information. In the case of the sensory aid, the **human/technology interface** is a **user display,** which portrays the sensory information for the human user. The processed information is presented to the user so that the alternative pathway can process it. For the visual pathway this is a visible display (e.g., a video monitor), for the auditory pathway it is an audio display (e.g., a speaker), and for the tactile pathway it is a vibrating pin or electrode array through which pressure or touch data are provided to the user.

## Augmentation of Existing Pathway

For someone who has low vision or is hard of hearing, the primary pathway (i.e., the one normally used for input) is still available, it is just limited. The limitation may be one of several types. The most common type of limitation is one of *intensity.* For visual information, this means that the size of the input signal is too small to be seen. Eyeglasses are the most common type of aid used for this problem, but we can also magnify in other ways. For auditory information, insufficient intensity means that the signals are too weak to be heard, and an amplifier (hearing aid or assistive listening device) is required.

The second type of impairment is referred to as a *frequency* or *wavelength* limitation. For visual input this is manifest in inadequacy discerning colors or the contrast between foreground and background, and we can address this problem with filters or by varying contrast (e.g., black on white rather than white on black). For people who are hard of hearing, certain frequencies may be more limited than others, and the hearing aid must be designed or specified to take this into account. For example, in aging there is usually a greater hearing loss in high than in low frequencies.

Finally, there are *field* limitations. This term is most commonly used in describing visual loss, and the field may be limited in several ways (see Figure 3-4). The most common approach to problems of this type is to use lenses that are designed to widen the field.

## Use of Alternative Sensory Pathway

When a sensory input modality is so impaired that there can be no useful input of information via that channel, we must substitute an **alternative sensory system.** Common examples of this approach are the use of braille for reading by persons who are blind (tactile substitution for visual) and the use of manual sign language by persons who are deaf (visual substitution for auditory). Tactile and auditory systems replace the visual system, and visual and tactile systems substitute for auditory input of information. When making this type of substitution, we must be aware of fundamental differences among the tactile, visual, and auditory systems.

**Tactile substitution.** The tactile system has been used as the basis for many visual substitution systems. Visual information is spatially organized (Nye and Bliss, 1970). This means that visual information is represented in the central nervous system by the relationship of objects to each other in space; that is, the left, right, up, down, far, and near features of objects are preserved. In contrast, the auditory system is temporally organized (Kirman, 1973). By this we mean that it is the time relationships in auditory signals that provide information. For example, it is the temporal sequence of sounds in speech that the auditory system uses to form words and derive meaning. Finally, tactile information is both temporally and spatially organized (Kirman, 1973), and sensory input via the tactile system requires both spatial and temporal cues. For example, the fingers are capable of distinguishing fine features such as those found on coins. However, in order to distinguish one denomination of coin from another, it is necessary to manipulate them in the hand. This movement of the coins provides temporal (time sequence) information that helps clarify the spatial information, and it is very difficult to distinguish two denominations of coins merely by placing a hand on top of them without movement. This combination of movement and texture is referred to as *spatiotemporal information.* The combination of tactile and kinesthetic or proprioceptive information is called the *haptic sensory system.*

Kirman (1973) presents an example that illustrates the differences between visual and tactile information for reading. Print on a page is organized spatially. We read by using saccadic eye movements, which jump from one group of letters to another. With each new point of focus, we take in new information. This allows the visual system (including the eyes, peripheral pathways, and central nervous system components) to use its spatial feature extraction to recognize shapes as letters, to assemble them into words, and to associate meaning with them. In contrast, a person reading with braille moves his hand across the line of raised dots, obtaining both spatial (the organization of the six braille cells) and temporal (the moving pattern under his finger) information. If the sighted person were to use the method employed with braille, the text would constantly move before the eyes, and this would result in a blurred image because the spatial information would be constantly changing. Thus we can say that the movement (temporal aspect) interferes with the visual input of information. On the other hand, if the braille user were to employ the approach used by the sighted reader, he would place his finger on a character, input the information, and then jump to the next character. This would severely limit the input of braille information because the movement required by the tactile system would be absent. Thus the visual and tactile methods of sensory input are very different, and we must take this into account when substituting one system for the other.

When vision is used for mobility rather than reading, there are some differences. In this case the visual image is constantly changing as the individual walks. The eyes scan the environment, and information is derived from the spatial arrangement of objects and people and from changes in the person's position relative to these objects as she moves. The visual system (including oculomotor components) functions to stabilize images on the retina for input of data, even during movement. This maximizes input of changing spatial information. We discuss ways in which persons with visual impairments use other senses and assistive devices for mobility in the section on mobility later in this chapter.

Substitution of tactile input for auditory information provides a different set of challenges. One major difference is that the rate at which the auditory information changes is relatively high compared with the time required for the tactile system to input information. Engineers refer to this as the relative *bandwidths* of the two systems. The auditory system has a broader bandwidth (more information can be handled in a given amount of time) than the tactile system. Because auditory information is a sequence of sounds, these must be translated into tactile information for presentation to the user. These tactile signals are then detected and assembled into meaningful units by the central nervous system. Because the tactile system requires spatial and temporal information, its rate of input is slower than for the auditory system. Another major limitation of the tactile system for auditory input is that it lacks a means of converting sound (mechanical vibrations) into neural signals. This is the function normally carried out by the cochlea.

The only tactile method for input of auditory information that has been successful is the *Tadoma method* employed by individuals who are both deaf and blind. In this method, used by Helen Keller, the person receives information by placing his hands on the speaker's face, with the thumbs on the lips, index fingers on the sides of the nose, little fingers on the throat, and other fingers on the cheeks. During speech, the fingers detect movements of the lips, nose, and cheeks and feel the vibration of the larynx in the throat. Through practice, kinesthetic input obtained from these sources is interpreted as speech patterns. One reason for the success of this method is that there is a fundamental relationship between the articulators (reflected in the movements of the lips, nose, and cheeks) and the perceived speech signal, and this relationship is at least as important as the acoustic information (pitch and loudness) in the speech signal for individuals using the Tadoma method (Lieberman, 1967).

**Auditory substitution.** The auditory system has been used to substitute for visual information in several ways. Some of these have been more successful than others, and the reasons for success or failure illustrate the challenges of substituting one sense for another. The least successful approaches have been those that converted a visual image of letters into a set of tones. One such device is the Stereotoner (Smith, 1972). The environmental interface for this device was a camera consisting of a set of horizontal slits. As the camera passed over a letter, a black area (i.e., a part of a letter) resulted in a tone being produced and a white area (no letter) resulted in silence. As the camera moved over a letter, a series of tones was heard as changing musical chords. Although some individuals were able to utilize this information at a reading rate of 40 words per minute, the device was generally unsuccessful. Cook (1982) cites several reasons for this. First, the device required the user to recognize a chord pattern, then to assemble that into a letter, and then to put the letters together into a word that was meaningful in the context of the whole sentence. This is a difficult and unnatural process for the auditory system. Second, the necessity to read letter by letter using this approach resulted in a slow input speed and placed additional memory requirements on the user. Finally, the Stereotoner was tiring to the user because of the intense concentration required. The major lesson to be learned from this example is that the auditory system is ideally suited to the receipt of language information in certain forms (e.g., speech), but it is poorly suited to complex signals that represent spatial patterns, as in the case of the Stereotoner. This is the primary reason that reading devices employing auditory substitution all use speech as the mode of presentation of information.

Devices for visual mobility have employed auditory substitution with greater success. This is because mobility depends much more on gross cues than on precise spatial information as in reading. In mobility the problem becomes one of identifying large objects as potential hazards.

**Visual substitution.** Visual displays of auditory information can take several forms. One example, sometimes used in speech therapy or as an aid to deaf individuals who are learning to speak, is to display a picture of the speech signal on an oscilloscope-like screen. Often a model pattern portraying the ideal is placed on the top half of the screen, and the pattern from the person learning to speak is placed on the bottom half of the screen. The learner attempts to match the model through practice. Some current devices also use computer graphics to make the process more interesting and motivating. This type of sensory substitution of visual for auditory information is a rehabilitative technology, and it is not practical for assistive technologies. The reasons that this is not an appropriate assistive technology parallel those presented for the Stereotoner in relation to auditory substitution.

Visual substitution for auditory information has been successful in several areas. These include visual alarms (e.g., flashing lights when a telephone or doorbell rings) and the use of text labels for computer-generated synthetic speech (see Chapter 8). Speech is the most natural auditory form of language. Likewise, written text is the most natural way of presenting visual language. Thus a major design goal for assistive devices that use visual substitution for auditory communication is to provide speech-to-text conversion. In this type of device, speech is received and converted by computer to text and displayed so that it can be read by the person with an auditory impairment.

## READING AIDS FOR PERSONS WITH VISUAL IMPAIRMENTS

Two of the major problems faced by persons with visual impairments are (1) access to reading material and (2) orientation and mobility (i.e., moving about safely and easily). In this section we first describe reading aids for people with low vision who still obtain information via the visual system. We then discuss tactile and auditory alternatives for people who are blind. The term *reading* is used here to include access to all print material, including text, mathematics, and graphical representations (e.g., maps, pictures, drawings, and handwriting). As we discuss later, some types of reading have very specialized alternatives (e.g., talking compasses in lieu of maps, talking bar code readers for medicines and food cans).

Dixon and Mandelbaum (1990) present an overview of technology-assisted reading aids for persons with visual impairments. One of the trends they describe is the availability of books on computer-readable disks. In this form a book can be loaded into a personal computer word processor (either Windows or Macintosh based) and displayed on the screen. The use of compact disk-read-only memory (CD-ROM) allows a great deal of information to be placed on a single disk. One CD can store a large amount of data. Reproduction costs are low. Because the CD-ROM is basically a storage medium for the computer (see Chapter 8), sophisticated search strategies can be used to find a particular item or place in the text. For persons with low vision or blindness, the availability of CD-ROM-based reading materials opens up many different options for obtaining access to print materials. For example, with an enlarged screen output, reading material on a CD-ROM can be accessed and presented to a person with low vision using a computer. More significant, however, is the use of either braille or speech output from the computer to allow individuals who are blind to read from the CD-ROM.

One of the challenges in any electronic format is standardization. Different countries have different recording formats for talking books on tape, and there are many formats for word processors in digital form. For this reason an international group, the **Digital Audio-Based Information System (DAISY) Consortium** (www.daisy.org) has developed an international standard for **digital talking books (DTBs)** (Kerscher and Hansson, 1998). This standard includes production, exchange, and use of DTBs. The goal of the DAISY Consortium is to promote the use of digital books that comply with an international standard. The members of the consortium are associations and organizations across the world that are involved in the provision of reading materials for individuals who are blind. The DAISY standard is hardware platform and operating system independent, and it makes use of the Web accessibility standards developed by the World Wide Web Consortium (W3C; see Chapter 8).

## Magnification Aids

Recall that there are three factors related to visual system performance for reading: size, spacing, and contrast. In Chapter 8 we describe how these three factors are accounted for in computer output displays for persons with low vision. In this section we discuss the principles of low-vision aids for reading print material. These devices are generally referred to as **magnification aids.** Magnification may be vertical (size) or horizontal (spacing) or both. We use the term *magnification* to also include assistive technologies that enhance contrast. There are three categories of magnification aids: (1) optical aids, (2) nonoptical aids, and (3) electronic aids (Servais, 1985). Examples of these are listed in Box 12-1.

| BOX 12-1 | Categories and Examples of Low-Vision Aids* | |
|---|---|---|
| **OPTICAL AIDS** | **NONOPTICAL AIDS** | **ELECTRONIC AIDS** |
| Handheld magnifiers | Enlarged print | Closed circuit televisions (CCTVs) |
| Stand magnifiers | High-intensity lamps | Portable CCTVs |
| Field expanders | Daily living aids | Slide projectors |
| Telescopes | High-contrast objects | Opaque projectors |
| | | Microfiche readers |

*Data from Servais SP, Visual aids. In Webster JG et al (eds): *Electronic devices for rehabilitation*, New York, 1985, John Wiley and Sons.

**Optical aids.** More than 90% of all individuals who have visual impairments have some usable vision (Doherty, 1993). Thus it is important to carefully choose low-vision devices to meet their needs. The National Institute on Disability and Rehabilitation Research has published a booklet describing clinical assessment methods, equipment, and tools needed for evaluating and matching of consumer's needs to low-vision devices (Doherty, 1993). With the use of **optical aids,** individuals with low vision may be able to see print, do work requiring fine detail, or increase the range of their visual fields.

The simplest of optical aids is the handheld magnifier. Among the advantages of these devices is that they require little training, they are lightweight and small (can fit in a pocket or purse), and they are inexpensive. Some also have a built-in light to increase contrast, and others have several lenses, which can be used alone or in combination, depending on the application.

Sometimes it is difficult to hold a lens and carry out a task (e.g., a two-handed task such as embroidery). In other cases it may be difficult to hold a magnifier steady (e.g., for someone who is elderly or in poor health). In these situations, stand magnifiers, some of which have a built-in light, are useful. Some magnifiers are mounted on eyeglass frames to free both hands.

One approach to limitations of visual field is the use of field expanders. These are generally prisms or special lenses built in to eyeglass frames. When magnifying lenses are used, the expansion of the field reduces the size of the image and a tradeoff occurs. The image is not reduced in size when prism lenses are used to expand the field.

Telescopes assist with distance vision. These may be either worn on the head or held in the hand, and they may be monocular or binocular (Mellor, 1981). They may be used, for example, by students who need to see a chalkboard or an adult who needs to monitor children playing outdoors. Telescopic aids provide an enlarged but narrowed visual field. Head-mounted units may be attached to eyeglass frames or have a separate frame. Head-mounted devices are particularly useful when long periods of wear are necessary, such as when watching television.

**Nonoptical aids.** This approach to magnification is based on changes in the actual material that is to be read (Servais, 1985). Common examples are large-print books or other materials such as menus, programs, and newspapers. High-intensity lamps can significantly increase contrast of reading materials, and high-contrast objects in the environment can aid in localization. For example, brightly colored furniture or dishes can help with visualization. A glass that stands out from a countertop is easier to find and fill with liquid. As Servais (1985) points out, nonoptical aids can be very useful under the right circumstances, but they are limited in application because they are specialized to one or a few tasks.

**Electronic aids.** There are limitations to the amount of magnification and contrast enhancement that can be obtained by optical approaches to magnification. Electronic devices can overcome these limitations. Many electronic low-vision aids are based on **closed circuit television (CCTV)** devices. Some manufacturers refer to these devices as *video magnifiers.* There are two primary advantages of CCTV devices. The first of these is that the image size can be increased much more than for optical aids. Equally important is that the image can be manipulated and controlled. For example, contrast can be dramatically affected by the use of color or reversed images (e.g., white type on black background). The overall brightness of an image can also be controlled in CCTV devices, further increasing contrast.

A typical CCTV is shown in Figure 12-2. The major components are a camera (environmental interface), a video display (user display), and a unit that controls the presentation of the image (information processor). The material to be read is placed on a scanning table, which easily moves both left to right and forward and back. There may be mechanical notches that help align the material, and some devices have adjustable margins. When the text is enlarged, the relative position of the material on the page is lost, and a spotlight of high intensity is sometimes used to show the user which part of the page is being imaged. Using a split video screen, CCTV devices can be operated in conjunction with enlarged computer video displays (see Chapter 8) to allow magnification of both computer data and the CCTV image of standard print material. Other contexts in which CCTV devices are used are to complete job-related tasks, to access educational materials at all levels, and for recreational reading.

All CCTV devices have the major features shown in Figure 12-2. An example of a CCTV device in use is shown in Figure 12-3. There is, however, a relatively wide range of features available in specific devices. The two broad categories of CCTVs are desktop and portable. The first category is by far the largest in terms of commercial products. Size and spacing are controlled primarily by two factors in desktop units: (1) size of the video monitor and (2) amount of enlargement provided by the electronics. Typical video monitors range in size from 12 to 19 inches, and maximal electronic magnification ranges from 45 to more than 60 times. There is a major tradeoff between monitor size and overall space required for the unit. Space requirements are often a significant limitation if a computer terminal, printer, and other office equipment must share space with the CCTV. A split-screen system overcomes this space problem to a large degree.

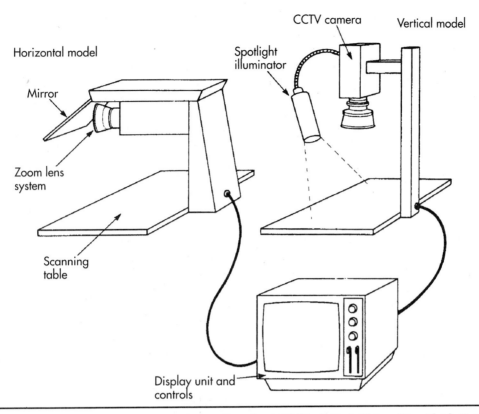

**Figure 12-2**    Closed circuit television system for low-vision assistance. (From Servais SP, Visual aids. In Webster JG et al [eds]: *Electronic devices for rehabilitation,* New York, 1985, John Wiley and Sons.)

Contrast enhancement is provided either by gray scale or color. In the former approach the foreground and background contrast is adjustable and may be reversed (e.g., black letters on white or white letters on black). Color adds significant contrast enhancement because the user can choose alternative background and foreground colors. Not all persons with visual impairments have the same color vision, and color vision varies with visual field. Having some control over the foreground-background color combination allows the display to be customized to the needs of an individual user. Another advantage of color displays is that the original color of the print material can be retained. Maps with colored areas can be imaged, a preprinted form that calls for a signature "on the red line" shows the line as red, and so on. The major tradeoff with color monitors is that the image is not as sharp as the black and white image, especially at large magnifications. Color CCTVs are also more expensive than their black and white counterparts.

Most desktop CCTVs are relatively large and heavy, primarily because of the video monitor. They also must be plugged into a wall socket for power. Thus it is difficult to transport them or to use them in contexts such as a classroom (unless a separate workstation is established—a common practice), and desktop units are generally kept in one physical location. Some desktop models have very small

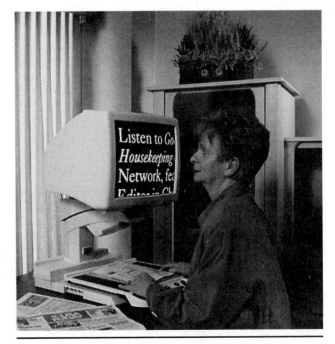

**Figure 12-3**    A CCTV device in use. (Courtesy NanoPac, Tulsa, Okla.)

cameras (e.g., 1-inch diameter, 3 inches long) that can be connected to any video monitor or television set. This facilitates transportation and use in different locations.

There are also fully portable CCTVs that are designed to be carried with the user. The most significant differences between these portable units and desktop CCTVs are size, weight, and battery power. Portable units weigh as little as 1.2 pounds and measure only about 9 × 3 inches for the display and 4 × 2 inches for the camera.* Portable units have a handheld camera that is moved over the page. Maximal magnification varies from 3 to 64 times, and it may be controlled by changing camera lenses or by electronic image enhancement. Some units allow the camera to be connected to a desktop video monitor or standard television set to display the CCTV output. This allows it to be used in a portable or stationary mode, depending on the needs of the user.† These cameras are extremely small (e.g., 2 inches × 2 inches × 4 inches, weighing 6 ounces). This flexibility is useful when greater magnification is needed for certain material (e.g., fine print) or at certain times (e.g., at the end of the day, when fatigue is greater), and when the user must travel to different settings during the day.

## Devices That Provide Automatic Reading of Text

Automatic reading of text requires the three components shown in Figure 12-1: an environmental interface, an information processor, and a user display. The environmental interface is a camera that provides an image of the printed page, and the user display can be either tactile (braille) or speech synthesis. A block diagram showing the major components of an automatic reading machine is presented in Figure 12-4. Device operation involves scanning, optical character recognition (OCR), and the translation of recognized characters and either text-to-braille or text-to-speech conversion (see Figure 12-4). Most reading machines provide speech output, and some provide braille or both braille and speech. Both software and hardware approaches are used for speech synthesis output in much the same way as those employed in screen readers for the blind* (see Chapter 8). Synthetic speech for automatic reading systems is available in a variety of languages. Some automatic reading devices utilize standard personal computers (PCs) with special software for information processing. The PC is interfaced to a scanner (camera with software) and display (refreshable braille or speech synthesis). Current stand-alone (scanner included in the basic system) automatic reading machines offer simple one-button operation to scan a document and have it read. These units also provide manual access to features such as cursor keys to move around in the text, storing and retrieving files, and transferring the text to a computer or floppy disk. Automatic reading systems can also be used in conjunction with the leading screen readers and Web browsers described in

*Liberty, HumanWare, Inc., Loomis, Calif.
†For example, OVAC Color-eye or Golden Eye OVAC, Cathedral City, Calif. (www.ovac.com); Vision Technology, Maryland Heights, Mo. (www.visiontech.com).

*For example, several versions of DECtalk (Digital Equipment Corp., Maynard, Mass); ViaVoice Outloud (IBM Special Needs Systems, Austin, Tex. (www.rs6000.ibm.com/sns).

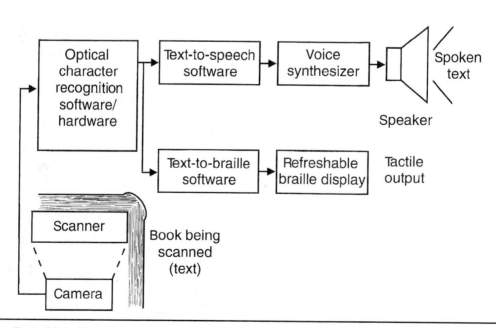

Figure 12-4 The major components of an automatic reading machine for persons with total visual impairment.

Chapter 8. Advances in OCR-based reading machines have led to reductions in price by as much as a factor of 10 during the 1990s (Scadden, 1997).

**Camera and scanner characteristics for automatic reading.** To input the information into the machine, reading devices may use a flatbed scanner, a handheld scanner, or a combination of the two (Fruchterman, 1991). Flatbed scanners have a glass plate 18 to 24 inches long and 10 to 14 inches wide. Scanners are usually defined as letter or legal size depending on the dimensions of the flat bed. This type of scanner, also called a *desktop scanner,* resembles a photocopy machine; however, the thickness is only about 3 to 4 inches. The material to be read is placed on the surface of the glass, and one advantage of this type of unit is that it can scan almost any kind of document, from a single sheet to a bound magazine or book. An automatic document feeder attachment can also be added to many flatbed scanners. This allows multiple sheets to be loaded and scanned. Scanners are widely used for home or business applications such as scanning photographs for use on Web pages or scanning documents for editing when an electronic copy is not available. For this reason the technology is improving and the prices are falling as a result of the general market demand (Grotta and Grotta, 1998). This has resulted in advances that benefit blind users of automatic reading systems. Handheld scanners vary in width from $2^1/_2$ to $8^1/_2$ inches (Converso and Hocek, 1990). For scanners narrower than the page, the camera must be moved across a line of text, then moved down to the next line, and so on all the way down the page. This can be difficult for a person who is blind, since there is no frame of reference to keep the scanner on one line or to move just one line down. Flatbed scanners overcome this problem. The handheld scanner can image most types of material, including single sheets and bound documents. An additional advantage is that it can be used with a laptop computer to create a portable reading machine.

All scanners consist of a light source and a camera, and some also contain lenses and mirrors to focus the image on the camera (Converso and Hocek, 1990). Grotta and Grotta (1998) describe both the use of charge coupled device (CCD) imaging electronics and an emerging technology called contact image scanners (CIS). CCD cameras use a lens and mirror arrangement that moves across the document with the light source (usually a fluorescent lamp) and is used to focus the image on the CCD detector. In contrast, CIS systems have a single row of sensors that is positioned just a few millimeters below the document and moves across it, together with an array of light sources, during the scan. The CIS systems draw less power; have a simpler mechanical design, making it possible to have thinner units; and eliminate the delicate optics of CCD devices. The resolution of CIS systems is not as good as that of CCD devices,

but it is rapidly improving. The CCD or CIS array serves as a camera that converts the areas of light and dark to an electronic format and computer software stores it in memory. Handheld types have only the camera and light source. The image that the camera stores consists of an array of black and white or color areas called pixels. The density of these pixels in the computer-stored image measures the quality of the scanner image. The units of measure are dots per inch (dpi). Scanners have resolutions from 300 to 4800 dpi (Grotta and Grotta, 1998). The other major specification that is used is gray scale levels (for black and white scanning) and color bit depth for color scanning. Typical gray scale values are 256 levels. Color bit depth varies from 24 to 36 bits (Grotta and Grotta, 1998). Some automatic reading systems have scanners built into them.* Other systems are designed to use external commercial scanners.†

**Optical character recognition.** The camera and scanner provide an image, consisting of an array of pixels. This image is black and white or color dots, and it is not in a form that can be translated into speech or braille. **Optical character recognition (OCR)** is used to carry out this conversion. Units, called OCRs, have been developed for scanning print documents into computer-readable form by businesses. They also are used in automatic reading devices for persons who are blind.

The OCR is a software program that runs on a standard PC. The primary function of the OCR is to analyze the raw pixel data and assemble it into letters, spaces (to delineate words), and punctuation. Graphics (pictures or drawings, as well as elaborate characters sometimes used to begin chapters in books) also must be removed from the text before output. There are a number of problems that OCR software must solve. The most significant of these is that letter recognition must occur with different print fonts. OCRs that accomplish this are called *omnifont OCRs.* Most scanners have an OCR product bundled with the scanner. These OCRs provide basic OCR capabilities, but they do not match stand-alone OCR products. Automatic reading systems use the professional stand-alone OCR products to achieve the best possible results. There are several general-purpose commercial omnifont OCR systems commonly used in reading machines for people who are blind. Some companies that provide automatic reading systems have their own proprietary OCR software, and others use professional-quality OCR software developed for business applications. The majority of the commercial software in-

---

*For example, the Aladdin Ambassador from Telesensory, Sunnyvale Calif. (www.telesensory.com), Galieo, Robotron Proprietary Limited, St. Kilda, Australia (www.robotron.net.au); Vera, Freedom Scientific, St. Petersburg, Fla. (www.freedomsci.com).
†For example, Open Book, Freedom Scientific, St. Petersburg, Fla. (www.freedomsci.com); Reading Advantage Telesensory, Sunnyvale, Calif. (www.telesensory.com).

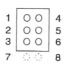

Standard braille cell

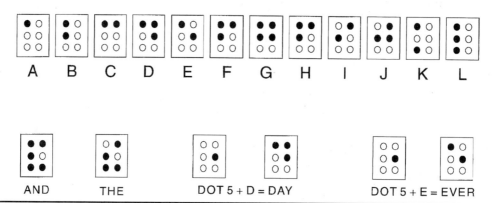

Figure 12-5　Examples of braille letters, word signs, and contractions.

corporated into automatic reading systems uses either the Xerox or Caere OCR software. Most current scanners use OmniPage LE,* the TextBridge Classic,† or proprietary OCR software. All the OCR software available separately is compatible with the Windows operating system, and several automatic reading systems utilize standard PCs, OCR software, and an external scanner. Converso and Hocek (1990) present some guidelines for selecting a scanner and OCR for specific applications. They also include a discussion of computer hardware and software (e.g., word processing) factors to consider when obtaining scanners and OCRs.

### Braille As a Tactile Reading Substitute

The most widely used tactile substitution device for persons with visual impairments is **braille**. Each braille character consists of a cell of either six or eight dots, as shown in Figure 12-5. The seventh and eighth dots are used to show cursor movement or to provide single-cell presentation of higher level ASCII codes. This is necessary because the six braille dots can only display 64 different combinations and there are 256 ASCII codes for characters (upper- and lowercase alphabet, numbers, special symbols and control characters like RETURN). Figure 12-5 shows examples of letters and numbers. When text is directly translated into braille letter by letter, it is referred to as *Grade 1*. Also shown in Figure 12-5 are some braille codes for words (called

*Caere Corp., Los Gatos, Calif.
†Xerox Corp., Peabody, Mass. (www.xerox.com).

*wordsigns*) and word endings. The use of these contractions significantly speeds up the rate of reading, and this type of braille is called *Grade 2* or *Grade 3*, depending on the number of contractions used. Reading rates with Grade 1 braille are about 40 words per minute (wpm). With Grade 3, reading speeds can approach 200 wpm (Allen, 1971). Traditionally, braille has been produced by embossing on heavy paper, and this method is still widely used. For persons who develop skill with it, braille can be a fast and efficient method for accessing print materials.

**Characteristics of braille.** There are several disadvantages to the use of braille, especially in embossed form. First, the embossed material is heavy and bulky, and each braille page has significantly less information than a printed page of the same size. For example, a braille version of a 400-page print book would fill four books, each the size of an encyclopedia volume (Mann, 1974). A second disadvantage is that the cost of producing braille in an embossed form is high compared with print materials. For this reason, only a fraction of the total print literature is available in braille form. A third limitation is related to the spatial orientation of visual (print) material. When we are scanning for a particular piece of information or editing text, we use this spatial orientation to find the particular piece of text we need. This process is difficult when using the embossed braille paper format. This is partially because of the bulky nature of the material, but it is also a result of the difficulty that braille readers have in scanning text quickly. Finally, braille embossers do not allow corrections to be made. Once

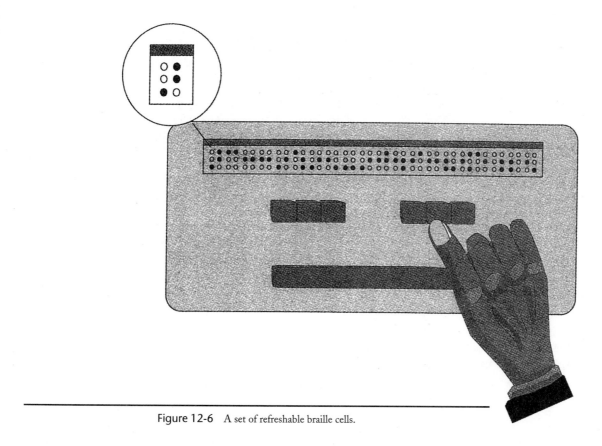

Figure 12-6    A set of refreshable braille cells.

the dot pattern is impressed into the paper, it is not possible to remove it.

Braille itself, regardless of format, has limitations as well. The most significant is that very few persons (less than 10%) with severe visual impairment learn to use it. This is partially because more than 65% of all persons who become blind do so after age 65 (Mann, 1974), and many of these cases are the result of diabetes, which also affects the tactile sense, making braille less desirable than other alternatives such as talking books. Despite all these disadvantages, braille is the modality of choice for many persons with severe visual impairment, and the use of a format other than embossed paper significantly enhances the effectiveness of this modality. One of the most widely used of these alternative formats is a refreshable braille cell.

**Refreshable braille displays.** Because braille is represented by a series of dots, raised pins can be substituted for the traditional embossed paper format. This approach, called **refreshable braille display,** is shown in Figure 12-6. There are several advantages of this format. The most significant of these is that the refreshable display is controlled by an electronic circuit that can be interfaced to computer displays or braille keyboards. This allows information to be stored electronically and greatly reduces the bulk compared with embossed braille. Second, because the text

material is in electronic form, it can be edited, searches can be made, and copies of braille material can be easily produced in electronic form (e.g., on floppy disk or CD). The refreshable braille cell (or cell array) can also be used as the output mode for an automatic reading machine.

Each refreshable braille cell has a set of small pins arranged in the shape of a standard braille cell. The pins that correspond to the dot pattern for a letter or word sign are raised. Both Grade 1 and Grade 2 braille can be presented on refreshable displays using software that converts text from ASCII format (see Chapter 8) to braille. Arrays of from 1 to 80 cells are available.

Stationary refreshable braille displays have arrays with multiple braille cells. Typically the array sizes are 20, 40, or 80 cells. These arrays, and the hardware and software to control them, typically cost in the range of $4500 for a 20-cell array.* As the number of elements in the array increases, the cost rises (about 25% for 40 cells). Generally the standard six-dot format is used for each cell. For an eight-dot cell, the price for a 40-cell array is 20% higher than for the six-dot format. The 80-cell format allows an entire line of a computer screen to be displayed at one time. An eight-dot, 80-cell refreshable display can cost as much as

---

*All Price Comparisons for Power Braille 40, 65, 80, Freedom Scientific, St. Petersburg, Fla. (www.freedomsci.com).

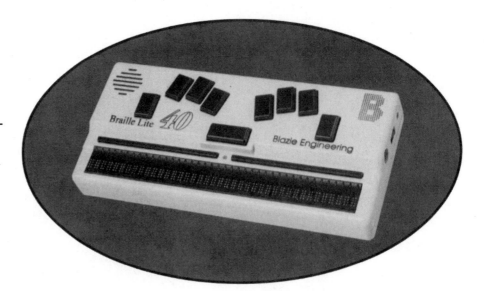

Figure 12-7   The Braille Lite 40 personal organizer with braille display and synthesized speech output. (Courtesy Freedom Scientific, St. Petersburg, Fla.)

$10,000, an increase of 123% over the cost of a 40-cell, eight-dot device. Thus price is a major consideration in refreshable braille displays. The refreshable braille arrays we have described generally can be used as an alternative to the screen in desktop computers. Most are designed for Windows- or Macintosh-based computers (see Chapter 8).

**Portable braille notetakers and personal organizers.**
These stand-alone data managers or personal organizers vary in size from a compact 4.5 inches square and about 1.5 inches thick to the size of a laptop computer (approximately 9 × 12 inches).* A typical model is pictured in Figure 12-7. Some models use a braille keyboard for input and others use a standard QWERTY keyboard. The braille keyboard has one key for each of the six dots in a braille cell. Additional keys are used for eight-dot braille and for control, editing, and data management. Output takes several forms. Synthesized speech is available in all units. Earphone and speaker output for the synthesized speech are also available. Some models include a refreshable Grade 2 braille display (from 8 to 18 braille cells) either alone or paired with synthetic speech. The speech synthesizer and refreshable braille display can also be used as outputs (replacing the output from the video monitor) in conjunction with screen reader software on a PC (see Chapter 8). Additional outputs available on selected models include computer file transfer, Internet and e-mail access via a modem (generally external to the notetaker), and print.

*For example, the 2000 Series, Freedom Scientific, St. Petersburg, Fla. (www.freedomsci.com); Ergo Braille, Braille Pad, SQWERT Family and TRANSTYPE Family, Artic Technologies, Troy, Mich. (www.artictech.com); Bookworm, Handy Tech Elektronik GmbH, Germany; Braille Companion, HumanWare, Loomis, Calif.; and Aria, Robotron Proprietary Limited, St. Kilda, Australia (www.robotron.net.au).

Some models also dial a telephone automatically from the data in the built-in address book. Built-in programs vary somewhat among various models. All include some sort of word processing for writing away from a computer (e.g., while sitting by the pool or riding a bus to work), editing documents developed on a PC word processor, and taking notes in class or at meetings. Other programs built into specific models, in various combinations, include a calendar, address book, calculator, timer or watch, e-mail access, Internet browser, and text (ASCII) to braille translation. Storage of data is in both random access memory (RAM) and flash read only memory (ROM). Removable flash memory cards increase both flexibility and growth potential as the capacity (currently about 2 to 20 megabytes) is continually being increased. Floppy disk storage, either built in or separate, adds to storage capability and provides an additional means of transferring files between the notetaker and a PC word processing program. Total storage varies from less than 1000 pages of text to more than 4000 pages. Storage of information may be in the form of braille or print or both. Control features may be via additional keys with specific functions or via a speech output menu of choices.

## Speech As an Auditory Reading Substitute

Because reading is based on visual language, it is logical that auditory substitution for reading also uses language—that is, speech. Audio technology is the primary method for information storage and retrieval used by individuals who are blind (Scadden, 1997). All the approaches discussed in this section have speech as the output mode.

**Recorded audio material.**   The oldest and still the most prevalent use of auditory substitution for persons with visual

## CASE STUDY 12-1

### BRAILLE NOTE TAKING IN SCHOOL

Jenny is an eighth-grade student. She uses many pieces of technology to assist her in being successful at school. She has been using a Braille 'n Speak since the fifth grade to take class notes, complete assignments, take tests, keep an assignment notebook, and maintain a personal phone and address book. Review the features of this device (www.freedomsci.com) and list those that are likely to benefit Jenny in each of these applications.

impairment is recorded material. Current technology used in recorded audio material is cassette tapes, CDs, and CD-ROMs.*

The major type of recorded material is cassette tapes. Several models are provided by The National Library Service for the Blind (NLS). The major features that are included on some or all of these are $15/16$-inch per second (ips) (nonstandard for longer play and copyright protection) and $17/8$-ips (standard used for music tapes) playback speeds, variable speed control, portability, automatic reverse or rewind, and frequency compensation to allow increased speed without a "chipmunk" sound. The variable speed allows the listener to review material faster than it was originally spoken. With practice, it is possible to understand speech at rates up to four times normal. Some people also use this type of machine to record lectures and then review the material in lieu of note taking. Cassette tapes can be produced by virtually any local library to make backup copies for distribution.

The major advantages of CDs for music are greatly increased fidelity resulting from greater frequency response, smaller size of both player and disks than phonograph records, and indexing, which can be used to find a particular track. These features are being exploited in recorded material for individuals who are blind (Scadden, 1997). The use of digitized audio information allows voice recordings to be mixed with headings that allow easier searching of the text. Multimedia presentations are also commonplace with CDs, allowing both visual and auditory presentation of information and thereby increasing the potential market and reducing price. Audio displays are also being used for the presentation of mathematical information using computers and speech synthesizers and as a substitute for data presentation (e.g., tables, charts) (Scadden, 1997).

**Synthetic speech output reading machines.** Auditory output from automatic reading machines is provided by synthetic speech devices. We discuss types of speech synthesis and conversion of ASCII text into speech (called *text-to-speech*) in Chapter 9. The use of speech synthesis in reading machines for persons with visual impairments or learning disabilities utilizes the standard types of speech synthesis. There are a variety of both hardware- and software-based speech synthesizers used with reading programs or aids (see Chapter 8). Because many reading devices are based on personal computers, screen readers (programs that provide synthetic speech output from the computer screen; see Chapter 8) can also be used as reading machines.

There are several ways in which information can be converted to ASCII form for use by a screen reading program. The most common is to use a scanner and OCR program as discussed in this section. A second approach is to obtain floppy disks or CD-ROMs that contain computer-readable written material (Dixon and Mandelbaum, 1990). There are services that make books on disk available to persons who are blind. The computer disks have files that can be loaded into a word processor and then read using a screen reader program. The CD-ROMs provide significantly greater storage than floppy disks, and they are made available to blind readers by publishers. Dictionaries, almanacs, and encyclopedias are among the many publications available in this format. A major advantage of this type of storage is the indexing and searching capability provided by CD-ROM technology. There is now a large and growing amount of literature (especially the classics) available on the Internet* in electronic form (called *e-text*). Many newspapers put their whole issues on the Internet, in addition to on-line news and sports services. Individuals who are blind can read this information using screen readers and accessible Web browsers (see Chapter 8).

### ■ MOBILITY AND ORIENTATION AIDS FOR PERSONS WITH VISUAL IMPAIRMENTS

The requirements of devices that aid mobility for persons with visual impairments differ significantly from those for reading. Mobility presents notable problems for persons with visual impairments, and the blind traveler uses many

---

*For example, Recording for the Blind and Dyslexic (www.rfbd.org); The Internet Talking Bookshop (www.orma.co.uk/intab); National Library Service for the Blind and Physically Handicapped, Library of Congress (http://lcweb.loc.gov/nls/nls).

*For example, The 1st Books Library (www.1stbooks.com); Gutenberg Project (http://promo.net/pg); BiblioBytes (http://www.bb.com); Camera Obscura (www.hicom.net/~oedipus/etext); Carrie (www.books.com/scripts/lib.exe); Electronic Library (www.books.com/scripts/lib.exe); Hanover College History (http://history.hanover.edu/texts.htm); Children's Literature Web Guide (www.acs.ucalgary.ca/~dkbrown/); Internet Public Library (Youth Division) (www.ipl.org/youth/); Project Bartleby (www.columbia.edu/acis/bartleby).

methods to orient herself to the environment and move safely within it (American Foundation for the Blind, 1978). Attention to sensory inputs of smell, sound, air currents, and surface texture alert the blind person to the terrain and environment, and a blind person can learn to pick up cues regarding objects. Sound cues are derived from reflections, sound shadows, and echo location. Temperature changes are also important. For example, passing a window on a cold day or passing under a canopy on a warm day provides information that is used in orientation. Odors from restaurants and crowds and other strong smells also provide information. Input regarding the texture of a sidewalk or grass is provided by the kinesthetic sense. Finally, persons with visual impairments also use travel aids, some of which are discussed in this section.

## Reading versus Mobility

There are several important differences between sensory input for reading and that for mobility (Mann, 1974). Inaccuracies in reading result in loss of information, but errors in **orientation and mobility** can result in injury or embarrassment. In a **reading aid** the input is constrained. By this we mean that the information to be sensed is always in a text or graphics form. Although there are differences in text fonts and reading needs, the differences across all reading material are relatively small. In mobility, however, the range of possible inputs is large. The blind traveler needs to avoid obstacles as varied as a roller skate and a tree. The environment changes frequently (e.g., a chair is moved to a new location), and the blind person must be able to sense these differences. Nye and Bliss (1970) point out that the obstacles of most concern to blind travelers are bicycles, streets, posts, toys, ladders, scaffolding, overhanging branches, and awnings. We define the environmental input required for mobility as being unconstrained because these changes are not predictable and cover a wide range of inputs. In order to be successful, the design and specification of mobility aids for blind persons must take into account these factors. *Orientation* refers to the "knowledge of one's location in relation to the environment" (Scadden, 1997, p. 141). There are several electronic travel aids that address this problem.

## Canes

The most common mobility aid for persons with visual impairments is the long cane, with as many as 40,000 users in the United States alone (Farmer, 1978). The standard cane consists of three parts: the grip, the shaft, and the tip. The entire cane is designed to maximize tactile and auditory input from the environment. The grip (which forms the handle) is made of leather, plastic, rubber, or other materials that easily transmit the tactile information to the user's

hand. The shaft and tip work together to sense and then relay the tactile information to the grip. The tip (especially a metal tip being used on a hard surface like concrete) is a major source of high-frequency auditory input used by pedestrians who are blind to detect obstacles and landmarks by echolocation. A careful balance is obtained between sufficient rigidity to resist wind and bending and adequate flexibility to transmit the tactile and auditory sense of the surface texture.

Many blind travelers use folding or telescoping canes, which offer the advantage of easy storage when not in use. Typically these are made of composite materials such as carbon fiber. When collapsed they can be placed in a pocket or purse.

The primary advantages of canes are the low cost and the simplicity of use. They have significant limitations, however. One of these relates to the range over which sensory information is obtained. In use the cane is moved in an arc approximately one step in front of the user. Any obstacles outside this range are not detected, and in some cases it is difficult for the blind traveler to adjust and avoid an obstacle within the space of only one step. A second limitation is that the cane only senses obstacles that are below waist level. In many cases, objects above knee level are not sensed until it is too late. For example, if there is a table in the path of the user, the cane may pass between the table legs, under the tabletop. The user will be unaware of the table's existence until he runs into it. Obstacles that are above waist height are also not sensed. Those of most concern are head-height obstacles such as tree branches.

## Electronic Travel Aids for Orientation and Mobility

**Electronic travel aids (ETAs)** have been developed to overcome some of the limitations of the long cane. These aids supplement rather than replace the long cane and guide dog. They are designed to provide additional environmental information over that which is sensed using a cane and to detect those obstacles typically missed by the long cane. ETAs also provide information that can assist with orientation for pedestrians who are blind (Scadden, 1997). We discuss both of these applications in this section. ETAs have the three components shown in Figure 12-1: an environmental interface, an information processor, and a user display. The environmental interface is typically both an invisible light source and a receiver (usually in the infrared range) or an ultrasonic transmitter and receiver. Both these technologies are similar to those used in television remote controls. The information processor may be a special-purpose electronic circuit or a microcomputer-based device. The user display may be either an auditory tone of varying frequency (e.g., higher as an object gets closer) or vibrating pins for tactile input.

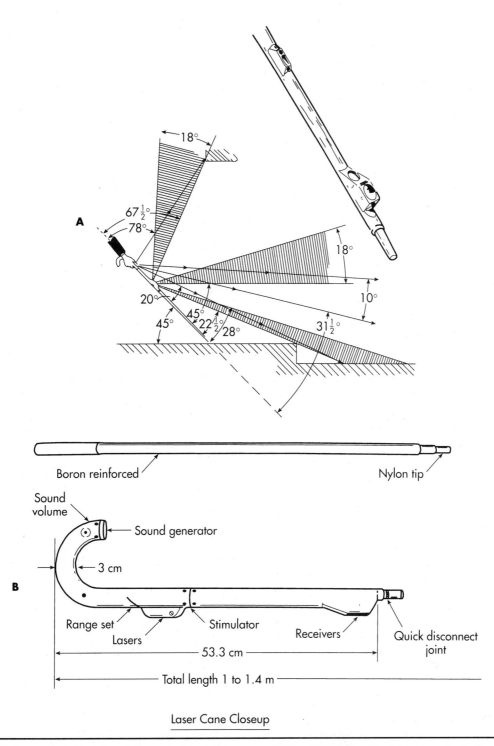

Laser Cane Closeup

Figure 12-8    The laser cane. **A,** The triangulation method employed. **B,** The major components. (From Nye PW, Bliss JC: Sensory aids for the blind: a challenging problem with lessons for the future, *Proc IEEE* 58: 1878-1879, 1970.)

**Laser cane.** The laser cane* extends the range of the standard cane and adds the capability of detecting overhangs. It also provides better sensing of drop-offs. Figure 12-8, *A,* illustrates the principle of operation of the laser cane. Three narrow beams of laser light are projected from the cane. One beam is directed upward, and it detects obstacles at head height about 2.5 feet in front of the cane tip. If an object is in the path of the beam, the light is reflected back to a receiver and a high-pitched tone is emitted. Another beam detects objects directly in front of the traveler at a distance of either 5 or 12 feet (depending on the setting of a switch on the cane handle). If an object is

*Nurion, Paoli, Pa.

encountered in this beam, the reflected signal causes the vibration of pins. The pins are located in the handle of the cane, where the fingers can comfortably rest on them (Figure 12-8, *B*). The final beam is aimed downward, and it is intended to detect drop-offs deeper than 5 inches (e.g., stairs or curbs) located about 3 feet from the cane tip. If the reflected beam is interrupted (because the drop-off does not reflect light back in the same way as a level surface), then a low-frequency tone is emitted.

Because each laser beam is only about 1 inch wide at a distance of 10 feet, it can be used to locate relatively small landmarks. The laser cane is used in the same way as the standard long cane. The user sweeps the cane in an arc in front of her as she walks. Although it is not quite as responsive as a standard long cane, primarily because of the added electronics in the handle, the laser cane can also provide conventional tactile and auditory information. One major advantage of the laser cane is that it is fail-safe; if the batteries run down or an electronic failure occurs, the cane can be used like a standard long cane.

The laser cane can also be used during mobility training, helping the trainee understand how to hold the cane correctly and move it in the correct arc (Mellor, 1981). After the training is complete, the trainee can choose either to use the standard cane or to continue with the laser cane. It can also provide important information for a congenitally blind child regarding the size of objects and their location in space.

There are several disadvantages to the laser cane. The most significant of these is the cost/benefit ratio. The laser cane is approximately 200 times more expensive than the long cane, and each individual user must decide how important the additional information received from the laser cane is to his work, lifestyle, or safety. In some cases the auditory and tactile signals from the laser cane can be misleading to the user (Mellor, 1981). For example, the laser beams may travel through a plate-glass door or window without being reflected, and the glass will not be detected. Nonglass portions of the door (e.g., frame or handle) will generally be detected, but they must be recognized as part of a door based on the laser cane signals. In other cases a shiny surface may be highly reflective and provide confusing reflections to the cane.

**Ultrasonic binaural sensing.** Several devices are intended for use as adjuncts to the long cane. One of these is the Sonic Pathfinder* This device has five ultrasonic transducers that are mounted on a headband. The two transmitters send out an ultrasound beam that covers the user's pathway. The three receivers (one pointing left, one right, and one straight ahead) receive echoes when the ultrasound beam is reflected from an object in the user's path. The

device is controlled by a microcomputer that processes the echoes and converts them to an audible output. The output is fed to the right, left, or both ear pieces, depending on the source of the echo. To simplify the information provided, only the echo of the nearest object is displayed to the user. Priority is also given to objects that are directly in front of the user. The output of the device can be explained by imagining walking toward a wall. The user hears in both ears the notes of the musical scale descending in order. For every 0.3 meters (1 foot), the pitch drops by one musical note. When the tonic note of the scale is reached, the user is within arm's length of the object. Likewise, if an object is to the right, a tone of constant pitch is played in the right ear piece as long as the user remains at the same distance from the object (say a wall). If the user moves closer to the wall, the pitch of the tone drops. The device is silent beyond a distance of 9 meters.

**Clear-path indicators.**    Another type of ETA is designed to be a **clear-path indicator;** that is, it provides signals to the user only if an object is detected in a field approximately 2 feet in diameter and 6 feet from the user (Farmer, 1978). The Polaron* is a device that is either worn on the chest or held in the hand. Ultrasound sensing is used to detect objects within 4, 8, or 16 feet. Feedback to the wearer is by either vibration of the unit or emission of a sound.

The device sends out an ultrasound (i.e., beyond the range of human hearing) beam that creates the clear-path cone for detection of signals. This signal is similar to those used in many television remote controls and in electronic aids to daily living. If an object is in the ultrasound beam path, some sound is reflected back to the device, where it is detected. The length of time it takes the reflected sound to be detected indicates how far away the object is. For objects at a distance of greater than 6 feet, a low-frequency audible sound is emitted from a speaker (the user display). For objects between 3 and 6 feet away, the Polaron emits a series of clicks and a vibration that is felt on the chest. The amplitude (intensity) of the signals is increased as the objects get closer. When an object is 3 feet away or less, the tactile vibration is transferred to the neck strap and a higher pitched beeping sound is heard. In contrast to other ETAs, the Polaron is totally silent when there is not an object in its path.

Because both hands are free, the clear-path indicators can be used in conjunction with the long cane, and they can be used by a person who requires a wheelchair and needs both hands free for pushing. The combination of auditory and tactile input makes these devices suitable for persons who are both deaf and blind. The simplicity of the feedback provided to the user increases the applicability of these devices, and they can be used by children and adults

*Perceptual Alternatives, Melbourne, Australia (www.ariel.ucs. unimelb.edu.au).

*Nurion, Paoli, Pa.

(Mellor, 1981). However, children may use them more for training and to learn spatial concepts than as travel aids, and they can use their free hands to reach out and touch objects they have detected. The simplicity of feedback also means that only limited information can be provided to the user, which can restrict the applicability of these devices. Mellor (1981) also points out that heavy clothing may make it difficult to feel the tactile vibration on the chest and to keep these devices aimed in the proper direction.

**Mowat sensor.** Whereas the clear-path indicators are intended to supplement the long cane, the Mowat sensor* can be used alone or with the cane. This device is about the size of a rectangular flashlight ($6 \times \frac{3}{4} \times 1$ inches) and is held in the hand (Farmer, 1978). It has an ultrasound transmitter and receiver located in rectangular windows at the front of the device; these emit and receive ultrasound pulses in an elliptical pattern. When an object is detected in the ultrasound beam, the device begins to vibrate gently in the hand. The vibrations become stronger for objects that are closer. The device may be set for one of two ranges: 3 feet and 13 feet. The normal use of the Mowat sensor is to scan the environment to locate specific familiar landmarks (e.g., a bus stop sign) or clear spaces such as doorways. It is small enough to be carried easily in a pocket or purse, and it is generally used to supplement other mobility and orientation devices. If two hands are used, it can detect overhangs with simultaneous use of the long cane. This may, however, be difficult for some persons. Mellor (1981) describes several unique uses of the Mowat sensor. For example, it can be used when reaching and touching may be dangerous or undesirable, such as in a machine shop or hospital. It can also be placed on the floor and slowly rotated to find an object that has fallen. Finally, it can be placed on a desk used by a blind receptionist to indicate when someone is standing in front of the desk. The simplicity and relatively low cost of this device make it functional as a supplement to other orientation and mobility devices.

**Wheelchair-mounted mobility device for blind travelers.** The clear-path indicator makes it possible for a person to use a wheelchair, but it is not designed specifically for this purpose. For example, it cannot detect walls to the side or drop-offs in front of the wheelchair. Because powered wheelchairs can move more rapidly than people normally walk, the range for detection of objects must be increased to allow adequate time to change direction or stop to avoid an obstacle. The Wheelchair Pathfinder† uses a combination of laser and ultrasound beams to sense objects, walls (or other obstacles to the side), and drop-offs. Feed-back is provided to the user through an audible tone, the frequency of which changes depending on the type of obstacle. There are two components, a master unit and a slave unit. These attach to brackets fastened on each side of the wheelchair. The frequency of the tone emitted by each unit is different, which allows the user to tell the direction of the obstacle.

As Owen (1990) describes, a device such as the Wheelchair Pathfinder can mean the difference between independence and dependence for a blind person who must use a manual wheelchair. Because it mounts on the wheelchair, it frees the hands and allows manual propulsion using the chair's push rims. Because it is optimized to detect obstacles relative to the chair, it provides the most important information to the user and takes into account the ways wheelchairs are used (e.g., how long it takes to stop or turn). Owen provides a description of her transition from being ambulatory and using a long cane with no ETA to using a wheelchair combined with the Wheelchair Pathfinder ETA. When she was ambulatory, she found that the ETAs did not provide her with sufficiently greater information than her long cane, and she felt that most ETAs were merely fancy gadgets. However, when she began to use a wheelchair and she could no longer use her cane because her hands were occupied pushing the wheelchair, she needed the drop-off sensing aid. This caused her to reassess the value of ETAs in general, and she found that they actually had a greater place in mobility and orientation than she had expected.

**Electronic orientation aids for people who are blind.** The simplest devices for assisting with orientation are adapted compasses. The braille compass has the major north, south, east, and west directions labeled in braille and the intercardinal points labeled with raised dots. The face opens, much like a braille watch, so that the direction can be felt. The Columbus Talking Compass* uses spoken output to help orient the user. The user points the compass in one direction and presses a button. The compass then speaks the direction as north, east, south, west, or intermediate directions (e.g., north-west). The compass can be purchased with two languages installed, and 20 languages are currently available.

Atlas Speaks† is a talking map on a personal computer (Scadden, 1997). A digital map is generated by software, and the user can navigate through the map by moving the cursor. Street names and other points of interest are spoken as they are encountered by the cursor. Personal points of interest may also be noted. These might include bus stops, favorite restaurants, frequently visited shops, friends' houses,

---

*Available from Pulse Data, Christchurch, New Zealand (www.pulsedata.co.nz).
†Nurion Industries, Paoli, Pa.

*Robotron Proprietary Limited, St. Kilda, Australia (www.robotron.net.au).
†Freedom Scientific, St. Petersburg, Fla. (www.freedomsci.com).

public buildings, landmarks, and museums. Pedestrians who are blind can use Atlas Speaks to plan trips. The user can also create points of interest by entering them into the computer. Several directional formats are available (compass, clock face, or degrees). Once a route is created, it can be saved on a tape recorder, copied to portable notetaker, or printed on a braille printer.

Strider* is an orientation device that consists of global positioning system (GPS) and differential GPS receivers, which provide input into a notebook computer running the Atlas Speaks software together with ETAK digital maps. The user's position is determined by the GPS information based on radio signals received from orbiting satellites. This GPS latitude and longitude information is used to establish the user's location on the ETAK maps. Once the location is determined, it is announced to the user via built-in speech synthesis. The prototypes of Strider have been packaged in a backpack. The combination of the Atlas Speaks and Strider technologies offer great potential for travelers who are blind (Scadden, 1997).

Another aid for travelers who are blind is Talking Signs.† Street signs and building signs provide a significant amount of our orientation as sighted travelers. Individuals who are blind or who have trouble reading require that same information in order to maintain their orientation as they travel. Developed at Smith-Kettlewell Eye Research Institute, Talking Signs voice message originates at the sign and is transmitted by infrared light to a handheld receiver at a distance. Because of the nature of infrared transmission, the transmission is directionally selective. As the user aims the receiver directly at the sign, the intensity and clarity of the message increases. This allows the user to focus the Talking Signs system and orient herself to her actual location. Talking Signs transmitters must be installed as adjuncts to all signs. This is a large task, but many signs have been installed. Talking Sign can also be used to label objects such as building entrances, drinking fountains, phone booths, or rest rooms (Scadden, 1997).

## ■ SPECIAL-PURPOSE VISUAL AIDS

In developing the HAAT model in Chapter 2, we defined three performance areas as part of the activity: self-care, work and school, and play and leisure. Persons with blindness or low vision may have needs in each of these areas, and there are special-purpose devices that can provide assistance. These devices are in addition to those serving needs for reading and orientation/mobility, which are used in all three performance areas. In this section we describe some of the special-purpose devices that serve these needs. Publications

and devices are available and the American Foundation for the Blind,* Sensory Access Foundation,† Smith-Kettlewell Eye Research Institute, Rehabilitation Engineering Center,‡ and the New York Lighthouse, Inc.§ are good sources of information regarding specific needs There are companies that sell large numbers of products for all three performance areas.‖

## Devices for Self-Care

Auditory or tactile substitutes can be used for many household tasks. For example, braille tape (similar to the tape used for labeling with raised letters) can be used to label canned foods and appliance controls. Another approach to identification of household objects is the use of bar codes and recorded speech (Crabb, 1998). Bar codes are typically used in supermarkets for checkout scanning. However, the codes used are stored in the grocery store computer, so they can't be read at home. Crabb developed a device, called the I.D. Mate,# that allows a sighted individual to sweep a reader over the bar code and then record a short spoken message describing the contents (e.g., "Campbell's tomato soup"). This information is then played back to the user who is blind when he scans a similar can at the grocery store. Other household items can also be scanned. Approximately 90% of the items sold in the United States have bar codes on them. This includes playing cards, cassette tapes, CDs, and many other items.

Voice output is also available on some appliances, such as microwave ovens. Kitchen timers, thermometers, and alarm clocks are available in both enlarged and auditory or tactile forms. Talking wristwatches are used by individuals who are blind. Electrical appliances often have controls marked with tactile labels to allow a blind person to adjust the control. Raised or enlarged print telephone dials can also be obtained from local telephone companies. There are also devices that read paper money and speak the denomination of the bill. These are similar to change machines or those used for automatic purchase of public transportation tickets in many cities. A portable paper money reader is shown in Figure 12-9.** When a paper monetary note of $1 to $100 value is inserted into the device, it automatically turns on and speaks the denomination of the note. Both English and Spanish voice outputs are available, and a headphone may be used for privacy. When the note is removed, the unit automati-

---

*Freedom Scientific, St. Petersburg, Fla. (www.freedomsci.com).
†Talking Signs, Inc., Baton Rouge, La. (www.talkingsigns.com).

*New York City.
†Palo Alto, Calif.
‡San Francisco, Calif.
§New York (www.lighthouse.org).
‖ LS&S Group, Northbrook, Ill. (www.Lssgroup.com); Maxi Aids, Farmingdale, N.Y. (www.maxiaids.com); Independent Living Aids, Inc, Plainsview, N.Y. (www.independentliving.com).
#En-Vision America, Normal, Ill. (www.envisionamerica.com).
**Note Teller, Brytech, Ottawa, Ontario, Canada.

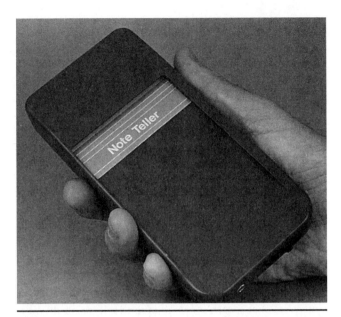

Figure 12-9   The Note Teller paper money reading device. (Courtesy Brytech, Nepean, Ont., Canada.)

cally turns itself off. Versions are available specifically for U.S. and Canadian currencies, as well as a universal model. More and more talking automatic teller machines (ATMs) are being installed. These will eventually replace all ATMs in the United States and Canada. Worldwide usage of this technology is likely to occur in the future. Banking over the Internet is also available for persons who are blind or have low vision.*

A leading cause of blindness is diabetes, and there are insulin injection devices that provide independence for blind users. Specially adapted syringes and holders for bottles are available. The holder guides the syringe into the bottle, and the syringe can be set to allow only the amount necessary for one dose to be drawn out of the bottle. Other home health care devices include thermometers with speech output and sphygmomanometers (for blood pressure measurement) that use raised dots on the pressure meter face or synthesized speech output.

## Devices for Work and School

The major needs within vocational and educational applications are for access to reading, mobility, and computers. The approaches and devices in the sections on reading and mobility in this chapter and computer access in Chapter 8 often meet these needs. In order to be operated as they were designed, many tools require the use of vision. It is possible to use either tactile or auditory adaptations to make these tools available to individuals who have visual impairments. A carpenter's level with a large steel ball and center tab has

*For example, Bradesco, Brazil (www.bradesco.com.br).

an adjustment screw on one end. The screw is calibrated with half a degree of tilt corresponding to one turn. To level the device, the carpenter adjusts the screw until the ball is at the center. She then knows how many degrees of tilt there are and can correct for the tilt. There is also a tactile tape measure with one raised dot at each quarter-inch mark, two at half-inch increments, and one large dot at each inch mark. Calipers, protractors, and micrometers use a similar labeling scheme. An audible device is used by machinists to determine depth of cut when using a lathe. There are also talking tape measures, calculators, scales, and thermometers. Many of these also have tactile versions.

Many electronic test instruments use digital (numeric) displays, and these displays are easily interfaced to speech synthesizers. The output of the meter (e.g., a voltage measurement by a technician) is heard instead of read. Oscilloscopes are also available in both auditory and tactile forms. Electronic calculators that have speech output provide an alternative to visual display-based devices. It is possible for a person with total visual impairment to perform virtually all the tasks required for electronic or mechanical design, fabrication, and testing using adapted tools and instruments.

## Devices for Play and Leisure

Almost any common board game can be obtained in enlarged form. There are also enlarged and tactually labeled playing cards, and braille or other versions exist for common board games and dice. Computer games that emphasize text rather than graphics can be used with computer screen reading software (see Chapter 8).

More active games include "beeper ball," in which auditory signals replace visual cues. In this softball-like game, the ball contains an electronic oscillator that emits a beeping sound. The batter can aim for the sound. Bases are also labeled with sounds. Similar approaches are available for playing Frisbee, soccer, and football. In each case the object to be thrown or kicked emits a beep and goals are labeled with auditory markers. Individuals who are blind can snow ski with the assistance of both sighted guides and auditory signals from barriers such as slalom poles and fences.

## ■ AIDS FOR PERSONS WITH AUDITORY IMPAIRMENTS

Helen Keller, who was both deaf and blind, is reported to have been asked whether she would prefer to have her vision or her hearing if she could have one or the other. She responded that she would prefer to have her hearing, since she felt that people who are blind are cut off from things, whereas those who are deaf are cut off from people. It is important to keep this concept in mind as we discuss aids

### CASE STUDY 12-2

#### CHANGING NEEDS FOR VISUAL AIDS

Ken has enrolled this fall semester as a student at the state college. He has retinitis pigmentosa. Retinitis pigmentosa is a midperipheral ring scotoma that gradually widens with time, so that central vision is frequently reduced by middle age. Night blindness occurs much earlier, and total blindness may eventually ensue. Ken has recently noticed that his vision seems to have deteriorated significantly. He would like to study to become a journalist. Ken lives alone in an apartment close to campus so he can walk to school or, when it is raining, take the bus. As Ken's retinitis pigmentosa advances, what types of assistive technology for sensory impairments might be useful to him in order to enable him to continue with his activities in the following areas: (1) school, (2) home/self-care, and (3) recreation/leisure?

for persons who are deaf or hard of hearing. Auditory impairment is often not as obvious as visual impairment, and society does not view it as having the same degree of significance as visual impairment. It is natural for a person to wear glasses as a part of the inherent process of aging. However, many people are embarrassed to admit hearing loss sufficient to require a hearing aid. Despite these considerations, hearing loss is significant, and it can be socially isolating. Assistive technologies can provide great improvement in the lives of persons who have either partial or total auditory impairments.

## Hearing Aids

**Hearing aids** are often conceived of as simple devices that amplify sound, primarily speech. Although hearing aids do contain amplifiers, hearing loss is rarely consistent across the entire speech frequency range. As discussed in Chapter 3, hearing loss is generally greater at some frequencies than others. This presents a problem in the design of hearing aids. If we amplify all frequencies the same amount, the sound will be unnatural to the user. An additional difficulty encountered in providing hearing aids of high fidelity is that the components are small, and this miniaturization can limit the frequency response of the microphone and speaker, further reducing the quality of the aided speech.

Approximately 60% of the *acoustic energy* of the speech signal is contained in frequencies below 500 Hz (Berger, Hagberg, and Rane, 1977). However, the speech signal contains not only specific frequencies of sound, but also the organization of these sounds into meaningful units of

auditory language (e.g., phonemes), and over 95% of the *intelligibility* of the speech signal is associated with frequencies above 500 Hz. For this reason, speech intelligibility rather than sound level is often used as the criterion for successful application of hearing aids.

**Electroacoustical parameters of hearing aids.** Hearing aid output is typically specified in decibels (dB) referred to a standard of 20 micropascals (see the discussion of sensory function in Chapter 3). Sound pressure level (SPL) is used to designate this parameter. Standards for hearing aid specification have been developed by the American National Standards Institute (ANSI) and the Acoustical Society of America (ASA). These standards allow for the comparison of hearing aids from different manufacturers, and they specify parameters that are used in this comparison.

Speech SPLs vary from 42 (softest) to 90 dB (loudest). Conversational speech is in the range of 40 to 50 dB SPL (Stach, 1998), and the maximal SPL that can be applied to the ear without damage is 130 to 140 dB. The maximal output for a hearing aid is typically specified as the saturation SPL (SSPL) and is usually measured at 90 dB (SSPL-90). An SSPL-90 saturated output curve is generated by applying a 90-dB input over the 500- to 2000-Hz range with the gain (volume control) of the hearing aid set to maximum. A typical curve of this type is shown in Figure 12-10. A second gain parameter is the full-on gain with 50-dB SPL input. This curve is indicative of the response of the hearing aid amplifier at a midrange of the speech SPL range, and a typical curve is also shown in Figure 12-10. Some hearing aids also have adjustable gain, and the SSPL and full-on gain are plotted for typical gain ranges. In Figure 12-10 this is illustrated by the three curves labeled *L* (low), *N* (normal), and *H* (high). Hearing aids have low gain at frequencies below 200 Hz, and the gain above 7000 Hz is sharply reduced. This corresponds to the frequency range of conversational speech described above.

**Types of hearing aids.** Conventional hearing aids are available in several different configurations (Stach, 1998). Figure 12-11 illustrates several commonly used types of aids. The major types are behind-the-ear (BTE), in-the-ear (ITE), in-the-canal (ITC), and completely in-the-canal (CIC).

BTE hearing aids fit behind the ear and contain all the components shown in Figure 12-12. The amplified acoustic signal is fed into the ear canal through a small ear hook that extends over the top of the auricle and holds the hearing aid in place. A small tube directs the sound into the ear through an ear mold that serves as an acoustic coupler. This ear mold is made from an impression of the individual's ear to ensure comfort to the user, maximize the amount of acoustic energy coupled into the ear, and

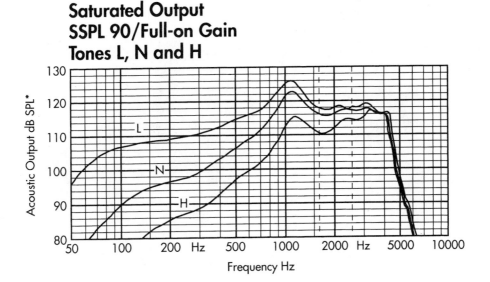

## Saturated Output
## SSPL 90/Full-on Gain
## Tones L, N and H

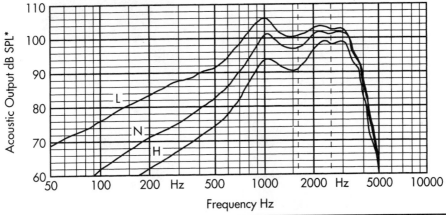

## Frequency Response
## 50 dB SPL Input/Full-on Gain
## Tones L, N and H

Figure 12-10   Specifications for a standard hearing aid. (Courtesy Phonic Ear, Petaluma, Calif.)

prevent squealing caused by acoustic feedback. When the mold is made, a 2-ml space is included between the coupler and the eardrum. A vent hole can also be added to an ear mold, which can add to acoustic feedback and distortion, as well as preventing the ear from being blocked. The vent hole allows sound to travel to the tympanic membrane directly. An external switch allows selection of the microphone (M), a telecoil (T) for direct telephone reception, or off (O). The MTO switch and a volume control are located on the back of the case for BTE aids.

The ITE aid makes use of electronic miniaturization to place the amplifier and speaker in a small casing that fits into the ear canal. The faceplate of the ITE aid is located in the opening to the ear canal. The microphone is located in the faceplate. This provides a more "natural" location for the microphone as it receives sound that would normally be directed into the ear (Stach, 1998). External controls on the ITE include an MTO switch and volume control. The ITC is a smaller version of the ITE. The CIC type of hearing aid is the smallest, and it is inserted 1 to 2 mm into the canal with the speaker close to the tympanic membrane. Because this type does not protrude outside the ear canal, it is barely visible. Any controls for the aid are fit onto the faceplate of the ITE, ITC, and CIC types of aids.

**Basic structure of hearing aids.** Figures 12-13, *A, B,* and *C,* illustrate the basic components of analog and digital hearing aids. The microphone is the **environmental sensor,** and it is the component that receives the speech signal. Overall fidelity of the hearing aid is directly related to the

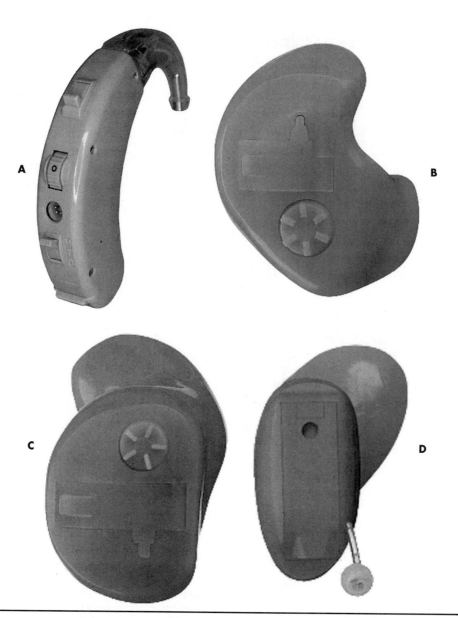

Figure 12-11    Types of hearing aids. **A,** Behind the ear (BTE). **B,** In-the-ear (ITE). **C,** In-the-canal (ITC). **D,** Completely in-the-canal (CIC). (Courtesy Siemans Hearing Instruments, Inc.)

quality of this component. Several types of microphones are employed in hearing aids (see Stach, 1998). The function of the microphone is to convert the acoustical speech waveform into an electrical signal, which is sent to the amplifier. Microphones may be omnidirectional (amplify sound from any direction) or directional. They also include noise reduction properties to obtain the best input signal possible.

The information processor (see Figure 2-1) in a hearing aid is the amplifier. It performs several functions. The first and most basic of these is amplification of the input signal with a frequency response (amplifier gain between the input and output, which is different at different frequencies) that is matched to speech signals. Amplifiers may be linear or nonlinear (sometimes called *curvilinear*) (Stach, 1998). Linear amplifiers increase the gain in signal from input to

output by the same amount for all intensities of input. This means that a small speech signal and a large noise signal are both amplified the same amount. Linear amplifiers restrict the output to a level that is not harmful to the ear by clipping the signals that are large enough to cause damage. This approach is called *peak clipping* (see below). In a nonlinear or curvilinear amplifier, the output signal does not have the same proportional relationship to the input as in a linear amplifier. The nonlinear approach provides for compensation for louder signals and greater amplification of speech signals through a variety of approaches. Nonlinear amplification is also more versatile in the processing options it allows. Second, the information processor limits loud input signals to prevent distortion and protect the user from damage to the peripheral auditory system. Finally, signal

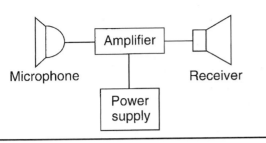

Figure 12-12    The major components of a hearing aid.

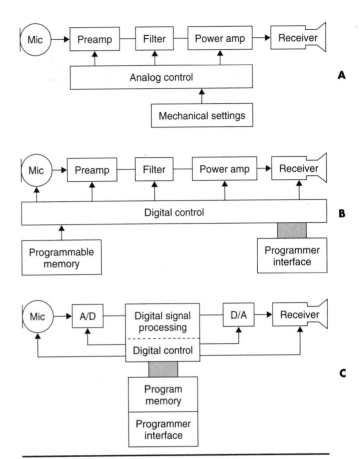

Figure 12-13    Three approaches to the electronic design of hearing aids. **A,** An analog hearing aid. **B,** A digitally controlled analog hearing aid. **C,** A digital signal processing hearing aid. (Modified from Stach BA: *Clinical audiology,* San Diego, 1998, Singular Publishing Group.)

processing is provided to minimize noise and maximize the speech signal.

In an ideal amplifier, all signals are amplified in such a way as to preserve the shape of the input curve at the output of the device. Because the input shape (SPL versus gain plot) is determined by the speech signals picked up by the microphone, maintenance of this shape is important to the signal's intelligibility. Any difference in the shape of the input and output signals is called *distortion.* Distortion can arise from several factors and can appear in several ways (Stach, 1998). Two of the most important types of distortion are frequency distortion and noise distortion. Frequency distortion results when certain frequencies are amplified more than others and when there are shifts in the relationship between different frequency bands in the input and output signals. Noise distortion is the result of nonspeech signals being introduced into the amplified output of the hearing aid, and it results in decreased intelligibility. Noise may originate within the components of the hearing aid or outside the aid. Examples of external distortion are skin or other materials rubbing against the microphone. The ANSI standard includes a specification for the maximal allowable noise level. This is measured as the SPL output with the input signal set to zero. Obviously the lower this noise level, the greater the fidelity and intelligibility of the output speech signal.

With the increase in capability and decrease in size of digital signal processing (including miniaturized computers), there have been significant advances in hearing aid design. The major advantage of using this type of signal processing is that it can be more exactly matched to the acoustic properties of the auditory system than the less sophisticated analog signal processing approach of Figure 12-13, *A.* Preves (1988) describes several of the digital signal processing approaches used in hearing aids (Figure 12-13, *B, C*). Among the advantages are lower distortion, less acoustic feedback, more precise compression of loud signals, and greater fidelity and intelligibility in the speech signal supplied to the ear.

As stated earlier, the maximal allowable acoustic input at the ear is 130 to 140 dB. One way of limiting this signal is to set a maximal value for the output and cut off any signals that exceed this value. This is referred to as *peak clipping.* The net result is that loud signals have the peaks of the

waveform cut off, or "clipped." Peak clipping often results in distortion and a decrease in intelligibility of the speech signal (Dillon, 1988). To reduce the negative effects of peak clipping, a concept known as *automatic gain control* is used in analog hearing aids to automatically decrease the amplifier gain whenever a loud signal is provided at the input. Figure 12-14 shows how this type of compression works. As the input signal is increased in amplitude, the amplifier senses this and reduces the gain. The amount of time that it takes for the amplifier to respond is referred to as the *attack time* of the circuit. When the input signal is reduced, the amplifier again responds as shown in Figure 12-14. The time it takes the amplifier to recover and increase its gain back to normal is called the *response time.* These two times are often part of a hearing aid specification. This type of hearing aid compression does not decrease intelligibility of the speech signal for large acoustic inputs (Dillon, 1988).

Nonlinear circuits allow for more complex compression methods to be employed (Stach, 1998). Nonlinear compression not only limits the effect of loud sounds as described above for analog compression, but it also provides nonlinear gain with various input levels within the user's dynamic

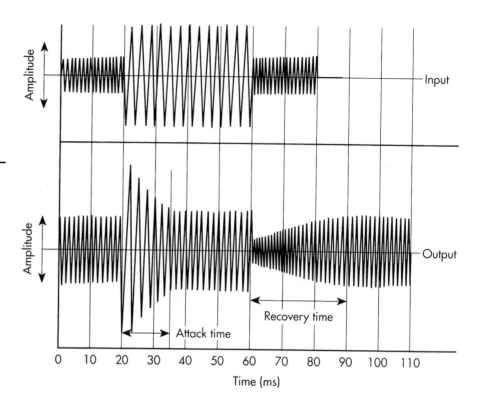

**Figure 12-14** The compensation response of a hearing aid to sudden changes in input (top waveform); sound intensity is shown in the bottom trace. (Modified from Staab WJ: *Hearing aid handbook,* Blue Ridge Summit, Pa, 1978, TAB Books.)

range. Dynamic range is the difference between the softest detectable signal and the loudness of input that causes discomfort. This varies from individual to individual. For individuals who have normal hearing, the dynamic range is up to 100 dB. An individual with significant hearing loss of 50 dB would have a dynamic range of only 50 dB. This might be further reduced if recruitment occurs in the cochlea and auditory nerve, resulting in an increase in the loudness of the signal. Recruitment is common in sensorineural hearing loss (see Chapter 3). One goal of nonlinear speech compression techniques is to fit the input speech into the user's dynamic range. Low-intensity signals are amplified to be in the user's range, and high-intensity signals above the user's comfort range are reduced. Because low- and high-intensity signals require different levels of amplification, a nonlinear approach is needed. This type of nonlinear processing is called *dynamic range compression* (Stach, 1998). Compression may be applied at the input or output of the hearing aid circuitry. With input compression, the microphone and preamplifier trigger the compression when a signal above a preset threshold is detected. Alternatively a high output level may be used to activate the compression. This is termed *output compression.* It is possible to adjust several of the compression parameters, which makes it easier to match the characteristics of the hearing aid to the needs of the user.

The user display (see Figure 2-1) for a hearing aid is the *speaker.* This component is often referred to as the *receiver,* and it converts the electrically amplified signal to an acous-

tical waveform that is coupled to the ear. The small size of these devices severely limits the frequency response of the hearing aid for signals above the range of speech. Most receivers are air-conduction types, which acoustically couple the speech signal to the ear canal. When the middle ear is damaged, bone-conduction receivers may be used. In these circumstances the case of the receiver is designed to fit against the head of the mastoid bone posterior to the auricle. When the device vibrates, it transmits through the skin and bone to the inner ear, where it produces the sensation of sound. These are also indicated in cases of outer ear damage that precludes the use of an ear mold, the absence of the pinna, drainage from the ear, atresia, or microtia. There are also bone implant hearing aids.

**Types of hearing aid signal processing.** Current hearing aids use one of the three design approaches shown in Figure 12-13 (Stach, 1998). Figure 12-13, *A,* illustrates the classical analog approach to hearing aid design. The majority of hearing aids made have been of the analog type. Analog hearing aids operate directly on the acoustic signal detected by the microphone; this signal is continuous. In an analog hearing aid, the time-varying input acoustic signal is amplified and filtered and compression is applied if necessary. The signal is then fed directly to the speaker.

The second type of hearing aid circuitry is referred to as *digitally controlled analog* or *hybrid* (Stach, 1998; Levitt, 1997). As shown in Figure 12-13, *B,* the signal path (amplification, filtering, and compression) is still analog, but

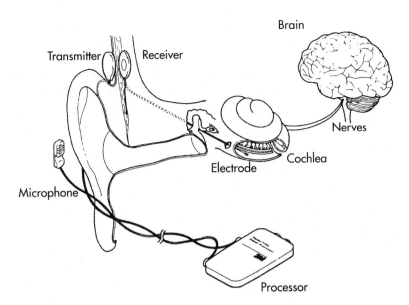

Figure 12-15   The components of a cochlear implant. (From Radcliffe D: How cochlear implants work, *Hearing J,* p 53, November 1984).

the control of these circuits is set by digital parameters. Because the digital parameters control the device and they can be stored in memory, this device is very flexible. Digitally controlled analog devices can be customized to meet the needs of the user with the parameters stored in the digital memory. Parameters that can be digitally controlled include gain, frequency response, compression parameters, and electroacoustical parameters. The primary reason for the development of the hybrid type of hearing aid was that early pure digital hearing aids were bulky and consumed larger amounts of power than corresponding analog aids. The hybrid approach gave increased flexibility without the larger size and greater power requirements.

With the development of low-power, small digital signal processing circuits, digital hearing aids (see Figure 12-13, *C*) are possible. This type of hearing aid uses stored control parameters like the hybrid type; the signal is converted to digital form and then processed. Even these hearing aids have analog preamplifiers to boost the signal to a level sufficient for analog-to-digital conversion. One of the advantages provided by digital circuitry is the capability of shaping the frequency response of the hearing aid. This provides the possibility of canceling acoustic feedback and increasing the signal-to-noise ratio of the hearing aid (Levitt, 1997). Digital aids also can use adaptive filtering to shape the frequency response based on the spectral characteristics of the incoming signal. Currently available digital hearing aids have the computational capability of a small computer. The major limitation at this time is not signal processing capability but rather our limited understanding of the most effective way to process speech signals for people who have hearing aids (Levitt, 1997). As in many areas of assistive technology application, we are limited by our understanding of the clinical and biological aspects of the problem, not by the available technologies.

## Cochlear Implants

If there is damage to the cochlea of the inner ear, an auditory prosthesis can provide some sound perception. The first reported use of electrical stimulation of the inner ear was made by the Italian physicist Alessandro Volta (for whom the volt is named) more than 200 years ago. He inserted wires into his ear and connected them to a 50-volt battery, and he experienced an "auditory sensation" when the voltage was applied. More recently, engineers and physiologists have developed sophisticated aids that accommodate lost cochlear function.

These devices, termed **cochlear implants,** have the components shown in Figure 12-15 (Feigenbaum, 1987). As long as the eighth cranial nerve is intact, it is possible to provide stimulation via implanted electrodes. Cochlear implants have been shown to be of benefit to adults and young persons who have adventitious hearing loss (i.e., hearing loss after acquiring speech and language) (Stach, 1998). Children who have congenital hearing loss may also benefit if the hearing loss is identified early and they receive a cochlear implant at an early age. The total number of implants over the past 10 years is less than 30,000 worldwide. Because the characteristics of cochlear implants are not precisely defined and agreed upon, there is a great deal of confusion when reading manufacturers' literature and claims. The guidance of an audiologist experienced in this area is crucial.

There are two major parts of most cochlear implants. External to the body are a microphone (environmental interface), electronic processing circuits that extract key parameters from the speech signal, and a transmitter that couples the information to the skull. The implanted portion consists of an electrode array (1 to 22 electrodes), a receiver that couples the external data and power to the skull, and electronic circuits that provide proper synchronization and stimulation parameters for the electrode array. Stimulation of an individual electrode results in auditory perceptions resembling clicks or hisses.

**Electrodes.** The three major considerations in design of electrodes are (1) biocompatibility of materials, (2) placement of electrodes, and (3) the number of electrodes in the array (Shallop and Mecklenberg, 1988). The stimulating portion of most electrodes in current devices is made of platinum because it is electrically stable and does not react with biological tissue. The "leads," wires that connect the stimulator to the platinum-tipped electrode, need to be flexible enough to curve around the cochlea, but they also must be rigid enough not to bend as they are inserted. The electrode array and the lead wires are coated with Teflon or silicone to insulate them from each other and from the tissue. If there are small holes or breaks in the insulation, the tissue near the break will be exposed to electrical current. This can damage both the wire and the tissue. The insulation material must also be impervious to leakage of ionic fluids in the body.

Electrode placement is either intracochlear (inside the cochlea) or extracochlear (adjacent to the round window in the middle ear). For intracochlear electrodes, the size is dictated by the microanatomy of the cochlea. The average cochlea is about 32 mm long, and electrode arrays can be up to 25 mm long for insertion into this cavity (usually the scala tympani). Stimulation is either monopolar or bipolar. Monopolar stimulation places one reference electrode outside the cochlea and an array of single electrodes inside the cochlea along the basilar membrane. This arrangement requires less power for stimulation but results in less specific and less focused stimulation in the cochlea. Bipolar stimulation places electrode pairs along the membrane. This results in much more localized and specific stimulation, but it requires more power. Greater power means larger size, and this dictates the type of external packaging. The external package may be in either a behind-the-ear or body-level type. The majority of the cochlear implants in use are body-level types. As technologies are perfected, behind-the-ear types will become much more common. The minimal spacing between electrode tips, based on electrical stimulation parameters, is 0.5 to 1 mm (White, 1987). This sets a practical limit of 22 electrodes in an array. Several different numbers of electrodes have been used in cochlear implants. Initially all devices used only one electrode. Currently available types of cochlear implants* have 8, 12, or 22 electrodes (Millar, Tong, and Clark, 1984). Although 22 electrodes is a significant technological accomplishment in cochlear implants, it is humbling to consider that the cochlea itself contains nearly 30,000 hair cells (organ of Corti), each of which generates neural signals in response to

*Clarion, Advanced Bionics Corp., Sylmar, Calif. (www.cochlearimplant.com/); Nucleus 24, Cochlear Inc., Lane Cove NSW, Australia (www.cochlear.com/).

auditory input. Thus the implant has only 0.07% of the number of active areas that the biological system has.

**Transmission of power and data.** Because the microphone and speech processing components need to be adjusted and because of their size and weight, they are placed outside the skull. The electrode array must be inside the cochlea, and there must be a connection through the skull. Initially this was done with wires that passed through the skull and a percutaneous plug that was used when the wires were removed. This type of percutaneous connection is subject to infection, and it has been replaced by a transmitter-receiver approach (Shallop and Mecklenberg, 1988). A small induction coil on the external skin surface is connected to the transmitter. This coil transmits through the skin to the receiving coil located directly opposite, under the skin. The receiving coil is connected to the internal electronics and the electrode array. Power for the internal electronics is also coupled through the skin. In some cases the internal circuitry is totally passive and merely passes the stimulation signal to the electrodes. In other cases (such as that shown in Figure 12-15), the internal circuitry processes the incoming signal and distributes it to the different electrodes in the array. This consumes power, which is normally coupled through the skin just as the data are.

**Speech processing.** The purpose of the cochlear implant is to provide an electrically triggered physiological signal that can be related to speech and environmental sounds. The process by which the cochlea, auditory nerve, and higher centers process speech is not well understood, and it is difficult to design an electronic speech processor that provides physiologically meaningful data to the electrode array. The area of speech processing or coding of the signals to be sent to the electrode is one in which great differences exist among different cochlear implants. Both digital and analog signal processing is employed in commercial units. Digital processing of the speech signal, by miniaturized computer systems built into the device, is aimed at extracting the relevant speech data from the microphone and converting it to a form that provides the most possible information to the user via stimulation of the basilar membrane. It is in this area that the most rapid changes in cochlear implants are occurring.

In order to recognize speech, it is necessary to encode frequency, intensity, and temporal patterns (Shallop and Mecklenberg, 1988). Frequency is encoded in the normal cochlea by location along the basilar membrane (referred to as *tonotopic organization*). A multiple electrode array can provide different frequencies at different locations along the basilar membrane, but the normal cochlea uses other, more sophisticated methods to further encode frequency (Feigenbaum, 1987). Intensity or amplitude or loudness can be encoded by the magnitude of the stimulus at any electrode location. However, the normal cochlea also uses "recruitment" of adjacent hair cells to reflect increased intensity. Recruitment can also happen with electrical stimulation of neural tissue as the intensity of the stimulus increases. Another approach that is used is called *continuous interleaved sampling* (CIS) (Wilson et al, 1993). This approach was designed to avoid some of the problems of channel interactions by delivering temporally offset trains of pulses to each electrode. This helps to eliminate overlap across channels. A key feature is a relatively high rate (greater than 800 pules per second) of stimulation on each channel. This provides the basis for tracking rapid variations in speech using pulse amplitude variations presented to the electrodes. Millar, Tong, and Clark (1984), Shallop and Mecklenberg (1988), and White (1987) describe several approaches to speech processing for cochlear implants.

Major cochlear implant manufacturers also provide software for Windows-based PCs that is used to program the signal processing characteristics of the implant to match the needs of the user. These are used after the surgery has been completed and healing has taken place. Signals are supplied to the implant and psychophysical measurements are made to determine the optimal type of signal (pulse or analog) and electrode combinations. This uses pure tone responses. Then speech input is evaluated and adjustments are made to maximize speech intelligibility.

**User evaluation results.** Cochlear implants also improve the accuracy of lip-reading by providing additional acoustic cues, which help to distinguish sounds that look the same on the lips. However, the speech signal is complex, and there is a large amount of encoding done by the cochlea and auditory nerves before sensory data are sent to the central nervous system (CNS). Cochlear implants cannot replace this sophisticated peripheral processing capability, and current devices do not significantly increase speech recognition; neither do they provide input that is anything like that received from normal hearing.

Multiple electrode devices also provide significant improvement in environmental sound recognition, including distinguishing such sounds as telephones, door knocks, and dogs barking. Some users of these devices have also reported limited use of the telephone when speaking with a familiar person and limited ability to understand face-to-face speech without lip reading.

## Telephone Access for Persons Who Are Deaf

The isolation imposed on deaf persons by the telephone is ironic given that Alexander Graham Bell was working on an aid for the deaf when he invented it. For some individuals, additional amplification is sufficient to make the telephone accessible. This may be built into the person's telephone or it may be an add-on unit that can be placed over the earpiece of any telephone. Both types of devices are available from local telephone companies. As discussed in the previ-

ous section, many hearing aids have a magnetic induction feature (telecoil) that allows the output of the telephone to be directly coupled to the hearing aid.

For many individuals with severe hearing loss, even increased amplification does not make the telephone signal audible. In order for these persons to obtain access to telephone conversations, a device that can visually send and receive telephone information is used. These individuals also often use master ring indicators, which either amplify the ringing of the telephone or connect the ringer to a table lamp that flashes when the telephone rings. These adaptations are also available from local telephone companies.

**Telephone devices for the deaf.** Originally, deaf individuals used teletype (TTY) devices designed for sending weather and news information over telephone lines to provide a "visual telephone." Many of these TTYs were donated by IBM and other companies to help deaf people talk to each other. The original TTY, now obsolete, consisted of a typewriter and electronic circuitry for converting the typed letters to pulses that could be sent over the telephone line to another TTY. The second TTY converted the pulses back into text that was typed on paper on the remote TTY. Because of their low cost, especially for surplus units, TTYs were very popular with deaf individuals, and some are still in use. A good source of information is the Gallaudet University Technology Assessment Program (http://tap.gallaudet.edu).

Electronic versions of earlier TTYs are still referred to as TTYs.* They use a keypad, a one-line visual display, a modulator-demodulator (modem) to convert the electronic signal to pulses, and an acoustic coupler to couple the pulses to the telephone handset. They should be thought of more as a phone than a data modem. An example of a TTY is shown in Figure 12-16. In some cases the telephone line is plugged directly into the TTY, instead of through an acoustic coupler. However, there are times (e.g., when calling from a pay telephone) when an acoustic coupler is required. In computer-to-computer telephone line communication, each computer can send and receive at the same time. Thus if one device is sending, the other unit can interrupt it. This type of operation is called *full-duplex*. Because of their design, TTYs are only able to send (originate) or to receive at one time, not both; this is called *half-duplex* mode. After each transmission, the user must type *GA* (go ahead) to indicate that he is finished and then wait for a response. Half-duplex is also useful when voice communication is occurring, since line discontinuities at

---

*For example, Ameriphone, Inc., Garden Grove, Calif. (www.ameriphoneinc.com); Krown Mfg., Inc., Fort Worth, Tex. (www.krowntty.com); Ultratec, Inc., Madison, Wisc. (www.ultratec.com); Lober & Walsh Engineering, San Luis Obispo, Calif. (www.lober-and-walsh.com).

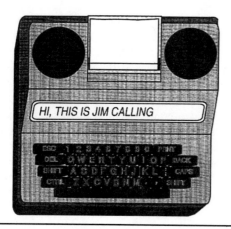

Figure 12-16 A typical TTY has an electronic display and a keyboard for typing messages.

switching stations or over long distance lines can result in a reflected signal that is heard as an echo by the speaker. Half-duplex switches the direction of transmission based on voice-activated sensors. Full-duplex operation requires that the sending and receiving computers solve the problem of echoes, but it is more rapid and it allows interruption of a long transmission if an error occurs. TTYs are extremely easy to set up and use in the basic configuration. Advanced TTY features include use with an answering machine, remote retrieval of messages, message notification via paging, and a printer. The printer function gives both a permanent record of the conversation and a chance to review messages before responding to them. Some TTYs plug directly into cellular and cordless telephones to allow mobile use.

The TTYs also employ a unique coding approach based on five bits of data, rather than the customary eight used in computer ASCII transmission. This code, called Baudot, is widely used by the deaf community, and it is still used in modern TTYs even though it does not match the standard for all other computer communication, which is based on the ASCII code. When data are in ASCII form they can be displayed on a computer screen, enlarged, combined with time or date information, and stored in files for later use. In contrast to ASCII, Baudot does not require a carrier signal, it uses only two frequencies (1800 and 1400 Hz), and it does not require "handshaking" protocols. As discussed in Chapter 8, communication between a computer and a peripheral or another computer is either parallel or serial. In serial transmission a rate of transmission, called the baud setting, must be the same for the receiving and the transmitting devices. TTYs typically use a rate of 110 to 300 baud. Computer modems typically use rates of 2400 baud or higher. The slower TTY speed offers an advantage when single-line displays are used, since it is slow enough to be read during the transmission and 300 baud is the maximum that can be used easily with an acoustic coupler.

There are two primary ways to use the TTY with the telephone. If both parties have a TTY, then each simply types her message, sends a "go ahead" (the letters *GA*) command to indicate that she is finished, and then waits for an answer. If the deaf person needs to talk to someone who does not have a TTY, then a relay operator is provided by the telephone company. The operator has a TTY, and he reads the message sent by the deaf person to the hearing person. The response is then spoken to the operator, who types the message to the deaf person's TTY. Under the provisions of Title IV (telecommunications) of the Americans with Disabilities Act (ADA), all the telephone services offered to the general public must include both interstate and intrastate relay services for persons who use TTYs. The Federal Communications Commission (FCC) issued the rules for Title IV, and this agency monitors compliance. These rules also require that both ASCII and Baudot capabilities are provided by the relay services. Approximately 95% of the calls through a relay operator use Baudot data format. Title IV regulations also specify the conduct of relay operators. The most important features of these rules are complete confidentiality and verbatim transmission of messages.

AT&T employs an interesting combination of the technologies described in this chapter in its relay services (Halliday, 1993). A blind operator serves as a relay communications assistant. Incoming voice messages are relayed by typing on a computer terminal that sends the message to the deaf person's TTY. Incoming TTY messages are converted to braille using a refreshable braille display and then relayed by voice to the hearing person. This is a unique combination of technologies for persons who are deaf and who are blind, and it takes advantage of the skills of each individual.

There are a large number of deaf persons who have and use TTYs (Baudot protocol), and there are also many individuals who have personal computers with modems that use the ASCII protocol. Therefore current TTYs often include both ASCII and Baudot, and some computer programs that convert from one code to another are available. To use a computer for TTY communication, the user must have both TTY software and a modem that can emulate a TTY (Baudot at 300 baud*). The TTY software generates the Baudot codes and sends information to the TTY modem (hardware plugged into the computer). The modem then communicates with a stand-alone TTY at 300 baud. The modem must meet all the transmission protocols (e.g., frequency, 5-bit code, half-duplex communication) of the Baudot TTY in order for the communication to be successful. These protocols are not available on standard computer modems, and that is the reason that a special TTY modem (with a setting of 300 baud to communicate in

---

*For example, Futura Wave Communications, Inc., Bowie, Md. (www.futuratty.com); Microflip, Inc., Glenn Dale, Md. (www.microflip.com); NXi Communications, Inc., Salt Lake City, Utah; Phone-TTY, Inc., Parsippany, N.J. (www.phone-tty.com); Ultratec, Inc., Madison, Wisc. (www.ultratec.com).

Baudot code with other TTYs) is required for successful communication with a TTY.

One of the major advantages of the Baudot-based TTYs is simplicity, since all have the same transmission protocol. Use of ASCII offers a variety of protocols that differ in significant ways, and a successful transmission depends on both the transmitting and the receiving parties having the same setup. This requires that the sender know the protocol of the receiver. A hearing person can obtain this information via voice, an option not available to the deaf caller.

Williams, Jensema, and Harkins (1991) compared the features of 11 ASCII-based TTY products to determine their compatibility with Baudot devices. To determine compatibility of ASCII-based TTYs with each other, Williams and co-workers used each of the 11 devices in their sample to call each of the others. This resulted in 110 calls. The purpose of this study was to determine the degree to which deaf people could place a phone call successfully to other TTY products. To parallel the use of Baudot-based TTYs, in which the user can turn on the unit and immediately begin sending and receiving, no adjustment was made in the ASCII protocol other than to set it at the default settings.

Of the 110 outgoing calls, 77 (70%) were unsuccessful (e.g., receiving unit automatically switched to Baudot, garbled or failed transmission). For incoming calls, 81 (74%) were unsuccessful. Combining incoming and outgoing results, only 12% of the total calls were successful on both ends. Many of the calls resulted in both ends being automatically switched to Baudot, eliminating all the advantages

of using ASCII. Also, not all units had automatic switching (three for outgoing, seven for incoming).

**Visual telephones for the deaf.** Because it requires typing of each utterance, TTY telephone transmission is slow, typically one third to one fourth the rate of human speech (Galuska and Foulds, 1990). Visual sign language, on the other hand, results in communication rates comparable to human speech, and it is the primary form of communication used by individuals who are deaf. It does, of course, require that both the speaker and the listener understand sign language or that an interpreter be available. If standard telephone lines could be used to send visual images of manual signs, it would significantly increase communication rates over those obtained using TTYs.

There are several difficulties with sending video information over standard telephone lines. The most significant of these is that video signals contain much more information than audio signals. The way in which this larger amount of information is accommodated is to allow a wider bandwidth for the signals. The bandwidth is a measure of how much information can be accommodated. Because the telephone is intended to serve only voice communication, its bandwidth is very narrow (as low as 3000 Hz). In contrast, television channel bandwidths are measured in megahertz. Thus we have two choices: (1) increase the bandwidth of the telephone or (2) decrease the bandwidth of the video signal. If video telephones come into widespread usage in homes, then the first option will be realized. However, in order to allow use over any existing telephone line, the second approach is most practical. Narrowing the bandwidth of the video signal is accomplished by data compression (Galuska and Foulds, 1990). In this process the video signal is sent with lower bandwidth, and the intelligibility of the visual signing is used as a criterion for acceptability. Using a test instrument designed to simulate different bandwidths, Harkins, Wolff, and Korres (1991) tested four rates of transmission (slower rates are analogous to lower bandwidths). They found that intelligibility decreased with decreasing bandwidth, and that a bandwidth about one third of the normal television signal provided was optimal. Decreases below this level resulted in significantly poorer intelligibility, but bandwidths greater than one third of the normal yielded only marginal improvement. Harkins, Wolff, and Korres (1991) also found that finger spelling at normal rates was less intelligible than whole words at normal rates or reduced-speed finger spelling.

In a work environment there is an alternative to the visual telephone that can provide many of the same benefits: the use of PCs and local area networks (LANs). LANs are typically used to transfer data and messages (e.g., electronic mail) from one PC to another within an office or over a wider network. When PCs and LANs are used in conjunction with a simple video camera and software, visual images can be sent from one computer to another (Galuska, Grove, and Gray, 1992). This allows two individuals with hearing impairments to communicate via sign language. Another, more far-reaching application is to use a LAN to provide interpretive services to a deaf employee or customer. The interpreter can be connected via video on the network to the employee. A speakerphone provides audio connection from the meeting to the interpreter and from the hearing impaired person (via the interpreter) to others at the meeting. The network video provides signed interpretation to the individual with a hearing impairment from the interpreter and from the hearing impaired individual to the interpreter for voice relay to the meeting.

SignWorks* is a project of the Deaf Studies Trust at the University of Bristol in Britain. The goal is to support deaf business within the United Kingdom. Because there is very little business activity in the United Kingdom by people who are deaf, SignWorks also helps new businesses get started and works with deaf entrepreneurs, managers, and professionals. A key element in this project is the use of multimedia information services. SignWorks utilizes on-line information services and visual telecommunications to create a system of advice for deaf people in business. SignWorks provides a range of services (e.g., job counseling and training support), as well as facilitating the development and application of telecommunications equipment. A key element of this project is the use of sign language on the telephone, allowing people who are deaf to conduct daily business on a equal standing with hearing people. The video telephone being used in the project is the mm220 by Motion Media Technology.† The videophone will be installed at libraries, schools, support organizations for the deaf, and companies that have deaf employees. The mm220 videophone is about the size of a traditional business telephone. It is one of the first videophones whose picture quality and speed can successfully transmit and receive sign language. It includes a built-in camera, microphone, and video screen. It can also be connected to a PC for two-way data sharing for documents, files, and interaction with Internet-based meetings software.

## Alerting Devices for Persons with Auditory Impairments

There are many environmental sounds other than speech about which a person who is deaf needs to know. Examples are telephones, doorbells, smoke alarms, and a child's cry. There are **alerting devices** available that detect these sounds and then cause a vibration, a flashing light signal, or both to call attention to the sound. Some devices are very specific. For example, one device is tuned to the frequency of a smoke alarm and it responds only to that sound. When

the smoke alarm auditory signal is detected, the visible smoke detector transmits a flasher, which can be connected to a standard lamp. The lamp flashes as long as the smoke detector is active.

Telephone alerting devices include amplified ringers that plug into a standard telephone jack and provide up to 95 dB of ringing sound (McFadden, 1996). Another approach is to use a flashing light that is connected to the telephone line. This can alert the person who is deaf that there is an incoming TTY call. Some systems have a strobe light connected to them; others use a table lamp plugged into the alerting device. The only modification required for these adaptations is a two-plug telephone adapter to allow plugging in of both the adapted alerting device and the telephone.

Doorbells can be both directly wired into a flashing light or detected by a microphone and then converted into a visible (typically a flashing light) or tactile (vibration) signal. For more general sound detection there are silent alarms that can detect any signal and then transmit to a wrist-worn receiver. This both vibrates and flashes a light to indicate that the sound has occurred. Some devices can accommodate 16 or more channels, and different lights flash for each sound. A microphone and transmitter can be placed in each of the locations where an important sound may occur. For example, one can be near the front door, another near the telephone, another in the baby's room, and a final one near the back door. When a sound is detected at any of these locations, the wrist unit vibrates and one light is illuminated to indicate which sound has been detected.

Alarm clocks for persons who are deaf generally are either visible (flashing light on a bedside table) or tactile (vibration under the pillow). They may either be built in to an alarm clock (e.g., the entire face of the clock flashes) or they may detect the clock's alarm and then cause the vibration or flashing light (or both).

One of the major difficulties faced by persons who are deaf is the lack of awareness of sounds associated with traffic. Sirens, horns, and ambient traffic noise all contribute to our ability to drive. Miyazaki and Ishida (1987) developed a device that detects specific sounds and displays a visible alarm to the driver. Traffic horns of different types (air horn on a truck versus a car horn), sirens, railroad crossings, and motorcycles are typical of the sounds detected and displayed.

## Assistive Listening Devices (ALDs)

All the devices we have discussed in this chapter have been designed for use by hearing-impaired individuals. There is also a class of assistive devices that are intended to be used in group settings, such as lecture halls, churches, business meetings, courtrooms, and broadcast television. These are called **assistive listening devices.**

---

*www.deafstudiestrust.demon.co.uk/text/Projects/sworksum.
†Bristol, U.K. (www.mmtech.co.uk).

**Small-group devices.** For many individuals who have auditory impairments, hearing aids are only effective for one-on-one conversations at close range (and possibly for telephone use). When they are in a group, even a small group of five or fewer persons, it is very difficult to understand what is being said, and *small-group* or *personal listening devices* are helpful (Williams and Snope, 1985). These devices consist of a microphone and a battery-powered radio transmitter that are worn by the speaker and a receiver that is carried by the person with an auditory impairment. The output of the receiver can either be fed into earphones (personal FM system) or coupled directly to the hearing aid (similar to the telephone aids described earlier). If the person does not normally use a hearing aid or the hearing aids used do not accommodate direct coupling of the signal, the earphones are used. The speaker uses a microphone and whatever she says is then transmitted to the listener with a high signal-to-noise ratio. For small-group meetings with several participants, the speaker and microphone can be placed in the middle of the conference table to pick up all the voices. Small-group devices can have multiple receivers for one transmitter if there is more than one person requiring amplification. Another approach used in classrooms and meeting rooms is a "sound field" FM system in which audio speakers are located around the room and the FM signal is presented through the speakers rather than through earphones to each listener.

Several manufacturers produce devices that combine a conventional BTE hearing aid with an FM system.* One manufacturer has developed a microminiature FM receiver that is mounted in a "boot" that fits over the bottom of the BTE device and directly couples the amplified sound to the hearing aid. A wireless FM microphone transmits the radio signal from the person who is speaking to the receiver attached to the BTE device. The FM receiver can be removed easily from standard BTE hearing aid.

**Large-group devices.** The problems addressed by small-group devices also exist in large meeting rooms such as concert halls, lecture auditoriums, and churches. Under the provisions of the ADA, these areas must be equipped with assistive listening devices. There are several approaches possible, all of which are directly coupled to the public address system of the facility being equipped. These are (1) hard-wired jacks for plugging in earphones, (2) FM transmitter-receiver setups similar to small-group devices, and (3) audio induction loops for transmission to hearing aids equipped with telecoils (Williams and Snope, 1985). Hard-wired systems have the advantage of privacy (there is no transmission over the air) and simplicity of technology.

---

*For example, the Extend Ear, AVR Communication Limited, Eden Prairie, Minn (www.avrsono.com); Microlink, Phonak Staeta, Switzerland (www.phonak.com).

There are two primary limitations of this approach, however. First, rewiring a facility has a high cost and, unless the wiring is done during construction, it is usually not feasible. Second, persons requiring the use of the assisted listening device are forced to sit in a few predetermined locations (where there are earphone jacks).

The audio induction loop devices have their roots in Europe. They require that the user's hearing aid have an induction coil (often called a *telephone coil*). The major limitations of the induction coil approach are the large amount of power required to drive the induction coil transmitter and susceptibility to interference. FM transmission has low levels of interference, a large transmission range, and a transmission band specifically for use by persons with hearing impairment (72 to 76 MHz). FM systems have the advantage that the listener can sit anywhere within range, and they can easily be wired into the normal public address system. Limitations of this approach include varying degrees of strength in the signals being received by telecoils in different hearing aids and a nonuniform transmission pattern resulting in unequal signal strength within the area served by the transmission loop.

Other ALDs have been developed for television viewing and for use as personal amplifiers (Stach, 1998). Personal amplifiers are hard-wired microphones connected to an amplifier and to earphones worn by the person who is hard of hearing. They are used in hospitals and similar situations for temporary amplification when hearing aids are not available or not worn. Television listeners are ALDs that connect directly to the audio of the television set and transmit the signal to a receiver via FM or ultrasound. The user has earphones connected to the receiver.

**Closed-captioned television and movies. Closed captioning** is a process whereby the audio portion of a television program is converted to written words, which appear in a window on the screen. It is called closed because the words are not visible unless the viewer has a closed-caption decoder. In the United States the Telecommunications Act of 1996 (see Chapter 1) resulted in FCC regulations requiring television broadcasters to provide closed captioning. New programming released after January 1, 1998, must be "fully accessible." *Fully accessible* means that 95% of the nonexempt programming must be closed captioned. A telecaption decoder can be connected to a television set, VCR, or cable TV receiver to decode the captioning signal and display the words on the screen. All television sets currently being produced have a built-in closed caption converter. It takes between 20 and 30 hours to close caption a 1-hour television program. The individual broadcasters make decisions regarding which programs are captioned consistent with the regulations described above. Some programs, such as live newscasts, are captioned on the fly, whereas others are captioned in postproduction. With approximately 20 million new TVs sold in the United States each year, every household was expected to have at least one caption-capable set by the year 2000.

More than 3000 titles of home videos and nearly 500 hours of network, cable, and independent programming a week are now available in closed-caption form. Closed captioning includes movies, network news, comedies, sporting events, dramas, and educational, religious, and children's programming. In excess of 550 national advertisers have closed captioned more than 13,000 commercials. The NCI can also caption live programs such as news broadcasts, presidential speeches, and coverage of the Olympics. Captions can aid those learning English as a second language and provide assistance in efforts to eradicate illiteracy.

People who are deaf or blind can enjoy first-run movies in theaters. A project carried out by the CPB/WGBH National Center for Accessible Media (NCAM)* in Boston has developed systems that enable these populations to access movies through closed captions (for deaf patrons) and descriptive narration (for blind patrons). Both these adaptations have been developed to avoid altering of the moviegoing experience for the general audience. Reversed captions are displayed by the Rear Window Captioning System on a light-emitting diode (LED) text display that is mounted in the rear of a theater. Deaf and hard-of-hearing persons use transparent acrylic panels attached to their seats to reflect the captions so that they appear to be superimposed on the movie screen. The caption users can sit anywhere in the theater, since the reflective panels are both portable and adjustable. Blind and visually impaired moviegoers can hear the descriptive narration on headsets using the DVS Theatrical system. The narration is delivered via infrared or FM listening systems. These descriptions provide information about key visual elements such as actions, settings, and scene changes. This makes the movies more meaningful to people with vision loss. Initially only available in specialty theaters, these technologies are being introduced into conventional movie theaters. The captioning and descriptive narration systems are integrated into the movie projection sound system using CD-ROM technology. A reader attached to the film projector reads a time code printed on the film. The caption and descriptive narration tracks are recorded on a separate CD-ROM, which plays alongside the other disks in the movie sound player. The information on the movie time code signals the CD sound player to play the audio descriptions synchronously with the film soundtrack. The CD player also sends the captions to the LED display and the descriptive narration to the infrared or FM emitter. WGBH is working with all the major studios and exhibitors to encourage them to adopt these technologies and make closed captions and descriptive narration available for movies on an ongoing basis.

*www.wgbh.org/wgbh/pages/ncam/.

## AIDS FOR PERSONS WITH BOTH VISUAL AND AUDITORY IMPAIRMENTS

Individuals who are both deaf and blind must use tactile input to obtain information about the environment and to communicate. There are two basic methods used by this group of people. The Tadoma method (see the section on fundamental approaches in this chapter) is used to understand speech; finger spelling, with the deaf-blind individual sensing the signs in his hand, is used when both persons in the conversation know signing or one person acts as an interpreter.

### Automated Hand for Finger Spelling

One of the difficulties for deaf-blind individuals who depend on finger spelling is that the speaker must be able to finger spell or there must be an interpreter present. A further limitation is that the deaf-blind person gives up her privacy when an interpreter is used. One approach, still under development, is the use of a mechanical hand connected to a keyboard (Gilden and Jaffe, 1987). The hand is fully articulated; that is, all joints of each finger are independently adjustable. The finger positions for each letter are stored in the computer and are generated when a letter is typed from the keyboard. The mechanical hand can also be connected to a TTY for telephone conversations and to a remote computer via a modem for bulletin boards. Because it is programmed to accept computer input from a keyboard, it can also accept alphabetic characters from a computer. This allows it to be connected to a text-scanning computer in place of the normal voice synthesizer. An evaluation of the second generation of this hand by a group of deaf-blind individuals showed that some could easily interpret the finger patterns, whereas others had great difficulty (Jaffe, Harwin, and Harkins, 1993). Based on these results, as well as advances in mechanical design, a third generation of this hand was developed (Jaffe, Harwin, and Harkins, 1993). This version is faster, smaller, and more portable. Finger positions are also more accurately portrayed. Because many deaf-blind individuals are born deaf and develop blindness over the course of their late teenage years, they learn to finger spell early but do not learn braille. Therefore by the time they become blind they desire a system they can use easily, and the mechanical finger meets this need.

## SUMMARY

For persons who have low vision, it is possible to improve performance by increasing size, contrast, and spacing of the text material. Low-cost magnification aids and filters can help in this regard, but electronic aids provide much greater flexibility. Reading aids for persons who are blind rely on either tactile or auditory substitution. The most effective of these are language based (e.g., speech or braille). Fully automated reading devices are capable of imaging print documents and converting them to speech using voice synthesis.

Electronic travel aids for persons who are blind serve a useful but limited purpose in aiding mobility and orientation for blind travelers. Just as reading aids use alternative sensory pathways of auditory and tactile input, so do ETAs. The basic structure of a sensory aid shown in Figure 12-1 applies to ETAs, as well as reading aids. The environmental interface is either a light (laser or infrared emitter and sensor) or sound (ultrasound), and the user display is either an auditory tone or series of tones of varying frequency and amplitude or tactile vibration. The information processor converts the reflected light or ultrasound information to the audible or tactile display information presented to the user. Current technology provides only limited substitution or augmentation for the long cane. Future developments will most likely be in the extraction of useful features from the visual image for display to the blind traveler (see Adjouadi, 1992, for example). By concentrating on achieving input that is more informative regarding obstacles and the orientation and location of objects in the environment, the utility of these devices will be greatly enhanced. Electronic aids that assist blind travelers with orientation are also available; some make use of global positioning satellite information.

Hearing aids provide assistance for persons whose hearing is inadequate for conversation. Recent trends in hearing aid design have focused on improved fidelity and digital speech processing. When an individual has damage to the cochlea, he may benefit from the use of cochlear implants. Emphasis on speech processing algorithms will continue in order to provide better understanding of how stimulation via cochlear implants can aid speech recognition.

Aids for persons who are deaf utilize either visual or tactile systems as alternatives. Speech-to-text (sound-to-visual display) devices are not as well developed as text-to-speech aids, and visual information is most commonly used for alarms rather than for communication. Exceptions to this are telephone communication using telephone devices for the deaf (TTYs).

Aids for persons who are both deaf and blind must use tactile substitution. The major approach is braille output with a text-based keyboard for communication between a sighted and a deaf-blind individual. A mechanical device that emulates finger spelling (commonly used by deaf-blind persons) and is driven by a computer with keyboard entry provides communication between a sighted person who does not know finger spelling and a deaf-blind person who does.

## Study Questions

1. What are the two basic approaches to sensory aids in terms of the sensory pathway used?
2. List the three basic parts of a sensory aid and describe the function of each part. Pick one example from visual aids, one from auditory aids, and one from tactile aids and describe the three parts that make up each aid.
3. Compare the visual, auditory, and tactile systems in terms of their basic function and as substitutes for each other.
4. What are the three types of scanners used in reading machines, and how do they differ?
5. What is an OCR, and what function does it perform in a reading machine for the blind?
6. List three output modes available for reading machines.
7. Computer disks or CD-ROMs with text stored on them can be used to provide access to reading material for persons who are blind. What components (e.g., adapted output devices) must be included in such devices, and what role does the computer play?
8. What are the major differences in the effects of errors in reading and in mobility devices?
9. What are the major limitations of the long cane for use as a mobility aid by persons who are blind?
10. What is an electronic travel aid?
11. List three advantages and three disadvantages of the laser cane.
12. What is a clear-path indicator, and how is it used in mobility for people who are blind?
13. What are the major assistive technologies applied to orientation for people who are blind?
14. Pick a tool or measurement instrument and figure out how to adapt it for both a person with low vision and one who is blind.
15. Discuss the major differences between blindness and deafness in terms of the effect on the individual's social, work or school, and private lives.
16. What are the two major acoustic parameters used to specify hearing aids, and how are they measured?
17. What are the major parts of a hearing aid, and what is the function of each?
18. What are the four types of hearing aids?
19. What is acoustic coupling, and how does it affect hearing aid performance?
20. List the major functions that a cochlear implant must accomplish.
21. What are the major differences among analog, digitally controlled analog, and digital hearing aids?
22. What is meant by *compression* in hearing aids?

23. What is the difference between linear and curvilinear amplification in hearing aids?
24. How are data and power coupled to cochlear implants?
25. What is the relationship between the number of electrodes and the functional performance for a cochlear implant?
26. What are the major differences between a channel and an electrode in cochlear implants?
27. Describe the major approaches to signal processing used in cochlear implants. What are the advantages and disadvantages of each?
28. What is a TTY, and why is the Baudot code used?
29. Compare a stand-alone TTY with a computer TTY modem using Baudot coding. What advantages does each offer to a deaf user?
30. Why can't a standard computer modem be used to communicate with a TTY?
31. What are the major limitations to the use of standard telephone lines for visual information transmission (such as for manual signing)?
32. What are "alerting devices"? For what purposes are they normally used?
33. What are FM transmission systems for group listening, and how are they typically used?
34. What are the three major assistive technology approaches used for deaf-blind individuals to obtain communication input? What are the relative advantages of each approach?

## References

Adjouadi M: A man-machine vision interface for sensing the environment, *J Rehabil Res Dev* 29(2):57-76, 1992.

Allen J: Reading aids for the severely visually handicapped, *CRC Crit Rev Bioeng* 12:139-166, 1971.

American Foundation for the Blind: *How does a blind person get around?* New York, 1978, The Foundation.

Berger KW, Hagberg EN, Rane RL: *Prescription of hearing aids: rationale, procedures and results,* Kent, Ohio, 1977, Herald.

Converso L, Hocek S: Optical character recognition, *J Vis Impair Blindness* 84(10):507-509, 1990.

Cook AM: Sensory and communication aids. In Cook AM, Webster JG, editors: *Therapeutic medical devices,* Englewood Cliffs, NJ, 1982, Prentice-Hall.

Crabb N: Mastering the code to independence, *Braille Forum,* pp 24-27, June 1998.

Dillon H: Compression in hearing aids. In Sandlin RE, editor: *Handbook of hearing aid amplification,* vol 1, Boston, 1988, Little, Brown.

Dixon JM, Mandelbaum JB: Reading through technology: evolving methods and opportunities for print-handicapped individuals, *J Vis Impair Blindness* 84(10):493-496, 1990.

Doherty JE: *Protocols for choosing low vision devices,* Washington, DC, 1993, National Institute on Disability and Rehabilitation Research.

Farmer LW: Mobility devices, *Bull Prosthet Res* 30:41-118, 1978.

Feigenbaum E: Cochlear implant devices for the profoundly hearing impaired, *IEEE Eng Med Biol Mag* 6(2):10-21, 1987.

Fruchterman JR: Reading systems for the visually and reading impaired, *Proc 1991 CSUN Conference,* 1991.

Galuska S, Foulds R: A real-time visual telephone for the deaf, *Proc 13th Ann RESNA Conf,* pp 267-268, 1990.

Galuska S, Grove T, Gray J: A visual "talk" utility: using sign language over a local area computer network, *Proc 15th Ann RESNA Conf,* pp 134-135, June 1992.

Gilden D, Jaffe DL: Speaking in hands, *SOMA,* pp 6-13, October 1987.

Grotta D, Grotta SW: Desktop scanners: what's now . . . what's next, *PC Magazine* 17(18):147-188, 1998.

Halliday J: How can braille help people who are deaf, *Human Awareness Newsletter,* Autumn 1993.

Harkins JE, Wolff AB, Korres E: Intelligibility experiments with a feature extraction system designed to simulate a low-bandwidth video telephone for deaf people, *Proc 14th Ann RESNA Conf,* pp 38-40, June 1991.

Jaffe DL, Harwin WS, Harkins JE: The development of a third generation finger spelling aid, *Proc 16th Ann RESNA Conf,* pp 161-163, June 1993.

Kerscher G, Hansson K: DAISY Consortium—developing the next generation of digital talking books (DTB), *Proc CSUN Conf,* 1998 (http://www.dinf.org/csun_98_065.htm).

Kirman JH: Tactile communication of speech: a review and analysis, *Psychol Bull* 80:54-74, 1973.

Lieberman P: *Intonation, perception and language,* Cambridge, Mass, 1967, MIT Press.

Levitt H: Digital hearing aids: past, present and future. In *Practical Hearing Aid Selection and Fitting,* Washington, DC, 1997, Department of Veterans Affairs, pp xi-xxiii.

Mann RW: Technology and human rehabilitation: prostheses for sensory rehabilitation and/or substitution. In Brown JHU, Dickson JF (eds): *Advances in biomedical engineering,* New York, 1974, Academic Press.

McFadden GM: Aids for hearing impairments and deafness. In Galvin JC, Scherer MJ (eds): *Evaluating, selecting and using appropriate assistive technology,* Rockville, Md, 1996, Aspen Publishers.

Mellor CM: *Aids for the '80s,* New York, 1981, American Foundation for the Blind.

Millar JB, Tong YC, Clark GM: Speech processing for cochlear implant prostheses, *J Speech Hearing Res* 27:280-296, 1984.

Miyazaki S, Ishida A: Traffic-alarm sound monitor for aurally handicapped drivers, *Med Biol Eng Comput* 25:68-74, 1987.

Nye PW, Bliss JC: Sensory aids for the blind: a challenging problem with lessons for the future, *Proc IEEE* 58:1878-1879, 1970.

Owen MJ: Close encounters of a technological kind: a personal transformation, *J Vis Impair Blindness* 84(10):491-492, 1990.

Preves DA: Principles of signal processing. In Sandlin RE, editor: *Handbook of hearing aid amplification,* vol 1, Boston, 1988, Little, Brown.

Radcliffe D: How cochlear implants work, *Hearing J,* p 53, November 1984.

Scadden LA: Technology for people with visual impairments: a 1997 update, *Technol Dis* 6:137-145, 1997.

Servais SP: Visual aids. In Webster JG et al (eds): *Electronic devices for rehabilitation,* New York, 1985, Wiley and Sons.

Shallop JK, Mecklenberg DJ: Technical aspects of cochlear implants. In Sandlin RE, editor: *Handbook of hearing aid amplification,* vol 1, Boston, 1988, Little, Brown.

Smith GC: The Stereotoner—a new sensory aid for the blind, *Proc Ann Conf Eng Med Biol* 14:147, 1972.

Stach BA: *Clinical audiology,* San Diego, 1998, Singular Publishing Group.

White RL: System design of a cochlear implant, *IEEE Eng Med Biol Mag* 6(2):10-21, 1987.

Williams NS, Jensema CJ, Harkins JE: ASCII-based TDD products: features and compatibility, *Proc 14th Ann RESNA Conf,* pp 41-43, 1991.

Williams PS, Snope T: *Assistive listening devices: professional practices,* Washington, DC, 1985, American Speech-Language and Hearing Association.

Wilson BS et al: Design and evaluation of a continuous interleaved sampling (CIS) processing strategy for multichannel cochlear implants, *J Rehabil Res* 30(1):110-116, 1993.

# The Contexts for Assistive Technology Applications

## CHAPTER 13

# Assistive Technologies in the Context of the Classroom

## Learning Objectives

Upon completing this chapter you will be able to:

1. Describe the context in which assistive technologies are applied in education
2. List the major assistive technologies that are used in educational settings
3. Describe how assistive technologies are used in the classroom to facilitate learning
4. List the major technological approaches used to assist individuals who have learning disabilities
5. Describe how soft technologies are utilized in education to enhance the use of hard technologies

In preceding chapters we have developed principles for assistive technology application based on the Human Activity Assistive Technology (HAAT) model (see Chapter 2). Two of the major settings in which assistive technologies are used are education and work, and each of these has features that make assistive technology applications unique. In this chapter we discuss educational applications. Vocational applications are covered in the next chapter. In both cases we will use the HAAT model as a framework around which to discuss assistive technology (AT) applications.

Assistive technologies can provide major benefits for children in educational settings from preschool through postsecondary levels (Todis and Walker, 1993). Postural support systems (see Chapter 6) allow children to be positioned for maximal participation in classroom activities. Often this positioning is necessary to allow access to computers for learning (see Chapter 8). Special-purpose input methods or control interfaces (see Chapter 7) are often necessary for use of computers and other electronic devices. Augmentative communication systems (see Chapter 9) play a major role in learning for children who have disabilities affecting speaking or writing. Research has also shown that independent mobility (see Chapter 10) has a significant benefit even to very young children (Butler, 1985). There is an increasing use of "manipulatives" in education. Some assistive technologies (e.g., electronic aids to daily living [EADLs] and robotics; see Chapter 11) can provide assistance to children who cannot independently manipulate real objects. Finally, children who have sensory disabilities (visual or auditory) are aided by the technologies described in Chapter 12. Thus the potential for achieving a positive educational effect is great. However, reaching that potential requires careful planning and policy making to ensure that opportunities and not barriers are created (Merbler, Hadadian, and Ulman, 1999).

Now that we have identified the individual tools for access to education that appear in previous chapters, we turn our attention to how they are combined and applied to maximize the opportunities for learning by children who have disabilities. That is the subject of the remainder of this chapter.

## ■ EDUCATIONAL ACTIVITIES THAT CAN BE AIDED BY ASSISTIVE TECHNOLOGIES

In order to discuss assistive technology applications in the classroom, we must first define the activities that characterize educational endeavors. Having done that, we can then begin to identify the ways that assistive technologies can contribute to those activities. In the following sections, each of the learning activities is described in terms of the tasks that must be accessed in order to complete the activity. Identification of these tasks will then help us to define both the human skills and the technologies required to successfully complete them.

In all these functional areas there are educational technologies (see Chapter 1) that aid in the acquisition of the necessary skills. In many cases the educational technologies are software programs that provide systematic skill development in the various activities.

For example, using CD-ROM-based educational software and the Internet, learners can access a much wider range of curriculum material, concepts, ideas, and lessons than are available by print materials and worksheets alone. Because all these sources require the use of a computer, the adaptations described in Chapter 8 are often necessary to ensure access for learners who have motor or sensory disabilities. Because schools often have computers available for general use by learners, it is necessary for the ATP to work with school staff to determine the appropriate access methods for individual learners. The ATP can also work with teachers to integrate appropriate software and hardware into the curriculum.

### Reading

Reading requires motor, sensory, and cognitive skills. For print materials, motor skills are primarily associated with positioning the reading material, turning pages, and similar tasks (e.g., picking up a book, opening it, using an index, thumbing through pages). As shown in Figure 13-1, an aide often assists with manipulation of the reading materials. For reading materials that use electronic media, the motor tasks include mouse or keyboard use to scroll through text, highlight a portion of text, search for particular words or topics, and print out part or all of a document.

Success in reading also requires that sensory tasks be completed. Typically we use the visual system to take in information via reading. For this function there must be sufficient visual field, visual acuity, and oculomotor function to scan text and recognize letters and words. If the visual system cannot support these functions, then an alternative format in either tactile (braille) or auditory (speech) form can be used instead.

Conversion between print and electronic forms and between visual and auditory or tactile formats can be aided by assistive technologies. Some of these are described in Chapters 8 and 12. The use of digital scanners to aid in this function is described later in this chapter.

Cognitive tasks are those associated with literacy; that is, word identification, spelling, and comprehension. Educational software for assisted reading includes programs that present very simple stories that the child can control, programs with multiple output modes (e.g., visual and auditory), interactive stories that the child can change by pointing and clicking the mouse, and on-line books (including current bestsellers, children's books, and the classics).

## Writing

In Chapter 9 we grouped the types of writing into three categories: note taking, messaging, and formal writing. Individuals who do not have disabilities may use handwriting for some or all of these. As we discuss in Chapters 8 and 9, there are also many alternatives to handwriting for

successful completion of these tasks. These include assistance provided by an aide (Figure 13-2), computer-aided writing using word processing, personal digital assistants that recognize handwriting on a screen and store it as text for editing, modified pens and pencils (e.g., enlarged grip or holder), and systems that recognize speech and translate it directly into text (automatic speech recognition).

Writing as a cognitive process has been described as consisting of four phases: (1) prewriting or brainstorming, (2) drafting or organizing and composing, (3) editing, and (4) publishing (Calkins, 1986). Technology can aid all four phases of this process and thereby positively affect the learner's writing skill development (Rocklage and Lake, 1997). As Rocklage and Lake point out, assistive technology for writing provides both a structure within which the learner can learn to write and a polished finished (or published) product.

Writing requires motor, sensory, and cognitive skills. The use of pencil or pen and paper requires fine motor control to hold the pen or pencil and to produce letters. When the learner's disability significantly affects these motor skills, it may be necessary to recognize that some skills will not be functional and develop alternative approaches to writing. This allows the learner to move on to other educational goals rather than working on the functional tasks of handwriting at the expense of these other goals. The assistive technology practitioner (ATP) must use her judgment as to when to make the transition from handwriting skill development to electronic alternatives, but in most cases it is desirable to accommodate in the short

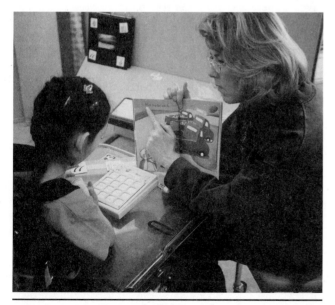

**Figure 13-1**    An aide often assists with manipulation of reading materials when it is difficult for the student to hold the book.

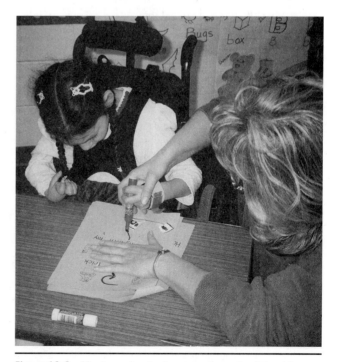

**Figure 13-2**    Hand-over-hand assistance can be used to help with writing.

term to enable learning, even if handwriting might be functional in the long term.

Assistive technology-based writing requires the ability to use a keyboard or mouse. As we discuss in Chapter 7, there are also many alternatives to keyboard/mouse entry, including automatic speech recognition. Sensory skills are primarily used for monitoring of what is being written. This is most commonly done visually, but auditory or tactile monitoring is also possible using various types of assistive technologies. Cognitive and language skills include spelling (spontaneous, first letter, recognition), grammar, and sequencing.

Writing may be aided by a personal assistant (e.g., peer, teacher, teacher's aide, parent) or through the use of assistive technologies. In many cases a combination of these approaches is utilized. The assistance provided by a human aide is often called **scribing**. Scribing is used for most children, at least initially, to help them keep up with written work. With this approach, children complete written assignments, but a question arises as to who is really doing the work, the learner or the aide? Scribing may also limit the development of other cognitive processing skills. The writing experience that we often take for granted is a critical thinking skill. Because scribing involves another person actually putting the thoughts on paper, it may change the process of writing as a complement to thinking and reasoning. In general the more we write, the better we get. For the learner who has significant motor disabilities, we can expect writing to be slow and difficult initially; however, persistence will pay off in most cases.

One type of writing, note taking, plays an important role in learning for many people. This type of writing requires the learner to process the information being given, isolate salient points, and translate between auditory and visual modalities. This active processing may be lost when a student uses the teacher's notes, or scribing. By providing assistance for independent writing, the student is more likely to have the opportunity to become an active learner in the classroom. Some alternative methods of writing using assistive technologies are slow, and learners may only generate a small percentage of the total written work. However, they should have the opportunity to develop this form of reasoning.

Educational software for assisting writing includes programs that allow the child to create his own story. Other programs provide monitoring through visual and auditory feedback. Word prediction and completion programs (see Chapter 9) can aid spelling and word finding. The use of abbreviations and macros (see Chapter 9) that reduce the number of keystrokes can increase the speed of text entry.

## Mathematics

In Chapter 9 we described many of the problems and solutions for manipulation of mathematical symbols and the

---

### CASE STUDY 13-1

#### COMPUTERS AS WRITING AIDS

A school-based occupational therapist has presented you, the ATP, with this question: "I know that written expression in schools can be done through scribing by a peer or aide or through teacher notes. At my school, a student is only considered for a laptop computer or a portable note-taking device if she is academically inclined and dexterous enough. Do you agree with this approach?" What would you tell her? Consider your answer in light of the discussion in this chapter about writing and the skills required.

---

completion of the mechanical aspects of mathematical operations for those who cannot use the traditional paper and pencil approach. A scribe can be used to assist in learning mathematics just as in writing. However, many of the same concerns and limitations described for writing apply to mathematics. For mathematics there is the added requirement that thinking mathematically almost always requires having a worksheet on which to solve the problem. Very few people can develop mathematical skills without some visual representation. When this is impossible (e.g., when the learner is blind), other strategies have to be developed. A learner may use an augmentative and alternative communication (AAC) device to instruct an aide who is scribing for the learner (e.g., "The answer is 5" or "Move the yellow one to the other pile").

Mathematical ability, including precursor skills (e.g., counting, sorting), is often developed using **manipulatives**. These are rods, blocks, buttons, beads, or other objects that vary by color, length, and weight and can be sorted, counted, and used to enhance concept development in mathematics. Piaget believed that learners use "concrete operations" (Box 3-1) to develop many cognitive concepts from 7 to 11 years of age (Brainerd, 1978). Others now believe that concrete operations using manipulatives of various types are an important part of learning for much older learners, including adults (Resnick et al, 1998). In order to fully benefit from concrete operations, the learner must have control over objects. For example, a simple task with manipulatives might involve being able to see that "I have two pieces in this pile, and I move two more pieces over and now I have four."

Although the learner typically manipulates real objects, there are also computer programs that substitute computer-generated graphics of manipulatives for persons who cannot use their hands. The computer mouse (e.g., click and drag) or keyboard (e.g., arrow keys) can be used to move these manipulatives. Conceptually this type of manipulation can develop the same skills as manipulation of real objects.

Manipulatives can also be switch controlled either by using software specifically designed for that purpose or by using computer adaptations such as SmartClick* (see Chapter 8) to create adapted access to standard software.

Mathematics differs from writing in several important ways. The cursor moves right to left rather than left to right for entering sums or differences. The functions of borrow and carry also require unique cursor movements. Higher mathematics requires Greek symbols, superscripts, subscripts, and mathematical symbols (e.g., integral sign, summation sign). Typical symbols are shown in Figure 9-4. Some AAC devices (see Chapter 9) have built-in math worksheet software including special symbols. These features of mathematics worksheets differ from calculator functions, and they are intended to facilitate the development of math skills. There is a use for calculators that are adapted for access by learners who have difficulties with the keys on standard calculators. Some enlarged key calculators are available, and some AAC devices also include calculator functions. Calculator functions are also built into Windows and Macintosh operating systems, and they can be used with any of the access approaches described in Chapter 8.

Word processing software often includes the special symbols required for mathematics but lacks the special cursor movements. The required symbol set is selected and inserted into a document or worksheet. This is useful for a teacher creating a worksheet or to a learner using a computer. However, these approaches do not address the special cursor movements required for mathematics. Those functions are available in special computer software (e.g., Math-Pad, FractionPad,† and Access to Math‡), as well as some AAC devices (see Chapter 9). The selection of characters can be left open as a window and the user can pick the desired symbol and insert it as necessary. This approach allows the learner to write out the equations, solve them, and print the results. Both direct and indirect (scanning and encoding) access are available to accommodate a variety of motor skill levels in learners (see Chapter 7).

Educational software that helps develop math skills from basic counting through higher mathematics is available for both the Windows and Macintosh environments. These programs address skill development through drill and practice, as well as concept development, through the use of computer graphics, games, and word problems integrated into an interesting illustrated story (see Case Study 13-2).

## Science

Educational activities in science are both theoretical and experimental. The latter is based on hands-on manipulation

---

---

### CASE STUDY 13-2

#### AT ASSISTANCE WITH MATHEMATICS

Ken is a young high school student who uses a single-switch scanner. In math skills he has never gone beyond number recognition and simple addition up to 10. He has no use of his hands to use manipulatives to assist him in higher calculations. Ken's team would like him to use a math worksheet program. Also, because he cannot add more complex sums in his head, they would like him to have access to a calculator that he would use only as needed. He should be able to transfer the calculator results to his worksheet. The built-in calculator on the computer is rather small, and he would be unable to carry the answer in his head to put it on his worksheet. What approaches would you suggest to Ken's team to help in this situation?

---

of objects in biology, physics, and chemistry. Sometimes these concepts and skills are taught with physical objects and laboratory experiments. However, with the increased quality and resolution of computer graphics, a lower cost alternative is computer simulation of experimental situations (e.g., frog dissection in biology, chemical reactions, laws of motion experiments in physics). There are also Internet-based sources from which experiments can be downloaded.

There are several ways in which learners with physical disabilities that limit reaching and grasping can participate in science activities that require manipulation. Instructions for manipulation can be given to a peer, aide, or teacher via natural speech or AAC devices. Independent manipulation of objects can be aided by EADLs or robotic systems. In Chapter 11 we describe EADLs, or environmental control systems (ECUs), in detail. The use of robotic arms to aid in science instruction is also described in Chapter 11. Finally, if suitable computer adaptations are available, learners with disabilities can participate equally in computer simulations, concept development software, and Internet-based science instruction.

## Music

Music instruction involves basic rhythm and group participation. Young learners use instruments and their voices to participate in music. Music appreciation through listening is also part of the curriculum. Adaptations (e.g., adapted handles, activation by head or foot movement) can be made for students who cannot use musical instruments as a result of disabilities. AAC devices that use digitized speech (see Chapter 9) can store musical sounds (i.e., an instrument) or a vocal song. Most computers can be equipped with a **musical instrument digital interface (MIDI).** This

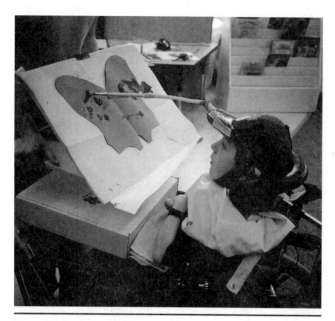

Figure 13-3   For assistance with painting in art class, we can attach the paintbrush to a head-pointing stick or baseball cap.

interface is a file that is used to store music as a series of notes with volume and duration attached. The file allows music to be played back through a sound card in a computer. If a digital musical instrument (e.g., a piano keyboard) is attached to the MIDI interface, it can be used to store the musical notes so they can be played back on the instrument or through the sound card (Merbler, Hadadian, and Ulman, 1999). With this arrangement, learners can create original songs, learn musical instruments, and explore sounds. With appropriate computer adaptations, the learner who has a disability can also access a MIDI-equipped computer.

## Art

Art activities help students develop fine motor control and an understanding of shapes and colors and provide a creative outlet for students. For students who lack the fine motor skill for drawing, adaptations can be provided. For example, a pen, pencil, or paintbrush can be attached to a head pointer or mouthstick (see Chapter 7). One example of such an arrangement is shown in Figure 13-3.

Handles on drawing instruments can be enlarged and adapted grips can be added (see Figure 11-3). Alternatively, the manipulation of digital images can be substituted for drawing with pencil and paper. This can present challenging art projects in a format accessible by learners with physical

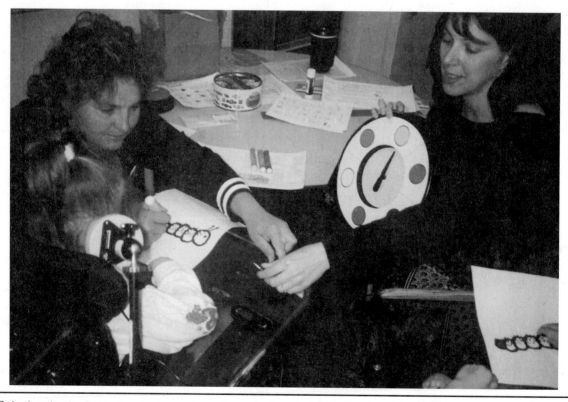

Figure 13-4   A student is selecting the color she wants to use by pressing her switch when the pointer is aimed at her choice. The teacher then uses that color to fill in a part of the picture.

disabilities (Merbler, Hadadian, and Ulman, 1999). Computer software for drawing is also used in educational settings. With the appropriate computer adaptations, this software is accessible to all learners regardless of disability.

Open-ended tasks such as drawing can also be carried out using single-switch scanning. In one approach the learner selects the color by scanning (Figure 13-4) and the teacher or aide then uses that color to fill in a part of the picture. A more independent method can be achieved using an adapted robotic system (Smith and Topping, 1996) such as the Handy 1, a robotic system specially designed for feeding (Topping, 1996). The Handy 1 is described further in Chapter 11. In the application for art, selection of the color of a pen, the position of the pen, the activity of the pen (move or draw), and its movement are accomplished using single-switch scanning. Using scanning for tasks such as these is cognitively demanding, and Smith and Topping (1996) reported widely different levels of success in the three subjects included in their study.

## IDENTIFYING STUDENT SKILLS AND NEEDS FOR ASSISTIVE TECHNOLOGY

The letter and response shown in the Case Study 13-3 were posted on the Rehabilitation Engineering and Assistive Technology Society of North America (RESNA) assistive technology listserv. They point out some of the issues in assistive technology assessment for education.

This exchange of letters points out the necessity for a team approach, including the learner and her family. It also illustrates the necessity of focusing on need rather than technology. In this section we describe several commonly employed approaches to assistive technology assessment in education. A general assistive technology assessment process is detailed in Chapter 4.

### Meeting Educational Goals: The Role of Assistive Technologies

We have defined the activities that are typically carried out in educational settings. Given these activities, it is important to determine the skills and abilities that the learner brings to the process. This evaluation of learner skills is obtained from a systematic assessment process. In Chapter 4 we describe both the essential information that must be obtained through an assessment process and the major approaches to service delivery in assistive technologies. AT assessment in education has some unique goals that we discuss in this section. We also describe the major approaches employed to obtain this assessment information.

The development of services and service delivery in the United States has been impacted significantly by federal legislation (see Chapter 1). The **Individuals with Disabilities Education Act (IDEA)** includes definitions of assistive technology devices and assistive technology services. It mandates that local educational agencies be responsible for providing assistive technology devices and services if these are required as part of a child's education, as well as related services and supplementary aid or service. These devices and services must be directly related to the child's educational program.

IDEA also mandates that an **Individual Education Plan (IEP)**, which incorporates the specialized program, be written for each student. The 1997 reauthorization of IDEA mandates that the IEP team must consider assistive technologies as a special factor when developing the learner's IEP (Merbler, Hadadian, and Ulman, 1999). A policy statement on the rights of a student with a disability to assistive technology under Public Law 94-142 was issued August 10, 1990 (Button, 1990). This policy statement describes a variety of services and devices that may be included in the IEP. The impact of this law has been far reaching, and devices ranging from sensory aids (visual and auditory) to augmentative communication devices to specialized computers have been provided to help children with disabilities access educational programs (Desch, 1986).

### The Assessment Team

The assistive technology assessment team usually includes a variety of disciplines (e.g., occupational therapist [OT], physical therapist [PT], speech-language pathologist [SLP], ATP, and pediatrician) (Todis and Walker, 1993). The classroom teacher and the local **resource specialist** in assistive technology may also be included, together with the family (parents and sibling) of the learner who is being assessed. If the assessment team is outside the learner's school, it is a greater challenge to develop sufficient understanding of the learner's needs. Ideally the assessment team would carry out their assessment in the school, community, and home, as well as any specialized assessment center (Todis and Walker, 1993). This approach allows the team to determine the preferences and goals (sometimes conflicting) of the learner, the family's values, and the short- and long-term goals of the educational program for the child.

As we have discussed in Chapter 4, there are many possible pitfalls and barriers in carrying out an assistive technology assessment. One potential problem in matching the assistive technology characteristics to the learner's needs is that the assessment team or the evaluator may have only a limited knowledge of assistive devices available. This will of course be driven by the experience of the evaluator, but it can severely limit the choices considered by the team or individual evaluator. This will result in the range of possible devices considered for a given learner being restricted (Todis and Walker, 1993).

## CASE STUDY 13-3

### ASSESSMENT FOR AT IN A SCHOOL SETTING

Dear Ms. A. T. Pea,

I am struggling with my school system on an assistive technology issue. I have a son with dyslexia, dysgraphia, moderate to severe attention deficit, a hearing loss that causes him to miss about half of what is said in his classes, and a tested IQ that falls just short of gifted.

This fall I requested an assistive tech evaluation to see whether he would benefit from greater use of a computer. I suggested that they consider providing a mid-range laptop and appropriate software for math and writing. I also requested someone to coach him in using it to compensate for his difficulties. I suggested that he be allowed to do scanned-in worksheets on it and maybe even take tests (under supervision so he couldn't make copies).

A few weeks later, without doing any sort of evaluation, the school provided an ancient black-and-white laptop with inadequate memory, no coaching, and no software other than an early word processing program, saying it was a test of whether a laptop would actually help him. Despite the laptop's inadequacy, there has been some improvement in his work. However, it's no good for math or science, and it has far too little memory to act as a "portable filing cabinet" for all his work, something he desperately needs.

I am desperate to find him some help now, so he can learn how best to use a computer before starting high school next fall. I can't resign myself to seeing a child with so much potential fall through the cracks. Even though it's the district's responsibility and the district can afford to meet his needs, I would buy him the computer and software myself if only the district would willingly provide a "coach" and make appropriate computer use part of his IEP. Right now, my only hope is to find material from other education professionals that can convince them that I'm not asking for something exotic. I am wondering whether you could point me to some sources of information. Thank you for any information you can offer.

Sincerely,

I. M. Concerned

The ATP wrote back to the mother:

Dear Ms. Concerned:

The school must provide any assistive technology that the IEP team determines necessary for your son in order to meet the IEP goals and objectives. You need to start with the IEP. Unfortunately, assistive technology is often requested after the IEP is in place, and there is no indication on the IEP that it is needed. The AT assessment should start with the student and what he needs to do, not with a piece of equipment. From a school's perspective, you are starting with a tool instead of analyzing the need first. Most administrators I know would balk at the request for a trial period of a piece of equipment before a thorough AT evaluation was completed.

I am beginning to see a willingness for school districts to provide more expensive assistive technology if (1) it is a team decision, (2) there is documentation of what has already been tried, (3) lower tech solutions have been tried and found to be inadequate, and (4) there is a trial period with the recommended system with clear documentation of benefit.

I also need to point out a laptop may not be the answer you hope for. Computer access for those with dysgraphia can be very helpful. However, for those with ADHD the computer is not necessarily an advantage. Depending on the level of ADHD and distractibility, the ability to "fiddle" that a word processor offers can actually slow down production over handwriting in some cases.

Your son does have a right to an AT assessment if he is currently unable to meet his IEP goals and objectives as a result of his disability; however, the outcome of that assessment should reflect a team decision. I think you have several choices:

1. Invest in a laptop and training for your son.
2. Approach the team from a slightly different angle, requesting a thorough assessment, not a specific solution.
3. Contact a special education resource center in your area for assistance in evaluation and some trial period of software or equipment.

I know that this is a difficult situation for you, and I hope that your son is able to obtain the assistive technology that will benefit him in his educational program.

Sincerely,

A.T. Pea, ATP

In Chapter 7 we present a detailed description of evaluation for access (e.g., use of a keyboard or alternative) to the assistive technologies. This is an area that is often overlooked until late in the assessment process, according to Todis and Walker (1993). Another area of potential concern is that the assessment may only address immediate learner needs and not pay enough attention to future growth and implications for new devices or expanded features (Beukelman and Mirenda, 1998). Assistive technology devices are often expensive, and funding sources will generally not purchase new technology repeatedly for the same child. The tradeoff is that the technology must have growth potential but not be too complicated or sophisticated for the learner to access it now (Todis and Walker, 1993).

As the letter from the mother in Case Study 13-3 illustrates, assistive technology procurement can sometimes become the goal rather than the process or means by which the goal can be achieved. This can place pressure on the assessment team to recommend assistive technology without adequate regard for the learner's goals.

Finally, the assessment process must carefully evaluate the potential impact of the new assistive technology on the classroom in which the learner's program is conducted. We discuss this further in the section on contexts of use for educational assistive technologies later in this chapter.

## Models for Educational Assistive Technology Assessment

There are only a few commonly used models of delivery for assistive technology devices and services. One set of models is built around an assistive technology expert or an expert team that is brought into the classroom. In some cases the assistive technology experience and expertise is not available in the local school, and external assistance is sought. Often a team of assistive technology specialists provides this assistance. In other cases a single external assistive technology consultant is called on to carry out assessment of a child. When a school or local education authority has experience in meeting the needs of a number of their students, they may build local assistive technology resources around this experience and not rely on external consultants. This is often an interdisciplinary team that works together within the local educational authority. Alternatively, a single well-qualified and experienced ATP may also take on this role for a local school district.

Another approach or model is to refer the child to the assessment setting in an evaluation center. Although this assessment is also carried out by a team, this model differs from the first model in that the child is typically seen in the center rather than in the classroom because they have a wide range of equipment to be demonstrated and they can involve specialized staff as the learner's needs dictate. Each of these delivery models is discussed in general in Chapter 4. In this chapter we focus on their use in educational settings.

As Todis and Walker (1993) point out, successful AT outcomes are dependent on a careful and thorough evaluation of the individual learner's needs. This is true regardless of the type and extent of disability or the format of the evaluation. If we are to ensure that there is "goodness of fit" between the learner's needs and the recommended assistive technology, then we are required to consider the full constellation of unique abilities and disabilities of the learner during the assessment process. Todis and Walker (1993) present two case studies that illustrate the importance of a thorough evaluation in order to achieve the desired outcomes for the learner.

**Specialist team.** A specialist or, more often, a multidisciplinary team is responsible for AT assessment. The team may be part of the school district or external to it. The role of the ATP in either case is as a consultant to the classroom team and family, not as a part of the learner's classroom staff. This role places limitations on what the ATP is able to do and how effective he is. As an outside consultant the ATP is able to make recommendations, offer expert advice, and provide information that may not be available to other team members. However, the implementation of assistive technology devices and services is out of his control. This means the ATP must carefully evaluate the educational context and take into account the resources, limitations, and expertise available in that setting before making recommendations for assistive technologies. This is especially important when considering soft technologies such as training of the learner and staff, strategy development for the use of the AT, and evaluation of outcomes of the AT intervention.

One of the most valuable contributions that the ATP can make to the school team is a perspective on what is possible, what is reasonable, and what is technologically feasible. Equally important is to be able to identify situations in which the available technologies are not suitable for the existing problems. Consumers may not appreciate the implications of new technological advances, many of which are reported in the popular press. Also, sometimes things that seem like they should be easy to do technically are really quite difficult and those that seem to a nontechnical person to be difficult may in fact be easy and inexpensive to accomplish. Thus a major role for the ATP as a consultative member of the school team is to provide a perspective on the question of what is and what is not technically possible. This perspective also helps to determine what *should* be done technologically, as well as what *can* be done.

In order to fill the need for technological information, the ATP needs specific skills. These include (1) an understanding of the special and regular educational systems, (2) knowledge of current assistive technologies used to improve access to education for children with disabilities, (3) understanding of the roles of other members of the team (teacher, resource specialists, OT, PT, speech pathologist, parents), and (4) technical knowledge and experience sufficient to apply the assistive technologies (hard and soft) effectively.

**Local resource specialist.** Many schools have resource specialists who provide expert advice on approaches, curriculum adaptation, and assistive technologies for learners who have special needs. The role of this individual is similar to the ATP role on the assessment team, but the range of experience with assistive technologies may be less extensive. Typically the resource specialist has a number of areas for which she is responsible. Her participation in assistive technology assessment is most effective as a member of the assessment team. Once an assistive technology plan is developed, the local resource person is valuable in helping to implement both the hard and soft technologies. This individual is also often involved in evaluating the success of the assistive technologies provided and in determining when reassessment is warranted.

**Referral to an evaluation center.** Referral to a center or clinic specializing in assistive technology applications has advantages and disadvantages. The center-based assessment teams may have a clinical orientation. This may make it more difficult for them to relate to the learner's specific needs unless they have experience with assessment and recommendation of assistive technology for children. However, a center of this type is more likely to have a broad knowledge of available assistive technologies for trial and loan, and their experience with a large group of clients provides a rich source of soft technologies such as strategies and approaches to training. It is important that a center-based assessment include the teacher and other school staff, as well as the learner and his family, in the evaluation process. The center-based assessment team needs to ensure that everyone's goals for the learner are identified. Typically assessments are carried out over several sessions, with some assessment taking place in the school (to focus on needs and the school environment) and some in the center (to allow access to a wide range of technology for trial and evaluation).

## ■ THE CONTEXT FOR EDUCATIONAL APPLICATIONS

The context portion of the HAAT model describes where the activity is being performed. In Chapter 2 we defined four types of context: setting, cultural, social, and physical. Each of these plays an important role in the ultimate effectiveness or ineffectiveness of an assistive technology system. In this section we examine each type of context from an educational perspective.

## The Educational Setting

Education for children who have disabilities used to be carried out in segregated, specially-equipped classrooms set up to meet the unique needs of children with disabilities. Increasingly this specialized classroom is a thing of the past, except in cases of children with severe multiple disabilities. The current practice is **inclusion** of students with disabilities in the regular educational programs. Even when there is a specialized classroom, children are integrated into regular classes for at least part of the school day. Under this model, resource specialists often provide support services related to assistive technology devices and services. However, even if a resource specialist is available, the knowledge and skills of the general classroom teacher must be expanded to include special services and assistive technologies necessary to support learners who have disabilities. One of the implications of inclusion is that there are fewer concentrations of assistive technologies in specialized classrooms and greater diffusion of these technologies throughout the educational system. When there were concentrations of assistive technologies in special education classrooms, relatively few teachers needed to have expertise in their application. With the changing, more diffuse educational model, any teacher may have contact with assistive technologies. The school is now to be adapted to the student, rather than the student adapting to the school (Baker, 1993).

Baker (1993) expresses the concern that some school districts may view the full inclusion policy as a way to deny "expensive" special education support services (e.g., speech pathology, occupational therapy) to students who need them. There are additional benefits that are possible with full inclusion, such as nondisabled peer tutors, cooperative learning, and team teaching (Baker, 1993).

Beukelman and Mirenda (1998) conceptualize **academic participation** as occurring at four levels. The first is *competitive,* in which the learner who has a disability has the same expectations as her nondisabled peer. The workload may be adjusted at this level, but the learner's academic progress is evaluated in the same way as it is for nondisabled peers. The second level is active participation, in which the workload is also adjusted and the evaluations based on individualized standards. At this level the academic expectations are less than for nondisabled peers. The third level is referred to as *involved.* At this level, academic expectations are minimal and inclusion occurs via alternative activities. Academic evaluation is based on individualized standards. At the fourth level there are no academic expectations and the student passively observes learning activities in the regular classroom. The role and nature of assistive technology devices and services vary across these four levels.

In considering the educational setting, it is also important to be aware of the **learner-teacher interactions** occurring in the classroom (Beigel, 2000). The way in which teachers present information can be an important factor when considering assistive technologies for the classroom. In settings that are primarily lecture based, note taking and writing take on greater importance. Teachers who place an emphasis on discussion value oral communication skills, and the assistive technology must support this type of interaction. **Learning styles** are also important. In settings in which small-group interaction is the focus, oral communication and social interaction skills are more important. If the teacher uses group or individual projects, the learner must also organize materials, communicate with peers, and develop time management skills. All these factors influence the type of assistive technologies that are recommended, as well as their effectiveness.

## Social and Cultural Contexts

In the context portion of the HAAT model, we use social and cultural contexts to describe important aspects of both interaction and acceptance of assistive technologies. These two contexts play important roles in the use of assistive technologies in an educational setting. Social and cultural factors also include local policies and attitudes toward technology and toward disability by school personnel. These factors can impose barriers to successful assistive technology application. For example, a policy that prevents school-purchased assistive technologies (e.g., AAC device or laptop computer) from being taken home will significantly compromise the opportunities the student has to complete homework and to apply his developing communication skills in the community. Likewise, if a teacher has a negative attitude toward a blind student's use of a computer to complete tests, then the student may be less independent because of dependence on a sighted reader and scribe to complete the test.

The Participation Model developed by Beukelman and Mirenda (1998) (see Chapter 4) provides a useful framework for the identification of potential barriers to educational access, especially those that can be addressed through the application of assistive technologies. Two types of barriers are identified: opportunity and access. The first refers to policies, practices, attitudes, and knowledge and skills of the school personnel (e.g., teachers, aides, and administrators). Access barriers include the learner's natural abilities, the use of environmental adaptations (discussed under physical context later in this section), and the capabilities or limitations of the learner.

Beukelman and Mirenda (1998) describe an assessment process that leads to identification of the relevant barriers for a learner through a systematic consideration of opportunity and access barriers. Once the barriers are identified, an intervention plan can be developed to overcome the barriers. This may involve changing a policy or attitude, training staff, altering the environment, or matching the needs of the learner to assistive technology characteristics based on a

---

### CASE STUDY 13-4

#### OPPORTUNITY BARRIERS

Joan is an elementary student. She has severe cerebral palsy that affects all her limbs and has resulted in dysarthric speech. Her assessment has shown that she has receptive language at her age level, but she is unable to speak intelligibly or to write independently. During the assessment, an AAC device (see Chapter 9) was recommended. The school has agreed to purchase it if it is kept at school. The teacher has indicated that she will work with Joan to learn to use it, but she does not have time to learn the device given the demands of the other 25 students in the classroom. The device has been purchased, but it is not being used by Joan, since she has not been given the necessary training at school and she cannot take the device home to practice because the school is concerned that this expensive ($8000) device might be broken or lost.

#### QUESTIONS:

1. Identify the barriers in this case.
2. Which of these are opportunity and which are access barriers?
3. What steps would you, as the ATP, take to try and remove the barriers so that Anita can gain access to the learning environment using this device?
4. What additional information would you require in order to carry out your plan?

---

capability assessment (see Chapter 4). Any specific situation will likely involve a combination of most or all of these.

Beukelman and Mirenda (1998) also present a categorization of **social participation** that parallels the academic framework presented earlier. The same four levels are used, but the criteria are participation and social influence rather than academic performance. A student at the competitive social level participates in social interactions and influences her nondisabled peers. At the level of active participation, the learner with a disability chooses whether to be involved in social contexts and does not directly influence the activities of the group. The student at the involved participation level also chooses whether to be involved in the social interaction or not, but her participation may be passive. At the fourth level the learner is not involved in social activities with her nondisabled peers. Depending on the type of disability and the level of social participation, assistive technologies may facilitate social interaction.

Another important factor in the cultural context is how willing the learner is to try new activities or tasks. This refers to the learner's personal style (Beigel, 2000). Individual learners and their families and teachers vary widely in their willingness and ability to cope with change and uncertainty. The use of assistive technologies can be intimidating, especially when there is insufficient training and opportunity to develop the necessary skills through practice. The socioeconomic status of the learner and his family also has an impact on the effectiveness of recommended assistive technologies and their ability to affect the learner's educational experience (Beigel, 2000). Although there are no specific research findings in this area, it is known that the socioeconomic status of a learner has an impact on how teachers view the learner and how the educational program is presented. Learners with low socioeconomic status often have an educational program that focuses on rote learning rather than higher level cognitive skills (Beigel, 2000). This bias can lead to difficulties when assistive technologies are introduced into the classroom, especially if they require practice and advanced level skills for operation.

## The Physical Context for Educational Use of AT

In an educational setting the physical context for assistive technology use includes a number of factors. Some of these are specific to the physical arrangement and layout of the classroom itself, including the type of furnishings and their locations, physical dimensions of doors, and absence of barriers. Another aspect of the physical context applies to the learner. Appropriate postural support (see Chapter 6) allows positioning of the child in a way that allows the child to attend to classroom activities. In addition to providing safety and comfort, proper positioning promotes independence and allows the child to function efficiently to manipulate objects and activate switches or other technical equipment. A recommended sitting posture is shown in Figure 13-5 (see Chapter 6 also). In this position the feet are supported on the floor or the footrest of the wheelchair; the hips are flexed to

90 degrees. The chair and seat provide adequate thigh support, back support, and lateral support. The ideal classroom work surface is 1 inch below the learner's bent elbow, with the most frequently accessed items within reach. If the learner uses a computer, the monitor should be located approximately at arm's length away from the face. The top of the monitor should be at or just below eye level and perpendicular to the light source. If there is a document holder, it should be positioned next to the monitor. For students with severe physical disabilities, learning may take place in other positions, such as side lying or in a stander. These positions may change throughout the day.

The physical environment also includes considerations related to the placement of the learner in relation to the teacher, to the other learners, to her equipment, and to the activity. Ideally the learner with a disability will be integrated into the classroom environment as shown in Figure 13-6. In order to provide access to furnishings and materials, it may be necessary to make room modifications that enhance learning opportunities by creating accessible classrooms. For example, it may be necessary to modify or rearrange a classroom to allow space for mobility devices (e.g., wheelchairs and walkers; see Chapter 10) by increasing the width of aisles or the space between desks. Table heights for wheelchair access are also different than for learners who use standard chairs, especially for younger children. A device such as an AAC system (see Chapter 9) mounted to the wheelchair may require even greater clearance, in addition to special considerations for transferring the child to

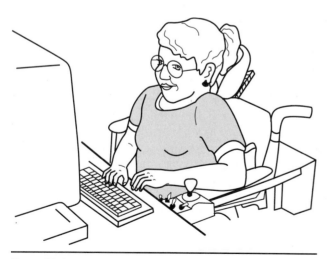

**Figure 13-5**  A proper sitting posture can promote independence and allow the child to function efficiently in the manipulation of objects or the activation of switches. (Courtesy www.Lburkhart.com.)

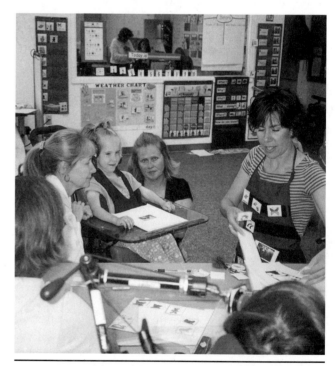

**Figure 13-6**  This classroom arrangement gives all learners access to the classroom activities. The student with a disability is integrated into the classroom environment.

ensure that the chair does not tip as a result of the weight of the mounted device.

For learners who are hard of hearing, FM antenna systems (see Chapter 12) may need to be installed. If automatic speech recognition (see Chapter 7) is used, the learner needs to be located in a place that does not disturb the other students. If the learner uses a computer workstation for completion of assignments, it needs to be located in the classroom, not a separate computer room, and it needs to be located with the other students, not off in a corner of the room. If a printer is used for completing computer-generated assignments, it must be located to reduce disturbance of other students as a result of noise.

Lighting is also important when students are using assistive devices in the classroom. If a room is too bright, glare may prevent the reading of computer screens or liquid crystal display (LCD) screens on laptop computers or AAC devices (Church and Glennen, 1991). Antireflective screens can be used when it is not possible to reduce sunlight or natural lighting sufficiently to avoid glare. On the other hand, individuals who have low vision may require special lighting to increase contrast (see Chapter 12). These modifications can enhance participation in class by learners who have physical or sensory disabilities. When modifications such as these are made, it can also encourage learners to participate in activities that involve groups of learners working together.

Important considerations when evaluating the physical context of the classroom include the following questions: (1) Is the student with the other children or physically isolated by his equipment, technology, or other factors? (2) What information or technology is needed to make the learning environment more accessible to the student? (3) How can the student participate? and (4) Who can assist in the learning?

## ■ HARD AND SOFT TECHNOLOGIES FOR EDUCATIONAL SUCCESS

The fourth component of the HAAT model is hard and soft assistive technologies. There are many characteristics of assistive technologies that we discussed in Chapters 1 and 2. When considering a unique environment such as education, some of these are more important than others. In this section we discuss the major characteristics of assistive technologies that can help ensure their successful application in an education setting.

### A Technological Description of the Modern Classroom

Assistive technology applications in the classroom include both hard and soft technologies (see Chapter 1) (Odor, 1984). Practitioners generally agree that success of assistive

technologies depends on a ratio of 10 to 1 (soft to hard technologies). Funds allocated by schools are likely to be earmarked for hard rather than soft technologies. (Blackstone, 1990). When assistive technologies (both hard and soft) were concentrated in a few classrooms with resident experts, development of soft technologies was easier. With diffusion of services throughout the curriculum, this process has become much more challenging. Of particular importance are the implications for how assistive technology training is carried out. Assistive technology service delivery in the classroom setting must address both hard and soft technologies.

Blackstone (1990) describes areas in which assistive technologies are being used in the classroom (Table 13-1). These include (1) positioning (e.g., seating inserts, side-lying frames), (2) access to electronic assistive devices (e.g., computers, communication devices), (3) environmental control, (4) augmentative communication (writing, speaking, drawing, mathematics), (5) assistive listening devices (e.g., hearing aids, FM systems, teletypes [TTYs]), (6) visual aids (for both print and computer-based text materials), (7) mobility aids, (8) recreation and leisure activities (e.g., hobbies, free time), and (9) self-care (e.g., feeders, aids for hygiene). Blackstone gives examples of equipment and specific classroom considerations for each of these areas. The hard and soft technologies in each area are described in earlier chapters.

### Considerations in the Use of Assistive Technologies in the Classroom

In Chapter 4 we discuss general characteristics of assistive technologies. When considering assistive technology use in education, some of these characteristics are more important than others. Beigel (2000) lists a series of questions to be asked when considering assistive technologies for educational application. Among the areas he discuses are durability; portability; availability of a trial or loan period; company reputation; and aesthetic acceptability to the learner, family, and teacher. Classrooms are active environments in which a device may be subjected to drops, bumps, spills, and other "insults." Durability in this environment is a high priority; this can affect a decision between a specially designed assistive device and the use of a commercially available device like a laptop computer. Learners move from place to place in the classroom and from classroom to classroom. A device that is not portable severely restricts the benefits to the learner in accessing the standard curriculum. Assistive technologies may be complex devices that require skill to operate and place unique demands on the learner and her environment. It is difficult to assess the impact of these devices in a brief assessment. A long-term (a few weeks to a month) trial of devices can disclose features that make them unsuitable. This should be determined before committing funds for purchase if at all possi-

**TABLE 13-1** Hard Technologies for Education

| Application | Goals | Equipment Examples | Classroom Considerations |
| --- | --- | --- | --- |
| Assistive listening devices (ALDs) | Appropriate signal-to-noise ratio so student's hearing is accessible | Hearing aids, personal FM systems, sound field FM systems, TTYs, closed-caption TV (see Chapter 12) | Hearing is a core activity leading to instructional access & learning. Signals deteriorate beyond 6 inches from the source; ALDs should be considered. Background noise can limit high pitch sound detection. |
| AAC | Independent means of expression | Symbols, communication displays, devices, word processing, fax (see Chapter 9) | Intervention begins early. Set up class for communication. Use digital recording for circle time, other sharing, communication displays located near activity areas. Integrate AAC devices into learning routine. |
| Access to computers and other electronic technologies | Enhancement of speed, accuracy, endurance, and independence in device use | Input device, head pointers, key guards, automatic speech recognition, input device-emulating interfaces, Internet access (see Chapters 7 & 8) | Access technologies are key to effective use of electronic devices. Optimal use requires consideration of best control sites, selection technique (direct or indirect), and acceleration approaches. |
| Environmental control | Positive control of the environment without assistance from aides | EADLs, robotics, appliance control adaptations, switch-controlled toys (see Chapter 11) | May be introduced in early infant programs. Appliance control can be incorporated into learning activities. EADLs can help develop sense of control and independence. |
| Mobility | Independent movement, exploration, social interaction, and learning | Self-propelled walkers and wheelchairs, powered wheelchairs, tricycles, and scooters (see Chapter 10) | Children move with intention at 4-5 months. Mobility aids can enhance socialization, communication, and environmental control. Independent mobility leads to increased interaction with peers. |
| Positioning | Increased function and participation through stable and comfortable positioning | Side-lying frames, floor sitters, chair inserts, trays, standing aids, bean bag chairs, etc. (see Chapter 6) | Positioning includes child's individual posture and position relative to other learners and teacher. Multiple positioning systems are often used at different times during the day and for different activities. |
| Recreation, leisure, play | Access to materials and activities allowing peer interaction, hobby development, effective use of free time | Outdoor adaptations (slides, swings), computer games, board games, adapted play materials (e.g., Velcro on toys) | Listening and viewing activities include music and taped reading, slide/ tape, and computer-based stories. Group games include music (adapted instruments, MIDI), art and craft projects with adaptations, dramatic play, adapted puzzles. |
| Self-care | Independent self-care activities | Electric feeders, adapted utensils, toilet seats, aids for tooth brushing, washing, dressing, food preparation (see Chapter 11) | Incorporate self-care activities and adaptations as they naturally occur in activities of feeding, dressing (coats, shoes), toileting, meal preparation. |
| Visual access | Enhancement or interpretation of visual information | Screen readers, screen magnifiers, braillers, high-contrast materials, thermoform graphics (see Chapter 12) | Vision is a major learning mode. Increase contrast, enlarge stimuli, and use tactile and auditory modes to enhance sensory information content. Develop screen reader and Internet navigation skills early. |

Modified from Blackstone SW: Assistive technology in the classroom, *Augment Commun News* 3(6):1-8, 1990.

ble. There are many companies that supply assistive technologies. Some have been in business for many years and provide high-quality support and service. Others do not. An experienced ATP knows which companies can be trusted to provide the necessary support and follow-up and how well repair and service are handled. Although our focus must be on functionality, it is also important to consider the aesthetics of assistive technologies. Motivation to use an assistive technology can be greatly affected by such things as color, overall pleasant design, size, and weight. As Beigel (2000) points out, one learner may prefer a mouse with a colored ball but another might prefer the traditional mouse. The color of the wheelchair frame can be of great importance to the child and affect his self-image when he is in the classroom. Devices that are well designed do not call as much attention to the user and do not seem to be so "different" from what other learners are using.

Merbler, Hadadian, and Ulman (1999) present another set of recommendations that apply to assistive technologies use in the classroom. They recommend that, whenever possible, open-ended devices that can be customized be used. This allows changes to be made to the device (e.g., in software or vocabulary) as the needs of the learner and her academic program change. They also recommend minimal technology solutions (see Chapter 1) that can meet the functional need with the least complexity. This can make acceptance more likely and will significantly affect the amount of training required.

## Student Workstations

Much of the technology on Blackstone's list is computer based, and she uses the term **student workstation** or life station to describe these computer-based setups. The workstation may provide specialized assistance with writing and conversation; an adapted access method for the classroom computer (for software that everyone else is using); access for wheelchair riders (manual or powered); and possible integration of controls for powered wheelchair, computer, environmental control, and augmentative communication device (Caves et al, 1991; Guerette, Caves, and Gross, 1992).

In general, productivity software (word processing, database, drawing, plotting, math) is included. For students with oral communication or visual access needs, voice synthesizers may be added. If the student is not independently mobile, a manual or powered wheelchair may be included and the workstation may be integrated into the wheelchair system for portability. In cases in which the student is ambulatory, portability can be more of a challenge, since the workstation must be carried or pushed from classroom to classroom. Blackstone describes a logical and systematic process for developing individualized workstations based on student needs.

Additional software commonly included in workstations

are programs for skill acquisition in the specific activity areas described earlier in this chapter (reading, writing, mathematics, science, music, and art). Software for desktop publishing (e.g., for a school newspaper, flyers, posters) and digital scanning is often also included (Merbler, Hadadian, and Ulman, 1999). The scanner can be very useful in the classroom. Worksheets can be scanned and then filled in using a computer workstation. Materials to be read can also be scanned and read back using the computer to enlarge print, convert to alternative form (e.g., braille or speech), or make turning pages easier, as noted earlier. This can be beneficial to learners who have sensory, learning, or physical disabilities. Scanners can also be used for other creative projects such as class newsletters, special customized awards with a picture of a student in the background, and similar activities using optical images (Merbler, Hadadian, and Ulman, 1999).

In developing workstations it is important to consider the concept of **functional equivalency.** For example, if a student has difficulty turning the pages on a book, a mechanical page turner (see Chapter 11) can be used. Alternatively, books available on computer disk can be loaded into a word processor and the pages can be "turned" electronically. Thus the same function is obtained in very different ways.

## Internet-Based Educational Resources

Many schools (some estimates are as high as 90%) have Internet access in the classroom. This provides a rich and exciting resource for learners to do research for class projects, use Web-based instructional materials, and develop effective information search skills. If appropriate consideration is given to accessibility of Web sties (see Chapter 8) and principles of universal design are incorporated (see Chapter 1), the success of Web-based instruction for all learners is enhanced (Romereim-Holmes and Peterson, 2000). Learners who use alternative methods of accessing the Internet must be accommodated in the instructional process when Web-based instruction is employed. The principles described in Chapter 8 apply to education, as well as to other environments. The use of Web-based instruction and the development of Web content by learners will increase as more and more schools are on-line and teachers develop instructional design principles that incorporate the use of the Internet. Adherence to the principles of accessibility and consideration of universal design during the curriculum process will greatly expand the opportunities for learners who have disabilities.

## Soft Technologies in the Classroom

There are two broad types of soft technologies (see Chapter 2) that have applications in education: training and strategies.

**Training in an educational context.** Training activities in assistive technologies for school personnel may be of two general types: (1) broad-based group or (2) individual study and training that apply to a number of learners or focused training that provides information regarding the use of an AT system for a specific learner (Church and Glennen, 1991). Carefully developed strategies allow the learner to maximize the effectiveness of his assistive technology.

In Chapter 1 we describe a number of approaches to in-service education. Many of these apply to educational staff (teacher, aide, therapist, speech-language pathologist). Conferences, journal articles, Internet sources, and on-site in-service presentations by ATPs or specialist teams are the major formats. Church and Glennen (1991) list a number of in-service topics presented in one school district. Shown in Box 13-1, these are examples of the types of presentations that are of interest to school staff.

The second type of training is individualized to meet the needs of the learner, parents and family, and those staff who will be working with the learner and the AT system. In earlier chapters we have described the nature of this training for specific technologies (e.g., AAC in Chapter 9). It is crucial that the training received by school staff be aimed at how the technology will achieve the goals set for the learner, rather than just focusing on the technical aspects of the device (Todis and Walker, 1993). In an educational setting it is also important that those who will work with the student are familiar with operation of the technology, how to troubleshoot the device in the case of operational difficulties, and specific features for individual technologies (Church and Glennen, 1991). In the latter category are such things as vocabulary selection for educational use of AAC, training in the use of specific educational software, and training related to skill development in such areas as powered mobility.

---

**BOX 13-1** | **Example of In-Service Topics in Assistive Technologies**

Overview of augmentative communication
Low-tech AAC aids and techniques
Make-and-take session for low-tech AAC displays
Overview of high-tech AAC aids
Vocabulary selection for AAC
Overview of AT in the classroom
Using assistive technology to make the classroom accessible
Computer adaptations for students with physical disabilities
Software selection and integration to facilitate educational activities
Word processing for students with disabilities
Technology applications for young children

---

Modified from Church G, Glennen S: *The handbook of assistive technology,* San Diego, 1991, Singular Publishing Group.

In education, peers also need to be trained. **Peer training** introduces the new technology to the classmates of the target learner. It also can be an opportunity to answer questions that peers have regarding the disability, as well as the technology. Another goal of this training is to establish the rules governing the use of the technology (Church and Glennen, 1991). School staff and the family of the learner may decide to implement a "hands-off" policy for other students so as to avoid damage to the assistive technology. As Church and Glennen (1991) point out, this can make the device more enticing and arouse the curiosity of the peers regarding how it works. For this reason, some families and teachers allow classmates to experience the device during the familiarization phase of training.

Church and Glennen (1991) suggest that the student who will be using the assistive technology be part of the in-class training session in which her technology is introduced to the rest of the class. This peer training session is also an opportunity for a presentation on how the peers can appropriately help the student who will be using the assistive technology. This is a chance to emphasize the need for the learner to be independent and to not have things done for him by his classmates, as well as to introduce the new technology. Rules can also be established regarding the new device and how much access the learner and his family want to give the peers. In all cases the target individual must have control over his new technology. This includes being able to decide who can try it out (if anyone) and when they can do so.

**Strategies for the use of assistive technologies in the classroom.** Educational strategies are really techniques that increase the effectiveness of assistive technologies in the classroom. There is no specific formula for their development. Rather, they arise from a thorough understanding of the educational goals and the skills of the learner. Most often strategies are based on innovative ideas generated from careful observation, experience, and consultation with other team members. In this section we describe several examples of specific strategies to illustrate how many different learning strategies can be used to meet the same educational goals. We also present some specific approaches to the generation of strategies.

One systematic approach is the **Technology Integration Plan** (Church and Glennen, 1991). The development of this plan begins with a team meeting in which an analysis of the student's daily schedule is carried out. Emphasis is placed on the identification of target activities for technology intervention. Church and Glennen suggest that activities meeting the following criteria be chosen (1991, p. 217):

1.   They occur frequently
2.   They are motivating and enjoyable
3.   They present opportunities for independence in one

of several areas (verbal or written communication, mobility, self-care, vocational skills, control of the environment)

4. They are activities that the student cannot effectively complete utilizing their current modes or methods

There are three parts to the Technology Integration Plan: (1) Preparation (Figure 13-7, *A*), (2) Action Plan (Figure 13-7, *B*), and (3) Review (Figure 13-7, *C*) (Church and Glennen, 1991). The Preparation form is designed as a framework to record the information developed by the discussion of target activities. A three-point rating scale is used to indicate the relative level (high, moderate, or low) for each activity in several areas (see Figure 13-7, *A*). The Action Plan (see Figure 13-7, *B*) is then completed for each identified activity. The Action Plan is a framework for recording target skills and objectives for each activity. It is also used to identify suggested materials, equipment, motivators, and strategies for each activity. In addition, the required preparation and the projected date for a review are included on this form. The final form, Review (see Figure 13-7, *C*), is used to record any modifications to the plan, as well as to record progress in meeting the goals set out in the plan. An organized format such as the Technology Intervention Plan can help a team to focus on the educational goals first, developing strategies for implementing both the hard and soft technologies required to meet the goals and then monitoring progress. Church and Glennen (1991) present two examples of the use of this approach.

Strategies to help a student accomplish learning tasks are often best developed by a team of professionals. Brainstorming and planning from several different points of view can lead to innovation as one idea triggers others. Merbler, Hadadian, and Ulman (1999) recommend that teachers share information regarding assistive technology application. With the myriad devices and strategies available, it is impossible for any one teacher to monitor them all, and sharing expertise can benefit all learners. Collaboration with parents can also ensure that assistive technology devices that go home are properly used and maintained. With the complexity of some current assistive devices, the teacher may place unreasonable demands on herself to completely master a device or software program before using it. This is often not necessary, and many applications can be successfully accomplished with the device as skill is developed. They also encourage teachers to experiment with the technology. This may lead to the discovery of new applications or strategies.

Even if you do not have a team locally, you can collaborate by using various online listservs. One that is often used is the RESNA assistive technology listserv (e-mail address: resna@maelstrom.stjohns.edu). As discussed earlier in this chapter, manipulatives (objects that can be counted, moved, and sorted) are often used in mathematics instruction.

When a child lacks the fine motor skills to manipulate the objects, alternatives are required if he is to access the same curriculum as his classmates. Here is an example of an on-line "virtual collaboration" involving the use of manipulatives (paraphrased):

One subscriber to the listserv (Y.T., a rehabilitation engineer from New York City) posted the following question:

> I'm working with a child with CP [cerebral palsy] in the 3rd grade. He can grasp and manipulate objects with his left hand, but he has extensor tone that makes it difficult to lean or reach forward, or bring his arm across his body. His right side is more involved and he doesn't use it much. I'm looking for ideas to assist him in using manipulatives in his math class. He has a desk that allows him to pull up close, and he can be placed on a slant. I'm going to give him a tray table to elevate the surface even more so he doesn't have to reach down. When using manipulatives, the students often have to organize counters into groups and arrange objects on their desk. I was thinking possibly little containers to help with that. Does anyone have any other suggestions?

K.P., an occupational therapist in Massachusetts, offered these suggestions:

> Use muffin tins of various sizes, paint palette trays, etc, which are easier to scoop from. More important, though, is whether his seating needs have been adequately addressed to maximize dynamic trunk balance and provide as much normalization of tone as possible.

R.G., a rehabilitation technologist in San Francisco, added his thoughts:

> I would encourage all involved to step back and look at the educational goals of the activity. Perhaps they can be achieved without using the same objects that are typically used (though he might be strongly motivated to use the same tools as all the other students). The example that comes to mind is the abacus that can help people learn math without requiring a lot of range of motion—though some fine motor ability is needed. Otherwise, plastic organizers for silverware drawers or pencil drawer organizers are two readily obtainable items. Use small containers velcroed to a flat board that can be rearranged as desired. Try putting the containers on a lazy susan to provide access to more items without reaching.

C.C., a speech-language pathologist from Nebraska, contributed other ideas:

> There are often easier physical methods to accomplish the educational tasks involved in the manipulatives. Manipulatives tend to be used educationally for two or three reasons: they make abstract concepts concrete, they help students make active problem solving decisions, and they are easy to manage for typically developing students. Because the latter is

Student:                                        Date:
Team Members:

<u>Typical daily schedule</u>

Directions: List all daily activities and rate each one for the listed characteristics using the following scale: 3 - high 2 - moderate 1 - low. Total the ratings for each activity and record the number in the Total column. Place a check in last column when the activity is included in the student's Technology Integration Plan.

**A**

| Daily Activities | Current Mode(s) of _____ | Motivation | Opportunities for Independence | Present Mode(s) Ineffective | Total | Included in Plan |
|---|---|---|---|---|---|---|
|  |  |  |  |  |  |  |
| Other routine events (at least once per week) |  |  |  |  |  |  |

Student's Name:                                 Date:
Team Members:

Target activity:

Target skills (objectives):


Suggested equipment:


Target vocabulary to be represented by___ Photos ___ Symbols ___ Words/Sentences

**B**   Suggested materials/motivators:

| Preparation needed | Person(s) responsible | Target date |
|---|---|---|
|  |  |  |

Suggested strategies:

Anticipated date of review:


Target activity:                         Date of initial Action Plan
Team Members revising Plan:

**C**

| Date of review | Modifications | Person responsible | Initiation date | Review date |
|---|---|---|---|---|
|  |  |  |  |  |

Figure 13-7   The Technology Integration Plan. **A,** Preparation sheet. **B,** Action plan. **C,** Review. (From Church G, Glennen S: *The handbook of assistive technology,* San Diego, 1991, Singular Publishing Group.)

not true for this child, we don't want him to be spending all of his educational time managing the mechanics of the task and missing the educational point.

I've seen this work well by students pairing together. The student with a disability makes decisions about which items go into which groups, and gets to control the physical division of the items by strategies like eye pointing or binary choice making [see Chapter 9] with a peer (i.e., which group?). The peer does the physical manipulation according to the student's direction, and by third grade most peers can be coached in strategies for getting the student's input without being directive. This embeds a communication strategy that is both more accessible and interactive for the student, as well as probably already established in other ways.

This example illustrates several points about strategies. First, there are many strategies for any one problem in the classroom. Often the possible strategies are very different. Our virtual team suggests a variety of approaches from making the manipulatives easier to reach and grab to using a peer partner to help with the task. Second, alternative strategies often involve different skills on the part of the student. In this example, the skills range from gross motor to fine motor to communication. The third general point is that strategies may or may not involve technology, and the technology may be high or low, depending on the strategy. In this example, low technologies such as muffin tins and a lazy Susan are suggested by two of the professionals. The third suggests communication, and this might be no-tech (i.e., speech) or a high-tech augmentative communication device. This example also illustrates the role of innovation and problem solving in the development of useful strategies.

A frequent concern of teachers and classroom aides is that there is not time to add assistive technology use to an already crowded day with many students in the classroom. The time demands of the classroom are high, and this is a legitimate concern; however, it is possible to use strategies for infusing technology into the classroom throughout the day (King-DeBaun, 1999). King-DeBaun suggests integrating assistive technologies into regular classroom activities throughout the day. One example described by King-DeBaun (1999) is Danny, an 8-year-old boy who attends a typical first grade classroom for 75% of his school day and spends 25% of his day in a resource room. Danny uses an AAC device and receives instruction and support from his regular education teacher and part-time classroom aide, as well as the resource room teacher and his speech-language pathologist. Danny's day begins with story group, and for the class discussion, he uses the IntelliKeys* keyboard (see Chapter 7) with an overlay containing simple words related to the story. His speech-language pathologist made the overlay using a computer program called Overlay Maker.† Using a talking word

processor, Danny is able to participate in the story group discussion. Students also participate in journal writing as an arrival activity. They record the day of the week, school activities, and special events at home or school. Danny uses his augmentative communication device to complete this task, making use of a posted "word wall" (an alphabetic list of words he uses frequently). Later in the day, Danny and his classmates create a story adventure based on a starting line from the teacher (e.g., "One day . . ."). The teacher bases the story on a familiar theme or a story that the children have often read. Students take turns participating in this activity, and each day one student is selected to help write a part of the class story. Once again Danny uses his augmentative communication device, but this time his aide has prepared a list of words related to the topic of the recent books the class has read, and she has stored them into his device so he can access them to participate in this activity.

King-DeBaun (1999) also describes another student, Anita, who is just learning how to scan (see Chapter 7). She uses her communication device in a circular scanning mode (see Chapter 7) to randomly select a student to be next. This places Anita at the center of attention as the class waits to see whom she will choose. In Dramatics, Danny and Amanda work together to use a drawing program on the computer to create masks for a talking mural. She creates a bird mask and he makes a lizard mask. They work together, with Danny picking a color and Amanda placing the cursor on that color. Amanda cuts out the mask for Danny and places both masks on the mural. For the presentation to the class the following day, Danny uses his augmentative communication device to speak his lines. Musselwhite and King-DeBaun (1997) describe many other activities and adaptations that can be used in the classroom.

There are many sessions at assistive technology conferences that include strategies for introducing and using assistive technologies successfully in the classroom. These are rich with new strategies. Several of the conferences have on-line proceedings. All have other resources available on their Web sites. Three of the most useful conferences are the California State University at Northridge (CSUN) Conference (held in March in Los Angeles; www.csun.edu/cod/center); Closing the Gap (held in October in Minneapolis; www.closingthegap.com); and RESNA (June, various locations; www.resna.org).

As the examples in this section illustrate, the most important factors in the development of assistive technology strategies are detailed familiarity with the educational task to be completed and innovative thinking. There are no basic principles or magic formula.

### ■ SUMMARY

In this chapter we have described the educational application of assistive technologies using the HAAT model as a

---

*IntelliTools, Petaluma, Calif.
†IntelliTools, Petaluma, Calif.

framework. Learners who have disabilities engage in reading, writing, mathematics, science, music, and art. The primary types of adaptations available in each of these areas involve both strategies and technologies. There are several assessment models utilized to determine the needs of learners for assistive technologies. Considerations in the cultural and social contexts include learner style, socioeconomic status, and other factors that can dramatically affect assistive technology effectiveness in the classroom. The emergence of inclusive settings in education has affected the way in which assistive technologies are applied and supported. The physical location of the learner in relation to other students and the layout of the classroom in general can affect on the success of assistive technologies. Many characteristics of hard and soft assistive technologies are important in ensuring that they are meeting the needs of learners and teachers.

## Study Questions

1. What are the major curricular areas (educational activities) in which assistive technologies are used?
2. What tasks must be accommodated for in order to ensure success in reading instruction?
3. Describe some of the differences between an assistive technology-based writing system and scribing.
4. How can an AAC system be used in mathematics instruction?
5. What are the two primary requirements in making adaptations for alternatives to pencil-and-paper mathematics instruction?
6. How can the concept of manipulatives be included in the mathematics curriculum for learners who lack the fine motor skill to work with physical objects directly?
7. What unique requirements do science, art, and music each place on the educational setting for assistive technologies?
8. List three factors that are essential to an effective assistive technology assessment to meet educational needs.
9. What steps are necessary to ensure that an assistive technology assessment focuses on the needs of the learner rather than the technologies to be employed in meeting those needs?
10. How are assistive technologies to meet educational needs incorporated into the IEP?
11. Who are the typical members of an educational assistive technology assessment team?
12. What are the primary models for educational assistive technology assessment, and what are the pros and cons of each?
13. What are the advantages of carrying out an educational assistive technology assessment in the school, family, and community environments?
14. What are the unique contributions that the ATP makes to an educational assistive technology assessment?

15. What are the advantages of an educational assistive technology assessment carried out in a center specializing in assistive technology evaluation and recommendation?
16. What are the implications for assistive technology application presented by an inclusive classroom?
17. What are the levels of academic and social participation defined by Mirenda and Beukelman (1998)?
18. List four aspects of the learner-teacher interaction that are important to the recommendation of assistive technologies for classroom use.
19. What are the major considerations in the social and cultural contexts as applied to assistive technologies use in education?
20. What social factors may affect the use of assistive technology in the classroom?
21. What cultural factors may affect the use of assistive technology in the classroom?
22. How does learning style affect the success of assistive technologies in the classroom?
23. List four factors that affect the physical context for the learner.
24. List the components that make up a student workstation.
25. What are the most important soft technology concerns in the educational setting?
26. What are the two major types of assistive technology training normally provided for school personnel? How do they differ?
27. What are the goals of peer training, and how can the learner who uses the technology. be included in this training?
28. What are the most important assistive technology characteristics when considering devices for classroom use?

## References

Baker LA: Educational challenges-strategies for the AAC student, *Commun Outlook*, pp 13-16, Spring 1993.

Beigel AR: Assistive technology assessment: more than the device, *Interven School Clin* 45(4):237-244, 2000.

Beukelman DR, Mirenda P: *Augmentative and alternative communication, management of severe communication disorders in children and adults*, ed 2, Baltimore, 1998, Paul H Brookes.

Blackstone SW: Assistive technology in the classroom, *Augment Commun News* 3(6):1-8, 1990.

Brainerd CJ: *Piaget's theory of cognitive development*, Englewood Cliffs, NJ, 1978, Prentice-Hall.

Butler C: Effects of powered mobility on self-initiated behaviors of very young children with locomotor disability, *Dev Med Child Neurol* 28(3):325-332, 1986.

Button C: Fast facts on individualized education programs, *AT Q RESNA* 2(5):5-6, 1990.

Calkins LM: *The art of teaching*, Portsmouth, NH, 1986, Heinemann.

Caves K et al: The use of integrated controls for mobility, communication and computer access, *Proc 14th RESNA Conf*, pp 166-167, June 1991.

Church G, Glennen S: *The handbook of assistive technology*, San Diego, 1991, Singular Publishing Group.

Desch LW: High technology for handicapped children: a pediatrician's viewpoint, *Pediatrics* 77(1):71-87, 1986.

Guerette P, Caves K, Gross K: One switch does it all, *Team Rehabil Rep*, pp 26-29, March/April 1992.

Hardman ML et al: *Human exceptionality: society, school and family*, Boston, 1990, Allyn and Bacon.

King-DeBaun P: Technology all day long: infusing technology into the curriculum, *Proc CSUN Conf 1999*, www.dinf.org/csun_99/session1008.html, December 1998.

Merbler JB, Hadadian A, Ulman J: Using assistive technology in the inclusive classroom, *Prevent School Fail* 43(3):113-118, 1999.

Musselwhite C, King-DeBaun P: *Emergent literacy success: merging technology and whole language for students with disabilities*, Park City, Utah, 1997, Creative Communicating Resources.

Odor P: Hard and soft technology for education and communication for disabled people, *Proc Int Comp Conf*, Perth, Australia, 1984.

Resnick M et al: Digital manipulatives: new toys to think with, *Proc CHI Conf*, Los Angeles, Calif, April 12-23, 1998 (http://www.acm.org/sigchi/chi98/cp/?show=252).

Rocklage LA, Lake ME: Inclusion through infusion, *Proc Closing the Gap Conf*, 1997 (http://www.closingthegap.com/cgi-bin/lib/libDsply.pl?a=1049&b=3&c=1).

Romereim-Holmes L, Peterson D: Instructionally sound web-based learning for diverse populations, *Proc CSUN Conf*, 2000 (http://www.csun.edu/cod/conf2000/proceedings/0032Romereim.html).

Smith J, Topping M: The introduction of a robotic aid to drawing into a school for physically handicapped children: a case study, *Br J Occup Ther* 59(12):565-569, 1996.

Todis B, Walker HM: User perspectives on assistive technology in educational settings, *Focus Except Child* 26(3):1-16, 1993.

Topping M: The Handy 1, a robotic aid to independence for severely disabled people, *Technol Disabil* 5:233-234, 1996.

# CHAPTER 14

# Assistive Technologies in the Context of Work

## Learning Objectives

Upon completing this chapter you will be able to:

1. Describe the vocational activities and related skills that can be aided by assistive technologies
2. Describe the context of vocational settings in which assistive technologies are applied
3. Understand the role of the assistive technology practitioner in addressing the vocational goals of the person with a disability
4. Understand the unique attributes of the assessment and implementation of assistive technologies in the vocational setting
5. List the major assistive technologies that are used in vocational settings
6. Describe the assistive technologies used to enhance the employee's function at the workstation

## Key Terms

Bidding Process
Essential Functions
Individual Written Rehabilitation
 Plan (IWRP)

Qualified Individual with a Disability
Reasonable Accommodation
Undue Hardship

Vocational Rehabilitation Agencies
Vocational Rehabilitation Counselor

Work is one of three basic performance areas (self-care, work and school, play and leisure) that many individuals participate in on a daily basis. As with the other performance areas, people with disabilities are confronted with barriers that make it difficult for them to participate in this important life role. Modifications to the work site and the provision of assistive technologies can help to eliminate some of these barriers and enable individuals with disabilities to carry out work-related functions.

The individuals served by vocational assistive technology are typically between 16 and 65 years of· age and have wide-ranging physical, sensory, and mental disabilities. There are two primary populations of persons who need assistive technologies for access to employment. The first group consists of individuals who are disabled and are interested in attaining employment. The disabilities typical in this population are spinal cord injury, arthritis, cerebral palsy, visual impairment, and hearing impairment. Individuals who are at high risk for injury or have been injured while working and will be reemployed at the company they were with before the injury comprise the second population. Disabilities most commonly seen in the second population are musculoskeletal disorders (MSD) such as back injuries, carpal tunnel syndrome, tendonitis, and shoulder injuries. For both these populations, assistive technology is one of many tools that can be used to help people become employed or reemployed. In this chapter we use the Human Activity Assistive Technology (HAAT) model as a framework around which to discuss vocational applications of assistive technology.

## ▓ VOCATIONAL ACTIVITIES THAT CAN BE AIDED BY ASSISTIVE TECHNOLOGIES

In order to discuss assistive technology applications in the work setting, we must first define the activities that characterize vocational endeavors. Having done that, we can then begin to identify the ways that assistive technologies can contribute to those activities. There are many different vocational activities to consider, each of which has much variability. We use the HAAT model and the three activity outputs of communication, manipulation, and mobility to provide a characterization of vocational activities. In the following sections, each of the activity outputs is described in terms of work tasks that an individual may potentially need to perform on the job. Identification of these tasks will then help us to define both the human skills and the assistive technologies required for successfully completing them. The assistive technologies, such as control interfaces, seating and computer access, apply across all these areas.

## Communication

Communication includes all the various information-handling activities in the workplace. Activities in this category include writing (pen/pencil or typing), reading, interacting with others in person, and using the telephone.

Interacting with others involves numerous skills, including oral motor skills required for speech; auditory function; cognitive skills, including receptive and expressive language; and social skills. Many of these skills are described in Chapter 3, and in Chapter 9 we describe the skills specifically needed to carry on a conversation. In some cases, individuals lacking these communication skills can use alternative modes of communication and an augmentative communication device. We discuss these devices in detail in Chapter 9.

A person with a disability may have trouble using the telephone to communicate as a result of deficits in communication, sensory, or motor skills. For someone who has difficulty holding the receiver of the phone, an alternative method of performing this activity is headphones and a computer (see Chapter 11). There are also low-tech adaptations that the person can use to facilitate grasping of the phone.

Reading requires motor, sensory, and cognitive skills. Many of the skills described in Chapter 13 for educational application apply in the workplace as well. For print materials, these include motor skills associated with positioning the reading material, turning pages, and similar tasks (e.g., picking up a book, opening it, using an index, thumbing through pages). In Chapter 11 we discuss devices to aid in the motor tasks involved with reading printed materials. For electronic media, the motor tasks to operate a mouse and keyboard are important (see Chapter 7).

Reading also requires sensory abilities such as visual field, visual acuity, and oculomotor function to scan text and recognize letters and words. If the individual lacks these capabilities, an alternative format in either tactile (braille) or auditory (speech) form can be used (see Chapters 8 and 12). Basic literacy skills are also required for reading. The level is determined by the specific job requirements. For example, a job as a stock clerk may only require the reading of simple labels, whereas a job as a paralegal or an attorney requires a higher level of skill for the reading of complex legal documents.

Whether writing is accomplished by handwriting or typing, it requires motor, sensory, and cognitive skills. The use of pencil or pen and paper requires fine motor control to hold the pen or pencil and to produce letters. In Chapters 9 and 13 we describe the use of different types of writing (note taking, messaging, and formal writing) as they apply to educational settings. Many of the considerations in the workplace are the same. There are also many alternatives to handwriting for successful completion of writing tasks (see Chapters 8, 9, and 11). These include assistance provided by a personal assistant, computer-aided writing using word processing, personal digital assistants that recognize hand-writing on a screen and store it as text for editing, modified pens and pencils (e.g., enlarged grip or holder), and systems that recognize speech and translate it directly into text (automatic speech recognition).

Keyboard or mouse use is required for all data entry tasks, including writing. There are many alternatives to keyboard/mouse entry, including automatic speech recognition (see Chapter 7). Sensory skills for monitoring what is being written include visual, auditory, and tactile approaches, some employing various types of assistive technologies. Cognitive and language skills for writing are described in Chapters 3 and 13.

## Manipulation

The activity output of manipulation also includes a number of different tasks. In general, manipulative activities in the workplace are those that have anything to do with handling of material. This includes filing; sorting; assembling; lifting and moving objects such as books, documents, and equipment; and using office machines such as copiers, adding machines, or fax machines. Besides requiring fine motor skills, these activities require sensory and cognitive skills.

The "paperless office" can substitute for the paper handling parts of this activity output by the use of electronic files. Material handling activities can also be carried out by a personal assistant. Controls on office equipment and machinery such as a forklift can be modified (e.g., with hand controls).

## Mobility

The activity output of mobility is characterized by activities that involve personal movement to and from the work site and within the workplace. In considering these activities it is important to determine what movements are required of the individual to complete the job and, if the individual lacks these movements, what alternative methods are available.

For many individuals, getting to work is the single largest barrier. Arranging wheelchair-accessible public transportation often means booking pickup times with a range of an hour or more, booking far in advance, and paying additional fees for the accessible service. If private transportation is used, the cost of a modified vehicle (see Chapter 10) is much higher than for a standard vehicle. Furthermore, finding a parking space at work that is accessible and close to the work site may also be a problem. Thus the options for transportation are significantly more challenging than for nondisabled workers.

Once at work, mobility and access in and around the work environment can be a challenge for some people with disabilities. Activities to consider are whether the person can enter and exit the building safely and in an emergency, open and close doors, and climb stairs. Sitting and standing requirements of the job also need to be considered. Sitting applies to the employee who requires seating technologies for postural control, pressure management, or comfort in order to be an effective employee (see Chapter 6). It is important that the employee have good postural alignment and postural support as needed to maximize function in the work environment, including the manipulation of objects and operation of assistive devices.

In addition to postural alignment and proper positioning, the employee needs to be free from pain while sitting and be able to perform pressure relief activities if needed. Persons who have had a back injury may have difficulty maintaining a static position in either sitting or standing for any length of time because of pain or fatigue. They may require modifications to the work area that enable them to alternate between the two positions. Other individuals may experience difficulty in coming to a standing position from sitting.

McNeal, Somerville, and Wilson (1999) conducted a study in which one of the purposes was to document the types of problems experienced by workers with spinal cord injury and workers with postpolio syndrome. The group of individuals with spinal cord injury reportedly experienced the greatest number of problems (39.8%) in the category of "using equipment/tools/furniture." More than one third of these problems had to do with desks, including an inability to get up to the desk because of the wheelchair, inability to access items on the desk, or a workspace that was too limited.

## Activities of Daily Living in the Context of Work

While an employee is at work, there are also a number of activities of daily living (ADLs) she may need to carry out. In that they are being performed in the work setting, these activities may have unique requirements. These activities include going to the bathroom, taking medications, and eating lunch or other meals. Accommodations for these activities can have as much of an impact as an accessible desk or workbench. If the workplace does not have accessible restrooms, then the worker who has a disability is at a significant disadvantage compared with his fellow workers. If assistance for taking medications is not available, the worker may not be able to perform the tasks of the job. Besides the requirements related to physical accessibility for completing these ADLs, time factors are also an issue. Some individuals may require additional time for toileting or eating. A flexible schedule with time off during the workday is needed. Issues of privacy and whether to ask co-workers for assistance also come into play.

# ■ THE CONTEXT FOR VOCATIONAL APPLICATIONS

The context portion of the HAAT model describes the environment in which the activity is being performed. In Chapter 2 we defined four aspects of the context: setting, cultural, social, and physical. It is critical that these aspects of context in the work setting are not ignored, because each plays an important role in the ultimate effectiveness or ineffectiveness of an assistive technology system. In this section we examine each aspect of the context as it relates to vocational settings.

## The Vocational Setting

The vocational setting is one of the four major settings (the others being residential, school, and community) in which individuals spend their time and perform activities. This setting has its own unique requirements. In Chapter 2 we described the setting as being more than the location in which the activity occurs. It also includes the surrounding environment, tasks to be done, a set of rules governing the tasks, and a level of comfort.

The type of setting dictates the characteristics of the assistive technology system, and a system that is successful in another setting may not be equally as successful in the work setting. Depending on the individual's circumstances, the assistive technology system may be used in a number of settings or its use could be limited to just the work setting. An augmentative communication device that is programmed appropriately can be successfully used by the individual in numerous contexts. On the other hand, a system that replaces the computer screen with a screen reader and speech synthesizer output (see Chapter 12) may be used in the home without affecting other people, but its use in a work setting may require that the operator use headphones to avoid disturbing her co-workers. Likewise, an individual may be able to propel a manual wheelchair in his home without difficulty but may require a powered wheelchair in order to effectively get around the work setting.

Normally the work setting is at a separate location from the person's residence; however, with technology and the advent of the Internet, more and more individuals are working out of their homes. The Internet and computer-related assistive technologies have made it possible for some individuals to "telecommute" or to start a home-based business when they would otherwise not have been able to seek employment. For an individual with a disability, being able to work out of the home has several advantages: (1) the workstation can be set up without interfering with others; (2) the individual is familiar with the home environment and likely to have a greater level of comfort; (3) the need to find transportation to and from a job site is eliminated; (4) the use of personal assistant services (PAS) may be less obtrusive; (5) ADLs may not have to be completed at all (e.g., putting on makeup to go to work) or may be easier to complete at home; and (6) equipment and modifications need only be provided once, not duplicated at a separate work setting (e.g., computer and control interfaces). There are also disadvantages to working out of the home. These include (1) the lack of social contact with other employees; (2) a lack of "group motivation" to complete work on time; (3) an employer who may perceive the worker as being less productive when working from home; (4) and resources that may only be available to the employee at the work setting.

For the new employee, the work environment is unfamiliar and requires some getting used to. Over time, as the person becomes familiar with the employment setting, maneuvering around the environment should be relatively easy as long as objects in the environment are fixed and travel paths are used repeatedly (e.g., from a workstation to the restroom or coffee machine). Otherwise this may pose a problem for certain individuals. For example, mobility by a person who is blind depends on the use of an assistive device (cane or electronic travel aid) to obtain some understanding of the type of terrain and the presence of obstacles (see Chapter 12).

In work settings, more than in other types of settings, there are rules that govern the setting and the tasks to be completed. For example, in a vocational setting there is usually a set time in which employees are scheduled to work and some type of productivity standards regarding the work that needs to be done. Most businesses are economically oriented, and in order to have a successful business, work needs to be completed in a timely and accurate manner. Fortunately, with the implementation of the Americans with Disabilities Act (ADA; see below), adjusting some of the rules in the work setting is considered a reasonable accommodation. For example, if Katie has multiple sclerosis and needs to see her doctor once a week, under the ADA it would be considered a reasonable accommodation for her employer to allow her to come in late and stay longer on the days she goes to the doctor. Assistive technologies are also considered a reasonable accommodation that can assist an individual with a disability to achieve these outcomes.

In terms of level of comfort (formal, informal, playful, serious), the work setting is considered to be more formal and serious than are other settings. This is particularly important to take into consideration for the programming of an augmentative communication device that is used in the work setting. Depending on the individual work setting, it is likely that the vocabulary programmed into the device will need to be more formal. This level of comfort may also change over time. During the job interview, the context may be very formal. Once the person is hired and gets to know her co-workers better, the atmosphere of the setting may become more informal. The employee must be able to change the vocabulary in the augmentative communication device as needed, whether this is done independently or with assistance from another person.

## Social and Cultural Contexts

In the context portion of the HAAT model, we use social and cultural contexts to describe important aspects of both interaction and acceptance of assistive technologies. Social and cultural factors also include policies and attitudes toward technology and toward disability by employers and fellow employees. For assistive technology use in a vocational setting, the social and cultural aspects of the context can be the most important.

In Chapter 2 we described three levels of environmental interaction and accompanying factors that affect decisions related to assistive technology implementation: macrosystemic, mesosystemic, and microsystemic (Fougeyrollas and Gray, 1998). The macrosystemic level is associated with issues of society as a whole. This includes policies relating to assistive technology use and funding levels (which can be a barrier to participation if a device is not funded). The mesosystemic level is the person's local environment, which includes those places in the community where the individual lives and functions. For purposes of this chapter, the mesosystemic level we focus on is the workplace. This includes the attitudes and policies of the employer, fellow employees, and customers with whom the worker may come in contact. At the microsystemic level the analysis is of the immediate environment of the person, including such factors as the existence of specific assistive technologies. This is the level at which the ATP typically functions in carrying out assessments, making recommendations, and supporting users of assistive technologies. This is also the level at which PAS are applied. For the remainder of this section we use these three levels as a framework to discuss the social and cultural contexts of the workplace.

**The macrosystemic level.** In the past, persons with disabilities who were interested in working were excluded from accessing the work environment or forced to work in sheltered workshops. With the passage of Rehabilitation Act of 1973, its amendments, and the ADA, these barriers are being challenged and persons with disabilities are being integrated into regular work settings.

The Rehabilitation Act establishes several important principles. One of the most important of these is the concept of reasonable accommodation in employment (see Chapter 1). The act mandates that employers receiving federal funds accommodate the needs of employees who have disabilities. It specifically prohibits discrimination in employment solely on the basis of a disability. This law originally described both reasonable accommodation and

least restrictive environment (LRE), a term relating to the degree of modification that is acceptable in a job.

As a result of the Rehabilitation Act of 1973, many employers made architectural changes to reduce barriers. These included installing elevators, placing ramps and curb cuts to accommodate wheelchair users, and adding voice and braille labels to signs (including elevators) to accommodate persons with visual impairment. Many of these efforts to achieve accommodation involved the use of assistive technologies.

The Rehabilitation Act Amendments of 1998, which are contained in the Workforce Investment Act of 1998 (Public Law [PL] 105-220), are the most recent amendments to the Rehab Act. These amendments include several provisions involving assistive technologies. First the amendments require that each state include within its vocational rehabilitation plan a provision for assistive technology (referred to in PL 99-506 as *rehabilitation engineering or technology* and in PL 105-220 as *rehabilitation technology*).

This plan is the basis by which states receive federal funding for vocational rehabilitation, and there is a strong incentive to provide these technology-related services in order to ensure continuation of the transfer of federal funds for rehabilitation programs. The Rehab Act also requires that provision for acquiring appropriate and necessary assistive technology devices and services be included in an Individual Written Rehabilitation Plan written for the individual. For individuals who are eligible for services through state vocational rehabilitation programs, the Rehabilitation Act has excellent provisions for the inclusion of assistive technology in all phases of the rehabilitation process, from evaluation through placement in employment. In its analysis of assistive technology policy in employment, The National Council on Disability (NCOD, 2000) identifies the following limitations in these provisions: (1) limits of funding for vocational rehabilitation and (2) implementation difficulties such as insufficient staff expertise with assistive technology and lack of service providers with this expertise.

Section 508 of the Rehab Act is an important provision because it ensures access to "electronic office equipment" by persons with disabilities who work for the federal government. Because the federal government is such a large purchaser of computers and other office technology, any purchasing specifications it makes take on the role of informal standards affecting all manufacturers of equipment and therefore all employers who purchase that equipment. Persons who are blind or have low vision and those with difficulty in accessing the keyboard have benefited from standards derived as a result of Section 508, and several manufacturers have included features in the basic designs of their computer systems technology that increases access (see Chapter 8). The provisions cover access to electronic office equipment and electronic information services provided to the public by the federal government. This includes ensuring that end users with disabilities (1) have access to the same databases and application programs as other end users, (2) are supported in manipulating data and related information resources to attain equivalent results as other end users, and (3) can transmit and receive messages using the same telecommunication systems as other end users.

As described in Chapter 1, the ADA is a federal civil rights law that is designed to prevent discrimination and enable individuals with disabilities to participate fully in all aspects of society. One fundamental principle of the ADA is that individuals with disabilities who want to work and are qualified to work must have an equal opportunity to work. Similar legislation exists in other countries, such as Thailand, the United Kingdom, and Germany.

Under Title I of the ADA the employer is required to provide reasonable accommodation to qualified individuals with disabilities who are employees or applicants for employment unless to do so would cause undue hardship. A **qualified individual with a disability** has the skills, education, experience, or other requirements needed for the job and can perform the essential functions of the position with or without reasonable accommodation (EEOC, 1996). The **essential functions** of a job are those job duties that are so fundamental to the position the individual holds or desires that he cannot do the job without performing them. An essential function of a nurse in a hospital would be to respond to a patient's call for assistance. An essential function for a painter might be to lift a 5-gallon bucket of paint weighing 42 pounds. An essential function for a clerical worker might be to type 75 words per minute. It is the employer who determines the essential job functions.

There are many individuals with disabilities who can apply for and perform job duties without any reasonable accommodations. However, there are barriers in the workplace that prevent other individuals with disabilities from doing the same thing unless they are provided with some form of accommodation. These barriers may be physical in nature (such as facilities or equipment that are inaccessible), or they may be procedures or rules (such as rules regarding when work is performed, when breaks are taken, or how essential or marginal functions are achieved). Reasonable accommodation can remove these barriers. **Reasonable accommodation** is "any modification or adjustment to a job or the work environment that will enable a qualified applicant or employee with a disability to participate in the application process or to perform essential job functions. Reasonable accommodation also includes adjustments to assure that a qualified individual with a disability has rights and privileges in employment equal to those of employees without disabilities" (EEOC, 2000). Reasonable accommodation is available to qualified applicants and employees with disabilities and must be provided regardless of whether the employee works part time or full time or is considered

---

> ### BOX 14-1    Categories of Reasonable Accommodation, with Accompanying Examples
>
> **MAKING EXISTING FACILITIES READILY ACCESSIBLE**
> Installing a ramp or modifying the rest room so that the facility is wheelchair accessible
>
> **JOB RESTRUCTURING**
> Reallocating or redistributing marginal job functions that an employee is unable to perform because of a disability; altering when or how a function, essential or marginal, is performed
>
> **MODIFIED OR PART-TIME SCHEDULE**
> Modified schedule may involve adjusting arrival or departure times, providing periodic breaks, altering when certain functions are performed, allowing an employee to use accrued paid leave, or providing additional unpaid leave
>
> **ACQUIRING OR MODIFYING EQUIPMENT**
> For example, providing alternative form of access to a computer, such as a head mouse, for someone who has fine motor problems or building up the controls on assembly line equipment
>
> **PROVIDING QUALIFIED READERS OR INTERPRETERS**
> Hiring sign language interpreters for someone who is hearing impaired or a reader for someone who is blind
>
> **MODIFIED WORKPLACE POLICIES**
> Allowing an employee with a disability to bring in a small refrigerator to store medication that must be taken during working hours
>
> **MODIFYING EXAMINATIONS, TRAINING, OR OTHER PROGRAMS**
> Allowing an applicant with a learning disability time and a half on an examination
>
> **REASSIGNMENT**
> Reassigning a current employee to a vacant position for which the individual is qualified

---

probationary. It is the responsibility of the individual with a disability to inform the employer that an accommodation is needed. The general types of reasonable accommodations that an employer may have to provide are illustrated in Box 14-1, along with examples of each type.

An accommodation is not required if the employer finds it would impose undue hardship on the operation of the employer's business. **Undue hardship** is defined as an "action requiring significant difficulty or expense" when considered on a case-by-case basis. In determining whether an accommodation would impose an undue hardship, the nature and cost of the accommodation in relation to the size, resources, nature, and structure of the employer's operation is considered. If the facility making the accommodation is part of a larger entity, the structure and overall resources of the larger organization is considered, as well as the financial and administrative relationship of the facility to the larger organization. Generally a larger employer with greater resources is expected to make accommodations requiring greater effort or expense than that required of a smaller employer with fewer resources. In situations where an accommodation would impose an undue hardship, the employer must try to identify an alternative accommodation that meets the employee's need and does not impose a hardship. The individual with a disability should also be given the option of paying for the cost (or a portion thereof) of an accommodation that would create an undue hardship.

There are also a number of modifications or adjustments that are not considered forms of reasonable accommodation. For example, the individual must be qualified for the position sought; there is no obligation to find a position for an applicant who is not qualified. An employer is not required to eliminate an essential function (i.e., a fundamental duty of the position). Although an employer may have to provide reasonable accommodation to enable an employee with a disability to meet quality or quantity production standards, they are not required to lower standards that are applied uniformly to employees with and without disabilities. Glasses and hearing aids are considered personal effects and are not included as reasonable accommodations.

There is a perception among employers that job accommodation is a complex and costly process. To the contrary, most accommodations are simple, inexpensive, and can reduce Worker's Compensation and other insurance costs (JAN, 2000). In addition, for qualifying small businesses, tax incentives are available to help cover the cost of providing accommodations. A survey conducted of employers by the Job Accommodation Network (JAN) for the period October 1, 1994 to September 30, 1995 shows that 69% of all accommodations cost $500 or less (Table 14-1). A cost analysis of work site accommodations completed by rehabilitation technology specialists was compared with cost information from JAN (Langton, 1996). This study found that the average cost for work site accommodations was similar between the two sources. More recent data from a study conducted by McNeal, Somerville, and Wilson (1999) indicate that 51.5% of the accommodations cost nothing and 79.9% cost less than $500. Other data collected by JAN show that employers who have established accommodations for people with disabilities have actually benefited financially, with 62% of employers surveyed reporting benefits in excess of $5000 (see Table 14-1).

In spite of the ADA and other legislation, barriers still exist when it comes to the employment of individuals with disabilities. In the United States the rate of employment among people with disabilities is still low (Frieden, 1997; NCOD, 2000). Similarly, there have been only small steps in the use of assistive technologies in the workplace as tools to level the playing field between workers with disabilities

## TABLE 14-1 Costs and Savings of Job Accommodation

### Costs of Job Accommodation*

| Costs | Percentages |
| --- | --- |
| No cost | 19% |
| Between $1 and $500 | 50% |
| Between $501 and $1000 | 12% |
| Between $1001 and $2000 | 7% |
| Between $2001 and $5000 | 9% |
| Greater than $5000 | 3% |

### Company Savings Because Accommodations Were Made

| Value | Percentage |
| --- | --- |
| Value unknown | 4% |
| Between $1 and $5000 | 34% |
| Between $5001 and $10000 | 16% |
| Between $10001 and $20000 | 19% |
| Between $20001 and $100000 | 25% |
| Greater than $100000 | 2% |

From President's Committee on Employment of People with Disabilities (PCEPD), July 1996, Washington, D.C.
*For the period October 1, 1994 to September 30, 1995, JAN received more than 80,000 calls from individuals and businesses in 50 states, the District of Columbia, and Puerto Rico. The above information is related to these calls for advice, as well as examples of accommodations that were implemented as a result of the advice.

and those without, particularly for workers from diverse backgrounds (NCOD, 2000).

In the United States, social security benefits provided to people with disabilities can act as a disincentive for people to work (Frieden, 1997). Often the income from jobs is only slightly more or the same as the Social Security benefits they receive. The loss of health care benefits is also a concern for individuals with disabilities once they become employed. People with disabilities want to work but frequently have difficulty trying to obtain health insurance when they leave the public health care system and enter the work force (NCOD, 2000). Because health care, including assistive technologies, is often a critically needed service, choosing between employment and health care does not take much in the way of deliberation. This issue is a significant barrier to participation in the work force by people with disabilities, and the ADA does not address it. The Work Incentives Improvement Act has the potential to provide better health care options for persons with disabilities wishing to work. This legislation gives states the option of allowing working-age adults with disabilities to "buy in to" Medicaid coverage if they leave the Supplemental Security Income program to work. However, depending on the state in which one lives and the assistive technology needs of the individual, the measures may be limited in improving access to assistive technology (NCOD, 2000). Because Medicaid coverage of assistive technology (AT) varies from state to state (see Chapter 5), a states decision to allow Medicaid buy-in may not result in improved access to AT needed by individuals who wish to enter the work force (NCOD, 2000).

**The mesosystemic level.** In considering the social context at work, we need to examine the policies and attitudes of employers and employees, the types of relationships the person has with people at work, and how they affect interactions and use of assistive technology. These factors can impose barriers to successful assistive technology application.

For example, a policy that prevents the use of automatic speech recognition because it interferes with other employees can prevent computer access for an individual with a high-level spinal cord injury. If there is also a practice that all employees are assigned to open cubicles, then the employee may not have any way to keep her voice from carrying to other cubicles and disturbing her co-workers. The attitude of the supervisor and manager will determine whether this employee can be accommodated or not. For example, if a cubicle out of the way of other workers or an enclosed office is available, that could reduce the disturbance of other workers.

Whether the person works alone or with the public is another consideration. For example, an individual who uses an augmentative communication device (see Chapter 9) both at home and at work needs to consider the differences in the social interactions in these two places and program the device with appropriate vocabulary for each setting. Over time the person's social interactions at work may change as he gets to know his fellow employees, and the vocabulary in his augmentative communication system may need to change as well. The social context directly affects total system performance. The effectiveness of his communication system will be measured by the degree to which it accommodates these varied needs. Effective assistive technology systems are flexible and accommodate these varying demands.

As described in Chapter 2, social influence on individuals is related to what is considered normal or expected, and individuals who have disabilities may be stigmatized because of their disability (Fougeyrollas, 1997). Unfortunately, the use of assistive technologies in the workplace can contribute to this labeling and lead to further isolation. In one study (McNeal, Somerville, and Wilson, 1999), some of the individuals surveyed reported that they deliberately tried to hide from their employer the fact that they were disabled or were having problems. Some were fearful that their employer would fire them if they learned about the problems related to the disability. This fear may prevent some individuals from requesting needed accommodations. The degree to which assistive technologies contribute to stigmatization differs (e.g., the stigma of a hearing aid as opposed to eyeglasses). Because the social context plays such a major role in assistive technology use in the workplace, it is important to consider the stigmatizing effect of any proposed workplace assistive technologies and to provide assistance to the worker in overcoming them. This may include awareness training for co-workers and strategies for assistive technology use by the worker.

**The microsystemic level.** At the microsystemic level, the analysis is of the immediate environment of the person, including such factors as the existence of specific assistive technologies. This is the level at which the assistive technology practitioner (ATP) typically functions in carrying out assessments, making recommendations, and supporting users of assistive technologies.

At this level it is important that the ATP have an awareness of different cultures and issues related to the provision of assistive technology devices and services (see Chapter 2). ATPs may have greater awareness and sensitivity to some cultures and populations than to others. Anecdotal evidence suggests that utilization of assistive technology is lower on Native American reservations than in urban areas (NCOD, 2000). It is suggested that the barriers include lack of knowledge of cultural issues by providers of assistive technology services, lack of knowledge about assistive technology services by the consumers who need them, and the fact that the ADA is not binding on Native American reservations because of their sovereign status.

### The Physical Context for Vocational Use of AT

In a vocational setting the physical context for assistive technology use includes a number of factors. These are specific to the physical arrangement and layout of the workplace itself, including the type of furnishings and their locations, physical dimensions of doors, and absence of barriers.

In order to provide barrier-free access in and around the work site, it is necessary that the ATP evaluate the work site and recommend modifications as needed. Shown in Box 14-2 are questions to consider when evaluating the physical context of the work site and the employee's personal workstation. The first consideration is the accessibility of the building in which the individual works. Does the building have an accessible entrance (e.g., no steps, or a ramp in addition to steps, and automatic electric doors)? Are the doors into the building wide enough? Is there an elevator to get to other floors? Are alternative format labels used (e.g., braille markings for room numbers and labels and restroom labels)?

The next consideration is the arrangement of the person's workstation. It may be necessary to modify or rearrange the work site to allow space for mobility devices (e.g., wheelchairs and walkers; see Chapter 10) by increasing the width of aisles or the space between desks. Table and desk heights may need to be modified if the employee uses a wheelchair. A device such as an augmentative and alternative communication (AAC) system (see

Chapter 9) mounted to the wheelchair may require even greater clearance.

Lighting is also important when a worker is using an assistive device in the workplace. If a room is too bright, the glare may prevent the reading of computer screens or liquid crystal display (LCD) screens on laptop computers or AAC devices. Antireflective screens can be used when it is not possible to reduce sunlight or natural lighting sufficiently to

avoid glare. On the other hand, individuals who have low vision may require special lighting to increase contrast (see Chapter 12).

## IDENTIFYING EMPLOYEES' NEEDS AND SKILLS FOR ASSISTIVE TECHNOLOGY

We have defined the activities that are typically carried out in vocational settings and the contexts in which they are carried out. Given these activities and contexts, it is important to determine the skills and abilities that the employee brings to the vocational setting. This evaluation of employee skills is obtained from a systematic assessment process. In Chapter 4 we describe both the essential information that must be obtained through an assessment process and the major approaches to service delivery in assistive technologies. The process for carrying out an assistive technology assessment for an individual with vocational needs follows the same general principles described in Chapter 4. Each assessment must be conducted on a case-by-case basis, with the first step being to define the problem. In defining the problem, it is essential to ask questions pertaining to the individual's specific situation. It is then necessary to identify the individual's skills and abilities and relate the information

---

| BOX 14-2 | Factors Related to the Physical Context of an Employee's Workplace |
| --- | --- |

What is the physical layout of the work site?

What equipment is used in the work setting?

What physical conditions are required for task completion (e.g., hot/cold, inside/outside, noise level, lighting, ventilation, etc.)?

How is the employee's workstation arranged?

How do workers obtain and discard equipment and materials?

How is the work organized?

Are there safety and quality control measures in place? Potential workplace hazards and the measures taken to eliminate them should be documented.

From Job Accommodation Network (www.jan.wvu.edu/media/ergo.html).

---

## CASE STUDY 14-1

### ASSESSMENT FOR ASSISTIVE TECHNOLOGY IN A VOCATIONAL CONTEXT

Your client, Roger, is employed by a company that has a governmental contract. Because the area in which he works is secured, the entrance, also used by other individuals, has a keypad at normal eye height, which currently requires punching in a code to gain entry. Roger has been diagnosed with amyotrophic lateral sclerosis (ALS). He began experiencing symptoms approximately 2 years ago and has lost leg function, requiring the use of a scooter for mobility. He is also rapidly losing shoulder function. Although his company is very interested in having him continue to work, they are concerned about what steps need to be taken, how these will affect his co-workers, and how much it will cost to make the necessary modifications for him to continue working. Roger is a client of the state vocational rehabilitation agency and has been assigned to a rehabilitation counselor. The goal stated in his Individual Written Rehabilitation Plan is for Roger, through the use of assistive technologies, to maintain employment in his current position for as long as possible. The vocational rehabilitation counselor has asked you to conduct an assessment to determine what changes must be made in the work environment in order to accommodate Roger. Although the company is

focusing on the problem of the security keypad, there are many other considerations as well. Read the section on assessment in this chapter and then answer these questions.

**QUESTIONS:**

1. What aspects of the work environment, in addition to the keypad issue, would you want to include in your assessment?

2. Because of security issues, you will not be able to see the actual keypad, but you will be able to see one similar to it. What type of assessment would you conduct to develop an alternative approach for your client to gain entry without interfering with other employees?

3. What policy and attitudinal issues would need to be addressed?

4. What is the role of the vocational counselor in this process?

5. What would you want to know in addition to the information provided here?

to the specific employment situation. In this section we describe approaches to assistive technology assessment that are unique to vocational services.

Case Study 14-1 points out some of the issues in assistive technology assessment for needs related to employment and illustrates the necessity for a team approach, including the employee, employer, and assessment team. It also illustrates the necessity to focus on need rather than technology.

## Meeting Vocational Goals: The Role of the Assistive Technology Practitioner

For an individual with a disability, assistive technology can have a major role in the ability to work. It is important to keep in mind that assistive technology devices and services are just part of an array of services involved in the successful employment of an individual with a disability. Making successful accommodations for an employee with a disability involves a multidisciplinary effort and collaboration among all involved parties. As with all other areas of assistive technology, the consumer is an integral part of the team. In order to achieve a successful outcome, it is necessary to seek the answers to accommodation questions and obtain input from the consumer. In addition to the consumer, the team may include a vocational rehabilitation counselor, a vocational evaluator, an employment specialist, therapy services, a rehabilitation engineer, the employer, and supervisors (if

the person already has a job). Fellow employees may also be included as part of the team if a workstation is shared or if they will be involved in training. Depending on the status of the consumer's employment and the nature of the disability, others who might be involved are a physician, a Worker's Compensation representative, and a job coach or trainer.

Each state has an agency designated to provide vocational rehabilitation services to individuals with disabilities who have employment as a goal. These services can include counseling, evaluation, training, and job placement. The **vocational rehabilitation agencies** are funded by a combination of state and federal appropriations. (Contact information for each state's vocational rehabilitation agency can be found at www.jan.wvu.edu/sbses/VOCREHAB. HTM). There are also private vocational rehabilitation agencies that provide similar services. The services that they provide are paid for on a fee-for-service basis by the consumer, the employer, or a third-party funding source such as Worker's Compensation insurance.

The publicly funded vocational rehabilitation agencies all use a standard process of providing services to the consumer (Flynn and Clark, 1995). There is no set period in the vocational rehabilitation process in which assistive technology services occur. In fact, there are several points in this process in which assistive technology services can be incorporated (Langton and Hughes, 1992). The Tech Points model, shown in Figure 14-1, provides a framework for

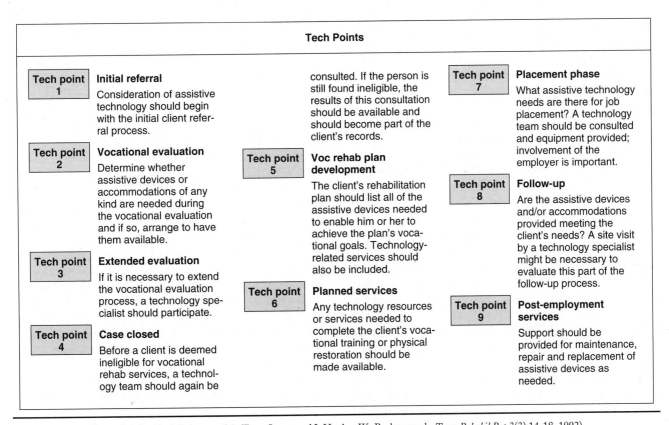

**Figure 14-1**   Tech Points model. (From Langton AJ, Hughes JK: Back to work, *Team Rehabil Rep* 3(3):14-18, 1992).

---

**BOX 14-3**    **Items for Inclusion in IWRP**

Employment goals and objectives

Intermediate objectives related to the attainment of rehabilitation goals; determined through assessment carried out in the most individualized and integrated setting (consistent with the informed choice of the individual)

Criteria, evaluation procedure, and a schedule for determining whether the goals are being met

A statement of the specific vocational rehabilitation services that will be provided and timelines in which the services will be provided

A statement of the specific rehabilitation technology services to be provided

A statement of the specific on-the-job related services, such as personal assistance services and training and supervision of the personal assistant

Assessment of the expected need for postemployment services

The name of any program or agency that will provide the vocational rehabilitation services and the process used to provide or procure such services

Client rights and information about the Client Assistance Program

A statement by the consumer describing how she was informed about and involved in choosing goals, objectives, services, agencies providing services, and any amendments agreed on with the counselor

The terms and conditions under which the specified vocational rehabilitation goods and services shall be provided to the individual in the most integrated settings

Information identifying other related services and benefits provided pursuant to any federal, state, or local program that will enhance the capacity of the individual to achieve the vocational objectives of the individual

---

integrating assistive technology into the vocational rehabilitation process. As this model demonstrates, assistive technology services may be considered at any time, from the consumer's initial referral to the vocational rehabilitation agency up through postemployment services.

A consumer receiving services from a vocational rehabilitation agency is assigned a **vocational rehabilitation counselor.** The role of the counselor is to assist the individual in identifying vocational goals and developing a plan to achieve those goals (Flynn and Clark, 1995). Upon a consumer's referral to a vocational rehabilitation agency, the first task carried out is the development of the **Individual Written Rehabilitation Plan (IWRP).** The purpose of the IWRP, which is developed jointly by the vocational counselor and the consumer, is to set in place a plan to achieve the consumer's employment objective. Items included in the IWRP are shown in Box 14-3. Each IWRP includes a statement of the consumer's long-term rehabilitation goals based on the assessment for determining eligibility and vocational rehabilitation needs, including an assessment of career interests. To the greatest extent appropriate, the goals should include placement in integrated settings. The IWRP

also specifies services that are to be provided to the consumer in order to achieve the goals. In addition to assistive technology services, this includes services such as occupational or physical therapy or speech-language pathology.

Some vocational rehabilitation agencies have ATPs on staff to provide services to their consumers. Other agencies obtain assistive technology services from an outside provider, either on a fee-for-service basis (where reimbursement is per hour of service provided) or through a contract (where *x* number of dollars are paid in exchange for evaluation and training of *y* number of consumers). In either situation it is the vocational rehabilitation counselor who can significantly affect the consumer's success or failure in acquiring assistive technologies for work. Therefore it is important that vocational rehabilitation counselors are educated about the assistive technology services and devices that are available to meet employment needs.

## Assistive Technology Assessment and Implementation for Vocational Needs

The assessment process should always start with an evaluation of the individual's needs and preferences. Background information available to the ATP before commencing a job site accommodation might include some of the following: physical capacity evaluation, functional capacity evaluation, workplace evaluations, and physician's report. It is preferable that the assessment of the consumer's technology needs and trials of the technology take place in the work setting in which it will be used. The employee being accommodated should be allowed to try out any assistive technology being considered, again preferably in the work setting. Some ATPs utilize mobile vans equipped with various technology and tools that are able to go to the employee's work site. The advantage of this is that the assessment and intervention is conducted at the employee's work site. The disadvantage is that the ATP may not have all the equipment needed in the van. This may necessitate a return visit to the work site with the desired equipment.

Generally the assessment process starts with a formal analysis of tasks associated with a specific job or group of jobs in order to identify what the worker does. In Box 14-4 we identify questions related to the person's occupation and job tasks for the ATP to ask during the assessment of an individual who needs accommodation in the workplace. It is important that the ATP ask as many questions as needed to get a clear picture of how the job is customarily performed. This includes information regarding equipment used, equipment that may be available, and methods of performing the tasks.

From the job analysis it can be determined what type of accommodations are needed. The ATP should explore with the employee the different types and ways of making

---

**BOX 14-4** Information Regarding the Person's Occupation and Job Tasks to Gather During Assessment

1. What is the occupation (e.g., clerical, laborer, sales, professional, medical, teaching) and employment status (e.g., full time, part time, temporary) of the individual?
2. What symptoms or limitations (sensory, motor, cognitive, psychosocial/psychological) is the individual experiencing?
3. What job tasks are performed, and how are they typically performed?
4. How do the person's symptoms or limitations affect job performance?
5. Is communication difficult?
   - Who does the individual need to communicate with (e.g., supervisors, co-workers, customers)?
   - How does communication typically take place (e.g., face to face, telephone, computer)?
6. Is mobility difficult?
   - How does the individual get to work?
   - Is access into and around the work site a problem?
   - Is sitting tolerated?
   - Is standing tolerated?
7. Is manipulation difficult, and in what ways?
8. Is there a need for and are there any difficulties performing ADLs at work?
9. What are the potential workplace hazards?
   - What measures have been taken to correct the hazards?
   - Have the *ADA Accessibility Guidelines* (ADAAG) been evaluated if appropriate?
10. What, if any, accommodations have already been implemented?
11. Is the person aware of any accommodations that are available to reduce or eliminate these problems? Are all possible resources being used to determine possible accommodations?
12. Has the employee been consulted regarding possible accommodations?
13. Do supervisory personnel and employees need training regarding disability or the Americans with Disabilities Act?

Modified from the Job Accommodation Network, Morgantown, WVa, www.jan.wvu.edu/media/ergo.html, May 2001.

---

**BOX 14-5** Responsibilities of the Assistive Technology Practitioner in Vocational Accommodation Assessment and Implementation

Understand referral and intake procedures of vocational rehabilitation agency.

Understand the counselor's role and their obligations to consumer and agency.

Be available to the counselor to address concerns from referral source.

Understand criteria that must be met for eligibility and policies and procedures that guide service delivery for the agency during evaluation to determine eligibility.

Understand it is the counselor's job to establish eligibility and the technologist's role to support the counselor, along with other team members, in offering information that relates to eligibility criteria.

Understand counselor and consumer expectations.

Consider all technology that facilitates evaluation and allows full participation of consumer in the evaluation process.

Explain clearly and specifically why and how technology is being considered when communicating with consumer.

Explain the technology processes, time frames, and options that assist in establishing a plan for services.

Use referral to assistive technology as an opportunity to educate the counselor on value of assistive technology services.

Agree on course of action and prioritize services if several are required.

Obtain all information about employment goals and objectives for consumer; review technology policies regarding provision of services to the consumer.

Identify major players in developing a team to make technology recommendations (e.g., consumer, rehabilitation professionals, caretakers, counselors, and vendors); communicate with team members to obtain information on effectiveness of technology recommendations and service delivery process.

Obtain all essential job functions information from counselor, employer, or employment specialist. All technology solutions considered should reflect back to vocational goals as identified on IWRP and communicated with counselor.

Follow up with vendor and consumer to ensure proper installation and use of assistive technology.

Modified from McAlees D, Oliverio M: *Achieving successful employment outcomes with the use of assistive technology.* Presented at the Alliance National Professional Development Symposium, March 1999, Dallas.

---

accommodations (see Box 14-1). Keeping any modifications simple using the least intrusive approach is important. The simplest approach may be to modify or revise the job task if possible. If technology is to be recommended, keep in mind the continuum of commercial to custom technology discussed in Chapter 1. Whenever possible it is preferable to recommend technology that is commercially available rather than custom made.

Once recommendations for equipment and modifications have been made, most state vocational rehabilitation agencies are required to go through a **bidding process** before making any purchases. In this process the recommendations are submitted to three outside vendors for pricing. Typically the lowest of the three bids is the one accepted, unless there is substantial justification to go with one of the other vendors. Alternatives to purchasing equipment immediately include the use of equipment loan programs. This way the employee can try out the device for a time before deciding on purchasing it. Once accommodations are in place, training and follow-up with the technology are essential (see Chapter 4). After the person has had some time to use the accommodations, it is beneficial to meet with her to evaluate the effectiveness of the accommodations and to determine whether additional accommodations are needed. Both the training and follow-up help ensure that the technology is being used appropriately and functioning as expected. A summary of the roles and responsibilities of the ATP during the vocational accommodation process is shown in Box 14-5.

An excellent resource for ATPs working in the area of workplace accommodation is the Job Accommodation Network (JAN). The President's Committee on Employment of People with Disabilities established JAN in 1984 as an information and consulting service. JAN has consultants who, via the phone and its Web site (http://janweb.icdi.wvu.edu/english/homeus.htm), provide information about job accommodations and the employability of people with disabilities. JAN provides the inquiring individual with suggestions and prices and can also give names and numbers of employers and workers who have made similar accommodations.

## ■ HARD AND SOFT TECHNOLOGIES FOR VOCATIONAL SUCCESS

The fourth component of the HAAT model is hard and soft assistive technologies. There are many characteristics of assistive technologies that we discussed in Chapters 1 and 2. When considering a unique environment such as the vocational setting, some of these are more important than others. As we have described earlier, accommodation includes both hard and soft assistive technologies.

Assistive technologies can provide major benefits for individuals in vocational settings. A range of workplace accommodations can be made, from inexpensive to costly, hard technologies to soft technologies, and simple to complex. Postural support systems (see Chapter 6) allow the individual to be positioned for maximal participation in work activities. The use of special-purpose input methods or

| TABLE 14-2 | Sample Workplace Accommodations for Persons with Visual Impairment |
|---|---|
| Job Activity | Workplace Accommodations |
| **Communication:** | Reduce glare by installing window coverings that allow for light adjustment and filtering |
| Writing | Increase lighting |
| Reading | Use nonglare lights with covers |
| Conversation | Use contrasting colors to define background and foreground (e.g., edge of steps and step surface, light switch plates, and walls) |
| | Use tactile indicators, raised letters |
| | Use large print on a background with high contrast |
| | Use visual aids such as closed circuit televisions, magnifiers, large-print computer monitors, talking devices, refreshable braille display |
| | Provide isolated workspaces for workers who use assistive technologies with automatic speech recognition or speech synthesis |
| | Use color acetate sheets over print materials to increase contrast |
| | Take frequent breaks to rest eyes when fatigue is a factor |
| | Use optical character recognition (OCR) to scan printed text and receive a synthetic speech output or save it to a computer |
| | Provide a qualified reader |
| **Manipulation:** | Use large-print labels on files and file folders |
| Filing/sorting | Provide magnification systems for assembly |
| Assembly | Enlarge print on office machines |
| Lifting | Provide talking office machines such as calculator, money sorter |
| Using office machines | |
| **Mobility:** | Eliminate clutter and obstacles |
| Sitting | Eliminate low-profile furniture or move it out of the way |
| Standing | Provide rest room and room labels in alternative formats (e.g., braille or large print) |
| Walking | Have visual alerting signal devices in case of emergency (AT) |
| Climbing stairs | Allow the use of a service animal |
| | Provide mobility and orientation training |
| | Mobility aid (cane, electronic aid, other) |
| | Install colored edges on stairs for improved color contrast |
| | Improve lighting in area |
| | Set up a traveling/evacuation partner |
| | Verbal landmark system |
| | Use public transportation or ride with co-worker to get to work |
| **Activities of daily living:** | Install bathroom grab bars of contrasting color from the wall |
| Toileting | Provide refrigerator for food and/or medications |
| Eating lunch | |
| Taking medications | |

control interfaces (see Chapter 7) are often necessary for use of computers and other electronic devices. In many employment situations the computer (see Chapter 8) is a valuable tool. Augmentative communication systems (see Chapter 9) play a major role for individuals who have disabilities affecting speaking or writing. Mobility devices (see Chapter 10) allow a person with motor deficits to get in and around the workplace. Some assistive technologies (e.g., electronic aids to daily living and robotics; see Chapter 11) can provide assistance to employees who cannot independently manipulate materials or objects. Finally, employees who have sensory disabilities (visual or auditory) are aided by the technologies described in Chapter 12. Thus the potential for achieving a positive vocational outcome using assistive technologies is great; however, reaching that potential requires careful planning to ensure that opportunities, not barriers, are created.

Strategies are also important to the success of assistive technology in the workplace. In Chapter 4 we discuss various types of strategies that also can apply to workplace applications of assistive technology. Simonds (2001) makes some suggestions of strategies that a person with a disability who uses assistive technology can use to attain employment. The ATP can impart these strategies to the applicant. Before going to a job interview or at the beginning of the interview, the applicant should inquire about the job's requirements. The person should then be knowledgeable about his own capabilities, such as how many words per minute he can dictate or how fast he can read text with a screen reader. A person who has range-of-motion deficits and uses assistive devices to enable her to reach and grasp

should know how far she can reach, how fast she can move, and how much weight she can lift. In some situations, such as with the use of speech-activated software, assistive technology may not only serve to level the playing field but may actually give the applicant a leg up on the competition because it enhances performance. Simonds also recommends that the applicant with a disability learn more than one version of whatever technology is available. If the applicant's assistive technology solutions only work on certain systems or with specific hardware, the question of adaptability arises, which can complicate the hiring process. Finally, it is suggested that the applicant be accepting of any assistive technology used and view it as part of the hiring package. The assistive technology should be presented as a bonus wherein the employer not only gets the applicant but gets this great technology as well.

Now that we have identified some of the tools that appear in previous chapters for access to vocational activities, we use case studies to demonstrate how they are combined and applied to maximize the opportunities for employment by individuals who have disabilities. That is the subject of the remainder of this chapter.

## Accommodating an Employee with a Sensory Impairment

Table 14-2 lists a number of sample modifications for persons with visual impairment. Read the following case study and use the information found in this table and in Box 14-4 to develop a plan for the assessment process and make recommendations for accommodations.

---

### Case Study 14-2

#### Vocational Accomodation for Sensory Impairment

Alyssa, a totally blind woman in her 20s, applied for a position as a reservations operator for a limousine service and was hired. The job requires that Alyssa access 15 to 20 different screens containing pertinent limo reservation information on the PC-based reservations system. Alyssa will need a number of shortcuts on the keyboard and screen to be able to effectively do the job. Because of the large volumes of information, speech output may need to be supplemented by braille. Fortunately, Alyssa has excellent braille-reading skills. You have been asked to conduct an assistive technology work assessment to determine the appropriate way to give Alyssa access to this system and to determine what other needs she might have for modifications to the work environment.

**QUESTIONS:**

1. List the areas that need to be evaluated and information you would want to gather during the assessment.
2. Identify the types of modifications to the work setting that might be appropriate.
3. Specify assistive technologies that might possibly be employed (refer to Chapters 8 and 12).
4. Describe any strategies that you would suggest to Alyssa to help her succeed in her new job.
5. Discuss the training that you would provide to Alyssa to help her adapt to the new job.

Modified from Gilson J: Assistive work technology—"the way Georgia does it," *Proc CSUN 15th Ann Conf*, www.csun.edu/cod/conf2000/proceedings/0157Gilson.html, March 20-25, 2000.

| TABLE 14-3 | Sample Workplace Accommodations for Persons with Motor Impairment |
|---|---|
| Job Activity | Workplace Accommodations |
| **Communication:**<br>Writing<br>Reading<br>Conversation | Provide telephone headsets, cordless headsets (no entangling cords), large-button phones, speakerphones, extendible holders, programmable and automatic dialing features, head or mouth pointing sticks<br>Provide writing aids for a person who cannot grip a writing tool: pen/pencil grippers, orthopedic writing devices, handle build-ups, weighted pens<br>Employ alternative control interfaces for computer entry to replace keyboard and mouse functions, control enhancers such as keyguards, typing aids, or head and mouth sticks<br>Provide page turners and book holders for a person who cannot manipulate paper |
| **Manipulation:**<br>Filing/sorting<br>Assembly<br>Lifting<br>Using office machines | Employ automated filing systems, carousels, lateral file cabinets, height-appropriate file cabinets (2-3 drawer), reduced number of files per drawer, ruler as a prybar and bookmark for tight files, hooks or tabs on file folders for easier grasping<br>Store office supplies and frequently used materials on most accessible shelves or drawers for a person who cannot reach upper and lower shelves and drawers<br>Use a lazy Susan at workstation for easy access to and manipulation of materials frequently used<br>Modify controls on office machines or use a pointing device |
| **Mobility:**<br>Sitting<br>Standing<br>Walking<br>Climbing stairs | Provide close, accessible designated parking and entrances to building<br>Have an accessible route of travel from the parking lot into the building<br>Offer opportunity to work from home if transportation to work is not available<br>Maintain unobstructed hallways, aisles, and other building egresses<br>Provide ramps and lightweight doors or automatic door openers<br>Provide elevators for multistory work sites<br>Provide large enough work area for wheelchair access, including turning<br>Provide accessible rest rooms, lunchroom, break room.<br>Assign workspace in close proximity to office machines with elevated access (e.g., a platform to allow access for those with restricted height) or lowered equipment (e.g., on a table rather than a countertop)<br>Modify workstation design and provide height-adjustable table or desk so a person who uses a wheelchair can get under it comfortably<br>Position filing cabinets and bookshelves at accessible heights for wheelchair users<br>Provide comfortable, supportive adjustable seating<br>Eliminate clutter, obstacles, and uneven surfaces<br>Allow the person to bring a service animal into the workplace<br>Develop a plan for safe evacuation, alerting the fire department of probable location of the individual with mobility impairments in case of emergency<br>Provide equipment for safe evacuation |
| **Activities of daily living:**<br>Toileting<br>Eating lunch<br>Taking medications | Allow the person to have a personal attendant at work to assist with toileting, grooming, and eating<br>Allow the person to have flexible scheduling and take periodic rest breaks for medications, repositioning, toileting, or grooming needs<br>Provide an office area within close proximity to rest rooms and an accessible rest room: commode lifts, commode seat risers, grab bars, appropriate height placement of mirrors, paper, soap, towels, lavatories. |

## Accommodating an Employee with a Motor Impairment

Throughout this chapter we have stressed the importance of ensuring that the employee's work site and workstation are fully accessible to the employee. Because this area most often relates to individuals with motor impairments, we describe these accommodations in this section.

A valuable resource for parameters on building or remodeling a work site to make it accessible is the *ADA Accessibility Guidelines as Amended, 1998* (ADAAG). This document, which can be found on the Internet at http://www.access-board.gov/adaag/html/adaag.htm, specifies the technical requirements for accessibility to buildings and facilities by individuals with disabilities under the Americans with Disabilities Act of 1990. Another useful publication on modifying the workplace is *The Workplace Workbook: An Illus-*

*trated Guide to Job Accommodations and Assistive Technology* (Mueller, 1990). This book contains detailed descriptions with accompanying illustrations related to three workplace topics: the universal workplace; seating, storage, and workstations; and computers, information displays, communication devices, and controls.

There are office products, such as adjustable-height desks, filing systems, and carousels, that are commercially available to meet the accommodation needs of someone with a motor impairment.* These modular workstation components can be assembled in configurations to meet a range of work-related needs of office employees with a disability. The modules can be controlled manually, by a motorized switch control, by computer, or by a computer-

---

*http://www.mouthstick.net/, http://techrehab.com/prod01.htm

controlled robotic arm. Components are available that allow the individual to manipulate files, store and retrieve books, refer to reference materials, open mail, staple papers, and answer the telephone.

Accommodations to the workstation and other types of accommodations for persons with mobility impairments are listed in Table 14-3. Read Case Study 14-3, and use the information found in this table and in Box 14-4 to develop a plan for the assessment process and make recommendations for accommodations.

## ■ SUMMARY

In this chapter we have described the vocational application of assistive technologies using the HAAT model as a framework. Employees who have disabilities engage in communication activities such as reading and writing; manipulation activities such as filing and assembly; and mobility activities such as sitting, standing, and lifting. The types of accommodations available in each of these areas involve both strategies and technologies. The four aspects of the context (setting, physical, social, and cultural) dramatically affect assistive technology effectiveness in the workplace. The emergence of the ADA and the Amendments to the Rehabilitation Act has affected the ways in which assistive technologies are applied and supported. The physical layout of the workplace can affect the success of the individual and his use of assistive technologies. Many characteristics of hard and soft assistive technologies are important in ensuring that they meet the needs of employees and employers.

---

### CASE STUDY 14-3

#### VOCATIONAL ACCOMODATION FOR MOTOR IMPAIRMENT

Larry was a CAD/CAM drafting specialist for a small design firm when he became quadriplegic. He uses a powered wheelchair with a chin-controlled joystick and has limited use of his upper extremities. The office he works in is on the ground floor, but there is a lack of accessible parking and the entrance is not accessible because of a large planter box in the way and a heavy glass door. His employer would like Larry to continue working with the company but is concerned with how Larry will access the building and operate the computer and CAD/CAM software. Larry was referred to you by the vocational rehabilitation agency for an assistive technology evaluation to determine accommodations so that Larry can return to work.

#### QUESTIONS:

1. List the areas that need to be evaluated and information you would want to gather during the assessment.
2. Identify the types of modifications to the work setting that might be appropriate.
3. Specify assistive technologies that might possibly be employed (refer to Chapters 8 and 12).
4. Describe any strategies that you would suggest to Larry to help him succeed in his job.
5. Discuss the training that you would provide to Larry to help him adapt to his job.

---

## Study Questions

1. What are the three major activities related to assistive technology use in the workplace?
2. What tasks are important in communication-related work activities?
3. What skills are required in order to ensure success in reading?
4. What tasks are important in manipulation-related work activities?
5. What tasks are important in mobility-related work activities?
6. What types of activities of daily living might an individual with a disability need to complete in the workplace, and what implications do they have for the work setting?
7. What categories of reasonable accommodations are made for people with disabilities?
8. What physical factors may affect the use of assistive technology in the work setting?
9. What social factors may affect the use of assistive technology in the work setting?
10. What cultural factors may affect the use of assistive technology in the work setting?
11. Describe the intentions of Title I of the Americans with Disabilities Act.
12. What does *essential functions of the job* mean and how is this concept applied to vocational access for persons who have disabilities?
13. What is meant by *reasonable accommodation* in the workplace?
14. List three factors that are essential to effective assistive technology service delivery to meet vocational needs.

15. What is the role of the vocational rehabilitation counselor?
16. What is an IWRP, and how are assistive technologies incorporated into it?
17. Who might be part of a team involved in job accommodation?
18. What are the advantages of carrying out a vocational assistive technology assessment at the work site?
19. Identify the roles of the ATP in vocational assistive technology service delivery.
20. What type of information should be gathered from the consumer during the assessment?
21. Identify modifications that might be made to an employee's workstation.
22. Identify potential accommodations for an employee who has a visual impairment and works as a paralegal.
23. Identify potential modifications for an employee with a motor impairment who works in an office setting.

## References

Flynn CC, Clark MC: Rehabilitation technology assessment practices in vocational rehabilitation agencies, *Assist Technol* 7:111-118, 1995.

Fougeyrollas P: The influence of the social environment on the social participation of people with disabilities. In Christiansen C, Baum C (eds): *Occupational therapy: enabling function and well-being,* ed 2, Thoroughfare, NJ, 1997, Slack.

Fougeyrollas P, Gray DB: Classification systems, environmental factors and social change. In Gray DB, Quatrano LA, Lieberman ML (eds): *Designing and using assistive technology: the human perspective,* Baltimore, 1998, Paul H Brookes, pp 13-28.

Frieden L: Disability policy in the United States. In National Institute of Disability Management and Research: *strategies for success: disability management in the workplace,* Fort Alberni, B.C., Canada, 1997, National Institute of Disability Management.

Job Accommodation Network (JAN): *Discover the facts about job accommodation,* www.jan.wvu.edu/english/accfacts.htm, March 13, 2000.

Langton AJ: Comparison of cost involved in making worksite accommodations, *Proc RESNA 1996 Ann Conf* 16:17-19, 1996.

Langton AJ, Hughes JK: Back to work, *Team Rehabil Rep* 3(3):14-18, 1992.

McAlees D, Oliverio M: *Achieving successful employment outcomes with the use of assistive technology.* Presented at the Alliance National Professional Development Symposium, March 1999, Dallas.

McNeal DR, Somerville NJ, Wilson DJ: Work problems and accommodations reported by person who are postpolio or have a spinal cord injury, *Assist Technol* 11:137-157, 1999.

Mueller J: *The workplace workbook: an illustrated guide to job accommodations and assistive technology,* Washington, DC, 1990, The Dole Foundation.

National Council on Disability (NCOD): *Federal policy barriers to assistive technology,* www.ncd.gov/newsroom/publications/1, May 31, 2000.

Simonds WS: AT, disability, and widgets: corporate priorities in the use of assistive technology, *CSUN 16th Ann Int Conf,* www.csun.edu/cod/conf2001/proceedings/0192simonds.html, March 2001.

U.S. Equal Employment Opportunity Commission (EEOC), U.S. Department of Justice Civil Rights Division: Americans with Disabilities Act: questions and answers, www.usdoj.gov/crt/ada/qandaeng.htm, July 1996.

U.S. Equal Employment Opportunity Commission (EEOC), U.S. Department of Justice Civil Rights Division, Social Security Administration: Americans with Disabilities Act—a guide for people with disabilities seeking employment, www.ssa.gov/work/workta2.html, October 2000.

**Abbreviation expansion:** an AAC or computer access technique in which a shortened form of a word or phrase (the abbreviation) stands for the entire word or phrase (the expansion); abbreviations are automatically expanded by the device

**Abductor:** a seating component used to keep the legs in a neutral abducted position; also referred to as *pommel* or *medial knee support*

**Academic participation:** a framework for considering four levels of participation in classroom activities: (1) competitive, (2) active, (3) involved, and (4) no academic expectations

**Acceleration vocabularies:** used by literate persons to increase the rate of communication through both selection of whole words and spelling

**Acceptance time:** a method used for selection of an item in a scanning system that is based on the user's pausing for a preset period, after which the entry is made

**Accessibility Options:** software adaptations included in Windows that address common problems that persons with disabilities have in using a standard keyboard

**Activation characteristics:** the method of activation, deactivation, effort, displacement, flexibility, and durability of a control interface

**Activity:** the portion of the HAAT model that defines the goal (e.g., cooking, writing, playing tennis) of the assistive technology system

**Add-on power unit:** a means by which a conventional manual wheelchair can be converted to a powered wheelchair

**Alerting devices:** sensory devices that detect sounds (e.g., alarm clock, doorbell, telephone ring) and then cause a vibration or a flashing light signal, or both, to call attention to the sound for a person who is deaf

**Alpha testing:** evaluation of a production prototype; in assistive technologies it is often one or two units

**Alternative:** in assistive technologies, a different way of accomplishing the same task

**Alternative sensory system:** the use of a different sensory channel to substitute for a nonfunctional one; common examples of this approach are the use of braille for reading by persons with visual impairment (tactile substitution for visual) and the use of manual sign language by persons who are deaf (visual substitution for auditory)

**Aphasia:** language disorder affecting both expression and reception of spoken and written language

**Appeals process:** the means whereby the ATP can appeal a funding denial

**Apraxia:** an inability to plan motor movements, wherein the peripheral components necessary to execute the motion are generally intact

**Assessment:** a process through which information about the consumer is gathered and analyzed so that appropriate assistive technologies (hard and soft) can be recommended and a plan for intervention developed

**Assistive listening devices:** a class of assistive devices that are intended to be used in group settings such as in lecture halls, churches, business meetings, courtrooms, and broadcast television to amplify sounds and broadcast them to receivers worn by persons who are hard of hearing

**Assistive technology:** a broad range of devices, services, strategies, and practices that are conceived and applied to ameliorate the problems faced by individuals who have disabilities

**Assistive technology practitioner (ATP):** a specialist in assistive technology application; typically has a professional background in engineering, occupational therapy, physical therapy, recreation therapy, special education, speech-language pathology, or vocational rehabilitation counseling

**Assistive technology service:** any service that directly assists an individual with a disability in the selection, acquisition, or use of an assistive technology device

**Assistive technology supplier (ATS):** one who provides enabling technology in the areas of wheeled mobility, seating and alternative positioning, ambulation assistance, environmental control, and activities of daily living

**Assistive technology system:** an assistive technology device, a human operator who has a disability, and a context in which the functional activity is to be carried out

**Augmentative and alternative communication (AAC):** approaches and systems that are designed to ameliorate the problems faced by persons who have difficulty speaking or writing because of neuromuscular disease or injury

**Augmentative manipulation:** assistance in doing a manipulative task in the same manner as it is normally done

**Automatic scanning:** items are presented continuously by the device at an adjustable rate, with selection of the choice made by activating the switch and stopping the scan; entry is by an additional switch press or acceptance time

**Belt drive:** a powered wheelchair in which the motor and wheel axle are coupled through a system of pulleys and belts

**Beta testing:** evaluation of a set of prototypes that form an initial production run

**Bidding process:** process used by third-party funding sources before making any assistive technology equipment purchases. Assistive technology, which has been recommended for an individual, is submitted to three outside vendors for a bid. Typically, the lowest of the three bids is accepted

**Braille:** raised dots that can be read by touch; a cell of either six or eight dots is used to portray letters and special computer symbols (e.g., cursor movement, uppercase and lowercase)

**Center of gravity:** the point in the body at which the acceleration caused by gravity is localized

**Central processing:** human functions of perception, cognition, neuromuscular control (including motor planning), and psychological factors

**Central processing unit (CPU):** the portion of a computer that executes a set of instructions assembled in the form of a program, accepts input (e.g., from keyboard or mouse), sends output (e.g., to a printer or speech synthesizer), and transfers data among the internal components

**Chain drive:** a powered wheelchair in which the motor and wheel axle are coupled through a drive chain with gears at each end

**CHAMPUS:** a federally funded program that provides medical benefits to active duty and retired members of the armed forces and their dependents

**Circular scanning:** an approach in which the selection set is organized in a circular pattern

**Clear-path indicator:** a sensory device that provides signals to the user only if an object is detected in a field about 2 feet in diameter and about 6 feet from the user

**Closed captioning:** a process whereby the audio portion of a television program is converted into written words, which appear in a window on the screen

**Closed circuit television (CCTV):** a video camera and monitor used to enlarge text and other print material; also called *video magnifiers*

**Cochlear implants:** an auditory prosthesis that provides some sound perception by directly applying electrical stimulation to the basilar membrane of the cochlea

**Coded access:** a form of indirect selection in which the individual uses a distinct sequence of movements to input a code for each item in the selection set

**Cognition:** the process of understanding and knowing which involves the skills of attention, memory, problem solving, decision making, learning, language, and other related tasks

**Command domain:** the set of assistive device functions available to the user

**Compact disk—read-only memory (CD-ROM):** optical storage of data and programs; uses lasers to read and write data to optical disks

**Compression:** occurs when forces act toward each other (pushing together), such as the force of the vertebrae on the disks in the spinal column

**Concept keyboard:** a keyboard in which the letters and numbers are replaced with pictures, symbols, or words that represent the concepts being used or taught

**Consumer:** the end user of the assistive technology system

**Contexts:** the portion of the HAAT model that includes four major considerations: (1) setting (e.g., at home, at work, in the community), (2) social context (with peers, with strangers), (3) cultural context, and (4) physical context (measured by temperature, moisture, light)

**Continuous input:** when the inputs to a device are ongoing, with an infinite number of possible values (e.g., volume control on a radio)

**Control enhancers:** aids and strategies that enhance or extend the physical control (range or resolution) a person has available to use a control interface

**Control interface:** the hardware (e.g., keyboard, joystick) by which the user operates an assistive technology system or controls a device

**Conversation:** AAC needs that would typically be accomplished using speech if it were available

**Coverage vocabularies:** a set of topics and concepts that can be used for basic communication by a person who cannot spell; may consist of pictures, symbols, or words

**Criteria for service:** the recognition of a need for assistive technology services that triggers a referral for services

**Criterion-referenced measurement:** a measurement in which the person's own skill level in using the system is used as the standard

**DAISY (Digital Audio-Based Information System):** an international consortium of organizations that produce reading material for the blind; has developed standards for digital books on tape

**Dampening:** the ability of a material to soften on impact

**Density:** the ratio of the weight of a material to its volume

**Dependent mobility:** mobility systems that are propelled by an attendant (e.g., strollers, geriatric wheelchairs, and transport chairs)

**Desktop robots:** general-purpose manipulators that create full access to an area dedicated to the performance of a specific job or activity (a workstation)

**Development:** the combination of growth and learning leading to changes in a child

**Device:** a piece of hardware or software used by an individual to accomplish a task

**Device characteristics:** general properties of the hard technology portions of an assistive technology system

**Diagnosis codes:** describe the person's condition or medical reason for the services being requested; the key to establishing medical necessity

**Digital recording:** human speech is stored in electronic memory circuits for later retrieval

**Digital talking books (DTBs):** reading material for individuals who are blind; produced on digital media (usually CD-ROM) and can be reproduced and read on a variety of hardware platforms and operating systems

**Direct consumer services:** assistive technology services provided to a consumer

**Direct drive:** a powered wheelchair in which the motor is directly coupled to the wheels through a gearbox

**Direct selection:** an approach in which the individual is able to use the control interface to randomly choose any of the items in the selection set

**Directed scanning:** an approach in which the user activates the control interface to select the direction of the scan, vertically or horizontally, and then sends a signal to stop at the desired choice; entry is by an additional switch press or acceptance time

**Disability:** results when an impairment leads to an inability to "perform an activity in the manner or within the range considered normal for a human being" (WHO ICIDH; termed *activity* in WHO ICIDH-2 [ICF] 2001)

**Discrete inputs:** control interfaces with a set of fixed values from which the user can choose

**Distributed controls:** an approach used when multiple devices are controlled and each has its own control interface

**Dynamic communication displays:** an input mode used in AAC in which the selection set displayed to the user is changed as new choices are made; can be altered easily depending on previous choices and allows reliance on recognition rather than recall

**Dysarthria:** a disorder of motor speech control resulting from central or peripheral nervous system damage; characterized by weakness, slowness, and incoordination of the muscles necessary for speech

**Easy Access:** software adaptations included in Apple Macintosh operating systems that address common problems that persons with disabilities have in using a standard keyboard

**Effectors:** the neural, muscular, and skeletal elements of the human body that provide movement or motor output

**Electrically powered feeders:** electrically powered devices that scoop food off a plate and raise it to mouth level; may also include rotation of the plate to position the food for scooping

**Electrically powered page turners:** devices that hold a book or other reading material and mechanically turn the pages when a switch or switches are pressed by the user

**Electronic aid to daily living (EADL):** device that allows control of appliances (e.g., radio, television, CD player, telephone) through the use of one or more switches

**Electronic travel aid (ETA):** sensory devices that supplement rather than replace the long cane or guide dog; designed to provide additional environmental information and to detect those obstacles typically missed by the long cane

**Emulation:** replacement of one type of computer input (typically the keyboard or mouse) with another more accessible form (e.g., head mouse or scanning input)

**Engram:** a preprogrammed pattern of muscular activity represented centrally

**Envelopment:** the degree to which the person sinks into a seating cushion and the degree to which the cushion surrounds the buttocks

**Environmental control units (ECUs):** see **electronic aid to daily living (EADL)**

**Environmental sensor:** the portion of a sensory device that detects the data that the human cannot obtain via her own sensory system

**Equilibrium:** the situation in which the force generated by one object is equal in magnitude and opposite in direction to the force generated by another object

**Ergonomic keyboards:** designed to reduce the strain placed on the hands and wrists during the repetitive motion of keying

**Essential functions:** those job duties that are so fundamental to the position that the individual holds or desires that he cannot do the job without performing them

**Expert systems:** computer-based software that assists in the decision-making process for assistive technologies

**Extrinsic enablers:** an equivalent term for *assistive technologies*

**Fee-for-service:** the traditional method of payment for health care under which providers are paid a certain rate per unit of service

**Fixed deformity:** a permanent change taking place in the bones, muscles, capsular ligaments, or tendons that restricts the normal range of motion of the particular joint and affects the skeletal alignment of the other joints

**Flexible deformity:** appearance of a deformity as a result of increased tone and muscle tightness causing the person to assume certain postures; externally applied resistance (passive stretch) in the opposite direction allows movement of the joint reduction in the "deformity"

**Follow-along:** the portion of the service delivery process in which a mechanism for regular contact with the consumer is established to see whether further assistive technology services are indicated

**Follow-up:** the portion of the service delivery process that determines whether the system as a whole is functioning effectively

**Force:** anything that acts on a body to change its rate of acceleration or alter its momentum

**Friction drive:** powered wheelchair systems that apply a driving force through a roller attached to the motor and pressed against the tire

**Frictional forces:** resulting forces from movement in opposite directions between two bodies in contact; may be static or dynamic

**Fulcrum:** the axis around which rotational movements occur

**Function allocation:** the allocation of functions in any human/device system in which some functions are allocated to the human, some to the device, and some to the personal assistant services

**Functional equivalency:** obtaining the same function in very different ways; for example, turning pages in a book can also be accomplished by a mechanical page turner or electronic books accessed by computer methods

**Functional performance measures:** measurements that address whether the individual can accomplish tasks that she could not do without the assistive technology

**Functional task position:** a forward-sitting posture in which the line of gravity runs just in front of the ischial tuberosities and then intersects the spine; can be obtained either with maximal flexion of the spine and little or no pelvic rotation or with a straighter spine and forward rotation of the pelvis

**General input device-emulating interface (GIDEI):** hardware or software adaptations to a computer that allow emulation of the mouse, the keyboard, or both

**General-purpose manipulation device:** designed to accomplish a variety of manipulative tasks; examples are robotic systems and EADLs

**Geriatric wheelchair:** a type of dependent manual wheelchair especially designed for elderly persons; also referred to as *geri chairs*

**Graphical user interface (GUI):** characterized by three distinguishing features: (1) a mouse pointer, which is moved around the screen; (2) a graphical menu bar, which appears on the screen; and (3) one or more windows, which provide a menu of choices

**Graphics:** AAC needs that are typically accomplished using a pencil and paper, typewriter, computer, calculator, or similar tools; includes writing, drawing, mathematics, and Internet access

**Gravitational line:** the axis of the body along which the force of gravity acts

**Group-item scan:** an approach that is used to increase the rate of selection during scanning by grouping the selection set and allowing the user to first select a group and then the desired item in the group

**Growth:** changes that occur in a child as a result of physical development of the central nervous system

**Handicap:** results when the individual with an impairment or disability is unable to fulfill his or her normal role (WHO ICIDH; termed participation in WHO ICIDH-2 (ICF])

**Head pointers:** devices that have a pointer attached to a headband and are used for direct manipulation

**Health-related quality of life:** the impact of health services on the overall quality of life of individuals; represents the functional effect of an illness and its consequent therapy

**Hearing aids:** sensory devices that provide amplification of sounds, including speech, for individuals who are hard of hearing

**Hoist lift:** a system for transporting a powered wheelchair in a van in which the wheelchair is attached with straps to an arm that swings out from the van door and lowers the wheelchair to the ground

**Human Activity Assistive Technology (HAAT) model:** a framework describing the major elements of an assistive technology system; consists of four parts: (1) activity, (2) context, (3) human skills, and (4) assistive technologies

**Human behavior:** the pattern of human actions leading to a result

**Human performance:** the result of a pattern of actions carried out to satisfy an objective according to some standard (Bailey, 1989, p. 4)

**Human/technology interface:** the portion of the assistive technology system with which the user interacts

**Icon prediction:** a feature of Minspeak-based devices that aids in recalling stored sequences

**Impairment:** any loss or abnormality of psychological, physical, or anatomical structure or function

**Implementation phase:** the portion of the service delivery process in which the recommended technology is ordered, modified, and fabricated as necessary; set up; delivered to the consumer; and initial training takes place

**Inclusion:** students with disabilities who are integrated into the regular educational programs for at least part of the school day

**Independent manual mobility:** systems in which the user has the ability to propel the device using body power only

**Independent powered mobility:** motorized wheelchairs that are controlled by the user

**Indirect selection:** an approach in which there are intermediary steps involved in making a selection; includes scanning and coded access; typically the control interface used is a single switch or an array of switches

**Individual Education Plan (IEP):** mandated by IDEA, the plan, written for each student, incorporates the student's specialized program. The IEP team must consider assistive technologies as a special factor when developing the learner's IEP

**Individual Written Rehabilitation Plan (IWRP):** A plan used by vocational rehabilitation agencies that is jointly developed by the vocational counselor and the consumer achieve the consumer's employment objective; the IWRP considers assistive technologies as part of the services received by the consumer

**Individuals with Disabilities Education Act (IDEA):** defines assistive technology devices and assistive technology services in an educational context; mandates that local educational agencies be responsible for providing assistive technology devices and services if these are required as part of a child's educational needs, related services, or as a supplementary aid or service

**Information processor:** the portion of a sensory aid that converts the raw sensory data from the environmental sensor to a form suitable for presentation via the user display

**Infrared (IR) transmission:** devices that use invisible light to remotely control an EADL; consists of a transmitter unit, which is either handheld or mounted on a wheelchair, and a set of receivers, one for each appliance to be controlled

**Input domain:** the number of independent inputs, or signals generated by the control interface; may be either discrete or continuous

**Integrated control:** an approach used when multiple devices are controlled with one control interface

**Internet:** worldwide computer network available via modem that connects users globally for electronic mail, file transfer, electronic commerce, and similar functions

**Intrinsic enablers:** general underlying abilities that individuals use to perform activities and tasks

**Inverse scanning:** an approach in which the scan is initiated by the individual's activating and holding a switch closed, with selection of the desired item indicated by releasing the switch; entry is by an additional switch press or acceptance time

**In-wheel motors:** an alternative to add-on power units in which electrical motors are integrated into the hub of wheels, which replace standard manual wheelchair wheels

**Learner-teacher interactions:** the way in which teachers present information to learners and the interaction expected of those learners in a classroom situation

**Learning:** changes that occur in a person because of contact with some environmental influence

**Learning styles:** the manner that is most appropriate for the acquisition of knowledge by the student; includes aural versus visual learning, types of problem solving used by the learner, and group interaction skills

**Least restrictive environment:** the degree of acceptable modification in a job or academic program

**Lever arm:** the distance from the fulcrum to the point that a force is applied

**Life roles:** positions in society with responsibilities and privileges

**Line of application:** the particular direction along which forces are applied, either pushing or pulling

**Linear scan:** an approach in which the selection set is organized in a linear (straight-line) format

**Low-shear systems:** systems in which the back hinges to the seat in a manner that reduces the movement of tissue across the seating surface during tilting or reclining of the seat

**Magnification aids:** low vision aids for reading print material

**Managed care:** any method of health care delivery designed to reduce unnecessary utilization of services and provide for cost containment while ensuring that high quality care or performance is maintained

**Manipulatives:** rods, blocks, buttons, beads, or other objects that vary by color, length, and weight and can be sorted, counted, and used to enhance concept development in mathematics

**Medicaid:** a health insurance program, established in 1965 by Title XIX of the Social Security Act, administered at the state level for persons who are unable to pay the costs of their medical care

**Medical necessity:** a specific criterion for funding under Medicare, Medicaid, and private health insurance that requires identification of a medical diagnosis or condition that is specifically coupled to the functional impairment being addressed by the device

**Medicare:** the health insurance program operated by the United States federal government; covers individuals age 65 and older and those adults under age 65 who are blind, are totally and permanently disabled, and have received Social Security Disability Insurance (SSDI) benefits or Adult Disabled Child benefits for at least 24 months

**Memory:** often considered to have three components: (1) sensory memory, (2) short-term memory, and (3) long-term memory, each playing a role in assistive technology use

**Mobile assistive robots:** devices that can move from one location to another to accomplish manipulative tasks under the control of a user who has a disability; two general classes: (1) wheelchair mounted and (2) mounted on a mobile base that is controllable by the user

**Modular power base:** a powered wheelchair design that maximizes power by attaching the motors directly to the wheels (direct drive); using small, heavy-duty wheels; and eliminating the cross-brace folding structure to increase strength and maneuverability

**Moment:** see **torque**

**Morphology:** the rules for organizing the smallest meaningful units of language, called *morphemes*

**Motivation:** any influence that gives rise to performance

**Motor control:** the result of the integration of sensory, perceptual, and cognitive components into a motor pattern that is executed by the effectors

**Mouthsticks:** devices that are held in the teeth and are used for direct manipulation

**Multitasking:** the capability of an operating system to pause while running one software program to run another program

**Muscle tone:** the resistance to stretch provided by neural activity, viscoelastic properties of muscle and joints, and sensory feedback to the CNS

**Musical instrument digital interface (MIDI):** a file used to store music as a series of notes with volume and duration attached; allows music to be played back through a sound card in a computer

**Needs identification:** the portion of the assessment during which more detailed specification of the consumer's assistive technology needs is made

**Norm-referenced measurements:** the ranking of the performance of the individual or system according to a sample of scores others have achieved on the task

**Numeric codes:** a number is used to stand for a word, complete phrase, or sentence; when the user enters the number, the device converts it into the word, phrase, or sentence

**On-screen keyboard:** emulation method that employs a video image of the keyboard on the video screen, together with a cursor

**Operational competence:** skills required for the individual and his aides to use the basic features of the assistive technology device

**Optical aids:** devices that allow individuals with low vision to see print, do work requiring fine detail, or increase the range of their visual fields

**Optical character recognition (OCR):** a software program that runs on a standard PC; its primary function is to analyze the raw video data and assemble it into letters, spaces, and punctuation for synthetic speech or braille output

**Optimal use:** the use of an assistive technology that is the greatest possible given the user's skill

**Orientation and mobility:** the process by which an individual who is blind is able to achieve independent movement in the environment

**Outcome measures:** used to evaluate the end result of the assistive technology intervention

**Parallel port:** a computer output used to send bytes of data as a whole; requires a larger number of wires and is faster than a serial port; commonly used in printers and some speech synthesizers

**Paralysis:** significantly reduced (or absent) muscle strength preventing the use of certain effectors; muscle weakness caused by partial paralysis that makes it difficult to move but does not prevent movement is called *paresis*

**Participation model:** A framework for the identification of potential barriers to educational access, especially those that can be addressed through the application of assistive technologies. Two types of barriers are identified: opportunity and access

**PASS (Plan for Achieving Self-Sufficiency):** a program that allows individuals to put aside income for equipment or services that will assist them in achieving a vocational objective

**Peer training:** instruction that introduces assistive technologies to the classmates of the learner who has a disability

**Pelvic obliquity:** one side of the pelvis is higher than the other when viewed in the frontal plane

**Pelvic rotation:** one side of the pelvis is forward of the other side

**Perception:** the interpretation and assignment of meaning to data received from biological sensors; involves an interaction between information derived from sensed data and information stored in memory based on previous sensory experience

**Performance aid:** a document or device containing information that an individual uses to assist in the completion of an activity

**Performance areas:** activities of daily living, work and productive activities, and play and leisure

**Phonology:** the sounds used in any particular language and the rules for their organization

**Planar:** flat seating components that support the body only where it easily comes into contact with the supporting system

**Platform lift:** the most common type of wheelchair lift for transporting powered wheelchairs in a van; consists of a platform on which the wheelchair sits while it is raised up or down

**Power assist:** a power system that only supplies power to the manual wheelchair when needed by the user, such as when going up an incline

**Pragmatics:** the relationship between language and language users

**Predictive selection:** a feature of scanning Minspeak-based AAC systems in which only valid following icons in a sequence are scanned after the initial icon is selected

**Pressure:** force per unit area

**Pressure ulcer:** a lesion that develops as a result of unrelieved pressure to an area and results in damage to underlying tissue

**Primary driving controls:** adapted driving system components that are used to stop (brakes), go (accelerator), and steer

**Primitive reflex:** characterized by immediate and automatic movement performed at a subconscious level, usually initiated by sensory stimulation

**Procedure codes:** a numerical system used to describe the services that the provider carried out and is billing for; the most commonly used procedure-coding system is the Common Procedure Coding System (HCPCS) of the Health Care Financing Administration (HCFA)

**Product liability:** exposure to legal action based on deficiencies in products or failure to warn of dangers to the user of a product

**Professional liability:** exposure to legal action based on professional services that are improperly provided

**Programmable controllers:** an EADL approach that is based on the storage, of user-selected codes that are appropriate to a wide range of appliances; entering the correct code into the controller allows control of the appliance by the user

**Propelling structure:** the portion of a manual wheelchair consisting of the wheels and an interface that the consumer uses to move the wheelchair; the portion of a powered wheelchair consisting of a wheeled mobility base with a power drive to the wheels, a control interface that the consumer uses to direct the movement of the wheelchair, an electronic controller, and powered accessories (e.g., recline, ventilator)

**Prototype:** the initial new device that is produced as the product of engineering development

**Psychosocial function:** consists of self-identity, self-protection, and motivation. These factors are related to the person's acceptance of a disability, the approach a person takes to the assistive technology, and the ultimate effectiveness of the assistive technology for the person

**Public funding sources:** government funding at the federal, state, or local levels

**Qualified individual with a disability:** a person who has the skills, education, experience, or other requirements needed for a job and can perform the essential functions of the position with or without reasonable accommodation

**Qualitative measurement:** a measurement in which an intelligible feature that can be used to characterize the thing under investigation is obtained, such as an observation of behavior (e.g., the user appears to be less depressed since beginning to use the device)

**Quality assurance:** involves a program of evaluation of the quality of services rendered and the effectiveness of the devices supplied

**Quality of life measures:** assess the effectiveness of assistive technology devices and services in the broader social context of the impact on the user's overall life

**Quantitative measurement:** a measurement in which an indefinite amount or number is obtained; for example, a numerical scale from 1 to 5 may be assigned to a given measurement, or the measurement may be in terms of a physical parameter such as weight

**Radio frequency (RF) transmission:** devices that use electromagnetic (radio) signals to remotely control an EADL; consists of a transmitter unit, which is either handheld or mounted on a wheelchair, and a set of receivers, one for each appliance to be controlled

**Random access memory (RAM):** used for temporary storage of data; only active when power is provided to the computer

**Range:** maximal extent of movement of an effector

**Rate enhancement:** AAC and computer access approaches that result in the number of characters generated being greater than the number of selections the individual makes

**Reacher:** a handle grip attached to a stem that is used to control the jaws of a device for grasping an object

**Reading aid:** a sensory device designed to provide access to print materials for an individual who is blind

**Read-only memory (ROM):** computer memory used for permanent commands and instructions that are required to allow the computer to function; cannot be erased and reprogrammed in normal operation

**Reasonable accommodation:** any modification or adjustment to a job or the work or educational environment that will enable a qualified applicant, employee, or learner with a disability to participate in the application process, perform essential job functions, or participate fully in the educational program; also includes adjustments to ensure that a qualified individual with a disability has rights and privileges in employment and education equal to those of employees without disabilities

**Recall:** the type of memory that relies exclusively on the person's abilities to retrieve information with no assistance

**Reclining back:** systems that allow a change in the seat-to-back angle of the wheelchair

**Recognition:** the type of memory that requires the person to identify the proper or desired item from a list

**Referral and intake:** the portion of the assessment in which the consumer, or someone close to him, has identified a need for which assistive technology intervention may be indicated and contacts an ATP; basic information is gathered and a determination of the match between the services provided and the identified needs of the consumer is made; funding is also identified and secured at this stage

**Refreshable braille display:** the use of mechanically raised pins to represent braille cells, organized in arrays of from 1 to 80 cells

**Reluctant users:** individuals who are unmotivated, intimidated by technology, embarrassed to use the device, impatient or impulsive, have low self-esteem, unrealistic expectations, or limitations in the AT skills needed

**Remote control:** the absence of a physical attachment between the various components of an EADL

**Resilience:** the ability of a material to recover its shape after a load is removed or to adjust to a load as it is applied

**Resolution:** the smallest separation between two objects that the effector can reliably control

**Resource specialist:** an individual associated with a local school that provides consultation regarding assistive technology applications

**Robotic systems:** electrically powered general-purpose manipulators that can carry out tasks under the control of a person who has a disability

**Rotary lift:** a system for transporting a powered wheelchair that has a post supporting a platform installed inside the van; in operation the platform rises a few inches above the height of the van floor and rotates on the post into the van

**Rotary scanning:** see **circular scanning**

**Rotational movement:** when the direction, distance, and time of a movement occur simultaneously, but the movement is through an angle instead of in a straight line

**Row-column scanning:** a form of group-item scanning in which the items are arranged in a matrix and the row is first selected by a switch press, then the item is selected from that row by a second switch press; entry is by an additional switch press or acceptance time

**Salient letter coding:** a technique for developing abbreviations in which the first letter of key words are included in the abbreviation (e.g., HJ becomes "Hi Jane")

**Scanning:** the most common indirect selection method, in which the selection set is presented by a display and is sequentially scanned by a cursor or light on the device, with the user selecting the desired choice by pressing a switch when it is indicated by the display; entry is by an additional switch press or acceptance time

**Scoliosis:** lateral curvature of the spine

**Scooter:** a powered wheelchair design featuring three or four wheels, a tiller steering system, and a bucket mounted to a single post coming up from the base; often used by marginal ambulators who need mobility assistance to conserve energy; often provided by grocery stores and shopping malls

**Screen readers:** systems that provide speech synthesis or braille output for blind users

**Scribing:** the assistance provided by a human aide for writing or mathematics pencil and paper work

**Secondary driving controls:** adapted driving system components that are needed for safe operation of a vehicle, including turn signals, parking brakes, lights, horn, turning on the ignition, temperature control (heat and air conditioning), and windshield wipers

**Selection methods:** an approach allowing the user to make choices from the selection set; includes scanning, directed scanning, and coded access

**Selection set:** the items available from which user choices are made; in an AAC device this is the component that presents the symbol system and possible vocabulary selections to the user

**Semantic encoding:** coding of words, sentences, and phrases on the basis of their meanings

**Semantics:** the relationship between words and their meaning

**Sensors:** intrinsic enablers that obtain data from the environment; characterized by sensitivity (minimal detectable levels of light, sound, or pressure) and range (allowable variation in size, amplitude, or magnitude of the sensory input)

**Sensory characteristics:** auditory, somatosensory, and visual feedback produced during the activation of a control interface

**Serial port:** a bi-directional computer output requires only two or three conductors; used to send bytes of data in sequence rather than as a whole; commonly used in assistive technologies (e.g., augmentative communication devices or powered wheelchair controllers and environmental control systems)

**Setting:** a combination of an environment, tasks to be done, a set of rules governing the tasks, and a level of comfort

**Shearing:** occurs when forces are parallel (sliding across the surfaces), such as the movement that occurs as the head of the femur moves across the acetabulum during hip movement

**Social participation:** a categorization of classroom participation that has four levels, whose criteria are participation and influence socially rather than academically; see **academic participation**

**Spasticity:** increased muscle tone; also referred to as *hypertonicity*

**Spatial characteristics:** the overall physical size (dimensions) and shape of the control interface, the number of targets available for activation, the size of each target, and the spacing between targets

**Special-purpose manipulation device:** a device designed to carry out only one manipulative task

**Speech synthesis:** the generation of human-sounding speech using electronic circuits and computer software

**Standard powered wheelchair base:** a powered wheelchair in which the base is similar in design to the conventional manual wheelchair frame, with large rear wheels and small front casters

**Step scanning:** an approach in which the user activates the switch once for each item to move through the choices in the selection set; entry is by an additional switch press or acceptance time

**Stiffness:** how much a material gives under load

**Strategic competence:** skills in the use of strategies that maximize the effectiveness of the assistive technology system

**Stress:** the resulting molecular change inside biological (e.g., soft tissue and bone) or nonbiological (e.g., metals, plastics, or foams) materials

**Student workstation:** computer-based setups that may provide specialized assistance with writing, conversation, and an adapted access method for the classroom computer; also includes access for wheelchair riders and possible integration of controls for powered wheelchair, computer, environmental control, and augmentative communication; also called *life station*

**Supporting structure:** consists of the frame of a wheelchair and its attachments

**Syntax:** the rules for organizing words into meaningful utterances

**System performance:** a combination of the human, the activity being performed, the context in which it is performed, and the assistive technology

**Tasks:** small elements into which activities can be broken

**Technology abandonment:** a situation in which the consumer stops using a device even though the need for which the device has been obtained still exists

**Technology Integration Plan:** systematic approach to the consideration of assistive technologies for classroom use

**Telephone controllers:** devices that allow a person with a disability to control a telephone using one or more switches; typically built around standard telephone electronics

**Telerehabilitation:** the use of telecommunications technologies to capture and transmit visual and audio information, biomedical data (e.g., electroencephalograms, x-rays, ultrasound data), and consumer information

**Tension:** forces that act in the same line but away from each other (pulling apart), such as the force applied on the antagonist muscle during contraction of the agonist muscle

**Text-to-speech programs:** programs that analyze a word or sentence and translate it into the codes required by a speech synthesizer

**Third-party payer:** a funding source that is public or private and covers the cost of devices and services

**Tilt-in-space:** wheelchair systems in which all seating angles (seat-to-back, seat-to-calf, calf-to-foot) are preset to consumer's needs and the entire seating system is tilted back as one piece

**Torque:** the product of the distance of the point of application of a force from a fulcrum; the magnitude of the force

**Traditional orthography:** the symbolic representation of language based on letters and words

**Trainable controllers:** devices that provide EADL functions by storing the control code for any specific appliance function

**Transdisciplinary team approach:** crossing over of professional boundaries and sharing of roles and functions in an assistive technology team, with all individual team members well-grounded in their profession but also comfortable extending their role beyond their profession

**Transitional mobility device:** powered mobility devices that can be used to augment a young child's independent locomotion without the complexity and expense of a powered wheelchair

**Translational movement:** when all parts of the body move in the same direction, at the same time, and for the same distance

**Transparent access:** two fundamental concepts that apply to all levels of computer adaptation: (1) 100% of the functions of the computer must be adapted if the user who has a disability is to have full access; and (2) all application software that runs in the unmodified computer must also run in the adapted computer

**Ultrasonic transmission:** devices that use high-frequency sound (above the range of hearing) to remotely control an EADL; consist of a transmitter unit, which is either handheld or mounted on a wheelchair, and a set of receivers, one for each appliance to be controlled

**Under-the-vehicle lift:** a system for lifting a powered wheelchair into a van; installed under the van and extends out from under the van when activated

**Undue hardship:** an accommodation requiring significant difficulty or expense on the part of the employer when considered on a case-by-case basis. In determining whether an accommodation would impose an undue hardship, the nature and cost of the accommodation in relation to the size, resources, nature, and structure of the employer's operation is considered

**Universal Access:** software adaptations included in Apple Macintosh operating systems that address common problems that persons with disabilities have in using a standard keyboard and in seeing characters on the screen; includes Easy Access and CloseView

**Universal design:** The design of products and environments to be usable by all people, to the greatest extent possible, without the need for adaptation or specialized design (NC State University, The Center for Universal Design, 2001)

**User agent:** software to access Web content; includes desktop graphical browsers, text and voice browsers, mobile phones, multimedia players, and software assistive technologies (e.g., screen readers, magnifiers, GIDEIs) used with browsers

**User display:** the portion of a sensory device that portrays the sensory information for the human user

**User satisfaction:** the consumer's perception of the degree to which the assistive technology system achieves the desired goals

**User satisfaction measures:** measures that address whether the assistive technology services and devices provided meet the consumer's needs from the consumer's point of view

**Visual accommodation:** the process by which the ciliary muscles change the curvature of the lens and hence the focal point of the eye

**Vocabulary expansion:** methods by which the available vocabulary is increased through the use of codes or levels

**Vocational rehabilitation agencies:** designated by each state to provide vocational rehabilitation services to individuals with disabilities who have employment as a goal; services include counseling, evaluation, training, and job placement; funded by a combination of state and federal appropriations

**Vocational rehabilitation counselor:** each individual receiving services through a state vocational rehabilitation agency is assigned a counselor who acts as a case manager and assists the individual in identifying vocational goals and developing a plan to achieve those goals

**Wheelchair tie-down and occupant restraint systems (WTORS):** a total system installed in a van, bus, or other vehicle that is designed to fasten the wheelchair and restrain the passenger in order to protect the passenger or driver who uses a wheelchair

**Windows:** generically, a portion of the computer screen that is devoted to a particular function; specifically, an operating system for computers developed by Microsoft Corp.

**Windswept hip deformity:** when one hip is adducted and the other hip is abducted

**Word completion:** a technique that displays stored words based on the sequence of entered keys; the user selects the desired word, if any, by entering its code (e.g., a number listed next to the word) or continuing to enter letters if the desired word is not displayed

**Word prediction:** a technique that displays stored words based on previous words entered

**Zero-shear systems:** wheelchair seating systems in which the seat back is attached to sliding mounts that move the seat back down as it is reclined, minimizing the movement of the seat across the body surface

The resources included here are all of a general nature. Some are professional organizations, some are assistive technology conferences, others are Web sites with assistive technology information, and still others are government agencies with information regarding assistive technologies. These resources supplement the many specific ones included in each chapter of this book.

**Abledata** (www.abledata.com): This Web site provides impartial information on assistive technology from the National Institute on Disability and Rehabilitation Research. The 7000-item database can be searched by keyword or phrase (such as "one-handed can-opener") to obtain product descriptions, manufacturers' contact addresses, and handy keywords for comparison shopping. More than 27,000 products are listed.

**Assistive Technology Industry Association (ATIA)** (www.atia.org/members.html): ATIA is a not-for-profit membership organization of manufacturers or distributors selling technology-based assistive devices for people with disabilities or providing services associated with or required by people with disabilities. An annual conference is held in Orlando, Florida, in January.

**Association for the Advancement of Assistive Technology in Europe (AAATE)** (www.fernuni-hagen. de/FTB/aaate.htm#resources): The goal of AAATE is to stimulate the advancement of assistive technology for the benefit of persons with disabilities, including the elderly. With memebership from countries throughout Europe, AAATE focuses on creating awareness of assistive technology, promoting research and development of assistive technologies, contributing to knowledge exchange within the field of assistive technology, and promoting information dissemination. One form of dissemination is the main conference every 2 years, with a multidisciplinary approach and a focus on scientific progress. AAATE also publishes a newsletter on assistive technology issues, meetings, and policies and publications and has special interest groups for specific areas of assistive technology application.

**Australian Rehabiliation and Assistive Technology Assocaition (ARATA)** (http://e-bility.com/arata): ARATA is an association whose purpose is to serve as a forum for information sharing and liaison among people who are involved with assistive technology. The focus of ARATA is on providing opportunities for sharing ideas to ensure the advancement of rehabilitation and assistive technology in Australia through activities as diverse as conferences, special interest groups, a Web site, listserv, membership directory, and a quarterly newsletter.

**Closing the Gap (CTG)** (www.closingthegap.com): CTG sponsors an annual conference held in October in Minneapolis. Conference topics cover a broad spectrum of technology as it is being applied to all disabilities and age groups in education, rehabilitation, vocation, and independent living. The conference attracts people with disabilities, special educators, rehabilitation professionals, administrators, service/care providers, personnel managers, government officials, and hardware/software developers. The CTG Web site also contains many links to assistive technology information, particularly related to educational applications.

**Communication Aid Manufacturers Association (CAMA)** (www.aacproducts.org): CAMA is a not-for-profit organization of the manufacturers of augmentative and alternative communication (AAC) software and hardware products. CAMA conducts 1-day workshops on AAC throughout the United States.

**CSUN Conference** (www.csun.edu/cod/center): This conference is a major international exhibit and scientific program covering a broad spectrum of assistive technology applications for sensory impairment, AAC, and computer access. The conference is held in March in Los Angeles. The Center on Disabilities at California State University, Northridge, sponsors the conference. The Web site contains other links and information regarding assistive technology applications.

**International Seating Symposium** (www.rst.pitt.edu/ iss/ISS2001HnT.html): This annual conference features presentations covering evaluation, provision, research, and quality assurance issues in seating and mobility for persons with disabilities. Scientific and clinical papers, in-depth workshops, panel sessions, and an extensive exhibit hall are featured. Attendees include assistive technology practitioners, assistive technology suppliers, educators, manufacturers, consumers, physicians, rehabilitation engineers, and vocational rehabilitation counselors.

**National Institute on Disability and Rehabilitation Research (NIDRR)** (www.ed.gov/offices/OSERS/NIDRR): The U.S. Department of Education's Office of Special Education and Rehabilitative Services (OSERS), through its National Institute on Disability and Rehabilitation Research (NIDRR), is the major U.S. funder of assistive technology research, including development of new devices, clinical studies of application, and outcome measures. The NIDRR-funded Rehabilitation Engineering Research Centers (RERCs) conduct research and development in specific areas of assistive technology application. NIDRR also sponsors research and related activities designed to maximize the full inclusion, social integration, employment, and independent living of disabled individuals of all ages. NIDRR's programs are balanced between the scientific and consumer communities.

**RehabCentral.com** (www.rehabcentral.com/index.cfm): RehabCentral.com includes a variety of resources on rehabilitation products and assistive devices, as well as applications notes written by clinicians.

**Rehabilitation Engineering and Assistive Technology Society of North America (RESNA)** (www.resna.org): RESNA is an interdisciplinary association of people with a common interest in technology and disability. Their purpose is to improve the potential of people with disabilities to achieve their goals through the use of technology. RESNA serves that purpose by promoting research, development, education, advocacy, and the provision of technology and by supporting the people engaged in these activities. RESNA's membership ranges from rehabilitation professionals to providers and consumers. All members are dedicated to promoting the exchange of ideas and information for the advancement of assistive technology. RESNA publishes the semiannual journal *Assistive Technology*, the bimonthly RESNA News, and RESNA Press and holds an annual national conference (held in June at various locations) and regional conferences that provide forums for the dissemination of information on the development and delivery of state-of-the-art technologies. Special interest groups and professional specialty groups provide additional forums for interaction with members who have similar interests in the various disciplines that comprise rehabilitation and assistive technologies.

**Special Needs Opportunity Windows (SNOW)** (http://snow.utoronto.ca): The SNOW Project at the University of Toronto is a provider of online resources and professional development opportunities for educators and parents of students with special needs. SNOW's tools and information, online workshops, curriculum materials, discussion forums, and other resources are available to assist assistive technology professionals in using new technologies.

**Web Accessibility Initiative (WAI)** (www.w3.org/WAI/WAI): In coordination with organizations around the world, WAI pursues accessibility of the Web through five primary areas of work: technology, guidelines, tools, education and outreach, and research and development.

Page numbers followed by f indicate figures; t, tables; b, boxes.